2022 Reimbursement Guide
Behavioral Health

Insurance & Reimbursement | Medicare | Compliance | Documentation
Diagnosis Coding Tips | Procedure Coding | Supply Coding

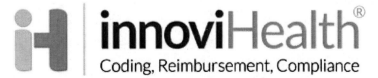

62 East 300 North Spanish Fork, UT 84660 USA
(801) 770-4203 | store.innoviHealth.com

Copyright Notice and Disclaimer

Published and copyrighted © by innoviHealth, Inc. 2021. All rights reserved.

No part of this publication may be reproduced, distributed, or transmitted in any form or by any means including photocopying, recording, or other electronic or mechanical methods, without the prior written permission of the publisher, except in the case of brief quotations embodied in critical reviews and certain other noncommercial uses permitted by copyright law. Some online resources may only be accessed by subscribers. Email info@innoviHealth.com for permission to reproduce or otherwise use this material other than as mentioned above.

This publication is distributed with the understanding that the publisher is not engaged in rendering legal or accounting or medical services. If legal advice or other expert assistance is required, the services of a competent professional should be sought.

innoviHealth assumes no liability for data contained or not contained herein. It does not directly nor indirectly practice law or give legal opinions. It assumes no responsibility for the consequences attributable to or related to any use or interpretation of any information or views contained in or not contained in this publication. Absolute accuracy cannot be guaranteed. innoviHealth is not responsible for informing the purchaser of any updates. Unless noted, the views expressed herein are that of innoviHealth and should not be construed as policy for any entity or insurance company.

2022 Reimbursement Guide for Behavioral Health is a registered trademark of innoviHealth, Inc.

Printed in the U.S.A.

ISBN: 978-1-64072-175-3

innoviHealth, Inc.
62 East 300 North
Spanish Fork, UT 84660 USA
Phone 801-770-4203

Visit innoviHealth.com for more information.

Current Procedural Terminology (CPT) codes and descriptions are copyright 2021 American Medical Association (AMA). All Rights Reserved. Fee schedules, relative value units, conversion factors and/or related components are not assigned by the AMA, are not part of CPT, and the AMA is not recommending their use. The AMA does not directly or indirectly practice medicine or dispense medical services. The AMA assumes no liability for data contained or not contained herein. CPT is a registered trademark of the American Medical Association.

Acknowledgments

Development of this annual edition requires extensive review and input. The contributions over many years from numerous physicians, assistants, consultants, and attorneys have made this book possible. Their efforts and professional input are sincerely appreciated but they are too numerous to list here. Special thanks also goes to all of the hardworking innoviHealth support staff.

President / Chief Executive Officer
LaMont Leavitt

Vice President / Chief Information Officer
David D. Berky

Chief Operations Officer
Tracy Young

Chief Financial Officer
John Davis

Chief Revenue Officer
Michael Hanahan

VP of Sales
Alan Crop

Director of Content Research
Wyn Staheli

Director of Content
Aimee Wilcox, CPMA CCS-P CST MA MT

Content, Design, Editorial, & Delivery
Alan Albright
Brandon Herman
Christine Woolstenhulme
David Lewis
DeVin Orton
Holly Michelsen
Jared Staheli
Jason Boogert
Jeff Lewis
Jonathan Mitchell
Justin Lewis
Kristy Ritchie
Melissa Hall
Raquel Shumway
Reed Larson

Special thanks to our third-party partners and reviewers

2022 Reimbursement Guide

The *2022 Reimbursement Guide* continues the innoviHealth tradition of providing helpful tools and resources for healthcare providers. This unique compilation of coding essentials makes it easier to get the job done.

When used properly, this book can not only save valuable staff and doctor time, but it can also build confidence and compliance in your practice's coding, documentation, reimbursement, and more.

Our Commitment is to provide current information in a manner that is easy to understand and implement in a healthcare setting.

Our Mission is to support healthcare providers seeking to navigate the complex and ever-changing world of insurance reimbursement through high quality products, services, and education.

Our Pledge is to help your practice survive and thrive with greater assurance.

We encourage you to take advantage of our free newsletter, sent by email. These alerts include the latest industry and coding news, notifications of helpful webinars, coding and reimbursement tips, and more. To register, visit www.FindACode.com/newsletter Your information privacy is assured – it is never shared with others.

Your opinions and suggestions are welcome and appreciated. With your feedback, we continue to improve year after year. Please send your comments and suggestions to info@innoviHealth.com.

Thank you for your continuing support.

LaMont J. Leavitt, President/CEO

Table of Contents

Introduction

Copyright Notice and Disclaimer ii
Acknowledgments iii
2022 Reimbursement Guide iv
Icon Legend viii

1. Insurance & Reimbursement   11

1.1 Insurance & Reimbursement Essentials 13
    Overview 13
    Billing Process Flowchart 24

1.2 Types of Insurance Plans 29
    Traditional Insurance (Individual or Group Health Plans) 29
    Managed Care Organizations (HMO, PPO, etc.) 31
    Consumer Driven Plans 32
    No-Insurance and the Cash Practice 34
    Government Programs 35

1.3 Claims Processing 39
    Overview of Claims Processing 39
    How to File Claims 42
    Filing Tips 43

1.4 Claims Management 63
    Claim Follow-up Procedures 63
    General Guidelines for Unpaid Claims 64
    Reducing Denials 66
    Refund Requests and Demands 67
    Managing Appeals 68

1.5 Establishing Fees 73
    About Fees and Fee Schedules 73
    Fee Schedule Methodologies 74
    Dollar Conversion Factors (DCF) 76
    Other Fee Schedules 77

2. Medicare   81

2.1 Medicare Essentials 83
    Introduction 83
    How Participation Works 87
    Impact of Secondary Insurance 89
    Non Part B Plan Information 91
    Medicare Administrative Contractors (MACs) 92
    Medicare Coverage and Billing 93
    Supporting Documentation 97
    Medicare Terms to Understand 99

Table of Contents (continued)

2.2 Medicare Fees 103
- Medicare Fee Schedule 103
- Understanding Medicare Fees 106

2.3 Medicare Appeals 113
- Medicare Appeals Process 113

3. Compliance — 121

3. Compliance Essentials 123
- About Compliance 123
- The Importance of Having a Compliance Plan 126
- OIG Compliance Programs 127
- Fraud and Abuse 128
- OSHA Compliance 132
- HIPAA Compliance 133
- Other Compliance Concerns 135
- Managing Audits 138

4. Documentation — 151

4.1 Documentation Essentials 153
- Introduction 153
- The Role of Medical Necessity 155
- Documentation and Recordkeeping Standards 156
- Transitioning from Active Care 167
- The Treatment Plan 168

4.2 Provider Documentation Training 173
- Provider Documentation Guides (PDGs) 174
- Diagnostic Statement 186
- Lessons from the Clinical Example 194

4.3 Documentation Tips 197
- Tips 200

5. Procedure Coding — 215

5.1 Procedure Coding Essentials 217
- Introduction 217
- Getting Started with CPT 219
- NCCI Coding Edits 222
- Evaluation and Management (E/M) Services 223

5.2 Procedure Codes & Tips 225
- Procedure Code Tips 225
- Common Procedure Codes 273

Table of Contents (continued)

5.3 Evaluation & Management Coding 311
The Basics 311
Office/Other Outpatient E/M Services 316
Coding Scenario 1: 2020 E/M Guidelines 324
Code Selection by Counseling Time (2020 Version) 341
Coding Scenario 2: Current Office E/M Guidelines 343
Evaluation and Management Codes 346

6. Supply Coding — 377

6.1 Supply Coding Essentials 379
About HCPCS Codes 379
Durable Medical Equipment (DME) 380

6.2 Supply Codes & Tips 383
Supply Tips 383
Common Supply Codes 392

Appendices — 399

Appendix A. NCCI Edits 401
NCCI Edits for CPT 404

Appendix B. Modifiers 419
Understanding Modifiers 419
Level I CPT Modifiers 420
Level II HCPCS Modifiers 434

Appendix C. Provider Documentation Guides 449
Introduction 449

Appendix D. Telehealth Services 459

Appendix E. Common Diagnosis Code Tips 467
Coding Conventions & Instructions 468
Tips 471

Appendix F. Coding Reference Tables 505

Appendix G. Glossary 519

Appendix H. Procedure Code Crosswalks 535

Indices — 543

General Index 545
Code Index 551

Icon Legend

The following icons are referenced throughout the book. Use this legend to understand how they are used.

Resources

Website/Book: This icon will direct you to online or print resources containing more information on a topic. Go to FindACode.com/books/bhrg for the full list of online resources.

Tips/Notes

Tip: This icon is used to point out useful tips, notes or special instructions. These are things that your office needs to review and include in your office policies and procedures where applicable.

Alerts

Alert: This icon indicates a warning or other important information that we really want to make sure you notice. These alerts could save you time, money and frustration.

Store

Store: This icon indicates helpful resources which may be purchased from our online store at store.innoviHealth.com.

Example

Example:
This icon highlights an example that will help you better understand a concept.

1. Insurance & Reimbursement

Chapter Contents

1.1 Insurance & Reimbursement Essentials 13
Overview 13
Billing Process Flowchart 24

1.2 Types of Insurance Plans 29
Traditional Insurance (Individual or Group Health Plans) 29
Managed Care Organizations (HMO, PPO, etc.) 31
Consumer Driven Plans 32
No-Insurance and the Cash Practice 34
Government Programs 35

1.3 Claims Processing 39
Overview of Claims Processing 39
How to File Claims 42
Filing Tips 43

1.4 Claims Management 63
Claim Follow-up Procedures 63
General Guidelines for Unpaid Claims 64
Reducing Denials 66
Refund Requests and Demands 67
Managing Appeals 68

1.5 Establishing Fees 73
About Fees and Fee Schedules 73
Fee Schedule Methodologies 74
Dollar Conversion Factors (DCF) 76
Other Fee Schedules 77

1.1 Insurance & Reimbursement Essentials

Overview

Billing and reimbursement are critical components to the success of your practice and therefore a thorough understanding is essential. The only way to ensure appropriate reimbursement (and keep it) is by knowing how to submit clean claims to payers with all the necessary information.

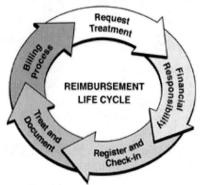

Reimbursement is cyclic in nature and has a life of its own. In this chapter, we refer to this complex process as the Reimbursement Life Cycle. In order to appreciate the complexities of this process and see the "big picture," the Reimbursement Life Cycle image will be referred to throughout this book. This enables you to see how each chapter relates to this cycle and how the entire reimbursement process works.

Concerns about avoiding false claims and allegations of fraud, along with expanding rules, regulations, and the associated paperwork required, can make this process challenging, but not impossible. This chapter teaches the concepts necessary for proper claims submission which leads to prompt and appropriate reimbursement.

Whether you do your own billing, use an outside billing service, or have your patients submit their own claims, every healthcare practice needs to understand and follow the proper documentation, coding, and billing protocols. It is the provider's responsibility to gather and submit the required information for reimbursement. This process of gathering and submitting information for reimbursement is what we refer to as the Reimbursement Life Cycle.

Step 1. Request for Treatment

The request for treatment most often begins with a phone call and the scheduling of an appointment. If this is a new patient, this is an excellent time to address your office policies regarding payment, scheduling, and cancellations. The remainder of this segment explains important information for effective intake of new patients. If this is an established patient, most of this segment is not necessarily applicable unless any pertinent office policies have changed since their last visit.

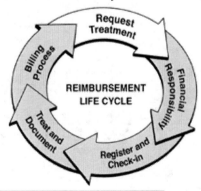

 Store: Be sure appointment reminders meet HIPAA compliance standards. See *Complete and Easy HIPAA Compliance* in the online store to learn more.

Before the Patient Arrives

When a patient calls to schedule an appointment, important office policies should be discussed with them. Briefly explain your office policies such as patient payment, insurance, and cancellation policies and collect any insurance coverage information for verification. Let the patient know that you would like to assist them by contacting their insurance company for coverage details prior to their scheduled visit. This will help avoid confusion or delays during their initial visit. Also, request that patients have all of your office's required documents (assignments, releases, etc.) signed by the appropriate parties. See the "Welcome Information" segment that follows for more information about these requirements. Explaining payment policies to your patients ahead of time will help reduce and eliminate confusion and anxiety. An easy transition is to simply as the patient if they would like to take a minute to learn about your office's payment policy.

Tip: When communicating by telephone, it may also be helpful to direct the patient to your website where they may review your written policies and download *Patient Information* and *Health History* forms.

Book: See "Step 2. Establishing Patient Financial Responsibility" on page 16.

Welcome Information

There are many forms that need to be completed before a patient is seen. With the increasing prevalence of computerized practice management systems, many of the tasks that used to be completed by hand may now be done online. This includes welcoming the patient to your practice. If you have a website, make it easy for them to find the information they need to complete before they arrive. Something like a [New Patients] or [Welcome Information] menu item or button on your website can be very helpful. If you do not have a website, or the patient isn't computer savvy, you could mail a welcome packet to patients so they can fill out these forms before they arrive. If there isn't enough time between the initial call and the time of the patient visit to mail your welcome information, either email it, or let them know that they need to arrive 20 minutes early in order to complete the forms before the doctor sees them.

Your welcome information typically includes the following:

- *Welcome Letter*
- *Patient Financial Responsibility Acknowledgment* form
- *Patient Information* form
- *Insurance Information* form
- *Medical and Health History* forms
- *Informed Consent* form
- *HIPAA Privacy Policy and Acknowledgment*

Tip: Although the *Verification of Insurance Coverage* form is not given to the patient, office personnel should begin to complete this form as soon as insurance information is obtained from the patient. For additional information see "Verification of Insurance Coverage" on page 19.

Resource: Sample forms can be found by visiting this *Reimbursement Guide's* resource page. See the introduction for more information about resource pages.

Welcome Letter

A *Welcome Letter* may be sent to all new patients before their first visit. Whether done by email or regular mail, be sure that the tone of this first correspondence with the patient is warm, friendly, and inviting. During this introductory phase, it is best to customize the letter for the patient instead of using a generic greeting such as "Dear Patient." This establishes the fact that your office views them as an individual, not just another number.

Resource: See Resource 140 for a sample letter.

Patient Financial Responsibility Acknowledgment Form

Patient financial responsibility is a major source of problems in the billing process. Some practices have found that an acknowledgment form outlining specific details about how the insurance process works reduces these problems by clearly outlining the insurance company's portion of the payment, as well as the portion for which the patient is personally responsible.

Resource: See Resource 141 for a sample form.
Book: See "Step 2. Patient Financial Responsibility" for additional information.

Tip — Insurance Coverage Communication: When communicating with patients about "insurance coverage," do not use the word "insurance" alone. Instead, use "insurance portion." This clarifies the true meaning for both the sender and listener as an effective checkmate to the false perception that "insurance" means total coverage. Always using both words together helps alleviate misunderstandings and avoids potential frustration.

Patient Information Form

A *Patient Information* form provides the basic information necessary for all types of healthcare practices. Be sure that the form you use works well with your practice management software and office procedures. Please note that now, before the patient arrives, is a good time to start verifying insurance coverage. See "Step 2. Establish Financial Responsibility" later in this chapter for more about obtaining insurance verification.

Resource: See Resource 143 for a sample form.

Insurance Information Form

An *Insurance Information* form provides the basic necessary information for insurance billing. Identifying the insurance type is critical for proper billing and appeals. For example, it is crucial to clarify if the insurance plan is "Employer Sponsored," which means that it will be governed by ERISA standards should you need to appeal. Two other important items to include on this form are:

- an "Authorization" portion which allows you to use "signature on file" on all future claims and
- a "Financial Responsibility" portion which clarifies what the patient is responsible for.

Resource: See Resource 142 for a sample form.

Medical History and Health History Forms

The *Medical History and Health History* forms are very important documents for the initial patient visit. Most patients dislike filling out forms when they arrive and sometimes they may not bring all the necessary information with them. By completing this form before arrival, the patient saves their time as well as yours. In addition, the healthcare provider will have the necessary information to meet documentation requirements for "Review of Systems" and "Health History."

Book: See also Chapter 4 — Documentation.
Resource: See Resource 144 for a sample form.

Store: See also innoviHealth's *Comprehensive Guide to Evaluation & Management.*

Informed Consent Agreement for Treatment

For appropriate risk management, every office needs to have a signed *Informed Consent Agreement* prior to treatment. Regardless of the services provided, the patient must demonstrate they are mentally capable of signing the form. If they are impaired (e.g., alcohol, medication) or their symptoms (e.g., dementia) indicate that they might not be considered legally competent, have an authorized representative (e.g., family member, legal guardian) sign the form. Additionally, this form should be available in other languages or have an interpreter available. It may also need to be available in large print for the elderly or those with a vision impairment.

Consult with legal counsel or your malpractice insurance carrier for any specifically recommended forms or state-specific requirements. Generally, there is no legally required expiration date on this consent, however, one year would be a good standard since a patient could forget details.

HIPAA Privacy Policy Form and Acknowledgement

HIPAA requires patients to receive a notice of the provider's (clinic's) privacy practices. Their individual medical record needs to contain their signed acknowledgement that they have received this notice and reviewed its contents. Such a statement is included on innoviHealth's sample *Patient Information* form; however an actual *HIPAA Notice of Privacy Practices* is not included in this publication.

 Store: For detailed information about HIPAA requirements and all necessary forms, see *Complete & Easy HIPAA Compliance* (Resource 116) and *HIPAA Notice of Privacy Practices* (Resource 262) in the online store.

Financial Hardship Policy and Application (Optional)

innoviHealth created an optional form for use when the patient appears to have a financial problem where they would be unable to meet their co-pays or deductibles. Having an official financial hardship policy and application is necessary and must be included in a patient's chart if you intend to waive all or part of their co-pay (patient portion) or deductible. Caution is advised when implementing hardship waivers. They should be used only in cases where hardship is clearly indicated and properly documented. If not done correctly, waiving deductibles or co-pays could violate several federal laws. Waivers and reductions for co-pays, co-insurances, and deductibles should not be routine and should not be advertised in any way. See the "Financial Hardship Discounts" segment in Chapter 1.5 — Establishing Fees for additional information.

Tip: Financial Hardship Agreements are not permanent financial arrangements and should be periodically reviewed to ensure they remain appropriate for the circumstances.

Step 2. Establish Patient Financial Responsibility

Establishing patient financial responsibility is not just about patient portion versus insurance payments. It is about eliminating surprises and establishing better communication between provider and patient regarding who pays for what. For many medical practices, it could also be about personal injury or workers compensation. It is up to the provider to obtain the necessary information for proper billing to third-party payers as well as the patient.

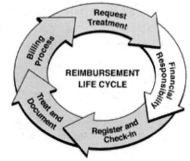

An *Insurance Information* form is an excellent tool for assisting in this process. Used in conjunction with a *Verification of Insurance Coverage* form, these tools establish the necessary financial requirements during the checkout process.

Informed Financial Consent Policy

An Informed Financial Consent Policy is the proper way to eliminate surprises and help the patient understand what their insurance may or may not cover. It should be used for noncovered or elective services, or at the beginning of a treatment plan. If you know that a service or item will not be covered, it is crucial to have an official written policy and to have the patient sign the necessary forms. For a patient, this policy is sometimes referred to as an "estimate."

Estimate of Medical Fees

For a third-party payer, using an estimate may be insufficient. Some payers have their own specific forms that must be used to notify the patient of their financial responsibility when supplies or services might be denied/noncovered. For example, UnitedHealthcare has a *Member Advance Notice Form for the Involvement of a Nonparticipating Provider* form and CMS has the *Advanced Beneficiary Notice (ABN)*.

Book: See Chapter 2 — Medicare for more about the *ABN* form and how to use it properly.
Resource: See Resource 147 for a sample form.

Cash/No Insurance

Even if your practice does not accept any insurance, financial policies need to be clearly documented. Your *Patient Financial Policy Letter* should clearly outline what payment options are available.

Book: See "Discounts" in Chapter 1.5 — Establishing Fees for information.
Book: See also "No-Insurance and the Cash Practice" in Chapter 1.2 — Types of Insurance Plans for additional information.

Personal Injury (PI)

Personal injury is for accidents pertaining to auto, home, or non work related business. Providers should be careful to gather all details of the incident including both personal injury and medical insurance coverage details. Situations involving "personal injury" (PI) *typically* involve medical conditions arising from three main accident scenarios:

- Motor vehicle involvement
- Accidents occurring in and around a home, which may include automobile related injuries occurring at a residence
- Accidents occurring on a business-site not related to the patient's work. See the "Workers Compensation" segment in Chapter 1.2 — Types of Insurance Plans for information about on-the-job injuries.

In each of these accident scenarios, there are potentially several different sources of payment: fault-based insurance coverages (e.g., liability, uninsured motorist coverage); no-fault coverages (e.g., medical payments benefits, personal injury protection); and attorneys.

If these sources are limited or exhausted, then health insurance could be a source. Additionally, patient payments could include cash, Health Savings Plans/Flex Spending, and Medical Cafeteria Plans.

Resource: See Resource 159 for additional information on personal injury.
Resource: See Resource 801 for help and information on personal injury cases.

Workers Compensation (WC)

Workers Compensation is for work related illness or injuries on the job. The employer pays for insurance which covers medical costs incurred, and replaces lost wages. Fees are based on their own specific fee schedule and vary by state.

There are three possible scenarios regarding workers compensation: the patient is covered by a WC carrier located in your own state, the patient is covered by a WC carrier located in another state, or the patient is covered by Federal Workers Compensation. The following information pertains to state based workers compensation claims. Please note that Federal Workers Compensation has very specific requirements. See the "Federal Workers Compensation" segment in Chapter 1.2 — Types of Insurance Plans for more information.

Resource: See Resource 468 for more information about Workers Compensation.

Health Insurance

Health insurance coverage is based on a payer's health benefit plan and is typically based on the concept of medically necessary services. There are several different types of health insurance and each one needs to be handled in accordance with their specific protocols. At this point in the visit, it is important to obtain copies of insurance cards and picture identification. If not done previously, contact the company to verify coverage. Obtain necessary pre-authorizations or referrals prior to the initial visit.

It is also important to understand that no matter what type of plan a patient may have, most payers only cover services to the point where the patient is considered stable or symptom free. Some therapeutic services may be clinically appropriate, but the third party payer does not consider them to be medically necessary.

Coverage

Coverage is outlined in the payer's health benefit plan. For payment to be made, services must be considered medically necessary and appropriately documented in the medical record.

Generally, medically necessary services or supplies are defined by payers as those that:

- Have been established as safe and effective
- Are consistent with the symptoms or diagnosis
- Are considered both necessary and consistent with generally accepted medical standards
- Are furnished at the most appropriate, safe, and effective level

Practitioners should contact their payers to discuss specific policies regarding the reasonable and necessary rationale of the services they provide, and to determine any coverage limitations. For example, many payers have a maximum number of visits on many types of services.

Tip: Routinely performing services that are not clinically indicated for that specific patient encounter are generally not considered to be medically necessary.

Handling Multiple Plans

If the patient's spouse or parents have an additional insurance plan, there could be multiple insurance plans which could cover the patient. It is very important to correctly determine which is the primary insurance and which is secondary. Generally, when both spouses have insurance coverage, the husband's insurance plan is the primary for him, and the wife's insurance plan is the primary for her. For dependents, the primary insurance company is determined by the insured's birthdate, which is referred to as the "birthday rule." The primary insured is the person whose birthdate (month and day) comes earliest in the year. For example, if the father's birthday is September 20 and the mother's birthday is February 5, the mother's insurance would be the primary plan for their dependents since her birthday is earlier. The year of birth is not applicable.

Book: See Chapter 2 — Medicare for specifics on Medicare coverage.

Verification of Insurance Coverage

If you will be billing insurance, coverage should be verified and all necessary pre-authorizations for treatment should be obtained. When you contact the insurer for coverage information, record the necessary insurance information using a *Verification of Insurance Coverage* form. This will help you to verify coverage for that individual. If they are enrolled in a particular insurance plan, it might require that the provider be a part of their panel for full coverage. Additional information on patient insurance coverage is found later in this chapter.

Alert: The marketplace plans available through Health Insurance Exchanges (HIE) can complicate the verification process. Even though you may be an in-network provider for a specific carrier, this does not mean that you are an in-network provider for that same carrier for insurance plans purchased through an insurance exchange.

Only fully compliant HIPAA offices may electronically verify coverage with health plans who offer that option. If your office is not HIPAA compliant, you may only verify insurance coverage by telephone or by regular mail (but not email). If there is other related information obtained about coverage during this verification process, record it on the *Verification of Insurance Coverage* form. See Resource 148 for some samples of this form.

Pre-authorization

Some payers may require pre-authorizations for certain types of services or for pre-approval of a specified number of visits. In some cases, you may need to have an official referral number before treatment begins. Pre-authorizations are commonly utilized in managed care situations.

Note: For some health plans, there may be situations in which additional benefits could be granted to patients who meet specific criteria. In such cases, it is important to document the clinical necessity for treatment beyond their usual limits. Your diagnosis should reflect the improvement or changes in your patient's condition as the case progresses. Providers should include all morbidities and prognostic factors in the assessment so that a clear picture is formed for the reviewer. Be aware of individual payer policies.

Book: See Chapter 4.1 — Documentation Essentials for more information about record keeping standards.

Step 3. Registration Process

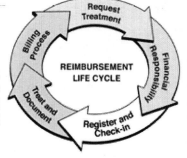

Step 3 of the Insurance Reimbursement Life Cycle covers the patient arrival, check-in and intake process. During this step, it is important to obtain patient demographics, verify insurance, obtain informed consent and financial responsibility forms, and take care of HIPAA Privacy requirements. Established patient registration is much simpler than that of a new patient.

Tip: Co-pays and deductible amounts should have been established during the insurance verification process. It is helpful to have these amounts noted on the superbill/charge sheet before the patient encounter takes place.

> **Alert:** Be aware of HIPAA regulations during this registration process. Simple sign-in sheets including patient name, arrival and/or appointment time, and date are permitted, but the reason for the visit or other protected health information cannot be included.

New Patient Initial Visit

When the patient arrives, it is important to ensure that all forms are properly completed and signed. If they have not already completed the forms online or in the Welcome Packet, give them time to fill them out. Pay particular attention to the following:

- Validate the information on the insurance card with another valid form of identification, such as a driver's license, to avoid security problems like patient misrepresentation and possible health care fraud. It is not necessary to copy the drivers license, just look at the name and address to ensure that the patient is who they claim to be. In fact, some states prohibit copying a driver's license, so be aware of your state law if you wish to make a copy.

- Referrals and/or pre-authorizations should have been obtained before the patient arrived. If not, call immediately to verify coverage.

- Make sure that all of the forms in the "Welcome Information" (see page 14) segment are properly completed.

- Obtain signed copies of other forms, such as the *Release of Information* or liens, where applicable.

 Store: See the *Complete & Easy HIPAA Compliance* (Resource 116) which includes authorizations such as the *Patient Authorization for Release of PHI* form.

Established Patient Subsequent Visits

One common problem in a medical office is not catching changes in demographic or insurance information when an established patient arrives for a visit. Be sure to ask the patient if anything has changed since their last visit. This could also be done by phone prior to the appointment. Verify the following:

- **Patient information/demographics.** This includes essential information such as address, phone, or employment.

- **Insurance plan change or coverage.** Remember that coverage can change, and the patient may not know about it or remember to tell you. Periodically ask, and document any changes using the Verification of Insurance Coverage (Resource 148) form.

- **Health history.** If there have been significant changes and/or it has been some time since the patient was last seen in the office, it might be beneficial to update the patient's health history with a new form. Otherwise, be sure to remind the patient to tell the provider of these changes so they are part of the medical record.

- **Evaluation.** If there have been significant changes, or after a specified number of days or visits, an updated evaluation is required by many third party payers. Verification of coverage is best done before the patient sees the provider.

Step 4. Treatment and Documentation

This step is the core of the patient encounter and drives the remainder of the Reimbursement Life Cycle. There are several tasks that need to happen beyond the actual treatment of the patient.

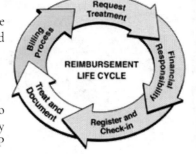

Document the Visit

As stated throughout this book, proper documentation of the visit is essential to payment. By properly following documentation protocol, you will appropriately capture the procedures and diagnoses which are required for billing. Your SOAP notes will be your supporting evidence. These notes show which systems were examined and which areas were treated. If there is any question when it comes time to bill, your billing specialist will need these records to ensure proper billing takes place.

Book: See Chapter 2 — Medicare for specific Medicare requirements pertaining to documentation and billing guidelines.
Book: See Chapter 4 — Documentation for more help with documentation.

Reminder: Diagnoses are dynamic, not static. As necessary, your documentation/diagnosis should reflect the improvement or changes in your patient's condition as the case progresses.

Create a Treatment Plan

The treatment plan must be fully documented and be part of the patient record. This is one of the most forgotten components of documentation and one of the most highly scrutinized areas by auditors. Additionally, it is also advisable to send written instructions of this plan home with the patient or caregiver. It is very easy for them to forget details about what they need to do when at home and before the next visit.

Book: See Chapter 4.1 — Documentation Essentials for more information about treatment plan standards.

Complete Fee Slip

Using a superbill is one way of providing all the necessary information for billing on one form. Superbills are also known as care tickets, charge-slips, or encounter forms. No matter what they are called, their purpose is to simplify both the checkout and coding processes. It makes it easier for the provider to let the billing staff know what codes to use and it can also make it easier to give the patient what they need.

If you have a computerized system, it is recommended that the items on your form be coordinated with the sequence in which data is entered in your computer. This will save time, frustration, and reduce the possibility of data entry errors.

Store: Find-A-Code's SuperBill Builder™ add on tool offers subscribers a way to create their own custom SuperBills using their own codes and descriptions or choose the standard code descriptions. SuperBills may be customized with practice name, provider name, NPIs and more. Go to FindACode.com/tools/superbill-builder to learn more.

Alert: Be aware that some automated billing systems review the documentation and select the billing codes based on internal EHR program settings. Auditors have found that in many cases, these systems may up-code to a higher billing level when they should not. If you have one of these systems, always review the selected code and make sure that the documentation appropriately justifies the code selected. You must be able to either approve or disapprove what the computer has chosen before it is billed. Understand what you are billing for, as you have ultimate responsibility for what is submitted for reimbursement. Remember, your documentation must support what is being billed.

Checkout Process

This is the final step in which the patient takes the super-bill to the front desk. At this time, it is important to not only schedule the next visit, but, even more importantly, to collect payment of the patient portion, if it has not already been done. The best time to collect the patient portion is when the benefit of the service is fresh in their minds and fully appreciated – during check-in or before they leave the office.

Step 5. Billing Process

As with all businesses, receipts and collections are an integral part of staying in business. Insurance payers can be slow and the collection equation could become a central issue for your office. Also, consider that overhead costs for billing and administration can be up to 30% of the fees. For this reason, some providers have chosen to either switch to a cash practice or else outsource their billing to an agency. Regardless of who does the work, the billing process has its own workflow. "The Billing Process Flowchart" in *Figure 1.1* outlines how this process can work.

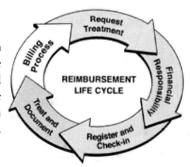

Resource: See Resource 819 and search on "outsourcing" or "billing agencies" for additional information.

This should be the end of the claims cycle, but there is one more thing to consider: post-payment problems such as audits, refund demands, and take-backs.

Prompt Filing

Both patients and insurance payers respond better to timely requests for payment. When insurance is involved, claims should be submitted promptly. Payers reject claims that exceed their claim filing time limits (usually 180 or 365 days, but some payers have shorter time frames). Know individual payer policies regarding timely submission of claims and their deadlines.

Book: See Chapter 1.3 — Claims Processing for more information.

Billing Managed Care

Managed care programs often have specific billing requirements. Obtain billing manuals and instructions directly from the carrier. Specific policies for referrals and coverage, along with claims submission requirements, are outlined within each carrier's billing manuals. Follow their guidelines carefully.

Tip: Routinely re-evaluate the costs of membership and payment benefits related to provider participation with all plans. These programs could be costing more than they benefit the practice. When calculating costs, include the cost of increased provider time and administrative costs incurred in dealing with managed care controls.

Benefit Notices and Payment Reports

Though you may receive a check from an insurance payer, that does NOT mean that the reimbursement process is complete. Carefully review their attached benefit notices to ensure that the appropriate payment has been received. The following segments explain some of these notices and what to expect.

Explanation of Benefits (EOB)

An *Explanation of Benefits (EOB)* is the explanation that accompanies either Medicare or private carrier disbursement or denial of healthcare benefits which are provided to the beneficiary. This document is the key to knowing what was paid or not paid and why. Knowing how to read an *EOB* will help a practice collect proper reimbursement. There are terms used on *EOBs*, such as, "applied to deductible," "usual and customary," "patient co-pay," "allowable," etc., which make it easier to determine what the patient is responsible for paying. Becoming familiar with these terms will allow you to process payments in a more efficient manner.

Remittance Advice (RA)

A *Remittance Advice (RA)* is similar to an *EOB*, in the manner that it is a notice of payments and adjustments sent to providers, billers, and suppliers. However, in this case, the healthcare provider is the recipient of the *RA*, which may serve as a companion to a claim payment or as an explanation when there is no payment. The *RA* explains the reimbursement decisions including the reasons for payments, adjustments, or denials.

The codes listed on the *RA* help the provider identify any additional action that may be necessary. For example, some *RA* codes may indicate a need to resubmit a claim with corrected information, while others may indicate whether the payment decision can be appealed.

It is very important that the *RA* be thoroughly reviewed. The *RA* features valid codes and specific values that make up the claim payment. If your claim has not been paid correctly, then it is necessary to carefully follow the appeals procedures and protocols for that payer.

Book: See Chapter 1.4 — Claims Management for more information on appeals.

Medicare Summary Notice

The *Medicare Summary Notice (MSN)* is a summary of all charges that providers and suppliers billed to Medicare over a 90-day period that is sent to the beneficiary. The *MSN* lists the details of the services received, Medicare payments and the patient portion or the amount a beneficiary may be billed for by the providers or suppliers. The *MSN* is mailed when claims are processed. Beneficiaries/patients should check this notice to be sure all the services, medical supplies, or equipment that providers billed to Medicare were actually received.

Billing Process Flowchart

The Billing Process Flowchart (see *Figure 1.1*) helps outline the decision process for maintaining an effective billing process. This is only a suggested work plan and is used for demonstration purposes to illustrate areas which may need more attention in your practice's policies and procedures. All billing begins when a service is completed and a payment is due. It doesn't end with the payment though. Often it is necessary to fight to keep that reimbursement.

Figure 1.1

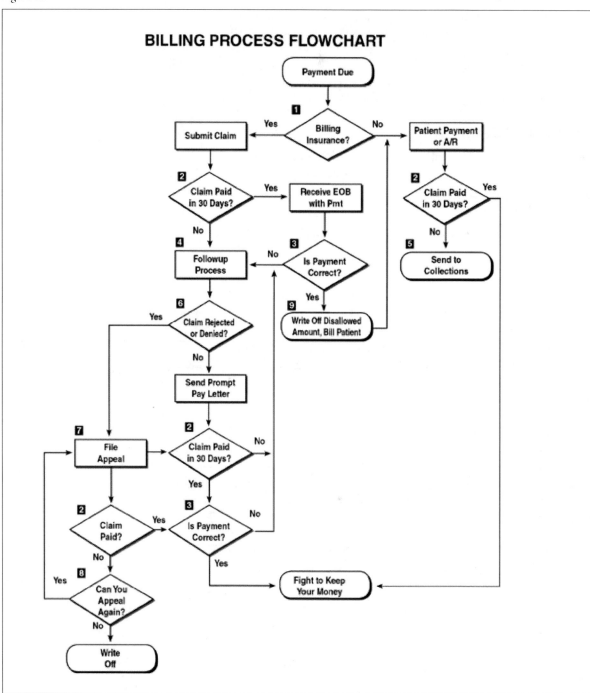

Flowchart Notes

Book: This segment only describes the flowchart in general terms. For a more comprehensive discussion on most of these items, See Chapter 1.4 — Claims Management for more information.

1. **Billing Insurance?**
   - If you are billing insurance, you will need to submit a claim. This can be either electronic or paper. Remember, the cleaner the claim, the faster payment will be received.
   - If you are NOT billing insurance, implement an effective accounts receivable procedure.

2. **Is the Claim Paid? Is It Paid in 30 Days?**
   - Unpaid claims must be reviewed at least every 30 days, more frequently if there is a known problem that is being addressed with a specific payer.
   - If payment has been received, carefully compare the *EOB* against the submitted claim to ensure that payments are correct.

3. **Is Payment Correct?**
   - If the payment is correct, then hopefully all is done and there are no post-payment reviews or audits to worry about. If the patient portion has not been collected, be sure to write off any disallowed amounts (if you are a contracted provider) and then bill the patient for the remaining balance.
   - If the payment is not correct, policies need to be in place to follow a specific procedure for both overpayments and underpayments. Overpayments will need to be paid back to the insurance company quickly to avoid allegations of fraud. Underpayments will need to be reviewed and may need to be appealed.

Resource: See Resource 195 for a sample *Voluntary Overpayment Refund Form*.
Book: See the "Handling Overpayments" and "Managing Appeals" segments in Chapter 1.4 — Claims Management.

4. **Follow-up Process**
   - Every office needs an established follow-up procedure. See the "Claim Follow-up Procedures" segment in Chapter 1.4 — Claims Management for more information.

5. **Send to Collections**
   - The decision to send an account to collections should not be an emotional decision. It should be clearly outlined in your office *Policies and Procedures*.

6. **Is Claim Rejected or Denied?**
   - If the claim has been rejected or denied, begin the claims appeals process. See the "Managing Appeals" segment in Chapter 1.4 — Claims Management for more about the steps that need to be taken.
   - If the claim is unpaid after 30 days and has not been rejected, then see the segment, "Prompt Pay Laws," in Chapter 1.4 — Claims Management for more about one possible option to encourage payment.

7. **File Appeal**
   - If the claim has been rejected or denied, begin the claims appeals process. See the "Managing Appeals" segment in Chapter 1.4 — Claims Management for more about the steps that need to be taken.

8. **Can You Appeal Again?**
   - Most payers have a limit on the appeals process, so follow individual payer guidelines carefully. If you have exhausted your appeal options with the payer, consider external appeals, making a complaint to the Department of Insurance, and notifying your state and/or professional association.
   - If these additional options are unsuccessful, then it may be necessary to write off the balance. In a limited number of cases, you may be able to collect from the patient. Be aware of individual payer policies about "balance billing." See the "Managing Appeals" segment in Chapter 1.4 — Claims Management for more information about appeal options.

9. **Write Off Disallowed Amount, Bill Patient**
   - Once the claim has been adjudicated and an *Explanation of Benefits (EOB)* has been received, the disallowed amounts (if required by contract or law) should be deducted from the patient account to accurately reflect their "patient portion." Only bill the patient the amount which you are legally allowed to bill. Do not write off patient co-payments or deductibles unless the patient has an approved and current *Financial Hardship Application* on file. See the "Financial Hardship Discounts" segment in Chapter 1.5 — Establishing Fees for more information.

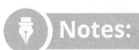

Notes:

1.2 Types of Insurance Plans

This chapter explains the different types of insurance plans that a healthcare practice may encounter. It is important to understand that there are a variety of insurance plans, each designed to meet the demands of consumers. These range from traditional fee-for-service health plans to managed care plans. Types of insurance administered by federal and state government include Medicare, Medicaid, Workers Compensation, etc., each of which serves a different purpose.

Although most payers use the universal *1500 Health Insurance Claim Form*, also referred to as the *1500 Claim Form*, for paper claims, or the *837(p)* format *(5010)* for electronic claims, some payers may have additional requirements or forms. Be aware of these differences.

The *1500 Claim Form* is used for professional services. Institutional or facility services are billed using the *UB-04 Claim Form (CMS-1450)* for paper claims, or the *837(i)* format for electronic claims.

Book: See Chapter 2 — Medicare for more information on Medicare.
Book: See Chapter 1.4 — Claims Management for more about claims submission requirements and help with managing denials and appeals
Resource: See Resource 458 for more information about the *UB-04 Claim Form*.

Traditional Insurance (Individual or Group Health Plans)

Traditional indemnity plans or fee-for-service plans are purchased by individuals or groups. In this model, after the service(s) are rendered, claim(s) are submitted and adjudicated before the provider is reimbursed by the payer. These types of plans are becoming less common as both employers and individuals switch to alternative payment models in an effort to save money. To help control the cost of medical care, traditional plans are increasingly adopting ideas from managed care plans, such as utilization review and prior authorization.

Alert — Healthcare Reform Entities Are NOT Insurance Plans
Led by provisions in the Affordable Care Act, three types of patient care and payment models do not adhere to traditional insurance protocols. Accountable Care Organizations (ACOs), Patient Centered Medical Homes (PCMHs) and Patient Centered Healthcare Homes (PCHCHs) are designed to improve the quality of patient care while simultaneously decreasing costs. As such, they are not fee-for-service insurance plans. Providers need to be aware of how these new entities function and become involved in this changing healthcare environment.
Resource: See Resource 803 for a more thorough review of the impact of healthcare reform

Typically, in a traditional insurance plan, the patient could use the service of any doctor or any other medical service provider. Either the patient or the provider forwards the bill to the insurer who reimburses the medical costs based on an established formula or fee schedule.

The formula for most of these types of plans begins with the "usual and customary charge" for covered medical service. The insurance plan pays a percentage (typically 80%) of these costs, after the patient has paid for services up to the deductible amount of the policy. The patient is responsible for the remaining 20%, plus any charges in excess of the usual and customary charges for services rendered by non-participating providers.

Annual and Lifetime Limits

Beginning January 1, 2014, the Patient Protection and Affordable Care Act (PPACA) changed the rules regarding annual and lifetime limits. Insurance companies can no longer set annual or lifetime limits on "Essential Health Benefits" (EHB) as long as the patient is enrolled in that plan.

Resource: See Resource 152 for additional information.

PPACA Essential Health Benefits (EHBs)

PPACA establishes the federal minimum standards for required health plan benefits. States have the flexibility to determine their own benchmarks for plans sold in the exchanges, as well as those sold in small group and individual markets. Most states plan to continue to define their essential health benefits much as they did originally.

Resource: See Resource 153 for additional information on Essential Health Benefits.

The following are the required federal essential health benefits categories for all health plans offered in the individual and small group markets, both inside and outside the Health Insurance Marketplace:

- Ambulatory patient services
- Emergency services
- Hospitalization
- Maternity and newborn care
- Mental health services and addiction treatment
- Prescription drugs
- Rehabilitative and habilitative services and devices
- Laboratory services
- Preventive and wellness services and chronic disease management
- Pediatric services, including oral and vision care

Alert — Federal vs State Minimum Standards:
The Patient Protection and Affordable Care Act (PPACA) is a federal statute which includes federal standards for essential health benefits. States can enact their own minimum standards which may be more stringent, but they must, at minimum, meet the requirements of PPACA. It is important for all providers to be aware of their own state's statutes and regulations in addition to federal requirements.

Out of Pocket Maximum

Once medical costs reach a given amount in a calendar year, the customary costs for the benefits covered would be met in full by the insurance firm, and the insured is no longer subject to any cost sharing (i.e., copays, coinsurance, deductibles). This concept is called an "out-of-pocket maximum." The allowed amount changes annually. For example, for plan years which began in 2021, the out-of-pocket limits were $8,550 for individuals and $17,100 for families (for in-network services).

Appeals

All payers have an appeals process if all or part of your claim is denied; however, these processes are not standardized throughout the industry. For example, Medicare has their own specific appeal guidelines which are different than the process required for employer sponsored plans which are governed by ERISA.

Book: See "Managing Appeals" in Chapter 1.4 — Claims Management for more information about appeals.

Resource: See Resource 804 for more information about ERISA appeals.

Managed Care Organizations (HMO, PPO, etc.)

Managed care was created as a way to contain costs and maintain quality care standards. Broadly speaking, managed care is any health care delivery system in which a party other than the physician or the patient influences the type of health care delivered. A managed care system also actively manages both the medical and financial aspects of a patient's care.

Defining managed care is difficult because it is an evolving concept made up of disparate organizations. The features once differentiating the various managed care plans have become less distinct as they move forward and adopt similar characteristics. The characteristics most common to Managed Care Organizations (MCOs) such as Health Maintenance Organizations (HMOs) and Preferred Provider Organizations (PPOs) include:

- Arrangements with selected providers who furnish a package of services to enrollees.
- Explicit criteria for selection of providers.
- Quality assurance, utilization review, and outcome measures.
- Incentives (financial or program coverage).
- Penalties to enrollees who do not use selected providers.
- Provider risk-sharing arrangements.
- Management by providers to ensure that enrollees or members receive appropriate care from the most cost-efficient mix of providers.

Note: Preferred Provider Organizations (PPOs) continue to be the most common type of health insurance plans in the marketplace today – far surpassing traditional insurance. However, according to one survey, Consumer Directed Health Plans (CDHPs) are a close second to PPOs. See page 32 for more about CDHPs.

To Participate or Not Participate

Reimbursement from these plans often requires a healthcare provider to be on their panel, or network of "preferred" providers. Sometimes this is known as "participating." If you are not on their panel, ask if the patient's plan has an "out-of-network" or "opt-out" benefit. The "out-of-network" percentage of coverage may be lower than if you were participating; however, if you were participating, you would be required to accept their fee schedule and you would not be allowed to bill the patient for charges above the contracted amounts for covered benefits (called "balance billing").

Also check their list of covered and noncovered diagnosis and service codes. Managed care systems typically will either not cover or will limit coverage for particular diagnosis codes or procedures. Providers should always review policy and contract guidelines for their specialty. Although a service might be covered by the plan, it might not be covered when rendered by certain types of providers.

Reminder: Coverage and limits are determined by both individual payers and the particular plan policy of the beneficiary. In other words, because a single payer typically has multiple types of plans, you cannot assume that a service will be covered in all circumstances for all patients covered by that payer.

Learn as much as you can about the MCO before signing up. What is their financial status? What is their reputation for paying bills? How stable is their contract with the employer? Know your local market. Is the company under pressure to compete? If they have potential problems, signing up might not be a good option. If an MCO goes bankrupt (and they do), your only recourse may be to hire a lawyer and go to court.

Note: Once you are a contracted in-network provider, changing network status can be extremely challenging. Carefully review the network's contract to understand this component in order to avoid problems changing your network status in the future.

Advantages of Participating

- **Increased Clientele:** Patient requests to their insurance carrier for the name of a provider in their area could be referred to you. This is free "marketing." Check to see how many providers are currently on their panel in your area. Note that the trade-off to this "free marketing" is that participating providers often have a slightly lower fee schedule than non-participating providers (if the plan includes coverage for out-of-network providers).

- **Direct Payment:** Payment comes from the HMO directly to the provider, eliminating the risk of the patient not forwarding it to you.

Disadvantages of Participating

- **Panel Costs:** Quite often, there are costs associated with becoming part of a panel. Ask what those costs are, along with their anticipated referral rate. The amount of "participating fees" for their referral rate might not be worth the effort. It may be less expensive to run your own marketing campaign.

- **Lower Fees:** By participating, you agree to accept their "allowable" amount and only bill the patient for the applicable patient portion or "co-pay" and/or deductible. Ask what the allowable amounts are up front to avoid any unpleasant surprises. Some have very low fee schedules.

- **Higher Overhead Costs:** There could be additional overhead costs in administering other plans in your office. For example, you would need to maintain separate fee schedules and/or write off disallowed amounts. Be aware of any additional overhead expenses.

Consumer Driven Plans

This segment covers Consumer Directed Healthcare Plans (CDHP), no insurance or cash, and medical discount plans for those who are uninsured or underinsured.

Resource: See Resource 819 and search on "CDHP" for additional information.

Consumer Directed Healthcare Plans (CDHP)

Consumer Directed Healthcare Plans (CDHPs) were developed as a way to shift the control of healthcare dollars from the insurance companies to the patient (consumer). The goal of these types of plans is to allow the patient to take a more active role in their own health and healthcare decisions in an effort to control costs. The Patient Protection and Affordable Care Act (PPACA) has fueled the growth of CDHPs.

Due to their growing market share, providers need to understand how these plans work. They must also be both willing and able to answer uncomfortable questions such as "How much is this going to cost?" or "Do I really need an MRI?"

CDHP Options

Here is a summary of major consumer driven health insurance options:

- **Health Savings Accounts (HSA).** These accounts permit eligible individuals to save and pay for healthcare expenses on a tax-free basis. HSA patients are empowered to spend their own dollars. Funds are held in a tax-exempt trust or custodial account with a qualified HSA trustee who pays or reimburses qualified health care expenses. Funds do not have to be used up at the end of the year and continue to accrue annually on a tax-exempt basis. To qualify for an HSA, there must be a high deductible health plan (HDHP).

- **Flexible Spending Account (FSA).** This type of account is similar to an HSA, but does not require an associated HDHP and can be used for purposes beyond health care, like child care. FSA funds also cannot be rolled over year-to-year like HSA funds and do not accumulate interest. These funds are owned by the employer, not the employee, so if an employee leaves the organization offering the FSA, they do not retain access to the funds.

- **Medicare Medical Savings Accounts (MSA).** This consumer-driven option for Medicare beneficiaries is a huge boon for beneficiaries because it eliminates the need for MediGap coverage and costs, provides a way of paying for Medicare noncovered services, limits out-of-pocket exposure, and offers the opportunity to save-up for future expenses. Unfortunately, not all states offer an MSA option for Medicare beneficiaries and Medicare MSA plans don't cover prescription drugs so a separate Medicare Part D policy may also need to be purchased.

- **Health Reimbursement Arrangement (HRA).** In these employer-sponsored health plans, the employee/patient has control of their funds. Plans can vary, and if specifically allowed, these personally controlled reserve funds can roll over from year to year and continue to grow. The result of which is a diminished need for major medical insurance and associated controls by others.

- **Voluntary Employee Benefit Associations (VEBA).** VEBA is a classification by law that permits employees within a geographic area to band together for a common good. For example, school teachers in the state of Washington organized themselves. As a result, a majority of the healthcare reserves are controlled by each member for their account within the VEBA, but only a minority of the funds are needed for outside catastrophic insurance.

- **Multiple Employer Welfare Arrangements (MEWA).** MEWA is a type of plan, established by ERISA and regulated by the PPACA, in which two or more unrelated employers, including those who are self-employed, may establish a health benefit plan. This can be done through an insurance plan or some other type of funding.

In concept, MEWAs are designed to give small employers access to low cost health coverage on terms similar to those available to large employers.

Alert — Affordable Care Act Limited Provisions:
The Affordable Care Act treats self-funded health benefit plans differently than fully insured plans. There are fewer regulations under the PPACA for self-funded plans and the new trend for employers appears to be moving towards the self-funded option. These differences make it essential for providers to verify coverage and plan information.
Resource: See Resource 804 for important information on self-funded plans.

Impact of CDHP on Patients and Practitioners

Beneficiaries enrolled in CDHP plans can now take a more active role in determining where their funds and benefits will be spent/utilized. Healthcare providers who give patients the best value-based care for dollars spent will be the most successful practitioners in the future. Providers will need to become more familiar with patient centered health care models, such as Patient Centered Medical Homes (PCMHs) and Accountable Care Organizations (ACOs) as regulations and guidelines under healthcare reform and quality improvement are implemented.

Resource: See Resource 803 for additional information.

No-Insurance and the Cash Practice

A growing number of healthcare practices offer some form of a cash practice, often as a result of frustrations due to inadequate reimbursement and excessive administrative requirements. Additionally, there are many individuals with a high deductible insurance plan (HDHP). These plans effectively make them a cash-paying patient until their deductible is met. For either situation, there are some unique challenges that must be addressed with written policies to ensure compliance.

No-Insurance

If you're a provider who desires to practice without third-party interference, while also getting a fair market value for your services, a no-insurance practice could be for you. This can be a positive business and financial decision. It provides an alternative to the labor-intensive health insurance reimbursement process. Healthcare providers and their patients can both benefit from this type of arrangement.

The benefits of having a no-insurance program or cash practice with payment in full at the time of service by cash, check, or credit card are:

- Hassle-free health care
- Elimination of administrative and other overhead costs
- Less paperwork
- No insurance forms or bills to send
- No referral approval or authorization
- Lower fees to patients

The risks of a cash practice include having fewer patients initially, having false illusions that quality is not important, and being a possible target of unfair fee allegations by third-party payers.

All who pay at the time of service should get the same benefit, whether they have insurance or no insurance. A patient sees a doctor for a non-catastrophic reason and the patient pays in full before leaving – it's just that simple!

Policies

- **Fees:** There needs to be transparency in pricing and your fee schedule should clearly define costs. In many cases, it is both feasible and beneficial to go over the projected costs with the patient prior to rendering the service. Many do not fully understand how much some procedures cost. Transparency in fee pricing reduces sticker shock and improves patient understanding.
- **Software:** Software systems need to be able to handle this type of pricing.
- **Staff:** Staff need to be trained on how to ensure that collections take place as outlined in your financial policy.
- **Non-covered services:** If you will be submitting to insurance, keep a listing of services that are non-covered by the payer. This way you know up front if this will be a cash situation.
- **Deposits:** Consider requiring deposits on lower-cost services. Include the process of how to issue a rebate on that deposit if the insurance does pay. This should clearly be outlined in your patient Financial Policy.

Book: See Chapter 1.5 — Establishing Fees for more information about discounting fee schedules.
Resource: See Resource 819 and search on "CDHP" for additional information.

Alert: If you have a "cash practice," you are still subject to rules regarding Medicare beneficiaries. See Chapter 2 — Medicare for more information.

Healthcare Discount Programs

Healthcare discount programs, also known as medical discount programs or Discount Medical Plan Organizations (DMPOs), are not medical insurance. Rather, they are member programs where a fee is paid in order to be part of the "group," which qualifies the buyer for discounted services. In many states, these types of programs are regulated, so be sure that any plan you are considering joining is approved in your state.

Benefits

There are many patients that are either uninsured or underinsured. Legal discount programs can help doctors enjoy the benefit of offering a discount (other than Time of Service) to patients that are part of their network of paid subscribers. Those plans which utilize the network concept and are approved and registered in your state can help to fill in those gaps. It has been compared to being in a PPO for your cash and underinsured patients. Some plans require you to accept discounts prescribed by the plan. Other plans may allow you to set your own level of discounts.

Unlike the Time of Service discount which must be paid in full at the time of service, some of these plans allow the patient to benefit from lower fees which can be paid over time.

Look Before You Leap

Not all healthcare discount programs are the same. The Federal Trade Commission (FTC) is warning consumers to carefully evaluate these programs. Providers need to exercise caution as well, as some programs are not as wonderful as they claim. Carefully review contracts, minimum requirements and exercise due diligence in evaluating these plans and any applicable state laws and regulations. In some cases, these programs have not really benefited the patient or provider.

For these reasons, some professional organizations have issued official policies regarding healthcare discount programs. Carefully consider the following:

- Carefully review state regulations to ensure compliance.
- Exercise caution using a discount program in conjunction with, or in lieu of, a patient's Medicare benefits.
- Caution should also be observed when using a discount program in conjunction with, or in lieu of, third party payers and managed care organizations.
- Providers should completely review contracts and investigate the policies in place for renewal and cancellation of membership by patients and participation by providers to determine their rights under the contract.

Resource: See Resource 110 to view additional comments, resources, networks, and opinions on discounts.

Government Programs

The Department of Health and Human Services (HHS) oversees all government health care programs. They are administered by various agencies such as the Centers for Medicare & Medicaid Services (CMS), the Veterans Administration (VA) and even on the state level. This segment gives a brief overview of these government services.

Book: See Chapter 2 — Medicare for information about the Medicare program.
Resource: See Resource 162 for additional information.

Federal Employee Plans

By law, Federal Employees are entitled to both workers' compensation benefits for work-related injuries and the Federal Employees Health Benefits (FEHB) program. These programs have caused some problems for healthcare providers in the past because they mistakenly bill the same as they would any other program like Medicare.

Federal Employees Health Benefits (FEHB) Program

The Federal Employees Health Benefits (FEHB) Program is a system of "managed competition" through which employee health benefits are provided to civilian government employees and annuitants of the United States government. Workers pay one-third of the cost of insurance; the government pays the other two-thirds.

The FEHB program, which is administered by the United States Office of Personnel Management (OPM), allows some insurance companies, employee associations, and labor unions to market health insurance plans to governmental employees.

Resource: See Resource 409 for more information.

Federal Workers Compensation

For all injuries that are work related, Federal employees are entitled to those services and supplies which are recommended by a physician which are likely to cure, give relief, reduce the degree or period of disability, or aid in lessening the amount of monthly compensation. Preventive care is not a covered benefit.

Note: To be paid for treating federal employees by the Federal Employees Workers Compensation Act (FECA), you must enroll with their bill consolidation contractor (ACS).

Resource: See Resource 14A for more information.

Military and Veterans

Military programs are offered through the Department of Defense (DOD) and the Department of Veterans Affairs (VA). The Department of Defense covers active duty service members and retirees from all branches of the military and their families. The Department of Veterans Affairs covers veterans and their eligible family members. Each program has different eligibility criteria and a variety of benefits packages.

Resource: See Resource 819 and search on "veterans" for more information.

TRICARE

TRICARE is the managed care program administered by the Department of Defense for active duty military, active duty service families, retirees and their families, and other beneficiaries. There are only a limited number of facilities. If your office is near a military facility, and you qualify, this could be a unique opportunity for your practice.

CHAMPUS and CHAMPVA

The Civilian Health and Medical Program of the Uniformed Services (CHAMPUS) and the Civilian Health and Medical Program of the Veteran Services (CHAMPVA) are not health insurance programs, but they do make payment for health benefits provided through certain affiliations with the Uniformed Services and the Veterans Administration. Similar to the Medicare program, the physician agrees to accept the charge determination as payment in full and the patient is responsible for any deductible, coinsurance, and noncovered services.

Those who are interested in positions or contracts should contact their nearest VA office. See Resource 407 for help in finding the nearest VA office.

Community Care Network

The VA Community Care Network (CCN) is a Veterans Health Administration (VHA) program created to provide eligible Veterans access to certain services when they are not readily available in the local VA. CCN has six regional networks who are managed by different third party adminators (TPAs) to provide services in those regions. Providers must be contracted (in-network) with the applicable TPA in order to provide services. The existing Patient-Centered Community Care (PC3) network is currently being phased in to the new CCN on a region-by-region basis. Note that Optum (part of UnitedHealth Group, Inc.) services Regions 1, 2, and 3. TriWest Health Care Alliance (TriWest) will manage Regions 4 and 5 and Region 6 does not currently have a TPA.

Resource: See Resource 136 for information about the CCN.

The Department of Veterans Affairs (VA) utilizes a process called a "standardized episode-of-care" (SEOC) which is a type of pre-certification to address the overall course of treatment for an illness or condition instead of a specific service. Employing SEOC aims to reduce the need for secondary authorization requests (SAR) for certain types of services (e.g., chiropractic care, maternity). It is anticipated that this will allow additional services to be more readily available to veterans.

Resource: See Resource 820 for more information about veterans healthcare programs.

Medicaid

Medicaid programs are available to anyone unable to afford private health insurance or unable to meet the requirements for Medicare benefits. Federal and state governments cooperate in financing the Medicaid program. Each state decides which Medicaid health services will be provided as covered benefits and how those benefits will be administered. There are distinct differences between the way Medicare and Medicaid programs are administered. Staff members involved with reimbursement must educate themselves regarding their own state's Medicaid policies.

Your local state health department or state professional association can provide more specific information about how Medicaid is administered in your area. Interested healthcare providers should contact their state health departments for detailed information on this program.

Note: Medicaid is the single largest payer for mental health services in the United States. All states offer some form of coverage for behavioral health services. Some through traditional fee-for-service arrangements and others through managed care programs.
Resource: See Resource 408 for more information.

Certified Community Behavioral Health Clinics (CCBHCs)

Certified Community Behavioral Health Clinics (CCBHCs) were established through Section 223 of the Protecting Access to Medicare Act (PAMA) to assist states in their efforts to improve access to and outcomes of behavioral healthcare by providing community-based mental and substance use disorder treatment. In 2015, it began as a demonstration program and ongoing legislative action keeps expanding the program. Some states (e.g., Minnesota, Nevada, Oregon) have been working to permanently fund these programs even without federal funding.

Resource: See Resource 466 for more information.

Notes:

1.3 Claims Processing

Proper claim processing is the keystone of the Reimbursement Life Cycle. Without claims payment or reimbursement, the practice will not survive. Although payment from an insurance company used to be the end of this process, that is no longer the case. Post-payment reviews and audits are placing an ever-increasing burden on all medical providers.

This chapter explains how to file claims correctly, using the *1500 Claim Form*.

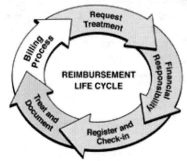

Book: See Chapter 2.3 — Medicare Appeals for information on appealing Medicare claims.
Book: See Chapter 3 — Compliance Essentials for more about post-payment audits & reviews.
Resource: See Resource 458 for more information about *UB-04 Claim Form* submission requirements for facility services.
Resource: See Resource 805 for additional resources including links, articles, & webinars.

Overview of Claims Processing

Submitting a clean claim is vital to the process of claims processing. Additionally, your treatment and documentation must meet medical necessity standards (establishing clinical need), and include all required elements for proper claims processing (e.g., proper claimant identification numbers). It may seem strange to include documentation in a discussion on claims processing, but claims auditors closely examine the medical record and thus it becomes an important, and often neglected, component of ensuring that claims are paid correctly without fear of recoupment.

Book: See Chapter 3 — Compliance Essentials for more information about this important part of claims processing and appeals.

Attend third party payer workshops or obtain and review their instructions for claims processing which are often accessible online. The specific written guidelines are typically found within the carrier or provider manual. Remember that not all insurance contracts and policies are alike. You need to understand the differences between companies and contracts.

Tip — Claims Adjudication:
This is the process by which the payer makes a determination about a claim based on internal edits, benefits and coverage information. When a payer receives a claim, adjudication follows a predetermined route before payment is either approved or denied.

Accurate Information Is Key

Pay particular attention to these items to ensure a clean claim.

- Place the beneficiary's name and ID number on each piece of documentation submitted. Always use the beneficiary's name exactly as it appears on their insurance card.

- Include all applicable National Provider Identifiers (NPI) on the claim, including the NPI for the referring provider.

- Indicate the correct address, including the valid ZIP code where the service was rendered to the beneficiary. Any missing, incomplete or invalid information in the Service Facility Location Information field will cause the claim to be rejected. Never use a post office box address in the field for the location where the service was rendered.

- Ensure that the number of units/days and the date of service range are not contradictory.

Resource: See Resource 175 for additional information about billing units.

Alert — Data Mining:
Computer information technology has made claims processing (adjudication) a science instead of a guessing game. Computerized data analysis, also called data mining, allows payers to profile physicians and review services and their billing patterns.

As Medicare analyzed these patterns to discover implications of fraudulent behavior, their fraud and abuse activities dramatically increased. It didn't take long for private payers to recognize the financial impact of Medicare's fraud and abuse initiatives. They also began to monitor and audit claims to verify the performance and necessity of billed services.

Book: See "Fraud and Abuse" in Chapter 3 — Compliance Essentials for more information.

Tip: Always verify that the codes reported on the claim are supported by the documentation in the clinical record. They must also support medical necessity requirements of the payer.
Book: See Chapter 4 — Documentation for more about documentation standards.
Book: See Chapter 3 — Compliance Essentials for more about medical necessity.

Diagnosis Code Pointing

Diagnosis code pointing is required by insurance companies in order to delineate which services were provided with which diagnosis. This is where the diagnosis listed in Item Number 21 on the *1500 Claim Form* is paired with a specific procedure code listed in Item Number 24D. Such pointing or pairing is standard within the insurance reimbursement industry. Since most claims are now processed by computer software programs which examine claim forms and transfer the information for processing in the carrier's system, there must be a valid diagnosis match (link) to each procedure or supply. The diagnosis is an essential part of the patient's medical record, and it is the driving force that justifies your treatment plan and payment.

Alert: When listing more than one diagnosis in the "diagnosis pointer box," (Item Number 24E), always have the procedure "point" to only the diagnosis that is most clinically significant for that particular service line.

It is important to ensure that the diagnosis pointing is consistent with the modifier(s) assigned to the service. For example, modifier 59 may be used to designate a different location or anatomic site.

Tip: The sequence, or order, of the codes that appear on the claim can be very important. For example, some conditions are considered 'secondary' and cannot be listed before other conditions. Also, some payers may require a specific order for reporting diagnoses. See Chapter 1 — Diagnosis Coding Essentials in innoviHealth's *ICD-10-CM Coding* books (available in the online store) for more information.

Multiple Diagnoses on a Claim Form

The paper *1500 Claim Form* is designed to match the electronic 5010 format and accommodate up to twelve diagnosis codes on a claim. Even though there is room for twelve codes, different insurance carriers have different requirements. Not all allow the maximum of twelve diagnosis codes on a claim so it is important to be aware of individual payer preferences. Notwithstanding the availability of space to report additional diagnoses, only include those which are relevant to the patient's treatment plan. It is also important to note that both the paper and electronic claim only allow four diagnosis codes to "point" to a single claim procedure line (see "Item Number 24E, Diagnosis Pointer" on page 59).

In the past, many payers wanted only one ICD diagnosis code: the primary code, which directly relates to the service/treatment. Although this protocol might fill the immediate processing needs of some payers (e.g., HMOs), it comes with big risks, because it fails to tell the complete story, which could lead to allegations of false claims. Always identify all applicable diagnosis codes on the claim, even if a payer will only look at one code. When you document services correctly, you protect your practice.

Book: See "1500 Claim Form Tips" on page 45 for additional tips about using the claim form.

Multiple Page Claims

The following general guidelines from the NUCC explain how to handle claims that span more than one page. However, be aware of individual payer requirements. Some may have different standards.

> "When reporting line item services on multiple page claims, only the diagnosis code(s) reported on the first page may be used and must be repeated on subsequent pages. If more than twelve diagnoses are required to report the line services, the claim must be split and the services related to the additional diagnoses must be billed as a separate claim."

Tip: Instead of using "Page XX of YY" for multiple pages, one way to avoid confusion is to simply split the claim. Bill related charges only on one claim form and put additional days of service on a separate claim form.

Timely Filing

Most insurance payers have a specific time period, commencing after the date of service, during which a health insurance claim must be submitted. If the claim arrives after this date, the claim is denied. Providers must obtain this information from each payer and make sure that claims are submitted within the time frame allowed.

To be eligible for Medicare reimbursement, claims must be filed with Medicare no later than one calendar year from the date of service or the claim will be denied.

Some payers follow the Medicare standard on the one calendar year filing deadline. However, it is always best to verify their standards by contacting their Provider Relations Department to find out about individual policies.

Late Filing Exceptions

Most providers are unaware that there are some late filing exceptions. Most payers allow claims to be filed late, but only under certain circumstances. Contact the payer to find out their particular policy regarding late filing. The following may be some accepted reasons for fighting a late filing denial:

- Errors on the original claim
- Claim filed with the incorrect carrier
- Missing authorizations or referrals
- Claims that were filed by the provider in the correct time frame, but lost by the carrier

Refiling/Resubmitting Claims

There are several reasons to refile or resubmit a claim. The carrier could lose them, they could be lost by the postal service, or there could be a problem during the electronic transmission. Whatever the reason, follow-up is important. Keeping a detailed log or printing reports of sent claims is essential. Some payers may have specific protocols which must be followed such as using a special form or printing "refiled claim" on paper claims. To avoid duplication errors, determine the insurer's policy before resubmitting a claim. Include this information in the *Daily Policies and Procedures Manual* for easy reference.

How to File Claims

Providers have only two options for filing claims: paper or electronic. There are pros and cons to either option. For example, electronic claims are paid faster, but you must meet all HIPAA requirements, which requires additional software and training costs. Evaluate both options to determine which one is an appropriate "fit" for your practice.

Other important factors to consider are state law and individual carrier contracts. Even though HIPAA does not require all claims to be submitted electronically (there are exceptions available), there are some states which do not allow any exceptions. Also, some payers require electronic claims submission. Pay special attention to your contract renewals to ensure compliance.

Paper Claims

Paper claims are submitted using the *1500 Claim Form* (or the *UB-04* for institutional claims). The form should be submitted using the red ink version that can be scanned by payers. A typical copy machine or printer cannot accurately duplicate the red ink used to print the *1500 Claim Form*. Therefore, if you attempt to print the red ink version of the *1500 Claim Form* from your printer, many payers will not be able to process your claims.

For those wishing to maintain exemption from HIPAA mandates (which is rare) and continue to bill paper claims, you must not send or receive any electronic transactions (eligibility, coordination of benefits, payments, payment reports, etc). However, be aware of any payer contracts that might require that you submit electronic claims. Medicare, for example, mandates electronic claims submission; however, small providers with less than 10 full-time equivalent employees may apply for an exemption. If you qualify for an exemption with any payer, follow-up and make sure they have your exemption status on file.

Resource:
- See Resource 194 for information about the Medicare electronic claims exemption.
- See Resource 178 for more information about *1500 Claim Form* submission requirements (requires a subscription to Find-A-Code and selection of the InstaGuide as an add-on).
- See Resource 458 for more information about *UB-04 Claim Form* submission requirements.

Electronic Claims

Electronic claims are *1500 claims* (or *UB-04* for facilities) in an electronic (837) format and are subject to all HIPAA standards for transactions, privacy, and security. When submitting an electronic claim, you automatically become a HIPAA entity. Make sure that your office, your software billing company, vendors, subcontractors, and the receiving payer are all HIPAA compliant.

The current official HIPAA transaction standard is version 5010. Version 5010 is the X12 standard (*837p* and *837i*) for all HIPAA electronic claims submission. HIPAA 5010 allows for the longer ICD-10-CM codes that were implemented in October 2015.

Tip — Version 7030:
The Accredited Standards Committee (ASC) has completed the public review and comment periods for the next proposed HIPAA X12 standard. At the time of publication, it was estimated that Version 7030 will be implemented in 2018 or 2019.

Paperwork Segment

The paperwork segment (PWK) was developed as a way for providers to ensure that additional documentation, which will be sent via fax or mail, is properly linked to an electronic claim. This is distinctly different than electronic submission of medical documentation (esMD) in which the supporting documentation is sent electronically. Instead, using the PWK segment on an electronic claim indicates that paper documentation will be submitted and links it to that specific claim. Most payers require the completion of a specific cover sheet to be included with documentation which is submitted via fax or mail. Generally, you only have 7-10 days to successfully submit the necessary documentation once the electronic claim has been filed.

When supporting documentation is linked to a claim, it helps to ensure that it is adjudicated properly the first time instead of going through an appeals process.

Even though PWK is voluntary and many payers are using it, be aware of individual payer requirements. For example, WPS Medicare requires PWK when electronic claims are submitted with modifiers 22 or 52.

Alert — Business Associates:
Your business associates and subcontractors, including your clearinghouse and billing software vendor, must be HIPAA compliant. The Omnibus Final Rule changed the definition of a business associate and updated Business Associate Agreements should have already been executed in accordance with that rule.
Store: For Business Associate Agreements see *Complete & Easy HIPAA Compliance* (Resource 116) available in the online store.

Filing Tips

General Filing Tips

The following tips apply to both paper and electronic claims.

Coding Tips

- Use current, valid diagnosis codes and code to the highest level of specificity (maximum number of digits) available. Also make sure that the diagnosis codes used are appropriate for the gender of the beneficiary.
- Use current, valid procedure codes as described in the Current Procedural Terminology (CPT) or Healthcare Common Procedure Coding System (HCPCS) manuals.

- Use current and valid modifiers when necessary.
- Follow the written guidelines of individual payers. If there is an issue with their policies, work with your professional association to resolve the problem. Professional associations are often successful in overturning incorrect coding policies.

Book: See Chapter 5 — Procedure Coding for current CPT and HCPCS codes for procedures.
Book: See Chapter 6 — Supply Coding for current HCPCS codes for supplies.

Store: See innoviHealth's *ICD-10-CM Coding* books for a list of specialty specific codes.

Common Errors to Avoid

- Using a patient name or address that is different than what the payer has listed for that beneficiary
- Incorrect patient ID number
- Incomplete patient information
- Incorrect or missing provider ID number(s)
- Incorrect dates of service
- Incorrect dates, or dates entered with an incorrect number of digits
- Insufficient information regarding primary or secondary coverage
- Invalid procedure, supply, or diagnostic codes
- Invalid or missing modifiers
- Unit of service errors (see Resource 175 for additional information)
- Invalid or missing Place of Service (POS) codes
- Invalid diagnostic codes that do not point to the correct procedure or service
- Failure to enter the fee (left blank); fees not itemized and totaled
- Missing patient and/or provider signatures
- Ineligible claims (expired or canceled insurance contract)
- Late filing errors

Alert — Lost Claims:
Lost claims are a dreaded but inevitable part of healthcare claims processing. The best way to avoid them is to file claims electronically. This removes a lot of pitfalls that can go wrong with paper, but it can still happen with electronic claims. If a claim is lost after being filed electronically then re-submit on paper. If you have talked to someone at the insurance company, ask to send it directly to their attention. To assure delivery, send the claim either by certified mail, with proof of service, or with delivery confirmation.

1500 Claim Form Tips

The following rules for the *1500 Claim Form* are excerpts from NUCC and Medicare instructions, but they are generally universal and apply to claims submitted either electronically or on paper. Please note that payment rules can change frequently for any payer, so consult with specific insurance payers for their adaptations.

The instructions included in this segment are excerpts from the following documents along with commentary by innoviHealth:

- *1500 Health Insurance Claim Form Reference Instruction Manual* for Form Version 02/12 (version 9.0 7/21), by the National Uniform Claim Committee (NUCC)
- Medicare instructions by CMS (Rev. 10341, 09-04-20)

Please note that this segment only contains instructions or information that should be paid close attention to when submitting claims. Complete instructions are available online.

Resource: See Resource 178 for the complete list of line items and their associated guidelines and revisions, including exclusive innoviHealth tips (requires a subscription to Find-A-Code and selection of the InstaGuide as an add-on).

Instruction Conventions

Item Number and Titles are in bold text.

NUCC descriptions are in italic text.

NUCC instructions are in regular text.

> Medicare instructions, as listed in the *Medicare Claims Processing Manual*, are in a style like this.

> Alerts and commentaries in this chapter by innoviHealth are in a style like this.

Overall Instructions

Each item number includes the title, instructions, description, and example. The examples provided in the instructions are demonstrating how to enter the data in the field. They are not providing instruction on how to bill for certain services. Note that form images may not be to scale.

Field Specific Instructions

Item Number 5, Patient's Address (multiple fields)

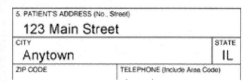

Description: The "Patient's Address" is the patient's permanent residence. A temporary address or school address should not be used.

Enter the patient's address. The first line is for the street address; the second line, the city and state; the third line, the ZIP code.

Do not use punctuation (i.e., commas, periods) or other symbols in the address (e.g., 123 N Main Street 101 instead of 123 N. Main Street, #101). Report a 5 or 9-digit ZIP code. Enter the 9-digit ZIP code without the hyphen.

If reporting a foreign address, contact payer for specific reporting instructions.

If the patient's address is the same as the insured's address, then it is not necessary to report the patient's address.

"Patient's Telephone" does not exist in 5010A1. The NUCC recommends that the phone number not be reported. Phone extensions are not supported.

For Workers Compensation and Other Property and Casualty Claims: If required by a payer to report a telephone number, do not use a hyphen or space as a separator within the telephone number.

Medicare: Enter the patient's mailing address and telephone number. On the first line enter the street address; the second line, the city and state; the third line, the ZIP code and phone number.

innoviHealth: Verify this demographic information. The patient's address is not always the same as the insured's address. Using the incorrect address is a common cause of delayed payment.

Item Number 9, Other Insured's Name

9. OTHER INSURED'S NAME (Last Name, First Name, Middle Initial)
Doe, Mary, A

Description: The "Other Insured's Name" indicates that there is a holder of another policy that may cover the patient.

If Item Number 11d is marked, complete fields 9, 9a and 9d, otherwise leave blank. When additional group health coverage exists, enter other insured's full last name, first name, and middle initial of the enrollee in another health plan if it is different from that shown in Item Number 2. If the insured uses a last name suffix (e.g., Jr, Sr), enter it after the last name and before the first name. Titles (e.g., Sister, Capt, Dr) and professional suffixes (e.g., PhD, MD, Esq) should not be included with the name.

Use commas to separate the last name, first name, and middle initial. A hyphen can be used for hyphenated names. Do not use periods within the name.

Medicare: Enter the last name, first name, and middle initial of the enrollee in a Medigap policy if it is different from that shown in item 2. Otherwise, enter the word SAME. If no Medigap benefits are assigned, leave blank. **This field may be used in the future for supplemental insurance plans.**

NOTE: Only participating physicians and suppliers are to complete item 9 and its subdivisions and only when the beneficiary wishes to assign his/her benefits under a MEDIGAP policy to the participating physician or supplier.

Participating physicians and suppliers must enter information required in item 9 and its subdivisions if requested by the beneficiary. Participating physicians/suppliers sign an agreement with Medicare to accept assignment of Medicare benefits for **all** Medicare patients. A claim for which a beneficiary elects to assign his/her benefits under a Medigap policy to a participating physician/supplier is called a mandated Medigap transfer. (See chapter 28.)

Medigap: Medigap policy meets the statutory definition of a "Medicare supplemental policy" contained in §1882(g)(1) of title XVIII of the Social Security Act (the Act) and the definition contained in the NAIC Model Regulation that is incorporated by reference to the statute. It is a health insurance policy or other health benefit plan offered by a private entity to those persons entitled to Medicare benefits and is specifically designed to supplement Medicare benefits. It fills in some of the "gaps" in Medicare coverage by providing payment for some of the charges for which Medicare does not have responsibility due to the applicability of deductibles, coinsurance amounts, or other limitations imposed by Medicare. It does not include limited benefit coverage available to Medicare beneficiaries such as "specified disease" or "hospital indemnity" coverage. Also, it explicitly excludes a policy or plan offered by an employer to employees or former employees, as well as that offered by a labor organization to members or former members.

Do not list other supplemental coverage in item 9 and its subdivisions at the time a Medicare claim is filed. Other supplemental claims are forwarded automatically to the private insurer if the private insurer contracts with the A/B MAC (B) or DME MAC to send Medicare claim information electronically. If there is no such contract, the beneficiary must file his/her own supplemental claim.

innoviHealth: Some payers may want the name entered without commas. Be aware of individual payer differences.

innoviHealth: For Medicare, Item Number 9 should only be completed when the provider is a participating physician or supplier, and when the patient wishes to assign his/her benefits under a Medigap policy to the participating physician or supplier. Participating providers sign an agreement with Medicare to accept assignment of Medicare benefits for all Medicare patients. A claim for which a beneficiary elects to assign his/her benefits under a Medigap policy to a participating provider is called a mandated Medigap transfer.

Other supplemental coverage should not be listed in Item Number 9 or its subdivisions at the time a Medicare claim is filed. Other supplemental claims are forwarded automatically to the private insurer if the private insurer contracts with the carrier to send Medicare claim information electronically. If there is no such contract, the beneficiary must file his/her own supplemental claim.

innoviHealth: This is an important item to properly complete because payers have been reviewing claims that were incorrectly paid as primary when it should have been secondary.

Items Number 10a–10c, Is Patient's Condition Related To:

Description: This information indicates whether the patient's illness or injury is related to employment, auto accident, or other accident. "Employment (current or previous)" would indicate that the condition is related to the patient's job or workplace. "Auto accident" would indicate that the condition is the result of an automobile accident. "Other accident" would indicate that the condition is the result of any other type of accident.

When appropriate, enter an X in the correct box to indicate whether one or more of the services described in Item Number 24 are for a condition or injury that occurred on the job or as a result of an automobile or other accident. Only one box on each line can be marked.

The state postal code where the accident occurred must be reported, if "YES" is marked in 10b for "Auto Accident." Any item marked "YES" indicates there may be other applicable insurance coverage that would be primary, such as automobile liability insurance. Primary insurance information must then be shown in Item Number 11.

Medicare: Check "YES" or "NO" to indicate whether employment, auto liability, or other accident involvement applies to one or more of the services described in item 24. Enter the State postal code. Any item checked "YES" indicates there may be other insurance primary to Medicare. Identify primary insurance information in item 11.

innoviHealth: Any item marked "YES" indicates there may be other insurance.

innoviHealth: The OIG and other payers are carefully evaluating claims they paid which may have been the liability of another party – secondary vs. primary.

Resource: See Resource 806 for more information.

Item Number 11, Insured's Policy, Group, or FECA Number

11. INSURED'S POLICY GROUP OR FECA NUMBER
A1234

Description: The "Insured's Policy, Group, or FECA Number" is the the alphanumeric identifier for the health, auto, or other insurance plan coverage. The FECA number is the 9-character alphanumeric identifier assigned to a patient claiming work-related condition(s) under the Federal Employees Compensation Act 5 USC 8101.

Enter the insured's policy or group number as it appears on the insured's health care identification card. If Item Number 4 is completed, then this field should be completed.

Do not use a hyphen or space as a separator within the policy or group number.

Medicare: THIS ITEM MUST BE COMPLETED, IT IS A REQUIRED FIELD. BY COMPLETING THIS ITEM, THE PHYSICIAN/SUPPLIER ACKNOWLEDGES HAVING MADE A GOOD FAITH EFFORT TO DETERMINE WHETHER MEDICARE IS THE PRIMARY OR SECONDARY PAYER.

If there is insurance primary to Medicare, enter the insured's policy or group number and proceed to items 11a - 11c. Items 4, 6, and 7 must also be completed.

NOTE: Enter the appropriate information in item 11c if insurance primary to Medicare is indicated in item 11.

If there is no insurance primary to Medicare, enter the word "NONE" and proceed to item 12.

If the insured reports a terminating event with regard to insurance which had been primary to Medicare (e.g., insured retired), enter the word "NONE" and proceed to item 11b.

If a lab has collected previously and retained Medicare Secondary Payer (MSP) information for a beneficiary, the lab may use that information for billing purposes of the non-face-to-face lab service. If the lab has no MSP information for the beneficiary, the lab will enter the word "None" in Block 11, when submitting a claim for payment of a reference lab service. Where there has been no face-to-face encounter with the beneficiary, the claim will then follow the normal claims process. When a lab has a face-to-face encounter with a beneficiary, the lab is expected to collect the MSP information and bill accordingly.

Insurance Primary to Medicare: Circumstances under which Medicare payment may be secondary to other insurance include:

- Group Health Plan Coverage
  - Working Aged;
  - Disability (Large Group Health Plan); and
  - End Stage Renal Disease;

- No Fault and/or Other Liability; and
- Work-Related Illness/Injury:
  - Workers' Compensation;
  - Black Lung; and
  - Veterans Benefits.

Note: For a paper claim to be considered for MSP benefits, a copy of the primary payer's explanation of benefits (EOB) notice must be forwarded along with the claim form. (See Pub. 100-05, Medicare Secondary Payer Manual, chapter 3.)

innoviHealth: The OIG and other payers are carefully evaluating claims they paid which may have been the liability of another party – secondary vs. primary.

Resource: See Resource 806 for more information.

Item Number 12, Patient's or Authorized Person's Signature

Description: The "Patient's or Authorized Person's Signature" indicates there is an authorization on file for the release of any medical or other information necessary to process and/or adjudicate the claim.

Enter "Signature on File," "SOF," or legal signature. When legal signature, enter date signed in 6-digit (MM|DD|YY) or 8-digit format (MM|DD|YYYY). If there is no signature on file, leave blank or enter "No Signature on File."

Medicare: The patient or authorized representative must sign and enter either a 6-digit date (MM | DD | YY), 8-digit date (MM | DD | CCYY), or an alpha-numeric date (e.g., January 1, 1998) unless the signature is on file. In lieu of signing the claim, the patient may sign a statement to be retained in the provider, physician, or supplier file in accordance with Chapter 1, "General Billing Requirements." If the patient is physically or mentally unable to sign, a representative specified in Chapter 1, may sign on the patient's behalf. In this event, the statement's signature line must indicate the patient's name followed by "by" the representative's name, relationship to the patient, and the reason the patient cannot sign. The authorization is effective indefinitely unless the patient or the patient's representative revokes this arrangement.

NOTE: This can be "Signature on File" and/or a computer generated signature.

The patient's signature authorizes release of medical information necessary to process the claim. It also authorizes payment of benefits to the provider of service or supplier when the provider of service or supplier accepts assignment on the claim.

Signature by Mark (X) – When an illiterate or physically handicapped enrollee signs by mark, a witness must enter his/her name and address next to the mark.

InnoviHealth: The signed agreement(s) should be kept with the patient's records in the provider's files. The authorization may be on a lifetime agreement. It need not specify a period of time and the patient can cancel it at any time. This agreement is effective from the date of signing, and is effective indefinitely unless the patient or the patient's representative revokes this arrangement.

During an audit, the payer may request that you provide them with the Signature on File or patient signature.

Item Number 14, Date of Current Illness, Injury, or Pregnancy (LMP)

```
14. DATE OF CURRENT ILLNESS, INJURY, or PREGNANCY (LMP)
    MM | DD | YY
    01 | 14 | 2020      QUAL. | 431
```

Description: The "Date of Current Illness, Injury, or Pregnancy" identifies the first date of onset of illness, the actual date of injury, or the LMP for pregnancy.

Enter the 6-digit (MM | DD | YY) or 8-digit (MM | DD | YYYY) date of the first date of the present illness, injury, or pregnancy. For pregnancy, use the date of the last menstrual period (LMP) as the first date.

Enter the applicable qualifier to identify which date is being reported.

    431 Onset of Current Symptoms or Illness
    484 Last Menstrual Period

Enter the qualifier to the right of the vertical, dotted line.

Medicare: Enter either an 8-digit (MM | DD | CCYY) or 6-digit (MM | DD | YY) date of current illness, injury, or pregnancy. For chiropractic services, enter an 8-digit (MM | DD | CCYY) or 6-digit (MM | DD | YY) date of the initiation of the course of treatment and enter an 8-digit (MM | DD | CCYY) or 6-digit (MM | DD | YY) date in item 19.

Additional information for form version 02/12: Although this version of the form includes space for a qualifier, Medicare does not use this information; do not enter a qualifier in item 14.

InnoviHealth: Not all payers accept or require a qualifier. Be aware of individual payer policies.

InnoviHealth: When there is a new course of treatment (e.g., exacerbations), this field may be used to indicate the new start date of the updated treatment plan. For injuries, this must be the date that the injury or accident occurred. This is for all types of injuries including home accidents. The only exception is when billing Medicare for chiropractic services, in which case, this field indicates the date the patient presented for care, not the date of current illness or injury.

Item Number 17, Name of Referring Provider or Other Source

```
17. NAME OF REFERRING PROVIDER OR OTHER SOURCE
    DN | Jane A Smith MD
```

Description: The name entered is the referring provider, ordering provider, or supervising provider who referred, ordered, or supervised the service(s) or supply(ies) on the claim. The qualifier indicates the role of the provider being reported.

Enter the name (First Name, Middle Initial, Last Name) followed by the credentials of the professional who referred or ordered the service(s) or supply(ies) on the claim.

If multiple providers are involved, enter one provider using the following priority order:

1. Referring Provider
2. Ordering Provider
3. Supervising Provider

Do not use periods or commas. A hyphen can be used for hyphenated names.

Enter the applicable qualifier to identify which provider is being reported.

    DN Referring Provider
    DK Ordering Provider
    DQ Supervising Provider

Enter the qualifier to the left of the vertical, dotted line.

InnoviHealth: If the name is very long, use the complete last name and as much of the first name as will fit in the remaining space.

Medicare: Enter the name of the referring or ordering physician if the service or item was ordered or referred by a physician. All physicians who order services or refer Medicare beneficiaries must report this data. Similarly, if Medicare policy requires you to report a supervising physician, enter this information in item 17. When a claim involves multiple referring, ordering, or supervising physicians, use a separate CMS-1500 claim form for each ordering, referring, or supervising physician.

Additional instructions for form version 02/12: Enter one of the following qualifiers as appropriate to identify the role that this physician (or non-physician practitioner) is performing:

Qualifier	Provider Role
DN	Referring Provider
DK	Ordering Provider
DQ	Supervising Provider

Enter the qualifier to the left of the dotted vertical line on item 17.

NOTE: Under certain circumstances, Medicare permits a non-physician practitioner to perform these roles. Refer to Pub 100-02, Medicare Benefit Policy Manual, chapter 15 for non-physician practitioner rules. Enter non-physician practitioner information according to the rules above for physicians.

The term "physician" when used within the meaning of §1861(r) of the Act and used in connection with performing any function or action refers to:

1. A doctor of medicine or osteopathy legally authorized to practice medicine and surgery by the State in which he/she performs such function or action;
2. A doctor of dental surgery or dental medicine who is legally authorized to practice dentistry by the State in which he/she performs such functions and who is acting within the scope of his/her license when performing such functions;
3. A doctor of podiatric medicine for purposes of §§(k), (m), (p)(1), and (s) and §§1814(a), 1832(a)(2)(F)(ii), and 1835 of the Act, but only with respect to functions which he/she is legally authorized to perform as such by the State in which he/she performs them;
4. A doctor of optometry, but only with respect to the provision of items or services described in §1861(s) of the Act which he/she is legally authorized to perform as a doctor of optometry by the State in which he/she performs them; or
5. A chiropractor who is licensed as such by a State (or in a State which does not license chiropractors as such), and is legally authorized to perform the services of a chiropractor in the jurisdiction in which he/she performs such services, and who meets uniform minimum standards specified by the Secretary, but only for purposes of §§1861(s)(1) and 1861(s)(2)(A) of the Act, and only with respect to treatment by means of manual manipulation of the spine (to correct a subluxation). For the purposes of §1862(a)(4) of the Act and subject to the limitations and conditions provided above, chiropractor includes a doctor of one of the arts specified in the statute and legally authorized to practice such art in the country in which the inpatient hospital services (referred to in §1862(a)(4) of the Act) are furnished.

Referring physician - is a physician who requests an item or service for the beneficiary for which payment may be made under the Medicare program.

Ordering physician - is a physician or, when appropriate, a non-physician practitioner who orders non-physician services for the patient. See Pub 100-02, Medicare Benefit Policy Manual, chapter 15 for non-physician practitioner rules. Examples of services that might be ordered include diagnostic laboratory tests, clinical laboratory tests, pharmaceutical services, durable medical equipment, and services incident to that physician's or non-physician practitioner's service.

The ordering/referring requirement became effective January 1, 1992, and is required by §1833(q) of the Act. **All claims** for Medicare covered services and items that are the result of a physician's order or referral shall include the ordering/referring physician's name. The following services/situations require the submission of the referring/ordering provider information:

- Medicare covered services and items that are the result of a physician's order or referral;
- Parenteral and enteral nutrition;
- Immunosuppressive drug claims;
- Hepatitis B claims;
- Diagnostic laboratory services;
- Diagnostic radiology services;
- Portable x-ray services;
- Consultative services;
- Durable medical equipment;
- When the ordering physician is also the performing physician (as often is the case with in-office clinical laboratory tests);
- When a service is incident to the service of a physician or non-physician practitioner, the name of the physician or non-physician practitioner who performs the initial service and orders the non-physician service must appear in item 17;
- When a physician extender or other limited licensed practitioner refers a patient for consultative service, submit the name of the physician who is supervising the limited licensed practitioner;
- Effective for claims with dates of service on or after October 1, 2012, all claims for physical therapy, occupational therapy, or speech-language pathology services, including those furnished incident to a physician or nonphysician practitioner, require that the name and NPI of the certifying physician or nonphysician practitioner of the therapy plan of care be entered as the referring physician in Items 17 and 17b.

Items Number 17a and 17b (split field)

```
17a. 0B ABC1234567890
17b. NPI 0123456789
```

Item 17a, Other ID#

Description: The non-NPI ID number of the referring, ordering, or supervising provider is the unique identifier of the professional.

The Other ID number of the referring, ordering, or supervising provider is reported in 17a in the shaded area. The qualifier indicating what the number represents is reported in the qualifier field to the immediate right of 17a.

The NUCC defines the following qualifiers used in 5010A1:

0B	State License Number	G2	Provider Commercial Number
1G	Provider UPIN Number	LU	Location Number (This qualifier is used for Supervising Provider only.)

Medicare: Leave blank

InnoviHealth: Other ID: Often providers ask which other ID number they should be using for a specific payer (e.g., State Farm, Cigna). Different payers have different requirements. Obtain this information directly from the payer.

InnoviHealth: Taxonomy codes are specific classifications for providers and are a component of NPI applications. The National Uniform Claim Committee (NUCC) is presently maintaining the Health Care Provider Taxonomy list. See Resource 197 for the taxonomy codes.

Item Number 19, Additional Claim Information (Designated by NUCC)

```
19. ADDITIONAL CLAIM INFORMATION (Designated by NUCC)

```

Description: "Additional Claim Information" identifies additional information about the patient's condition or the claim.

NUCC Instructions

Please refer to the most current instructions from the applicable public or private payer regarding the use of this field. Report the appropriate qualifier, when available, for the information being entered. Do not enter a space, hyphen, or other separator between the qualifier and the information.

For the Claim Information (NTE), the following are the qualifiers in 5010A1. Enter the qualifier "NTE", followed by the appropriate qualifier, then the information. Do not enter spaces between the qualifier and the first word of the information. After the qualifier, use spaces to separate any words.

ADD	Additional Information
CER	Certification Narrative
DCP	Goals, Rehabilitation Potential, or Discharge Plans
DGN	Diagnosis Description
TPO	Third Party Organization Notes

```
19. ADDITIONAL CLAIM INFORMATION (Designated by NUCC)
NTEADDSurgery was unusually long due to scarring
```

For additional identifiers (REFs), the following are the qualifiers in 5010A1. Enter the qualifier "REF", followed by the qualifier, then the identifier. Do not enter spaces between the qualifier and identifier.

0B	State License Number
1G	Provider UPIN Number
G2	Provider Commercial Number
LU	Location Number (This qualifier is used for Supervising Provider only
N5	Provider Plan Network Identification Number
SY	Social Security Number (The social security number may not be used for Medicare.)
X5	State Industrial Accident Provider Number
ZZ	Provider Taxonomomy (The qualifier in the 5010A1 for Provider Taxonomy is PXC, but ZZ will remain the qualifier for the 1500 Claim Form.)

The above list contains both provider identifiers, as well as the provider taxonomy code. The provider identifiers are assigned to the provider either by a specific payer or by a third party in order to uniquely identify the provider. The taxonomy code is designated by the provider in order to identify his/her provider grouping, classification, or area of specialization. Both, provider identifiers and provider taxonomy may be used in this field.

Taxonomy codes or other identifiers reported in this field must not be reportable in other fields, i.e., Item Numbers 17, 24J, 32, or 33.

```
19. ADDITIONAL CLAIM INFORMATION (Designated by NUCC)
REFG21234567890
```

When reporting a second item of data, enter three blank spaces and then the next qualifier and number/code/information.

For Supplemental Claim Information (PWK), the following are the qualifiers in the 5010A1. Enter the qualifier "PWK", followed by the appropriate Report Type Code, the appropriate Transmission Type Code, then the Attachment Control Number. Do not enter spaces between the qualifiers and data.

REPORT TYPE CODES

03	Report Justifying Treatment Beyond Utilization		HC	Health Certificate
04	Drugs Administered		HR	Health Clinic Records
05	Treatment Diagnosis		I5	Immunization Record
06	Initial Assessment		IR	State School Immunization Records
07	Functional Goals		LA	Laboratory Results
08	Plan of Treatment		M1	Medical Record Attachment
09	Progress Report		MT	Models
10	Continued Treatment		NN	Nursing Notes
11	Chemical Analysis		OB	Operative Note
13	Certified Test Report		OC	Oxygen Content Averaging Report
15	Justification for Admission		OD	Orders and Treatments Document
21	Recovery Plan		OE	Objective Physical Examination (including vital signs) Document
A3	Allergies/Sensitivities Document			
A4	Autopsy Report		OX	Oxygen Therapy Certification
AM	Ambulance Certification		OZ	Support Data for Claim
AS	Admission Summary		P4	Pathology Report
B2	Prescription		P5	Patient Medical History Document
B3	Physician Order		PE	Parenteral or Enteral Certification
B4	Referral Form		PN	Physical Therapy Notes
BR	Benchmark Testing Results		PO	Prosthetics or Orthotic Certification
BS	Baseline		PQ	Paramedical Results
BT	Blanket Test Results		PY	Physician's Report
CB	Chiropractic Justification		PZ	Physical Therapy Certification
CK	Consent Form(s)		RB	Radiology Films
CT	Certification		RR	Radiology Reports
D2	Drug Profile Document		RT	Report of Tests and Analysis Report
DA	Dental Models		RX	Renewable Oxygen Content Averaging Report
DB	Durable Medical Equipment Prescription			
DG	Diagnostic Report		SG	Symptoms Document
DJ	Discharge Monitoring Report		V5	Death Notification
DS	Discharge Summary		XP	Photographs
EB	Explanation of Benefits (Coordination of Benefits or Medicare Secondary Payor)			

TRANSMISSION TYPE CODES

AA Available on Request at Provider Site
BM By Mail

```
19. ADDITIONAL CLAIM INFORMATION (Designated by NUCC)
PWK03AA12363545465
```

When reporting multiple separate items, enter three blank spaces and then the next qualifier and followed by the information.

```
19. ADDITIONAL CLAIM INFORMATION (Designated by NUCC)
NTEADD Surgery was unusually long due to scarring PWK0BBM1213141
```

Alert: This "additional claim information" box can be very useful. This is the one place on the 1500 Claim Form where explanatory information can be given. The new NUCC guidelines provide additional information on how to appropriately use qualifiers to help ensure proper claim adjudication. If there is not enough space, check with the payer to determine their requirements. Some may allow using "REF" with the appropriate "Report Type Code" along with the attached report. Providers typically use this box to provide clarifying information (such as rationale for modifiers to procedure codes in Item Number 21).

Note that supplemental information relating to a specific procedure code should use the shaded area of Item Number 21 instead of this field.

Medicare Instructions

Enter either a 6-digit (MM | DD | YY) or an 8-digit (MM | DD | CCYY) date patient was last seen and the NPI of his/her attending physician when a physician providing routine foot care submits claims.

NOTE: Effective May 23, 2008, all provider identifiers submitted on the CMS-1500 claim form **MUST** be in the form of an NPI.

Enter either a 6-digit (MM | DD | YY) or an 8-digit (MM | DD | CCYY) x-ray date for chiropractor services (if an x-ray, rather than a physical examination was the method used to demonstrate the subluxation). By entering an x-ray date and the initiation date for course of chiropractic treatment in item 14, the chiropractor is certifying that all the relevant information requirements (including level of subluxation) of Pub. 100-02, Medicare Benefit Policy Manual, chapter 15, is on file, along with the appropriate x-ray and all are available for A/B MAC (B) review.

Instructions for Not Otherwise Classified (NOC) Codes – Any unlisted services or procedure code. **Note:** When reporting NOC codes, this field must be populated as specified below. Enter the drug's name and dosage when submitting a claim for Not Otherwise Classified (NOC) drugs.

Enter a concise description of an "unlisted procedure code" or a NOC code if one can be given within the confines of this box. Otherwise an attachment shall be submitted with the claim.

When billing for unlisted laboratory tests using a NOC code, this field **MUST** include the specific name of the laboratory test(s) and/or a short descriptor of the test(s). Claims for unlisted laboratory tests that are received without this information shall be treated according to the requirements found in Pub. 100-04, Medicare Claims Processing Manual, Chapter 1, Section 80.3.2 and "returned as unprocessable." Section 216(a) of the Protecting Access to Medicare Act of 2014 (PAMA) requires reporting entities to report private payor payment rates for laboratory tests and the corresponding volumes of tests. In compliance with PAMA, CMS must collect private payor data on unique tests currently being paid as a NOC code, Not Otherwise Specified (NOS) code, or unlisted service or procedure code.

Enter all applicable modifiers when modifier -99 (multiple modifiers) is entered in item 24d. If modifier -99 is entered on multiple line items of a single claim form, all applicable modifiers for each line item containing a -99 modifier should be listed as follows: 1=(mod), where the number 1 represents the line item and "mod" represents all modifiers applicable to the referenced line item.

Enter the statement "Homebound" when an independent laboratory obtains a specimen from a homebound or institutionalized patient. (See Pub. 100-02, Medicare Benefit Policy Manual, Chapter 15, "Covered Medical and Other Health Services," and Pub. 100-04, Medicare Claims Processing Manual, Chapter 16, "Laboratory Services," and Pub. 100-01, Medicare General Information, Eligibility, and Entitlement Manual, Chapter 5, "Definitions," respectively, for the definition of "homebound" and a more complete definition of a medically necessary laboratory service to a homebound or an institutional patient.)

Enter the statement, "Patient refuses to assign benefits" when the beneficiary absolutely refuses to assign benefits to a non-participating physician/supplier who accepts assignment on a claim. In this case, payment can only be made directly to the beneficiary.

Enter the statement, "Testing for hearing aid" when billing services involving the testing of a hearing aid(s) is used to obtain intentional denials when other payers are involved.

When dental examinations are billed, enter the specific surgery for which the exam is being performed.

Enter the specific name and dosage amount when low osmolar contrast material is billed, but only if HCPCS codes do not cover them.

Enter a 6-digit (MM | DD | YY) or an 8-digit (MM | DD | CCYY) assumed and/or relinquished date for a global surgery claim when providers share post-operative care.

Enter demonstration ID number "30" for all national emphysema treatment trial claims. Note: Effective May 23, 2008, all provider identifiers submitted on the CMS-1500 claim form MUST be in the form of an NPI.

Method II suppliers shall enter the most current HCT value for the injection of Aranesp for ESRD beneficiaries on dialysis. (See Pub. 100-04, chapter 8, section 60.7.2.)

Individuals and entities who bill A/B MACs (B) for administrations of ESAs or Part B anti-anemia drugs not self-administered (other than ESAs) in the treatment of cancer must enter the most current hemoglobin or hematocrit test results. The test results shall be entered as follows: TR= test results (backslash), R1=hemoglobin, or R2=hematocrit (backslash), and the most current numeric test result figure up to 3 numerics and a decimal point [xx.x]. Example for hemoglobin tests: TR/R1/9.0, Example for Hematocrit tests: TR/R2/27.0.

InnoviHealth: This "additional claim information" box can be very useful. This is the one place on the *1500 Claim Form* where explanatory information can be given. Supplemental information relating to a specific procedure code should use the shaded area of Item Number 24.

If there is not enough space, attach a report. Providers typically use this box to provide clarifying information (such as rationale for modifiers to procedure codes in Item Number 21).

Item Number 21, Diagnosis or Nature of Illness or Injury

```
21. DIAGNOSIS OR NATURE OF ILLNESS OR INJURY  Relate A-L to Service Line Below (24E)   ICD Ind. |0|
  A. S13121A        B. G441           C. S134XXA        D. V4351XD
  E.                F.                G.                H.
  I.                J.                K.                L.
```

Description: The "ICD Indicator" identifies the version of the ICD code set being reported. The "Diagnosis or Nature of Illness or Injury" is the sign, symptom, complaint, or condition of the patient relating to the service(s) on the claim.

Enter the applicable ICD indicator to identify which version of ICD codes is being reported.

    9   ICD-9-CM
    0   ICD-10-CM

Enter the indicator between the vertical, dotted lines in the upper right-hand area of the field.

Enter the codes left justified on each line to identify the patient's diagnosis or condition. Do not include the decimal point in the diagnosis code, because it is implied. List no more than 12 ICD-10-CM or ICD-9-CM diagnosis codes. Relate lines A - L to the lines of service in 24E by the letter of the line. Use the greatest level of specificity. Do not provide narrative description in this field.

Medicare: Enter the patient's diagnosis/condition. With the exception of claims submitted by ambulance suppliers (specialty type 59), all physician and nonphysician specialties (i.e., PA, NP, CNS, CRNA) use diagnosis codes to the highest level of specificity for the date of service. Enter the diagnoses in priority order. All narrative diagnoses for nonphysician specialties shall be submitted on an attachment.

Reminder: Do not report ICD-10-CM codes for claims with dates of service prior to implementation of ICD-10-CM, on either the old or revised version of the CMS-1500 claim form.

For form version 08/05, report a valid ICD-9-CM code. Enter up to four diagnosis codes.

For form version 02/12, it may be appropriate to report either ICD-9-CM or ICD-10-CM codes depending upon the dates of service (i.e., according to the effective dates of the given code set).

- The "ICD Indicator" identifies the ICD code set being reported. Enter the applicable ICD indicator according to the following:

Indicator	Code Set
9	ICD-9-CM diagnosis
0	ICD-10-CM diagnosis

  Enter the indicator as a single digit between the vertical, dotted lines.

- Do not report both ICD-9-CM and ICD-10-CM codes on the same claim form. If there are services you wish to report that occurred on dates when ICD-9-CM codes were in effect, and others that occurred on dates when ICD-10-CM codes were in effect, then send separate claims such that you report only ICD-9-CM or only ICD-10-CM codes on the claim. (See special considerations for spans of dates below.)
- If you are submitting a claim with a span of dates for a service, use the "from" date to determine which ICD code set to use.
- Enter up to 12 diagnosis codes. Note that this information appears opposite lines with letters A-L. Relate lines A- L to the lines of service in 24E by the letter of the line. Use the highest level of specificity. Do not provide narrative description in this field.
- Do not insert a period in the ICD-9-CM or ICD-10-CM code.

InnoviHealth: Up to 12 diagnosis codes can be accepted by Medicare and most payers. Remember that the primary diagnosis code submitted on a claim should be the main reason for the patient encounter AND that all services rendered must have adequate supporting diagnoses. Remember to record any non-billed diagnostic codes in the the patient's chart.

InnoviHealth: The following are common diagnosis coding problems that could possibly cause delay or denial of payments:

- Not coding to the highest level of specificity
- The code does not establish medical necessity
- Using a chronic diagnosis as the primary diagnosis when it is not the reason for the encounter
- Using an ICD-10-CM manifestation code alone or as the primary diagnosis, when coding guidelines instruct you to list an etiology code first.
- Using an external cause code alone or as the primary diagnosis

Book: See Chapter 5.1 — Diagnosis Coding Essentials for instructions on proper ICD-10-CM code selection.

Item Number 22, Resubmission and/or Original Reference Number

```
22. RESUBMISSION
      CODE              ORIGINAL REF. NO.
       7                ABC1234567890
```

Description: "Resubmission" means the code and original reference number assigned by the destination payer or receiver to indicate a previously submitted claim or encounter.

List the original reference number for resubmitted claims. Please refer to the most current instructions from the public or private payer regarding the use of this field.

When resubmitting a claim, enter the appropriate bill frequency code left justified in the left-hand side of the field.

    7 Replacement of prior claim
    8 Void/cancel of prior claim

This Item Number is not intended for use for original claim submissions.

Medicare: Leave blank. Not required by Medicare.

Item Number 23, Prior Authorization Number

23. PRIOR AUTHORIZATION NUMBER
1234567890A

Description: The "Prior Authorization Number" is the payer assigned number authorizing the service(s).

Enter any of the following: prior authorization number, referral number, mammography certification number, or Clinical Laboratory Improvement Amendments (CLIA) number, as assigned by the payer for the current service.

Do not enter hyphens or spaces within the number.

> **Medicare:** Enter the Quality Improvement Organization (QIO) prior authorization number for those procedures requiring QIO prior approval.
>
> Enter the Investigational Device Exemption (IDE) number when an investigational device is used in an FDA-approved clinical trial. Post Market Approval number should also be placed here when applicable.
>
> For physicians performing care plan oversight services, enter the NPI of the home health agency (HHA) or hospice when CPT code G0181 (HH) or G0182 (Hospice) is billed.
>
> Enter the 10-digit Clinical Laboratory Improvement Act (CLIA) certification number for laboratory services billed by an entity performing CLIA covered procedures.
>
> For ambulance claims, enter the ZIP code of the loaded ambulance trip's point-of-pickup.
>
> **NOTE:** Item 23 can contain only one condition. Any additional conditions should be reported on a separate CMS-1500 Claim Form.

> **InnoviHealth:** This item can only contain one authorization code for one condition. Any additional conditions and authorization should be reported on a separate *1500 Claim Form*.

Section 24

Supplemental information can only be entered with a corresponding, completed service line. The six service lines in section 24 have been divided horizontally to accommodate submission of both the NPI and another/proprietary identifier and to accommodate the submission of supplemental information to support the billed service. The top area of the six service lines is shaded and is the location for reporting supplemental information. It is not intended to allow the billing of 12 lines of service.

The supplemental information is to be placed in the shaded section of 24A through 24G as defined in each Item Number. Providers must verify requirements for this supplemental information with the payer.

Medicare: The six service lines in section 24 have been divided horizontally to accommodate submission of supplemental information to support the billed service. The top portion in each of the six service lines is shaded and is the location for reporting supplemental information. It is not intended to allow the billing of 12 service lines.

When required to submit NDC drug and quantity information for Medicaid rebates, submit the NDC code in the red shaded portion of the detail line item in positions 01 through position 13. The NDC is to be preceded with the qualifier N4 and followed immediately by the 11 digit NDC code (e.g. N499999999999). Report the NDC quantity in positions 17 through 24 of the same red shaded portion. The quantity is to be preceded by the appropriate qualifier: UN (units), F2 (international units), GR (gram) or ML (milliliter). There are six bytes available for quantity. If the quantity is less than six bytes, left justify and space-fill the remaining positions (e.g. UN2 or F2999999).

InnoviHealth: Additional instructions and supplemental examples are included in Resource 178.

Item Number 24E, Diagnosis Pointer [lines 1–6]

Description: The "Diagnosis Pointer" is the line letter from Item Number 21 that relates to the reason the service(s) was performed.

In 24E, enter the diagnosis code reference letter (pointer) as shown in Item Number 21 to relate the date of service and the procedures performed to the primary diagnosis. When multiple services are performed, the primary reference letter for each service should be listed first, other applicable services should follow. The reference letter(s) should be A – L or multiple letters as applicable. ICD-10-CM or ICD-9-CM diagnosis codes must be entered in Item Number 21. Do not enter them in 24E.

Enter letters left justified in the field. Do not use commas between the letters.

Medicare: This is a required field. Enter the diagnosis code reference number or letter (as appropriate, per form version) as shown in item 21 to relate the date of service and the procedures performed to the primary diagnosis. Enter only one reference number/letter per line item. When multiple services are performed, enter the primary reference number/letter for each service.

When using form version 08/05, this reference will be either a 1, or a 2, or a 3, or a 4.

When using form version 02/12, the reference to supply in 24E will be a letter from A-L. Otherwise, the instructions above apply.

If a situation arises where two or more diagnoses are required for a procedure code (e.g., pap smears), the provider shall reference only one of the diagnoses in item 21.

InnoviHealth: Even though 12 diagnosis codes are allowed in Item Number 21, only four diagnosis pointers may be entered in Item Number 24E.

InnoviHealth: It should be noted that in addition to avoiding the use of commas between letters, the use of spaces or dashes should also be avoided.

Item Number 27, Accept Assignment?

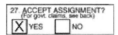

Description: The accept assignment indicates that the provider agrees to accept assignment under the terms of the payer's program.

Enter an X in the correct box. Only one box can be marked.

Report "Accept Assignment?" for all payers.

Medicare: Check the appropriate block to indicate whether the provider of service or supplier accepts assignment of Medicare benefits. If Medigap is indicated in item 9 and Medigap payment authorization is given in item 13, the provider of service or supplier shall also be a Medicare participating provider of service or supplier and accept assignment of Medicare benefits for all covered charges for all patients.

The following providers of service/suppliers and claims can only be paid on an assignment basis:

- Clinical diagnostic laboratory services;
- Physician services to individuals dually entitled to Medicare and Medicaid;
- Participating physician/supplier services;
- Services of physician assistants, nurse practitioners, clinical nurse specialists, nurse midwives, certified registered nurse anesthetists, clinical psychologists, and clinical social workers;
- Ambulatory surgical center services for covered ASC procedures;
- Home dialysis supplies and equipment paid under Method II;
- Ambulance services;
- Drugs and biologicals; and
- Simplified Billing Roster for influenza virus vaccine and pneumococcal vaccine.

InnoviHealth: These are mandatory Medicare assignment situations. When billing any of the above services/supplies, the "Yes" box should be checked.

InnoviHealth: Medicare *Participating* providers have signed an agreement with the Medicare program to accept assignment of Medicare Part B payment for all covered services provided to Medicare patients. *Non-participating* providers may accept or decline assignment of Medicare benefits on a claim-by-claim basis. However, they cannot accept assignment in Item Number 27 if it is not authorized in Item Number 13.

Note: It is very important to complete this field in accordance with Medicare requirements. Participating providers should always check 'yes.' Non-participating providers have the option to check 'yes' or 'no' unless the supply/service is a mandatory assignment situation. If the provider does not make an entry in Item Number 27, the carrier will automatically assume the following:

- Participating providers will be a "yes."
- Non-participating providers will be a "no."
- Mandatory assignment situations will be a "yes" (e.g., labs, physician assistants, etc.)

Book: See Chapter 2 — Medicare for detailed information regarding accepting assignment on Medicare claims.

InnoviHealth: Only when assignment is **authorized** by the patient in Item Number 13 can it be accepted (or rejected) by the provider in Item Number 27.

InnoviHealth — Non-Medicare Claims: By choosing to accept assignment, you know that the payment should come directly to your office without going through the patient. The provider may then bill the patient for the allowable "Patient Portion."

Tips for Error-Free Paper Claims

Troubleshooting Basics

- Use only an original *1500 Claim Form* (or the *UB-04* for institutional claims) that has red print on white paper.
- Use dark ink for entering claim information.
- Do not print, hand-write, or stamp any extraneous data on the form.
- Do not staple, clip, or tape anything to the claim form.
- Remove pin-fed edges at side perforations.
- Use only lift-off correction tape to make corrections.
- Place all necessary documentation in the envelope with the claim form.

Format Hints

- Do not use italics or script.
- Do not use dollar signs, decimals or punctuation.
- Use only uppercase (CAPITAL) letters.
- Use 10- or 12-pitch (pica) characters and standard dot matrix fonts.
- Do not include titles (e.g. Dr., Mr., Mrs., Rev., M.D.) as part of the beneficiary's name.
- Enter all information on the same horizontal plane within the designated field.
- Follow the correct Health Insurance Claim Number (HICN) format. No hyphens or dashes should be used. The alpha prefix or suffix is part of the HICN and should not be omitted. Be especially careful with spouses who have a similar HICN with a different alpha prefix or suffix.
- Ensure data is in the appropriate field and does not overlap into other fields.
- Use an individual's name in the provider signature field, not a facility or practice name.

Notes:

1.4 Claims Management

This chapter includes guidelines for dealing with denied or unpaid claims and is an important component of the Billing Process of the "Reimbursement Life Cycle." One of the most important factors for reducing the volume of unpaid claims is establishing effective office standards to minimize errors before the claims are submitted and follow-up policies to address situations when payment is not received as expected. When payments come in, carefully review the claim and the *EOB* to make sure that all items are accounted for. If any part of the claim is erroneously denied, then the appeals process should begin.

Resource: See Resource 805 to access additional resources including links, articles, and webinars.

Claim Follow-up Procedures

Every office should have a policy to review and keep track of claims that are unpaid as well as reviewing claim payments that are received. Designate a time each week for making appeals. At a minimum, all outstanding claims more than 30 days old should be reviewed to find out why they remain unpaid.

Some software programs automatically address this accounts receivables issue. However, specialized software is not a requirement for a good claims follow-up procedure. Some offices simply use a paper filing system with the days of the month. Regardless of the system used, if payment comes in, carefully review the claim and the EOB and make sure that all items are accounted for. If any part of the claim is denied, and you believe it should have been paid, then the appeals process should begin.

Review Payment Reports

Failure to review payment reports (e.g., *EOBs*) is a common oversight, however, this task must be done routinely. Some consultants suggest having at least one hour each week set aside for reviewing claims and filing appeals. This will help identify potential problems and increase cash flow. When claims are denied in whole or in part, it is important to evaluate the reason. If it is a valid denial, learn from it and improve your billing. If it is an invalid denial, an appeal should be made.

Carefully review all denials to ensure that the same errors are not being repeated, which could indicate a pattern of bad billing. These patterns are precisely what the insurance carrier "data mining" programs are looking for. If there is a problem on your end, recognize and remedy it quickly in order to avoid potentially negative profiling.

Handling Overpayments

When a provider's office discovers an overpayment or an error which could or may have resulted in incorrect reimbursement, they should sumbit a corrected claim with a letter describing the error to the payer. Mark the claim "CORRECTED BILLING – NOT A DUPLICATE CLAIM." Include any additional documentation needed along with any refund for overpayments. Check each payer's website to see if they require their own special voluntary *Overpayment Refund Form* to accompany all submitted overpayments.

Resource: See Resource 195 for a sample voluntary *Overpayment Refund Form* which could be used for payers not requiring the use of a specific form.

Not returning an overpayment within 60 days of the ***discovery*** of the overpayment is considered fraud and could result in prosecution. It may be possible to quickly resolve an overpayment issue with a telephone call, but this may vary by payer.

Alert — 60 Day Rule:
As of 2016, failure to report and subsequently return an overpayment within 60 days after the overpayment to Medicare or Medicaid was "identified" is a violation of the False Claims Act. Providers now have an obligation to exercise "reasonable diligence" through "timely, good faith investigation of credible information."

Resource: See Resource 202 for more information about this ruling.

Note: During a discussion with healthcare attorneys regarding overpayments, it was suggested that UNLESS you believe that there is evidence of fraud, it should be considered an administrative error and refunded to the insurance company along with the letter explaining why the money is being returned. Administrative errors are common and not an admission of fraudulent behavior. By following this process, it is less likely penalties will be applied. If the payer responds negatively, then it would be wise to consult an experienced healthcare attorney.

For Medicare overpayments, CMS is requiring the use of a new Voluntary Self-Referral Disclosure Form. This new form was made available on March 27, 2017 and made effective June 1, 2017. As a provider or supplier with CMS, every party is subject to audits, investigations, and routine oversight activities. Therefore, the self-referral disclosure form is used to report information to CMS to resolve potential liabilities. Do not send payments of presumed overpayments to CMS for any Federal Health Care programs, until it has been determined valid by CMS.

Prompt Pay Laws

If a claim is unpaid due to a delayed response from a payer, you may be able to seek recourse through your state's prompt pay laws which outline specific deadlines that insurance companies must meet in regards to processing claims. As long as your claim is "clean" and there are not errors which prevent it from being processed by the carrier, then they are required to respond before these state deadlines or face penalties. Use a *Prompt Pay Letter* to follow up with claims which have been filed for more than 30 days, or what your state allows. Be prepared to include documented proof that the claim was filed promptly and cleanly.

Resource: See Resource 196 for a sample *Prompt Pay Letter* which can be modified for your specific state law.

Unprocessable Claims

An unprocessable claim does not mean that the payer will actually return the claim by mail. The remittance advice will have a brief message identifying the problem so that the provider can correct the mistake and submit a corrected claim, either electronically, by fax, or by mail. Be sure to respond and correct unprocessable claims promptly. Do not appeal a claim when it has been denied because of incomplete or invalid information. Simply make the correction and submit a "corrected claim" for reconsideration.

Unprocessable claims are most often not processed at all and therefore have no remittance advice sent out. Responsibility for monitoring and properly managing this lies with the provider. First, with proper evaluation of claims to ensure they are correct and clean before submission and second, with regular accounts receivable evaluation and follow-up protocols for claims where processing details (remittance advice) have not been received.

General Guidelines for Unpaid Claims

These general guidelines are for dealing with unpaid claims with commercial payers. Note that specific payers may have their own unique appeals processes that must be followed.

1. **Review your contract.** Your contract may outline when the provider should expect to receive payment. Specifically review the part about payment obligations. Be able to answer the following questions:

    - Do you have the right to appeal?

- Do you have the right to represent the patient?
- Do you have the right to litigate if the appeals process is unsuccessful?
- Does accepting assignment limit your right to pursue an appeal?
- Are there specific guidelines about their appeals processes or how to contact people about problems with claims?

Tip — Evergreen Contracts: If your payer contracts are automatically renewed each year, consider the last time you reviewed your contract. There could be changes, new clauses, or additional conditions in it which could limit your appeal rights.

Alert:
Providers should be careful when signing payer contracts and if possible have a healthcare attorney who specializes in insurance contracts review the contract prior to signing it. Often there are catch phrases hidden in the text that allow major changes or alterations to the contract by the payer but limit the provider's options for a remedy. Some providers make the mistake of just reviewing the fee schedule amount for the main services they provide and verifying that all the codes they bill for are included in their fee schedule and simply agree to the rest. This can put a provider at a serious disadvantage when there is a disagreement.

2. **Ask questions and remain professional.** There could be many reasons why your claim has not been paid – do not assume that the delay is deliberate. Ask about the status of the claim first. If the delay is simply an administrative error, the person answering the phone may be able to correct the situation quickly.

   Please keep in mind that the first person you talk to on the phone may not know the solution, however, they may be able to steer you in the right direction. If the person you are speaking to cannot correct the situation or tell you who can, you will need to follow the chain of command to find someone who can help, therefore you may need to ask to speak with one or more of the following.

   - Supervisor or Benefits Supervisor
   - Provider Relations
   - Director of Provider Relations and/or the Medical Director

   Remember, it is important to fully document your calls. In the patient record, write down the contact individual's first and last name, date and time of the call, a reference number (if applicable) and the information given to you.

3. **Register complaints.** If it becomes necessary, send a written complaint to the director of provider relations. Read through it to ensure that the tone of the letter is professional and factual, not personal.

4. **Contact agencies and associations who advocate for providers and patients.** The following are some groups that may be willing to help with unresolved issues. Understand who the key players are in your state, as they may be able to point you in the right direction. If your appeal efforts are unsuccessful, you may want to try one or all of the following:

   - **Local Associations.** Your local professional association can be an important resource for information. They may collect and aggregate data on local reimbursement problems. Legislative representatives will be able to tell you the status of recent legislation. Insurance representatives may be able to assist you with local payer issues. They may even be able to contact the payers on your behalf.

   - **National Associations.** National associations are also collecting written reports of problems their members are encountering, and one of their targeted issues is reimbursement. Send them a summary of your problem with supporting documentation. Remember to follow HIPAA rules to protect patient privacy.

   - **State Insurance Commissioner.** Depending on your state, the state insurance commissioner may take complaints from both providers and patients (consumers), or only from the patient. If they are unable to help, ask them if there is some other department (i.e., the Department of Health or the Department of Labor) that can help.

> **Resource:** See Resource 204 to find state-specific insurance commissioner information.

- **State Attorney General.** Like the insurance commissioner, some attorneys general are proactive when it comes to health care. It doesn't hurt to call or write them to find out. In fact, it might be helpful.
- **Consumer Advocacy Groups.** Patients can register complaints with the local chapters of these groups. A simple internet search for "patient advocacy" can help direct a patient to the appropriate resource.
- **Media.** Many state and national television broadcasters have consumer advocacy departments, and the media can be particularly sensitive to health care issues.
- **Congressional Representatives.** A sympathetic congressperson can be very effective on your behalf. Contact their local office by letter or phone to describe the problem and ask if they would be able to intervene on your or your patient's behalf.

5. **Stay informed.** Information is power. Your professional association and organizations such as Find-A-Code may have newsletters or other forums designed to help their members stay current.

6. **Keep your patient (or a responsible family member) informed.** For employer sponsored health benefit plans, your patient should also inform their employer's Human Resources Department. In this situation, insurance carriers are under contract to employers to deliver medical services, and employers review these contracts periodically. If enough employees are dissatisfied, the employers may select another plan or advise the carrier to correct problem areas.

Reducing Denials

Basic Steps to Reduce Denials

Here are some basic proactive measures for healthcare providers to consider in order to reduce denials when billing third party payers:

1. Use the most current versions of the CPT, ICD-10-CM, and HCPCS code sets. Many healthcare providers still bill codes that haven't been in use for years. This is easily remedied: subscribe to Find-A-Code, update your codebooks annually, and use them!
2. Ensure the proper usage of modifiers on your claims where appropriate. Many coding situations require that modifiers be used.
3. Utilize the National Correct Coding Initiative (NCCI) edits in your defense if your billing standards are supported by these edits. Correct coding and billing typically matches the NCCI standards. Thus, in the event of an appeal, these NCCI guidelines can demonstrate that correct billing protocol was followed.
4. Stay current on payer policies and coverage by signing up for their newsletters or email notifications. Changes in policies are often announced in these publications. Many payer websites also allow you to search for billing and coding policies.
5. Review the OIG reports and change your billing policies as appropriate to avoid known coding problems.
6. Review documentation requirements and update as necessary to ensure that your records meet high standards.

> **Book:** See Chapter 4 — Documentation for more about meeting necessary requirements.
> **Book:** See Chapter 5.1 — Procedure Coding Essentials for more about NCCI edits and Appendix A — NCCI Edits for a specialty-specific list.

Downcoded Denials

Downcoding is the practice of using a lower level code when a higher level should have been either 1) billed on a claim or 2) paid by a third-party payer. On the part of the payers, a lower level code is paid rather than the one that was billed. On the part of the providers, a lower level of service is billed than what was actually provided. Regardless of the reasons why the provider may decide to bill a lower level code, it is important to always select the code which most accurately describes the services rendered. *Downcoding is not an effective strategy for avoiding audits.*

One issue with the practice of downcoding is that it results in an inaccurate record of the patient encounter. If the documentation supports the code that was correctly billed, and it was downcoded by the payer, be sure to appeal. Failure to do so may imply that you intended to bill the wrong code, and of course, it results in lower reimbursement.

Many providers are unaware that insurance companies use specialized software that analyzes submitted claims. This software can determine frequency of codes billed by a provider, by professional classification, or even within a geographic area. Those providers who consistently downcode their own claims, create a false picture of the actual care that was needed and over time, this can distort statistical averages. It is essential for providers to always bill appropriate codes, and support billed charges with detailed documentation.

Book: See Chapter 4 — Documentation for required information to support the codes billed.

Refund Requests and Demands

There is a growing trend of postpayment audits by payers and their claim recovery contractors in the form of either a refund request or demand. Providers need to carefully examine the exact wording in the letter. Is this a polite request or is it a demand which has severe implications? In many cases, providers are experiencing forced paybacks where the payer simply "takes" money that they feel they are owed and are calling it a "payment offset." Providers need to examine each payer request/demand carefully and determine the validity of the claim and then respond accordingly. Be advised that third-party payer errors do not give a practice the right to keep money that may have been paid erroneously. As a general rule, if it isn't yours, give it back.

Alert: Carefully watch *Explanation of Benefits (EOBs)* and *Remittance Advices (RAs)* for lost revenue due to payment offsets.

Providers can and should refuse to pay inappropriate demands for refunds in many situations. Unless your contract prohibits such action, an appropriate response such as a letter could be of great value. Prior to making the decision to refuse a refund request, professional assistance from an experienced biller/coder or attorney should be considered. The letter should include the following components:

- A review of your records indicates that their request is wrong. You have properly billed, documented, and rendered the services.

- Your contract with that payer specifically states that they are contractually bound to honor your payment because you met the policy requirements. You did what you were asked, met their requirements at that time and thus qualify to be paid.

- The payer incorrectly covered a service that it now says is not covered. The letter will often say that this was a mistake on their part and now they want the money back.

A response letter to refund demands for payer payment errors is ideal for most events wherein the claim was submitted in good faith and paid in good faith. Additionally, if you had recorded the verification of coverage with the payer, they could be held guilty of misrepresentation.

Resource: See Resource 309 for a sample *Response Letter to Refund Demands* for insurance payment errors.

Third-Party Refund Demands

Some payers have begun to use third-party companies to request recoupment of fees. This can be confusing as to where the payment refund should really go. Is the provider supposed to send the refund to the payer or the third-party company? Carefully review your payer contract to see if this recoupment method is specifically mentioned. If not, you may be able to respond with a letter informing them that you will pay any fees directly to the contracted party and ONLY them.

Resource: See Resource 308 for a sample *Third-Party Refund Demand* letter.

Fighting Payment Offsets

Payment offsets are placing a financial burden on healthcare providers. The problem is that the situation is not as black and white as providers would like it to be. To effectively fight payment offsets, providers need to understand the requirements of their state prompt pay laws, as well as audit and recoupment laws, and also the insurance company's internal claim and dispute appeals process.

Just as prompt pay laws assist in getting claims paid, they also outline the time limits in which payers can request refunds. If their request occurs after those deadlines, then technically, they are not legally entitled to take the money even though they might take it anyway. If this happens, immediately begin an appeals process and specifically quote the language of the prompt pay/audit and recoupment law in your appeal. You have the law on your side; however, it may be necessary to consult an attorney.

Every insurance payer has clearly defined procedures for claim disputes and this includes refunds. Read your contract or contact the provider relations department to obtain the specific rules regarding disputes. If you do not meet their timelines for an appeal, you may be waiving your right to dispute a payment offset.

Managing Appeals

An essential component of any effective claims management plan is the appeals process. The ability to successfully appeal a denied claim is an important skill set for providers in today's health care reimbursement landscape. No single strategy will prove successful every time. Success will often lie in a combination of approaches, depending on the case at hand.

Too often, practices think they are the ones who made the mistake when they get a denial from a payer, so they don't appeal, fearing further denials. That is just not the case. Providers who follow proper appeals processes actually demonstrate to the payer that they understand proper billing procedures.

Here are three basic rules to help with your claim denials:

1. Understand the payer's rationale for the denial.
2. Determine the jurisdiction (who has the authority to decide your appeal).
3. Understand the appeal process for each type of claim.

Denials and appeals are subject to state or federal laws, and all payers have an appeals process if all or part of your claim is denied. Be aware that appeal protocols can vary by payer types.

Tip: According to Government Accountability Office (GAO) data on the outcomes of appeals filed with private insurers in four states, 39% to 59% of appeals resulted in the insurer reversing its original coverage denial in favor of the health care provider. However, only a small percentage of practices appeal denied claims.

Why Appeal?

The typical practice loses thousands of dollars in reimbursements that are denied or paid incorrectly. Unpaid claims can be a challenge and an opportunity for every practitioner. Unfortunately, many write-off the loss as a cost of doing business rather than make the effort to collect fees that are rightfully and legally due. The American Medical Association recommends that providers utilize the appeals process for all inappropriate denials.

You should appeal all denials and adverse benefit determinations. Realize that it's not just an issue of one case, but it's about the value of all the similar procedures you will perform during the next several years. It will quickly become evident that the cost of additional hours by a staff member could be offset by successful appeals.

Use Appeals to Your Advantage

Know your appeal rights and the various steps involved with the process. Also, it is important to know state and federal insurance laws and regulations, so that your appeal is based on the regulatory environment in addition to billing guidelines. Individual plan documents regarding utilization review (UR) criteria are often available on their websites.

It is also critical to meet all appeal deadlines. If you do not, the merits of your case may not matter. Denials due to 'administrative noncompliance' are rarely overturned. If the case is denied on an administrative basis (i.e., a request for continued certification was not made within the specified time, pre-certification procedures were not followed, or there were benefit coverage exclusions), you will need to explain any extenuating circumstances in your appeal.

Under certain circumstances, a phone call to the payer requesting that the claim be reprocessed may be all that is needed to correct a denial or improperly processed claim. Carefully document the details of the call so that you can cite a reference if a written appeal or additional phone call is necessary. If the phone call is not effective, then proceed with a formal, written appeal.

Here are a few additional appeals tips:

- Regularly follow up on written appeals with a phone call.
- Record all communication with the payer: dates, names, titles, telephone numbers, reference numbers, and what was stated.
- If your appeal is denied, appeal again to the next highest level. Most payers offer at least two levels of appeal. Some states also require that payers have an external appeal process. Exhaust all levels of appeal before initiating litigation.
- Remember, it is required to get permission from your patients to release their information if authorization is not already on file.

Resource: See Resource 188 for more information about becoming an authorized representative.

- Ask the patient to contact his or her employer's Personnel/Human Resources Department with their concerns. Payers are often more responsive to employer complaints than to complaints from healthcare providers or patients.

Book: See Chapter 2.3 — Medicare Appeals for information on appealing for Medicare claims.

- Seek professional and experienced help if necessary. The appeals process can become complex and in some cases, may be more successful and less cumbersome if experienced guidance is sought.

Expedited Appeals

In an emergency or urgent care situation, it may be possible to request an "expedited appeal" over the telephone with a qualified specialist. The majority of payers have such services. If possible, have them fax their approval later for inclusion in the medical record.

These types of appeals are not common because they only apply in emergency situations. According to the requirements of the Patient Protection and Affordable Care Act (PPACA), these would only be situations in which delays could seriously jeopardize the life or health of the claimant, or jeopardize the claimant's ability to regain maximum function. Depending on your type of practice, these types of appeals might rarely be used.

Resource: See Resource 205 for more information regarding appeals under PPACA.

Appeal Letters

Write letters routinely and create templates or keep copies of various types of appeals to reuse the language.

When submitting an appeal, there is no substitute for an effective cover letter. Keep this letter to a single page as much as possible and direct it to the appropriate address. Specific appeals templates or forms required by the payer often include the proper mailing address.

Be sure your letter includes the following:

- Request for a reviewer that is trained in your specialty.
- Be specific, with a clear and compelling case for medical necessity.
- Clarify any information from the chart as needed.
- Correct any diagnostic or procedural coding or other information on the claim form.

Additional Appeal Letter Tips

- Documentation is extremely important. Send supporting information such as test results and other clinical evidence. Refer to objective measurements, not opinions. Also outline how the patient's episode of care progressed from beginning to middle to end.
- Keep communications professional, not personal. Remember that the employees at the payer's office are just trying to do their jobs.
- If you are appealing on the basis of medical necessity, be sure to include a report(s) that includes outcome assessments which indicate why treatment was necessary and have the healthcare provider sign the letter.

Book: See Chapter 4.1 — Documentation Essentials for information on outcome assessments.

Letters for Continued Care

If your claim is denied due to visit limits, time screens or other reasons, an appeal for continued care must establish medical necessity. Here are some concepts to help in that process.

- Be candid about the patient's condition. Describe any changes in diagnosis, comorbidities, progression, or regression of the patient's condition. Using objective measures such as Outcome Assessment Tools (OATs) are very helpful in establishing necessity of care.
- Describe the next phase of treatment, providing goals and an approximate time frame for the completion of treatment. This will demonstrate that you have an action-oriented approach.

- Present evidence of similar cases where the care was approved.
- Include any literature that supports your case, including references to practice guidelines. This may help convince the reviewer that the requested or updated treatment plan will result in the desired outcome.

Book: See Chapter 4.1 — Documentation Essentials for more about objective measures and treatment plans.

Consumer Health Plan Appeals

As part of the Patient Protection and Affordable Care Act (PPACA) of 2010, patients have expanded appeal rights in all states. These regulations grant the right to both an internal appeal through the insurance plan, as well as an independent external appeal.

Some states already have some consumer protection laws; however, the PPACA sets the minimum standard. Other provisions of this law also further extend patient protection in the following ways:

- Requiring insurance plans to give consumers detailed information about the denial along with information on how to appeal.
- Expedited appeals for urgent cases such as emergency room visits.
- Restricted appeal costs for the consumer. The health plan is responsible for the remainder of the appeal costs.

Plans that were in existence before implementation of this PPACA policy, that have not undergone substantial changes, are "grandfathered," and will not be covered under the new rules. Nevertheless, you should still follow every appeal possibility.

Resource: See Resource 804 for more information on ERISA.
Resource: See the "Grandfathered Plans" segment of Resource 156 for additional information.

External Appeals

External appeals may be available with the health plan or insurance company payer with whom you or the patient is contracted. All states have various review boards to protect the public interest. External appeals or reviews refer to a formal dispute-resolution process that has the authority to evaluate and resolve disputes involving health care. Outside review panels are mandated to have no connection to the health plan. Each side in the dispute agrees to abide by the board's decision, although in some states, patients may still sue a company if they're not satisfied with the decision. You can check with your local association to find out how review boards operate in your state.

An external review is not a substitute for first following the "internal" appeals process established by individual third-party payers. Never consider using external appeals until after exhausting all internal appeal levels.

Patients and providers might be hesitant to use the external review process; however, patients and their healthcare providers should take advantage of this process for resolving disputes that arise in obtaining appropriate care. Although this is still a relatively new concept, external review programs are popular with consumer advocacy groups. Some state laws encourage such a mediation process.

Notes:

1.5 Establishing Fees

About Fees and Fee Schedules

The establishment of appropriate fees for services is one of the greatest challenges in health care. The old concept – that you charge a fair amount based on your own costs and expected return on your investment – has given way to government controls and insurance mandates.

One of the more challenging tasks in a medical practice is to arrive at a fair and equitable fee that also meets all the requirements of the insurance industry. The objective of this chapter is to help providers obtain a better understanding of how fees are evaluated and established. It explains different fee methodologies (e.g., UCR and RVU), conversion factors, and how to appropriately discount your fees.

The most important thing to remember when setting fee schedules is that you must have only one standard schedule. This concept may seem odd considering the number of payer contracts your office may have; however, you must set one fee for each procedure code and that is your actual fee. Period. Once your fee is set, that fee is only changed in the following situations:

- Contractual obligations with third-party payers such as insurance companies or medical discount plans
- Prompt Pay/Time of Service (TOS) discounts
- Financial Hardship Discounts

Book: See "Discounts" on page 77 for more information.

Always bill your standard amount on submitted claims for reimbursement – not the contracted amount – unless your contract specifically states that your claim must only show the contracted amount. This is important for the following reasons:

- **Do you really want to get paid less?** What if the wrong fee amount/schedule is listed in your system and you are getting paid far less than you should? It has happened to many providers.
- **Do you want to lower national fee perceptions?** When claims data is used as part of the process to establish UCR limits, claims which have contracted amounts instead of the real value for the service will cause the averages to lower over time. See the segment "Usual, Customary and Reasonable (UCR)" for more about keeping national fees realistic.

Book: See Chapter 2 — Medicare for information about billing and fees for Medicare.
Website: Go to FindACode.com for comprehensive fee information available by subscription.
Resource: See Resource 807 for additional resources including links, articles, & webinars.

Alert — Price Fixing Warning: It is illegal for providers/physicians to discuss fees with each other and agree upon dollar conversion factors or fees. To do so is price fixing, and a violation of federal anti-trust laws.

Fortunately, there is information regarding fees available through a variety of sources, including FindACode.com. Fees should be studied to better understand the market forces affecting them. Additionally, many payers will disclose their fee schedules when asked (it is appropriate to limit your request to only the codes relevant to your practice).

Fee Analysis

Fees can and should be reviewed annually to make appropriate and informed decisions on pricing. To avoid improprieties, do not discuss fees with other providers. At a minimum, be sure to review fee schedules from contracted payers to ensure billing compliance. Find-A-Code includes comprehensive fee analysis information (available by subscription) for codes including:

- Medicare Allowed, billed/reported amounts
- UCR data (see below for more about UCR)
- Workers Compensation

Store: Find-A-Code offers both fee analysis services and tools which can be added to a subscription. Choose either the single Specialty Fee Report to review this information or the Unlimited Fee Reports Tool with comprehensive fee comparisons. Go to FindACode.com/fee-analysis to learn more.

Fee Schedule Methodologies

There are two methodologies used to determine fees. One method is the "usual, customary, and reasonable" (UCR), which is based on billed charges. Another method is the RBRVS system which is based on the actual value of the work, practice expense, and malpractice expense of the procedures/services.

Usual, Customary, and Reasonable (UCR)

"Usual, customary, and reasonable" (UCR) refers to the base amount a third-party payer may use to determine how much will be paid for services that are reimbursed under a health insurance plan. This amount is determined based on a review of the prevailing charges made by peer physicians for a particular health service within a specific geographical area. Typically, fee surveys are done by publishers and/or researchers through questionnaires for practitioners. Respondents report the fees which they are currently charging.

The UCR amount is generally set at different percentiles (e.g., 50th, 70th, 90th, etc.) which are mathematical formulas utilizing a comparison of all submitted fees by providers and thereby establishing fee ranges. Think of the "bell curve" where results tend to group in the center – the very center of this curve would be 50%, which means half of providers would have higher fees than at this point, while half would be lower. When a payer says they pay at the 70th percentile of the UCR, they mean that their "approved" fee is higher than what 70% of providers charge in that region and would be a higher fee than one who is in the 50th percentile. When a payer reduces a fee by using a UCR schedule it is important to know which percentile they are using.

Federal law does not regulate how UCR reimbursements are calculated; however, the Centers for Medicare and Medicaid Services (CMS) provides general guidelines that the insurance carriers must follow. Ultimately, the insurance company has flexibility when setting their maximum reimbursement fee.

Fee Schedules and UCR

When a healthcare provider creates a fee schedule, evaluating UCR data can be helpful to review prevailing charges in their area, however, it should not be the deciding factor. It should be noted that your fee schedule can impact the UCR as well. As you submit claims, you are contributing to the future data pool payers use to evaluate their fee schedules. Therefore, you should never set your fees to the contracted rates of your payers. Doing so will result in a continued reduction in fees. You need to keep your fees at a fair and marketable rate and then accept the payer reduction when you are a participating provider.

Opponents of this method feel that the UCR method used by insurance companies is less meaningful than the RVU methodology because the claims database has been polluted with inaccurate information (e.g., a provider submits fees that are mandated under contract in which fees are arbitrary and low).

Tip: Do not confuse UCR percentiles with the patient portion. If you are not a contracted provider with a specific payer, and if that plan covers 80 percent of UCR charges, then the patient is responsible for both the remaining 20 percent, and for the difference between what is charged by the provider and what the plan considers UCR.

UCR Example

Statistically, 30% of providers in your geographic area charge at least $100 for a particular service. This means that if ABC Insurance wants the UCR at the 70th percentile, they will set the UCR at $100 for that service. John Smith has met his deductible for ABC Insurance and comes in for that service. You are an out-of-network provider and you bill ABC Insurance $110 for that service. ABC Insurance pays $80 based on their UCR and the 80 percent of the covered service. John Smith is responsible for the $30 balance ($20 coinsurance and $10 for the amount over ABC Insurance's UCR).

If you were an in-network provider, you would need to discount the patient's bill by $10 to meet the contracted UCR amount.

Relative Value Units (RVU)

The second fee calculation methodology is the Resource-Based Relative Value Scale (RBRVS). The intent of RBRVS is to establish a consistent and rational basis for assessing the resources that go into providing any health care service. RBRVS utilizes Relative Value Units (RVUs) as the basis for establishing the value of services. These RVUs are based on quantifiable factors associated with a specific service (e.g., work, practice expense, malpractice expense).

RBRVS is the official methodology used to create the Medicare Physician Fee Schedule (MPFS) and it is also used by Medicaid and a significant number of third-party payers.

The RVU system is composed of two parts:

1. **Resource-Based Relative Value Unit (RVU):** An intrinsic value of one procedure or service as it relates to another. It is a mathematical expression, not a dollar amount. See the "RBRVS Components" segment for more about how this number is calculated.

   Example:

Code	Description	RVU
99212	Office or other outpatient services, established patient, level 2	1.70
99213	Office or other outpatient services, established patient, level 3	2.71

2. **Dollar Conversion Factor (DCF):** A dollar amount, which when multiplied by the RVU converts the RVU into a fee.

   Example:

Code	RVU		DCF		Fee
99212	1.70	x	$36.09	=	$61.35
99213	2.71	x	$36.09	=	$97.80

For every procedure or service (as defined by current CPT and HCPCS codes), RBRVS defines the physician's work, practice expense, and malpractice insurance costs. A percentage multiplier then adjusts them for variations in expenses between geographic areas. Finally, a dollar conversion factor, based on a provider's or payer's financial objectives, is applied to yield a dollar-based fee schedule.

RVUs are not perfect and not every code has an RVU. However, they do represent a high degree of integrity. It is the most widely used payment system with providers and carriers. Whether addressing pricing, contracting, strategic and financial planning or productivity, RBRVS has become the most credible method available to fairly evaluate pricing and compensation for healthcare providers.

Note: Not all codes are subject to RVUs and their calculations (e.g., laboratory services, supplies, and quality measure reporting). When there is resource data regarding fees other than the RVU, the fee is shown in this *Reimbursement Guide* as a dollar amount with the dollar ($) sign (e.g., $36.20).

RBRVS Components

The three RVU components in the RBRVS methodology are:

1. **Work (W):** the relative time and intensity associated with furnishing the service
2. **Practice Expense (PE):** the costs to provide the service (e.g., equipment, supplies, and overhead costs such as rent, phones, and support staff)
3. **Malpractice Expense (ME):** malpractice or professional liability insurance costs

For each component, there is a Geographic Practice Cost Index (GPCI) for each specific geographic area. The relative costs of the physician's work, practice expenses, and malpractice insurance in an area is compared to the national average for each component, and is adjusted accordingly with a GPCI. After the RVU is adjusted, it is multiplied by a Dollar Conversion Factor (DCF) as determined by the payer.

RVU Formula

In summary, the general formula for calculating RVUs for a given service in a geographic area can be expressed as:

$$\left. \begin{array}{l} (\text{RVU physician work} \quad \times \quad \text{GPCI for physician work}) \\ + (\text{RVU practice expense} \quad \times \quad \text{GPCI for practice expense}) \\ + (\text{RVU malpractice} \quad \times \quad \text{GPCI for malpractice expense}) \end{array} \right\} \times \text{DCF} = \text{Fee}$$

Updates to RVUs

The RVUs are updated on five year review cycles. The Relative Value Update Committee (RUC) makes recommendations to CMS for their review and endorsement/correction. CMS makes the final determinations for all RVUs.

Dollar Conversion Factors (DCF)

A dollar conversion factor (DCF) is a number that is multiplied by the RVU to arrive at a fee for a healthcare service or supply. It is a pivotal component in the fee calculation process for any payer utilizing the RVU methodology. Without a proper DCF, fees will be depressed.

Medicare's dollar conversion factor is set by law. Non-federal health plans have widely varied DCFs and theoretically, a single payer could have multiple dollar conversion factors based on the plan or even the type of service. For example, there could be one DCF for laboratory services, and another for surgery.

Resource: See Resource 807 for additional information and resources.

Medicare Dollar Conversion Factor Changes

Historically, Medicare's DCF was based on the Sustainable Growth Rate (SGR) formula and resulted in widely varying conversion factors and last minute legislative corrective actions. The Medicare Access and CHIP Reauthorization Act of 2015 (MACRA) repealed the SGR and replaced it with a conversion factor that was supposed to be frozen until 2026. However, the Budget Neutrality and sequestration rules have led to annual reductions which have been held off by congressional action.

Book: See "Quality Payment Program Adjustments" in Chapter 2.2 — Medicare Fees for more information about this legislation

Other Fee Schedules

Most healthcare providers try to remain competitive in the marketplace and keep the cost of their care affordable to their patients. However, depending on their fee reduction methods, they may get into trouble. For example, some providers may have developed a varying scale of fees, with numerous types of discounts: maybe a pastoral discount, a child discount, a friend discount, etc. Each of these discounts is different. Not every state has a rule regarding this practice, but some do. If your state does not have a specific rule as to how you can charge for your care, you need to make sure you are justified in your action. If your argument is purely financial then the legality is, at best, questionable.

Many allegations of fraud and abuse come from having more than one fee schedule. Medicare policy mandates that payment is determined by the lowest of either the Medicare Physician Fee Schedule (MPFS) or the lowest fee schedule in the provider's office. For example, if the MPFS for a specific service is $30 and the provider's lowest schedule is $15, Medicare could claim the $15 as their proper fee. Conversely, if a non-participating healthcare provider in the Medicare program charges more than the limiting charge, it is considered aberrant and subject to fines and penalties for fraud and abuse.

Alert: Usage of the term "cash discount" in a fee schedule is inappropriate and discouraged because it is about more than just cash. Most payments come in the form of checks or credit cards, so the safest method is to entirely eliminate the words "cash discount" from your vocabulary. Cash discounts could invite allegations that you are increasing the fees billed to insurance carriers.

Instead of offering a cash discount, offer patients and insurance companies your Time of Service (TOS) fee schedule. Payment at time of service reduces costs for all parties. Under this scenario, the patient chooses to submit their charges to their insurance carrier. The amount submitted must reflect the TOS fee schedule, and not your regular fee schedule.

If you are a participating provider, you may be precluded from collecting anything other than deductibles and co-payments directly from the patient, and you may be required to file claims on their behalf. Refer to your Provider Agreement for applicable rules.

Discounts

An unprecedented shift is occurring in health care. Deductibles are increasing and insurance is paying less. Even with healthcare reform, the number of underinsured and uninsured Americans continues to be problematic. The line between insurance and patient responsibility is clearly moving, with patients shouldering more of the costs for their care. Additionally, more patients are now in control of their healthcare dollars with Health Savings Accounts (HSA), Medical Savings Accounts (MSAs), Flexible Spending Accounts (FSAs), and Health Reimbursement Arrangements (HRAs) with their employers.

Because of this shift, patients are increasingly asking important financial questions, such as:

- How much is my insurance going to pay (insurance portion)?
- How much is this care going to cost me (patient portion)?
- What payment arrangements can you make for me?
- Can you discount your fees?

Tip: For patients concerned about prescription drug prices, discount prescription services (e.g., GoodRx, FamilyWize) might be an option to help them to reduce the price of their medications.

Alert — TOS Warning: Some professional organizations strongly discourage the use of TOS discounts due to the possibility of violating state and/or federal law. See the "Prompt Pay Discounts (PPD)" segment for a better way.

Can You Discount Your Fees?

The question "Can I discount my fees?" is applicable to any practice that provides covered health care to insured patients, especially those practices that might describe themselves as "out-of-network." The answer to this question is dependent upon properly following official guidelines and documentation protocols. Fees may be appropriately discounted in two ways, both of which are clearly recognized by the federal government: financial hardship or prompt payment. Although they have different requirements, both must be properly documented in order to avoid allegations of fraud or abuse.

There may be other types of discounts which are permitted under federal and/or state laws, such as healthcare discount plans in which the provider is an 'in-network' provider.

Alert: Blanket waivers for coinsurance, co-pays and deductibles violates many federal statutes, as well as third-party payer contracts.

Financial Hardship Discount

It is improper and illegal to waive co-payments and/or deductibles. For this reason, if you wish to offer some sort of financial assistance to a patient, the proper way to do so is through an official "Financial Hardship Policy."

Caution is advised when implementing hardship waivers. For example, waivers and reductions for co-pays, coinsurances, and deductibles should not be routine and should not be advertised in any way. Hardship waivers should be used only in cases where hardship is clearly indicated and documented. Clinics should have a written policy regarding determinations of financial hardship and a clear guideline on what qualifies as a hardship (e.g., by using federal poverty guidelines). innoviHealth created a *Financial Hardship Policy and Application* form which provides both the official policy, and the application which is completed by the patient.

Alert: Hardship waivers are a temporary courtesy arrangement which must be periodically reviewed with current financial information from the patient. Your policy must clearly communicate to the patient/responsible party that this arrangement is not permanent and has an end date.

As a reminder, routine waivers or reductions of the patient's responsibility can violate the federal False Claims Act, Medicare Exclusion Statute, Anti-Kickback Statute, and the Civil Monetary Penalties Law. Additionally, many commercial insurers have provisions within their provider contracts that prohibit routine waiver or reductions of co-pays, deductibles, or coinsurances.

For years, federal and state authorities have stated that providers can discount their fees based on patient financial need (hardship). These discounts (hardship policies) must be in writing and consistently applied. innoviHealth has created the necessary template to create your own *Financial Hardship Policy and Application*. This form should be used sparingly and only in accordance with your Financial Hardship Policy.

Resource: See Resource 146 for a full-size version of this form, with instructions.
Resource: See Resource 173 for more information from the Health Resources and Services Administration (HRSA).

Prompt Pay Discounts (PPD)

Prompt Pay Discounts (PPD) or Time of Service (TOS) discounts are different than hardship discounts. Whereas a hardship discount refers to a discount granted for a documented financial need, the "prompt pay discount" refers to situations where the provider is seeking to avoid the costs of debt collection.

According to the Office of Inspector General (OIG), a prompt pay discount is "designed to reduce the health system's accounts receivables and costs of debt collection, and to boost its cash flow." It's a discount that "bear(s) a reasonable relationship to the amount of collection costs that would be avoided."

The time frame for payment on PPDs can and should be defined by the individual office. This could mean that care is either pre-paid, paid immediately, or within a specified number of working days. The OIG advisory included an example of a greater discount for those that pay before leaving than for those that pay within 30 days. Whereas, as the name implies, a TOS discount generally means that payment is made at the time of service.

Tip: To avoid any allegations of impropriety, avoid the term TOS unless your policy specifically states that you only offer a discount if payment is made at the time of service.

To make it legal, the Prompt Pay or Time of Service discount is available to all sources of payment, which includes third party payers, personal injury, and Workers Compensation. Some of these payers will not meet your established deadline for this discount, but nonetheless it should be available to them.

Once you have created your standard rate, you then choose your discount percentage for your Prompt Pay or Time of Service discount. Keep in mind that you cannot have different discounts for different procedures. The discount rate you select is your choice; however, it must be considered "reasonable," and it must be a flat percentage of your standard rate.

Alert: Be aware of any applicable state laws and regulations regarding this practice. Some states have established laws such as an upper limit on the percentage of a PPD. Also, some third-party payer contracts prohibit this type of discount.

This system will simplify your fee schedules and eliminate any accusation that you are discriminating against any specific payer.

Resource: See Resource 174 to review the OIG advisory on prompt pay discounts.

Plan

1. Establish a standard fee schedule for the current year. This standard fee includes routine practice overhead expenses for the additional costs associated with claims processing, collecting, and follow-up.

2. Establish a Prompt Pay or Time of Service discount. This discount should never be lower than the Medicare allowed amount and is available to all who pay in full according to your official PPD or TOS policy.

3. Make your Prompt Pay or TOS discount available to all. Treat patients and insurance companies alike. All have an equal opportunity to participate in reducing healthcare costs and to share in the savings. Payments can be made in any form: check, cash, credit card, debit card, etc. However, all must meet the same expectation and standard: prepayment, payment at time of service, or within a specified number of working days.

4. Determine if there are any local state laws or advisories that may apply. Consult with an experienced healthcare attorney specializing in contract law or your professional association.

5. Review your contracts with third-party payers to ensure that you are not legally prohibited from offering this type of discount.

6. Consider participating in a medical discount program. These programs can promote doctor-patient relationships without third party hassles and costs. However, be aware of specific state requirements.

Resource: See Resource 100 for additional comments, resources, networks, and opinions on discounts.

Notes:

2. Medicare

Chapter Contents

2.1 Medicare Essentials 83
Introduction 83
How Participation Works 87
Impact of Secondary Insurance 89
Non Part B Plan Information 91
Medicare Administrative Contractors (MACs) 92
Medicare Coverage and Billing 93
Supporting Documentation 97
Medicare Terms to Understand 99

2.2 Medicare Fees 103
Medicare Fee Schedule 103
Understanding Medicare Fees 106

2.3 Medicare Appeals 113
Medicare Appeals Process 113

2.1 Medicare Essentials

Introduction

The Medicare program is administered by the Centers for Medicare and Medicaid Services (CMS), a division of the U.S. Department of Health and Human Services (HHS). It is the country's largest health insurance plan and provides coverage for millions of Medicare beneficiaries. As the baby boomer population continues to age, it will cover, and your practice will likely treat, an increasing number of Medicare patients. To be eligible for Medicare, U.S. Citizens must meet one or more of the following criteria:

- 65 years of age or older
- Disabled people of any age who have received Social Security benefits for at least two years
- People with End Stage Renal Disease (ESRD) or Amyotrophic Lateral Sclerosis (ALS-Lou Gehrig's disease)

Alert: As of January 1, 2020, you must use the new Medicare Beneficiary Identifier (MBI) on claims submitted to Medicare. Be sure that you have the correct identification number for your patients. Note that the dashes in between the digits of the Medicare Beneficiary Identifier (MBI) are ONLY for display purposes. Do NOT include dashes on submitted claims.

If a patient you are treating meets any of the above criteria, you must bill Medicare for covered services as either a participating provider or a non-participating provider. See the segment "How Participation Works" on page 87 for more information on participation.

There are four different "parts" to the Medicare program, each of which covers specific services.

- Medicare Part A covers expenses incurred at hospitals, some Skilled Nursing Facilities (SNF), home health, and hospice care.
- Medicare Part B covers physician and other healthcare provider services, outpatient care, durable medical equipment, and home health care.
- Medicare Part C is also known as Medicare Advantage and offers Part A and Part B benefits, and may offer prescription drug coverage (Medicare Part D), through private health plans. Some plans offer additional benefits that Medicare does not generally cover.
- Medicare Part D covers prescription drugs. Beneficiaries may need to pay a separate monthly premium for Part D unless it is included as part of a Medicare Advantage plan.

Outpatient services are generally covered under either Part B or Part C.

Alert: There are situations where a Medicare beneficiary will have Part A, but NOT Part B coverage. In these cases, the patient is responsible for Part B services. For this reason, it is important to carefully review their insurance card to ensure coverage of services.

Warning: ALL providers must understand Medicare rules regarding eligibility. Failure to follow the rules can result in allegations of fraud. If you do not plan on being a Medicare provider, you must officially "OPT OUT" of the Medicare system. See "Opt Out" in the "Medicare Terms to Understand" segment at the end of this chapter for additional information.

eHealth Initiative: The CMS eHealth initiative aims to improve the quality and efficiency of the Medicare program "by simplifying the use of electronic standards and the adoption of health information technology."
Resource: See Resource 212 to be linked to the CMS eHealth page.

Resource: See Resource 808 for the latest articles and webinars.
Book: See Chapter 4 — Documentation for best practice standards for medical record documentation.

The Need for Understanding

A major issue facing healthcare providers is that many practices do not fully understand Medicare regulations. A review of any Medicare Improper Payment Report clearly indicates that a significant percentage of claims that they consider improperly paid were due to insufficient documentation. As part of any ongoing efforts to reduce the potential for claims reviews, healthcare providers need to understand where they are falling short and improve.

Book: See Chapter 4 — Documentation for best practice standards for medical record documentation.

In addition to professional credibility, there are two other very important reasons why every provider needs to understand how Medicare works. First, Medicare is frequently used as a standard in the insurance industry. Decisions and regulations implemented by CMS are carefully observed, and often adopted by other payers and state agencies. Second, you must carefully adhere to rules and regulations in order to avoid federal allegations of fraud and/or abuse.

Alert: If you treat a Medicare beneficiary, you are required to bill Medicare for all covered services – this is true whether you are a participating or a non-participating provider. In addition, you are also required to submit a claim for noncovered services, when requested by the patient.

Participation status is a major source of confusion regarding Medicare. The terms **participating** and **non-participating** apply mostly to payment methods, NOT whether or not you want to be a Medicare provider. See the "Provider Enrollment" segment that follows for more information.

Provider Enrollment

To bill services for Medicare beneficiaries, you must enroll with CMS. In order to streamline the enrollment process, CMS has established an internet-based Provider Enrollment, Chain and Ownership System (PECOS) for physicians, non-physician practitioners, and provider and supplier organizations. PECOS allows providers to electronically enroll, revalidate, and make changes to their Medicare enrollment.

If you do not know if you are enrolled in PECOS, check the national listing of PECOS providers or call your local A/B Medicare Administrative Contractor (MAC) provider enrollment line. See page 92 for more information about MACs.

Although you may **treat** Medicare patients up to 30 days prior to your enrollment application being officially *received* by your MAC, you cannot **bill** Medicare until you have received all of your numbers. Before treating a Medicare beneficiary, contact your A/B MAC to 1) confirm that they are processing the enrollment application and 2) ascertain their official policy on when an applying provider may begin treating Medicare beneficiaries. You may also monitor the status of your application online from your individual MAC website enrollment status link. See Resource 213 for more information about provider enrollment.

Tip 1: One common enrollment mistake is when the provider's Provider Transaction Access Number (PTAN) does not match the NPI expected by CMS. This generally happens when the provider has more than one NPI number (i.e., a group NPI and an individual NPI). This can significantly delay the enrollment process so pay close attention if you have more than one NPI.

Tip 2: There is no cost to a healthcare provider for either enrollment or revalidation. However, facilities are charged a fee. See Resource 221 for more information.

Tip 3: Students preparing to graduate may want to create log-in accounts for the National Plan and Provider Enumeration System (NPPES) and PECOS systems. This may speed up the enrollment process once graduation is complete.

Note: At the time of enrollment, providers are required to disclose any affiliation (direct or indirect) with any provider/supplier that has or has had (within the last five years) certain problems with CMS (e.g., suspension, uncollected debt). Penalties for non-compliance are severe. See Resource 217 for more information.

Revalidation

Every five years, providers are required to revalidate their enrollment information or risk being removed from the system. As part of the revalidation process, providers are required to switch to Electronic Funds Transfer (EFT) for payment, if they have not already done so. This includes submitting form CMS-588 to your MAC.

Resource: See Resource 390 for more information about revalidation.

Screening Process

All new applicants, as well as those going through the revalidation process, are required to go through Medicare's on-going screening process. Most providers, unless they have had problems in the past, will have a limited screening which includes license verification and database checks. However, "moderate risk" providers will also have unscheduled/unannounced site visits. Because the screening also happens during the revalidation process, your ongoing compliance efforts are critical.

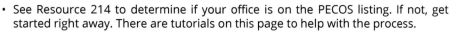

Are you properly registered with Medicare? Check the following:
- See Resource 214 to determine if your office is on the PECOS listing. If not, get started right away. There are tutorials on this page to help with the process.
- If you have been seeing patients who qualify as a Medicare beneficiary, and you have not been billing Medicare, then you are in violation of Medicare regulations as defined in the *Medicare Benefit Policy Manual* "Chapter 15, Section 40." Get enrolled today.
- Many providers have found that their NPI taxonomy designation is incorrect. This leads to payment problems. First, see Resource 197 to review current taxonomy codes and their definitions. Then go to Resource 215 and do a provider search on your own practice to review your taxonomy code(s).

Opt Out

"Opt Out" is an official designation for a provider who agrees to operate outside the Medicare system. When a provider opts out of Medicare, he or she opts out of all Medicare programs and plans for a two year period. This option is only available to the following:

- Physicians who are:
  - Doctors of medicine or osteopathy;
  - Doctors of dental surgery or dental medicine;

- Doctors of podiatry; or
- Doctors of optometry; and
- Who are legally authorized to practice dentistry, podiatry, optometry, medicine, or surgery by the State in which such function or action is performed

• Practitioners who are:
- Physician assistants;
- Nurse practitioners;
- Clinical nurse specialists;
- Certified registered nurse anesthetists;
- Certified nurse midwives;
- Clinical psychologists;
- Clinical social workers; or
- Registered dietitians or nutrition professionals; and
- Legally authorized to practice by the State and otherwise meet Medicare requirements.

If you are **not** one of the above provider types, if you wish to treat anyone eligible for Medicare, you must be enrolled as either a PAR or NON-PAR provider.

Why Opt Out?

By law, you cannot provide outpatient services for any Medicare Part B beneficiary unless you are a Medicare provider OR you have opted out of the system. If you do, you will be charged with fraud.

How to Opt Out

To Opt Out, submit a *Private Contract Opt-Out Affidavit* to Medicare. This affidavit must be filed with Medicare for 10 days before a private contract can be entered into with the first Medicare beneficiary. Do NOT provide any items or services until that time.

Have the patient read and sign a *Private Contract*. A copy of this contract must be given to the beneficiary or the beneficiary's legal representative. Keep the original in their medical record. A private contract is not required for an item or service not covered or statutorily excluded by Medicare.

Do NOT submit any claims to Medicare! Medicare considers this fraud.

Prior to the Medicare Access and CHIP Reauthorization Act of 2015 (MACRA), healthcare providers that wished to renew their opt out status were required to file new valid affidavits with their MACs every 2 years. However, Section 106(a) of MACRA changed that requirement. Opt out affidavits filed after June 15, 2015 will now *automatically* renew every 2 years. There is no need to re-file.

If a healthcare provider wishes to opt back in, the automatic renewal must be canceled by notifying their MAC in writing at least 30 days before the start of the new two-year opt-out period.

Resource: See Resource 201 to download a sample *Medicare Private Contract or Opt-Out Affidavit*.
Resource: See Resource 208 to review information by CMS regarding opting out.

Emergency Situations

When there is an emergency situation, providers who have opted-out and do not have a private contract with the beneficiary may submit claims for covered services with modifier GJ.

Resource: Review the *Medicare Benefit Policy Manual*, Chapter 15, Section 40.28 (Resource 209) for additional information on emergency situations.

How Participation Works

Medicare payment for covered services is dependent on many factors beyond provider participation status, including whether or not assignment is accepted, geographic factors, the current Medicare Physician Fee Schedule, the type of plan being billed and penalties or incentives as defined by quality measure programs.

Book: See Chapter 2.2 — Medicare Fees for information about fees.

Provider Participation Status

Every healthcare provider has an annual choice regarding their participation status in the Medicare program. You can change your status only once a year, during the "open enrollment period" which is generally from mid-November through December 31. This is the only time providers are given the opportunity to change provider status. Providers should contact their local Medicare Administrative Contractor (MAC) to learn where to send the agreement, and get the exact dates for their open enrollment period.

See *Figure 2.1* for a general comparison between Participation and Non-Participation in Medicare.

Figure 2.1

PAR/Non-PAR Comparison	
Participating Providers	**Non-Participating Providers**
Signed agreement/contract with Medicare	No signed agreement with Medicare
Accept assignment on ALL claims	May choose to accept or not accept assignment on a claim-by-claim basis
Payments are made directly to the provider	Non-assigned payments go to the patient
Medigap insurance automatically billed	Medigap insurance billed by provider or patient (Item Number 27 on the *1500 Claim Form*) Note: Some MACs automatically bill Medigap, be aware of individual payer policies/contracts.
Secondary insurance is automatically billed (if it is contracted with Medicare)	Secondary insurance is billed by provider or patient
Allowed Fees are 5% higher than Non-PAR assigned claim Allowed Fees	Charges cannot be more than the Limiting Charge

Participation

Participating (PAR) providers are those who are eligible to participate and have signed an agreement to participate. They are required to take assignment on every Medicare claim. Medicare sends 80% of the Allowed Amount directly to the provider, once the Part B deductible has been met. The patient portion under Part B, which is the annual deductible and then 20% of the Allowed Amount, should be collected at the time of service or it will have to be collected later.

It is the provider's responsibility to collect the deductible, as well as the coinsurance, from the patient. Remember that the patient portion should not be routinely waived. Exceptions can be made, but they *are rare* and must be documented as bona fide financial hardship cases.

Tip: Some supplemental policies pay the annual Part B deductible. Be sure to verify coverage before billing the patient erroneously.

Book: The "Financial Hardship Discounts" segment in Chapter 1.5 — Establishing Fees discusses the proper way to implement a *Financial Hardship Policy* (Resource 146) for your office. Without a policy and its proper use, it is improper and illegal to waive co-payments and/or deductibles.

The inducements for being a participating provider are many, such as more patients coming to the physician because they have fewer hassles with Medicare, lower out-of-pocket costs for your patients, the physician receiving direct payment from Medicare for the 80% portion of the allowed amount, and having an automatic cross over (transmittal) of claim information for qualified Medigap policies (supplemental insurance).

One very important benefit of being a participating provider is that you can bill your usual fee to Medicare. When you bill your usual fee to Medicare, you are paid 80% of the Medicare allowed amount, you collect 20% from the patient and you write off the balance.

One down side to participation is that PAR physicians receive about 9% less reimbursement overall than NON-PAR providers who do not accept assignment.

Figure 2.2, Medicare Fees Participation vs. Non-Participation Comparison Table clarifies this concept of payment for both types of providers.

Tip: Although the *Verification of Insurance Coverage* form (Resource 148) is not given to the patient, office personnel should begin to complete this form as soon as insurance information is obtained from the patient.

Non-Participation

Non-Participating (NON-PAR) providers are those who are **eligible** to participate (e.g., physician, non-physician practitioners) and are enrolled as a provider, but who have not signed the Medicare Participation agreement. They are only a registered provider with a number. With Medicare NON-PAR status and an unassigned claim, the maximum a physician can charge the patient for covered services is an amount known as the "Limiting Charge." It is a little more than the Allowed Amount for participating providers. Exceeding the "Limiting Charge" could result in a $10,000 fine per occurrence.

With NON-PAR status, you may elect to accept assignment (or not) on a claim-by-claim basis. NON-PAR offices typically do not take assignment, but might have reason to make exceptions. Either way, you must still file the claim with your Medicare Administrative Contractor (MAC). NON-PAR providers are subject to the same rules, regulations, and penalties as participating providers. Therefore, please note that being a NON-PAR provider will not keep you from being reviewed or audited or from refunding overpayments.

Tip: Non-participation is NOT the same thing as "opting out." See the segment "Opt Out" on page 85 and in the "Medicare Terms to Understand" segment at the end of this chapter for more information.

Book: See Chapter 3 — Compliance Essentials for further information on reviews, audits, and refund requests.

Figure 2.2

Medicare Fees Participation vs. Non-Participation Comparison Table

Example: Assignment impact if regular fee is $100 and the Medicare Allowed Amount is $50.

Usual Fee	Amount Billed	PARTICIPATING Assigned Claims			NON-PARTICIPATING Assigned Claims			NON-PARTICIPATING Unassigned Claims			Provider Loss
		Allowed Amount	Medicare Portion (80%)	Patient Portion* (20%)	Allowed Amount (95% of Par Allowed)	Medicare Portion (80%)	Patient Portion* (20%)	Limiting Charge (115% of Non-Par Allowed)	Medicare Portion (80%)	Patient Portion* (20%)	
$100	$100	$50.00	$40.00	$10.00							$50.00
$100	$54.63				$47.50	$38.00	$9.50				$52.50
$100	$54.63							$54.63 ‡	$38.00 §	$16.63	$45.37

*Supplemental insurance could apply if there is coverage for the 20% patient portion.
§ Paid directly to the patient.
‡ Patient pays provider $54.63 (both the Medicare Portion and the Patient Portion).

ALERT: *Figure 2.2* is a comparison table and is for general comparisons only. It does NOT take into account the impact of MIPS adjustments (see "Quality Payment Program" in Chapter 2.2 — Medicare Fees).

Impact of Secondary Insurance

Insurance Secondary to Medicare

If a patient has insurance coverage under more than one plan (or "payer"), "coordination of benefits" rules decide which one pays first. The one that is responsible for paying first is called the "primary payer" and the one that pays second is called the "secondary payer." Bill the primary payer first; they will process your claim(s) and issue to you a *Remittance Advice (RA)* along with any payment due. In cases where claim information is not automatically forwarded by the primary payer, to the secondary payer, a copy of the *RA* is then submitted to the secondary payer for processing of the beneficiary's benefits.

In some cases, there may also be a third payer (tertiary plan) in which the same protocol for billing a secondary payer should be followed. Each subsequent carrier following the primary needs a copy of the previous payer's *RA* or *Explanation of Benefits (EOB)* in order to correctly process the claim(s).

Tip: When billing the secondary or supplemental payer, the primary remittance needs to be included with the secondary claim. This allows the claim to be processed properly, thus minimizing the possibility of problems with overpayments/underpayments, etc.

Every office must stay alert to a patient's insurance status and conditions which could change the primary payer, especially with Medicare. There are different types of policies which are secondary to Medicare and they may need to be treated differently. Correctly identifying the type of secondary policy potentially reduces errors in billing as well as the amount collected from the patient.

Note: Providers who are not eligible (this is not the same thing as being a non-participating provider) to participate in Medicare (e.g., licensed marriage family therapist) might be able to send a claim directly to the secondary plan as if they were the primary payer. Be sure to obtain and follow any official written policies from the secondary payer regarding the billing of services rendered by Medicare-ineligible providers.

Medigap (Supplemental)

A Medicare supplemental insurance policy is commonly referred to as a Medigap policy and is used to help pay some of the costs not paid by original Medicare, such as copays, coinsurance, and deductibles. It fills in the payment "gaps" of original Medicare. In addition, for a PAR provider, if all the appropriate information is included on the claim form, once Medicare has finalized its payments, the claim may be automatically forwarded to the Medigap policy carrier along with any applicable explanation of benefits. The Medigap policy payer then reviews the claim and pays its portion of the charges. On assigned claims, this kind of insurance provides timely payment to the healthcare provider and can eliminate the patient's immediate out-of-pocket costs.

Other Secondary Insurance

Another type of secondary insurance policy is independent from Medicare and is often a group health plan supplied by a patient's employer. These types of policies may pay for services which are not normally covered by Medicare, such as exams and x-rays. A secondary insurance plan only pays if there are covered costs that the primary insurer did not cover. However, it is possible that a secondary insurance includes coverage and benefits that extend beyond that which is covered by Medicare. As a result, patients with a secondary policy may have more payable benefits. Therefore it is essential to understand individual payer policies.

Tip: When a patient indicates that there is a secondary insurance or if the benefits of the secondary coverage are unknown, it is prudent to verify benefits to ensure that the claim is properly billed.

Qualified Medicare Beneficiary (QMB) Program

Those who qualify for both Medicare and Medicaid, also known as Medi-Medi, are called "dual eligibles." The QMB program is similar to the Medi-Medi program. Providers may not bill the patient for any co-insurance, co-pays, or deductibles on covered services. Noncovered services may be billed as long as the patient understands, prior to providing the service, that it is not covered by their insurance and they agree to be personally responsible for the charges. Use the *ABN* for this notification.

Resource: See Resource 235 for more information about Medi-Medi. See Resource 236 for more about QMB.

Medicare as the Secondary Payer (MSP)

Medicare Secondary Payer (MSP) is the term generally used when the Medicare program does not have primary payment responsibility – that is, when another entity has the responsibility for paying before Medicare. MSP concerns are complex and involve a thorough understanding of both patient and provider responsibilities, rules for PAR vs. Non-PAR, conditional payments, and more. It is important to note that over the last several years, the Medicare program has increased its efforts to recoup payments when Medicare was billed in error as the primary payer.

Resource: See Resources 218, 219, and 806 for more info and for forms that will help clarify this important concept.

Non Part B Plan Information

Part C – Medicare Advantage

Medicare Advantage (MA) is also known as Medicare Part C. An MA plan is an alternative to original fee-for-service Medicare (Parts A and B). MA plans are sponsored by Medicare, which pays private insurance companies to provide coverage for health services to beneficiaries enrolled in these plans.

In order to join an MA plan, the patient must be enrolled in both Medicare Part A and Part B, and must continue to pay the Part B premium. Beneficiaries who elect to enroll in an MA plan are still on Medicare and retain the full rights and protections entitled to all beneficiaries; however the private insurance company's billing policies and procedures apply.

MA plans may give coverage and cost sharing options for beneficiaries beyond the traditional Part A and Part B fee-for-service program. Patients can have more benefits than Parts A and B but not less. Each plan is different, so it is important to verify the coverage and the patient cost-sharing for each patient. Please note that CMS does not process Part C claims. Those claims are processed directly through the Medicare Advantage insurance payer. Part C patients will have a different card from traditional Medicare which usually has the word "Advantage" somewhere on it.

There are four main types of Medicare Advantage Plans:
- Health Maintenance Organization (HMO) Plans
- Preferred Provider Organization (PPO) Plans
- Private Fee-for-Service (PFFS) Plans
- Special Needs Plans (SNP)

Other less common types of Medicare Advantage Plans include:
- Medical Savings Account (MSA) Plans – A high deductible plan combined with a bank account. Medicare deposits funds to this account and the beneficiary uses the money from that bank account (a medical savings account) to pay for health care services. See Resource 222 to learn more about MSAs.
- HMO Point of Service (HMOPOS) Plans – A HMO plan in which you may be able to obtain some services out-of-network for a higher cost.

Most of the plans have doctor networks, and sometimes patients must stay in the network in order to have coverage – except for emergencies. However, they may need to be an in-network provider with the Medicare Advantage payer (Resource 315). Call the payer listed on the card and verify the in-network/out-of-network (whichever applies to you) coverage as well as any applicable patient cost-sharing, prior to treating the patient.

Tip: Healthcare providers do not need to be enrolled in Medicare to provide treatment to Part C beneficiaries, however, be aware of plan limitations such as the requirement for referrals or in-network status.

Accountable Care Organizations (ACOs)/Shared Savings Program

As part of healthcare reform, some new types of patient care models with unique forms of reimbursement are emerging in the marketplace. ACOs are groups of doctors, hospitals, and other health care providers who voluntarily come together to provide coordinated high quality patient care. As these new types of integrated healthcare models are being explored, it is important for there to be services provided beyond the typical office visit, which show a coordinated effort to treat the overall health of the patient. Ancillary services, such as behavioral health and physical therapy, have been shown to assist in improving the overall health status of patients suffering from certain conditions or injuries, leading to reduced overall costs for the patient's care. For example, properly managed mental health conditions improve both patient compliance and outcomes for chronic pain management with reduced aberrant behaviors associated with medication management. Be prepared to see an increased number of Medicare ACOs. According to CMS, there are multiple types of Medicare ACOs, including:

- Medicare Shared Savings Program — a program that helps Medicare fee-for-service program providers become an ACO.

- Advance Payment ACO Model — a supplementary incentive program for selected participants in the Shared Savings Program.

- Pioneer ACO Model — a program designed for early adopters of coordinated care.

Resource: See Resource 126 for more information.

Resource: See Resource 803 for a more thorough review of the impact of healthcare reform.

Medicare Administrative Contractors (MACs)

Medicare has divided the country into jurisdictions, each with its own A/B Medicare Administrative Contractor (MAC) – formerly known as "intermediaries" and "carriers" – to process Part A and Part B claims. Most MACs publish a Local Coverage Determination (LCD) for the jurisdiction(s) they serve. According to "Chapter 13" of the *Medicare Program Integrity Manual*:

"The LCDs specify under what clinical circumstances a service is considered to be reasonable and necessary. They are administrative and educational tools to assist providers in submitting correct claims for payment. Contractors publish LCDs to provide guidance to the public and medical community within their jurisdictions. Contractors develop LCDs by considering medical literature, the advice of local medical societies and medical consultants, public comments, and comments from the provider community."

"...Contractors shall consider a service to be reasonable and necessary if the contractor determines that the service is:

- Safe and effective.

- Not experimental or investigational.

- Appropriate, including the duration and frequency that is considered appropriate for the service, in terms of whether it is:

  • Furnished in accordance with the accepted standards of medical practice for the diagnosis or treatment of the patient's condition, or to improve the function of a malformed body member.

  • Furnished in a setting appropriate to the patient's medical needs and condition.

  • Ordered and furnished by qualified personnel.

  • One that meets, but does not exceed, the patient's medical need.

  • At least as beneficial as an existing and available medically appropriate alternative."

Note: In 2019, Medicare stopped publishing the ICD-10-CM, CPT, and HCPCS codes within the LCDs and now only publishes them withing the Medicare articles.

Resource: See Resource 396 for more information on MACs, including an interactive tool to review state specific information.

Medicare Coverage and Billing

Coverage is not the same thing as payment, although it does determine if payment will be made. Actual coverage depends on the answers to the following questions:

1. Is the patient a Medicare Beneficiary? If so, to which Plan(s) do they belong?
2. What services were rendered?
3. Is there sufficient supporting documentation to justify coverage of the services?

Establishing Eligibility

The first step in determining coverage is establishing eligibility. You need to find out if your patient has Medicare coverage as well as which type of coverage they have. Not all Medicare Beneficiaries have Part B, which is what covers outpatient services. Carefully review the patient's Medicare card. For them to have coverage, it should specifically state that they have Part B or a Medicare Advantage plan (also known as Part C). Also, since Medicare is not always the primary payer, it is your responsibility to ask about other coverage and determine which plan is the primary policy.

Alert: Medicare is carefully reviewing claims to recover funds when Medicare was billed as the primary when they should have been billed as the secondary payer.

Book: See "Establish Patient Financial Responsibility" in Chapter 1.1 — Insurance & Reimbursement Essentials for more information.

Resource: Routinely use the *Medicare Status Questionnaire* form (Resource 220) to help identify Medicare as a Secondary Payer (MSP) and avoid billing errors.

Covered Services

Coverage is based upon the medical necessity (see "Establishing Medical Necessity" segment that follows) as defined within the *Medicare Benefits Policy Manual* and the Local Coverage Determinations (LCDs). It should also be noted that not all types of providers may perform all Medicare covered services. These limitations are typically outlined in the LCDs.

Establishing Medical Necessity

Medical necessity, from a Medicare perspective, is defined as "No payment may be made under Part A or Part B for expenses incurred for items or services which are not reasonable and necessary for the diagnosis or treatment of illness or injury or to improve the functioning of a malformed body member."

This official statement does not address specific situations, but rather a generalized thought process on how they approach this topic. It is left up to the MACs to establish individual policies based on the National Coverage Determinations (NCDs). These policies are called Local Coverage Determinations (LCDs) and whenever a provider seeks to determine coverage, reviewing LCDs is the best source of information.

The following segments from a CGS Local Coverage Determination (LCD) for behavioral health services is a good example. It is included here because all other medical services follow the same set of guidelines pertaining to medical necessity. Document the reasons why the service is to be performed, the goals for improvement hoped for by performing the service, and the results achieved (either positive or negative) from performing the service. Obviously, if no improvement comes from the service(s)/procedure(s) performed, it would not be considered medically necessary to continue to perform such services.

Reasonable Expectation of Improvement. Services must be for the purpose of diagnostic study or reasonably be expected to improve the patient's condition. The treatment must, at a minimum, be designed to reduce or control the patient's psychiatric symptoms so as to prevent relapse or hospitalization, and improve or maintain the patient's level of functioning (CMS Publication 100-02, Medicare Benefit Policy Manual, Chapter 6, Section 70.1).

It is not necessary that a course of therapy have as its goal restoration of the patient to the level of functioning exhibited prior to the onset of the illness, although this may be appropriate for some patients. For many other psychiatric patients, particularly those with long-term, chronic conditions, control of symptoms and maintenance of a functional level to avoid further deterioration or hospitalization is an acceptable expectation of improvement. "Improvement" in this context is measured by comparing the effect of continuing treatment versus discontinuing it. Where there is a reasonable expectation that if treatment services were withdrawn the patient's condition would deteriorate, relapse further, or require hospitalization, this criterion would be met (CMS Publication 100-02, Medicare Benefit Policy Manual, Chapter 6, Section 70.1).

Some patients may undergo a course of treatment which increases their level of functioning, but then reach a point where further significant increase is not expected (CMS Publication 100-02, Medicare Benefit Policy Manual, Chapter 6, Section 70.1). When stability can be maintained without further treatment or with less intensive treatment, the psychological services are no longer medically necessary.

Frequency and Duration of Services. There are no specific limits on the length of time that services may be covered. There are many factors that affect the outcome of treatment; among them are the nature of the illness, prior history, the goals of treatment, and the patient's response. As long as the evidence shows that the patient continues to show improvement in accordance with his/her individualized treatment plan, and the frequency of services is within accepted norms of medical practice, coverage may be continued (CMS Publication 100-02, Medicare Benefit Policy Manual, Chapter 6, Section 70.1).

When a patient reaches a point in his/her treatment where further improvement does not appear to be indicated and there is no reasonable expectation of improvement, the outpatient psychiatric services are no longer considered reasonable or medically necessary.

Tip — Purpose of the Visit: To meet coverage requirements, the purpose of the visit plays an important role. Services are only covered as long as the treatment is expected to improve the health status or function of the patient – also known as Maximum Therapeutic Benefit.

Incident To Services

Incident to services are a Medicare-specific option that allows physicians to extend the availability of services through the assistance of a Qualified Healthcare Professional (QHP) such as a Physician Assistant (PA), Advanced Practical Registered Nurse (APRN), or Family Nurse Practitioners (FNP). There are very strict guidelines for billing "incident to" services and Medicare often audits these services to ensure that the guidelines have been adhered to. It is important to ensure documentation supports the fact that all incident to rules have been met.

Some of the conditions that must be met for billing "incident to" include:

- The service is typically provided in the office/clinic setting (there are a few exceptions such as a rural setting).
- The service is for an established patient who already has a plan of care established by the MD or DO under whose name the service is billed.
- Both the MD or DO and qualified healthcare provider are employed by the same entity
- Services are furnished under the physician's direct supervision (physician is in the designated office area and immediately available to provide assistance and direction, or take over the performance of the service if needed).

- The MD or DO, under whose name the service is billed, remains involved in the care of the patient by performing subsequent services of a frequency which reflects his/her active involvement in the management of the plan of care (POC).
- If the patient presents for follow-up but has a new problem, "incident to" no longer applies and the MD or DO must perform the service to meet "incident to" requirements. However, the QHP may perform the service as long as the service is billed with the QHPs identification and not the MD or DO. Follow-up visits for this encounter would also be ineligible for "incident to" billing.

Other Payers

Commercial payers follow their own individual company policies when it comes to delegation of services by a physician to a non-physician (e.g., PA). Their guidelines pertaining to credentialing and billing for these delegated services must be carefully followed. "Incident to," as noted above, is particular to Medicare and unless specifically stated as acceptable by another payer, would not apply to commercial payer policies. It is strongly suggested to contact the commercial payer representatives to determine if specific services are payable under your individual contract in a delegated (incident to) situation.

Tip: If your practice will be billing incident to services to Medicare beneficiaries, enroll the practice as a group practice and obtain a group provider number and group NPI number. Then, enroll each employee eligible to provide incident to services (e.g., PA, NP) with Medicare using their own unique NPI number.

Resource: See Resource 819 and search on "incident to" for more information on how to properly bill these services.

Medicare Overpayment/Provider Recoupment

There may be situations when a healthcare provider realizes they have received an improper Medicare payment. Voluntary refunds should be reported to CMS and made within 60 days of when the provider discovers the error on their own. Solicited refunds are refunds requested from providers by Medicare. In the case of voluntary refunds, it is best to follow the guidelines and use the forms found on your local MAC website. It may be called a *"Voluntary Refund Form"* or an *"Overpayment Refund Form."* For refunds requested by Medicare, follow the guidelines received from them.

Resource: See Resource 819 and search on "60 day rule" for important information on ensuring compliance.

Billing Help

This section identifies some problem areas and offers guidance on billing both covered and noncovered services. Carefully review the following segments and pay close attention to the proper use of modifiers to appropriately bill Medicare and avoid allegations of fraud and/or abuse.

Book: See Chapter 4 — Documentation for medical necessity guidelines.

Tip: As a reminder, a Local Coverage Determination (LCD) is an excellent resource for reviewing covered diagnoses, treatments, and payment rules for proper claim submissions. Some may also include guidelines regarding the preferred order of diagnoses on claims.

Assignment Violations

When a healthcare provider accepts assignment, they are agreeing to accept Medicare's reasonable charge as the full charge for the service. Therefore, if the practice either collects or even attempts to collect anything from the patient other than coinsurance, the cost of noncovered charges or unmet deductibles, it is in violation of the agreement. Assignment violations are assessed penalties based on the severity of the violation. See Resource 450 for more about assignment violations and penalties.

Alert: It should be noted that statutorily noncovered services can be charged directly to the patient at the health care provider's usual and customary fee.

Tip: Once a claim is filed with an "assigned" status, Medicare treats that claim as assigned even if the assignment was billed in error.

Medicare Modifiers

It is critical for every office to clearly understand the proper use of modifiers. Here are some basics for coding and billing using modifiers GA, GX, GY and GZ.

GA: ABN signed for not reasonable and necessary services

Modifier GA must be used to indicate that Medicare will probably deny a service as not reasonable and necessary and that an *ABN* has been properly delivered to the beneficiary. Use modifier GZ when the *ABN* has NOT been properly delivered.

A signed waiver should also be obtained for these services (e.g., any investigational or experimental services or supplies). These services should be billed to Medicare with modifier GA appended to the procedure code(s). Modifier GA certifies that a signed waiver statement was obtained from the patient and permits the appropriate beneficiary liability to be calculated on the patient's Explanation of Medicare Benefits (EOMB) or Medicare Summary Notice (MSN).

For most services, the provider performing the service will obtain the waiver statement. However, for certain referred services (e.g., independent laboratory receiving a specimen for testing) the rendering provider (lab) may not see the patient or have the opportunity to obtain a signed waiver. In this instance, the referring entity should obtain the waiver statement as a courtesy and forward it with the lab requisition form. The laboratory may then bill the service(s) with modifier GA to indicate that a signed waiver was obtained.

Additionally, if the diagnosis code is known to be noncovered, append modifier GA to the procedure or supply code.

GX: ABN Delivered for Noncovered Service

Modifier GX indicates that the *ABN* was used to voluntarily inform the patient that Medicare will not pay for a service because it is excluded from coverage by statute. Since the GX modifier is used only with noncovered services, it should be used in combination with the GY modifier. Check your LCD to determine if your MAC accepts or requires this modifier.

GY: Noncovered Service:

Modifier GY must be used on all statutorily noncovered items or services (as defined in the *Program Integrity Manual (PIM)* Chapter 1, Section 2.3.3.B). It must also be appended when the item/service is not a Medicare Benefit (as defined in the *PIM*, Chapter 1, Section 2.3.3.A).

When billing for services requested by the beneficiary that are statutorily excluded by Medicare, report an ICD-10-CM code that best describes the patient's condition and the GY modifier (items or services statutorily excluded or does not meet the definition of any Medicare benefit).

GZ: ABN not Signed not Reasonable and Necessary Services

Modifier GZ indicates that it is expected that Medicare will deny an item or service as not reasonable and necessary and that an *ABN* has not been properly delivered to the beneficiary.

Tip: The GX and GY are often reported together. The GX is used to state that the *ABN* was used, and the GY to clarify that the services are excluded.

Alert — Modifiers GX and GA

The GX modifier is used to signify that the *ABN* was voluntarily given to a patient to inform them that they will be financially liable for statutorily noncovered services. Since the GX modifier is used only with statutorily noncovered services, it should be used in combination with the GY modifier. Contact your Medicare Administrative Contractor (MAC) for usage instructions.

The GA modifier should be used when the Waiver of Liability Statement Issued as Required by Payer Policy has been provided to the patient. The GA modifier should be used in conjunction with CPT codes only when appropriate.

Direct Submission to Secondary Insurance for Medicare Noncovered Services

When a secondary insurance plan is contracted with Medicare and the secondary information is correctly included, claims submitted by a participating provider are automatically submitted to the secondary payer. If these conditions are not met, the provider must either directly submit to the secondary payer themselves or the patient must do so. Some, but not all, billing software programs have the capability to submit secondary claims.

In situations where a secondary claim will be submitted manually, innoviHealth has created a sample letter which could be used along with the *EOB* for direct submission to these payers. Use this letter for services that are not covered by Medicare but will be covered by a secondary payer. However, be aware that most payers require a denial letter from the primary before they will make a payment.

Resource: See Resource 397 to download this sample letter with instructions.

Supporting Documentation

Properly documenting the service can include more than just the typical visit documentation. It can also include other compliance-supporting forms such as Medicare's *Advance Beneficiary Notice of Noncoverage (ABN)*.

Book: See also Chapter 4 — Documentation for medical record documentation requirements.

Advance Beneficiary Notice of Noncoverage (ABN)

Alert — New ABN Form Mandated:

As of June 21, 2017, a new *ABN* form is mandated for use. There were no significant changes to the form itself. There were, however, some new guidelines regarding non-participating providers.

Resource: See Resource 231 for more information.

The *Advance Beneficiary Notice of Noncoverage (ABN)* is one of the most critical Medicare forms that you can utilize. It is mandated for use when any of the following criteria are met:

- You believe Medicare may not pay for an item or service,
- Medicare usually covers the item or service,
- Medicare may not consider it medically reasonable and necessary for this patient in this particular instance.

It can also be used voluntarily to notify patients of their financial responsibility for statutorily noncovered services and items. See the segment "Voluntary Use of ABN" that follows for more information.

The *ABN* is proof that you have told the patient that these services/supplies will most likely not be reimbursable by Medicare. As an informed consumer they can then decide whether or not to receive your services as an out-of-pocket expense, or through other insurance, if they have it.

Alert: It is a requirement to provide a completed copy of the *ABN* to the beneficiary or their representative. The original must be kept on file by the provider. It is a requirement to provide a completed copy of the *ABN* to the beneficiary or their representative. The original must be kept on file by the provider.

Resource: See Resource 232 for frequently asked questions and answers regarding the use of an *ABN*.

If you use it properly, you will be able to collect your full fee from the patient if Medicare determines that the care you provided is not reasonable or necessary. Without a properly executed *ABN* on file for that patient, you will have to refund any money that Medicare and/or the patient paid.

Tip: Two commonly overlooked *ABN* instructions are those regarding 1. Non-participating providers (see Resource 231) and 2. the frequency and duration for repetitive or continuous noncovered care (see Resource 234). These are important so be sure to review your policies to ensure that your organization is aware of these instructions, where applicable.

Voluntary Use of ABN

The *ABN* may also be used voluntarily as a way to inform a patient of their financial responsibility regarding statutorily noncovered services and items or *most care* that fails to meet a technical benefit requirement (i.e., lacks required certification). When using the *ABN* this way, the beneficiary does not check an option box or sign and date the notice.

Using the *ABN* for voluntary purposes, as a courtesy to the patient, can more clearly communicate to them that those expenses are not covered by Medicare and thus are the financial responsibility of the patient.

Tip: Medicare does not permit patient signatures for voluntary use of *ABN* forms, therefore, it is better to use your own *Notice of Medicare Coverage* (Resource 227) that identifies Medicare noncovered items/services and have the Medicare beneficiary sign and date this accordingly.

Routine Use of ABN Prohibited

"Routine use" means giving *ABNs* to beneficiaries where there is no specific, identifiable reason to believe that Medicare will not pay. According to Medicare, a "reasonable basis" must exist for using the *ABN*. Healthcare providers are prohibited from using an *ABN* routinely just to avoid a potential problem. There must be evidence to support your use of the *ABN*.

There are some exceptions to the "Routine Use Prohibition." For example, an *ABN* may be used routinely for experimental items/services as well as items/services with frequency limitations for coverage.

Extended Treatment and the ABN

Generally, it is acceptable to issue a single *ABN* to cover an extended course of treatment as long as that *ABN* clearly identifies ALL items and services for that course of treatment. However, there are some notable exceptions:

- If the treatment goes beyond one year, a new *ABN* must be issued.
- If an item or service is needed which is not on the current *ABN*, then a new *ABN* must be issued to include that new item/service.

Resource: See Resource 451 for more about using an *ABN*.

Medicare Terms to Understand

Medicare often uses terms or phrases that may differ from the rest of the medical insurance industry. This segment explains some of the common terms that could be encountered while working with Medicare claims:

Abuse. Abuse describes practices that, either directly or indirectly, result in unnecessary costs to the Medicare Program. Abuse includes any practice that is not consistent with the goals of providing patients with services that are medically necessary, meet professionally recognized standards, and are fairly priced.

Examples of Medicare abuse may include:
- Misusing codes on a claim,
- Charging excessively for services, and
- Billing for services that were not medically necessary.

Accept Assignment. Assignment means that the provider is paid the Medicare-allowed amount as payment in full for all Part B claims for all covered services for all Medicare beneficiaries.

Actual Charge. The amount of money a healthcare provider or supplier charges for a certain medical service or supply. This amount is often more than the amount Medicare approves. It is also referred to as the usual and customary charge or fee.

Allowed Amount. The maximum amount on which payment is based for covered health care services. This may be called "eligible expense," "payment allowance," or "negotiated rate." It is usually less than the provider's actual charge.

Claims Submission Mandate. By law, Medicare claims for covered services must be submitted by providers - this includes both PAR and NON-PAR providers.

Coinsurance. The patient portion of the Medicare Allowed Amount after the deductible has been met.

Coordination of Benefits. When a beneficiary is covered by more than one type of insurance that covers the same health care services, one pays its benefits in full as the primary payer and the others pay a reduced benefit as a secondary or tertiary (third) payer. When the primary payer doesn't cover a particular service but the secondary payer does, the secondary payer will pay up to its benefit limit as if it were the primary payer.

Copayment. Though not common for Medicare Fee-for-Service plans, a copayment is a fixed amount (for example, $30) the patient pays for a covered health care service, usually when they receive the service. The amount can vary by the type of covered health care service.

Deductible. The amount that the beneficiary is responsible for during each calendar year before Medicare benefits begin to apply. This applies only to services and supplies covered by Medicare. The amount is based on the Medicare-approved amounts and not necessarily the charges billed by the provider. Deductible amounts are reviewed annually by CMS and can vary between Part A, Part B, Part C and/or Part D. Verify deductible amounts when you verify insurance coverage for the patient.

Exacerbation. An exacerbation is a temporary, but marked, deterioration of the patient's condition that is causing significant interference with activities of daily living, due to an acute flare-up of a previously treated condition.

Fraud. When someone intentionally executes or attempts to execute a scheme to obtain money or property of any health care benefit program which they are not entitled to.

Limiting Charge. A cap on how much Non-Participating physicians may bill Medicare patients on non-assigned claims. The limiting charge is 115% of the allowed amount for Non-Participating physicians (which is 95% of the Participating provider allowed amount).

MAC. Medicare Administrative Contractor. A MAC is a private health care insurer that has been awarded a geographic jurisdiction to process Medicare Part A and Part B (A/B) medical claims or Durable Medical Equipment (DME) claims for Medicare Fee-for-Service (FFS) beneficiaries.

Medigap. A Medigap policy is offered by a private company to those entitled to Medicare benefits and provides payment for Medicare charges not payable because of the applicability of deductibles, coinsurance amounts, or other Medicare imposed limitations.

Non-Participating Provider. A provider who chooses not to sign the Participation agreement. These providers can choose to accept assignment on a claim-by-claim basis; however, services that are unassigned are subject to the "Limiting Charge" restriction.

Offset. The recovery by Medicare of a non-Medicare debt by reducing present or future Medicare payments and applying the amount withheld to the debt incurred.

Opt Out. An official designation for a provider who agrees to operate outside the Medicare system. When a provider opts out of Medicare, he or she opts out of all Medicare programs and plans until such time as they request to opt back into the Medicare program. A Medicare beneficiary may be treated under a private contract. See the segment "Opt Out" on page 85 for additional information.

Overpayment Assessment. A decision that an incorrect amount of money has been paid for Medicare services and a determination of what that amount is.

Part A Hospital Insurance Benefits (Fee for Service). Hospital insurance covers institutional services for inpatients that are then billed by the hospital to the Medicare contractor. Individual providers do not submit claims for Part A services.

Part B Medical Insurance Benefits (Fee for Service). Medical insurance coverage which helps to pay for all physician services that are medically necessary, outpatient hospital care, and some other medical services that Part A does not cover.

Part C Medicare Advantage Health plans run by Medicare-approved private insurance companies. Medicare Advantage Plans include Part A and Part B benefits, and usually additional coverage like Medicare prescription drug coverage, sometimes for an extra cost. With this program, there could be overall lower costs and extra benefits for the beneficiary.

Part D Medicare Prescription Drug Plan. Sometimes called "PDPs," these plans add drug coverage to original Medicare, some Medicare Cost Plans, some Medicare Private Fee-for-Service (PFFS) Plans, and Medicare Medical Savings Account (MSA) Plans.

Participating Provider. A provider who agrees to "accept assignment" for all covered services provided to all Medicare patients for the following year. The provider signs a Participation agreement and accepts the Participating provider fee schedule.

Patient Portion. For participating providers, the beneficiary pays 20% (i.e., coinsurance) of the allowed amount plus any deductible. For NON-PAR, the beneficiary pays up to the limiting charge, or 20% of the NON-PAR allowed amount plus any deductible.

Private Contract. A contract between a Medicare beneficiary and a provider who has **opted out** of Medicare. The beneficiary agrees to give up all Medicare payments for services furnished by the provider and to pay the provider directly without regard to any limits that would otherwise apply to what the provider could charge. The contract must be in writing and must be signed before any service is provided. See the segment "Opt Out" on page 85 for additional information.

PTAN. The MAC's Provider Enrollment department issues Medicare Providers a Medicare Transactions Number called the Provider Transaction Access Number (PTAN). The PTAN is the same number as a previously issued Provider Identification Number (PIN).

Recoupment. The recovery by Medicare of Medicare debt by reducing present or future Medicare payments and applying the amount withheld to the debt incurred.

Recurrence. A return of symptoms from a previously treated condition that has been quiescent for a period of time.

Secondary Payer. When coordinating benefits, the health plan that pays benefits only after the primary payer has paid its full benefits. It will pay the lesser of a) its benefits in full, or b) an amount that when added to the benefits payable by the primary payer equals 100% of covered charges.

Unassigned Claim. NON-PAR providers can charge more than the Medicare-approved amount but no more than the limiting charge. If it is a covered service the physician is required to submit the claim to Medicare, but the program pays the patient.

Notes:

2.2 Medicare Fees

Medicare Fee Schedule

Medicare fees have become more complex over the years as new systems are implemented to improve quality while reducing costs. The majority of healthcare providers are paid through either the Prospective Payment System (PPS) or the Medicare Fee-for-Service (FFS) system. Medicare's shared savings programs have very different reimbursement systems which are not discussed in this chapter.

Resource: See Resource 803 for more about fees as they relate to the new healthcare reform systems.

Prospective Payment System (PPS)

A Prospective Payment System (PPS) is a method of reimbursement in which Medicare payment is made based on a predetermined, fixed amount. The payment amount for a particular service is derived based on the classification system of that service (e.g., diagnosis-related groups for inpatient hospital services). CMS uses separate PPSs for reimbursement to acute inpatient hospitals, home health agencies, hospice, inpatient psychiatric facilities, inpatient rehabilitation facilities, long-term care hospitals, federally qualified health centers, and skilled nursing facilities.

Note: As of January 1, 2014, Federally Qualified Health Centers (FQHC) began using their own payment system – FQHC PPS. Rural Health Clinics remain on their all-inclusive, per-visit payment schedule.

Resource: See Resource 334 for information by Medicare regarding these programs.

Medicare Fee-for-Service (FFS)

The FFS system is for payments to providers, including physicians, other practitioners, and suppliers. CMS develops fee schedules for physicians, ambulance services, clinical laboratory services, and durable medical equipment, prosthetics, orthotics, and supplies. The remainder of this chapter discusses fees for these types of services.

Medicare Physician Fee Schedule (MPFS)

Every participating healthcare office should receive its annual Medicare Physician Fee Schedule (MPFS) from its Medicare Administrative Contractor (MAC) prior to the new year. The MPFS is also available on individual MAC websites as well as the CMS website. Providers should be aware of the local Medicare allowed amounts and limiting charges for the coming calendar year in order to properly assess their current fee schedule.

Alert: As of 2019, new payment models based on the MPFS will have an impact on the fees paid to your practice by Medicare. See the segment "Quality Payment Program Adjustments" on page 109 for more information.

The MPFS lists the allowed amounts for participating providers and non-participating providers, as well as the **limiting charges** for non-participating providers not accepting assignment. Fees for all codes in your MPFS are already adjusted by the Geographic Adjustment Factor (GAF) for your area. These published fees become an excellent basis for evaluation and calculation of your other fees. Non-PAR are not allowed to exceed the limiting charge for Medicare covered services by any amount for any reason.

Your Medicare fee schedule is probably a good minimum standard. Traditionally, a majority of payers across the nation use the MPFS as a baseline and then add a percentage to it to set their own fee schedules. For example, some states (e.g., Florida), mandate that auto claims are paid at a set percentage above the Medicare fee schedule. The rationale behind this practice is that Medicare fees are known to be far below a provider's usual and customary fees. Unfortunately, a few payers have fee schedules that are less than the Medicare fee schedule.

Fee Calculations for Medicare

Medicare fees are calculated annually. They are a combination of:

- An adjusted Relative Value Unit (RVU) assigned by CMS to each procedure for each area/locality.

- The adjusted RVU is multiplied by the Medicare Physician Fee Schedule (MPFS) Conversion Factor (CF) to calculate the MPFS into a dollar amount, which is the allowed amount for participating providers. Non-participating providers have a different payment rate which is called the limiting charge.

- Physicians who qualify are paid at 100% of the applicable fee schedule. Other types of qualified healthcare providers are paid at a lesser rate. For example, Nurse Practitioners (NP), Clinical Nurse Specialists (CNS), and Physician Assistants (PA) are paid at 85% of the fee schedule while other types of providers may be paid even less.

- Adjustments are then applied based on the level of participation in the provider's chosen payment program. The result is that final payments may go up or down depending on how well the provider meets threshold requirements.

Website: Fees are shown with payment adjustments at FindACode.com (subscription is required).

If there are questions or concerns about whether or not Medicare has assigned the appropriate fee schedule to your practice, contact the local MAC to have this verified.

Alert: In April of 2015, the Sustainable Growth Rate (SGR) formula which is used to calculate the MPFS Conversion Factor was repealed as part of the Medicare Access and CHIP Reauthorization Act of 2015 (MACRA). The conversion factor will be frozen until 2026, after which it will increase by 0.75% per year for APM participants and 0.25% per year for MIPS participants, in addition to any bonuses and penalties based on performance.

Tip — Impact of Submitted Fee Amounts: Always submit your usual and customary fee on claims UNLESS you are a Non-Par provider who is not accepting assignment. Not using your standard rate can lead to overall lower national fees. See the "UCR" segment in Chapter 1.5 — Establishing Fees for more information.

CMS (Medicare) Conversion Factor

The annual Medicare Conversion Factor (CF) is the pivotal component in the fee calculation process. Without a proper conversion factor, fees will be depressed. See Resource 251 for current Medicare CF information.

Participation Status

Participating (PAR): This means that a provider has signed an agreement with Medicare to bill them directly with assignment on all claims for direct payments, according to the allowed amount on the Medicare fee schedule. Names of participating providers are published by Medicare for patients to use.

The fee amount submitted on a claim is not bound by law to be the Medicare allowed amount. PAR providers may bill whatever they wish on the claim. However, only the allowed amounts for covered services may actually be collected. Therefore, anything beyond the allowed amount must be written off and never billed to the patient!

Alert: Failure by PAR providers to attempt collection of either the patient's 20% co-insurance portion, or the annual deductible, could be considered fraud.

Non-Participating (Non-PAR): This means that a provider has not signed the participation agreement to take assignment on all claims. Assignment is an option. Non-PAR providers can collect from a patient at the time of service, up to the **limiting charge** amount, when not accepting assignment.

If a healthcare provider does not accept assignment on the claim, Medicare will reimburse the patient 80% of the Non-PAR fee allowance. If a non-participating provider accepts assignment, they must accept the Non-PAR fee allowance as payment in full.

Tip: When a Non-PAR provider does NOT accept assignment, the fee amount on a submitted claim cannot be more than the limiting charge.

Limiting Charge Warning: Not understanding the limiting charge could be costly. The following warning has been issued by Medicare (Resource 455):

"Submission of a non-par, non-assigned Medicare Physician Fee Schedule (MPFS) service with a charge in excess of the Medicare limiting charge amount constitutes a violation of the limiting charge. A physician or supplier who violates the limiting charge is subject to a civil monetary penalty of not more than $10,000, an assessment of not more than 3 times the amount claimed for each item or service, and possible exclusion from the Medicare program. Therefore, it is crucial that EPs are provided with the correct limiting charge they may bill for a MPFS service."

Alert — Limiting Charge Pricing Exception:
It is illegal for non-participating providers to bill the patient more than the limiting charge. However, there is one exception to the rule which states that Non-PAR providers may round the Limiting Charge to the nearest dollar without penalty, as long as they round consistently.

Understanding Medicare Fees

The Medicare Unadjusted Fees Flowchart (*Figure 2.3*) includes examples and helps outline the decision process for billing the appropriate fees for Medicare patients. Be aware that the fees included here are only examples which are used for demonstration purposes only.

Flowchart Notes

The following numbered points are used to explain *Figure 2.3*. They are not intended to explain every possible Medicare fee scenario since fees are impacted by participation in Medicare quality programs. Rather, it is used to help explain how Medicare calculates the basic unadjusted fee before any payment adjustments are applied.

Caution — This is an Unadjusted Fee Example Only:
Medicare fee calculations are now affected by a wide variety of factors. As explained in the "Fee Adjustment" segment earlier in this chapter, participation or non-participation in federal quality programs will either increase or decrease the final amount paid to your practice.

1. **Is This a Covered Service?**
   - Maintenance care does not go through the standard claims process. Since it is a noncovered Medicare service, you cannot bill the patient unless you have a properly delivered *ABN* on file. See Step 2 for more information on the *ABN*.

2. **Verify ABN and IF Appropriate Provide the Treatment Service**
   - Treatment may only be provided if the patient has a current, properly delivered *ABN* on file, and they have chosen either option #1 or #2. If they have chosen option #3, no treatment may be provided.
   - If you have an *ABN* on file, it must be less **than a year old** to be valid (see alert below).
   - You **cannot** bill the patient if Medicare decides that the service/supply (which is usually covered) is medically unnecessary unless you have a properly delivered *ABN* on file.
   - The *ABN* is only mandatory for services/supplies usually covered by Medicare that they deem not reasonable or necessary (e.g., maintenance care). It can also voluntarily be used as a method to explain statutorily noncovered services/supplies for which the patient will be required to pay out of pocket.

Alert: Once an *ABN* has been signed for the purpose of noncoverage, that *ABN* is valid for one year, until there is any change in the patient's condition which would then make the service/supply covered. Once there is an exacerbation or change in patient status, a newly delivered *ABN* is necessary.

Book: See Chapter 2.1 — Medicare Essentials for more information about when an *ABN* is needed and when it should be used.

3. **Collect Your Usual Fee From Patient**
   - You may collect your usual and customary fee from the patient for covered services performed during the maintenance phase of care, as long as you have a properly delivered and current *ABN*. Medicare Allowed Amounts and Limiting Charges do not apply. Note that some practices elect to charge the patient the same amount they would have received from Medicare instead of their usual and customary fee. If this is your policy, it must be clearly outlined in your Policies and Procedures manual.

Figure 2.3

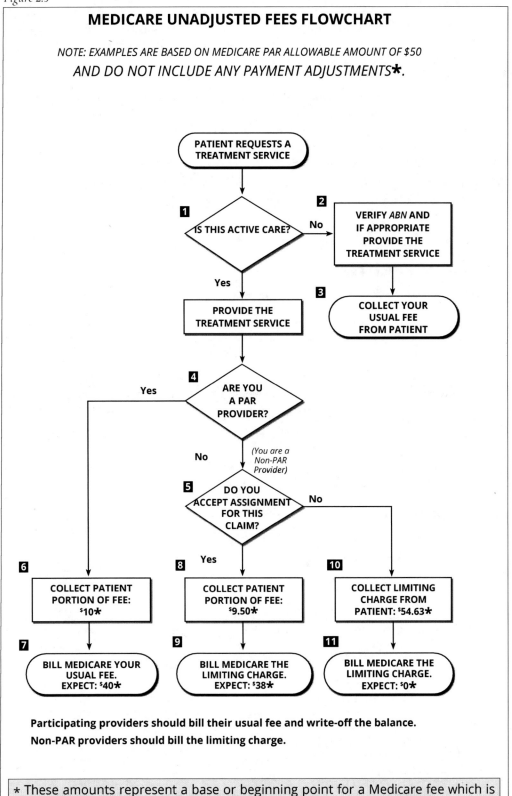

4. **Are You a Par Provider?**
   - A participating provider (PAR) takes assignment on all Medicare claims and accepts the Medicare allowed amount as payment in full.
   - Payment for Non-Participating (Non-PAR) Providers is 95% of the unadjusted allowed amount on assigned claims and up to the limiting charge (115% of the Non-PAR unadjusted allowed amount) on unassigned claims.

5. **Do You Accept Assignment?**
   - If you are Non-PAR and accept assignment, you can expect 80% of the unadjusted allowed amount from your MAC. If you are Non-PAR and do not accept assignment, you can charge the patient up to the limiting charge which is 115% of the Non-PAR unadjusted allowed amount.

6. **Collect the Patient Portion of the Fee**
   - When collecting the patient portion, if there is an unmet deductible, this amount would be more than the unadjusted amount of $10*.
   - The patient coinsurance, for a PAR-provider, is 20% of the unadjusted allowed amount for assigned claims. Medicare pays the other 80% directly to the provider.

7. **Bill Medicare Your Usual Fee**
   - Anticipate an unadjusted fee of $40*, unless the patient deductible has not been met.
   - Bill your usual fee and write off any difference over the PAR allowed amount. Expect 80% of the Medicare allowed amount less any adjustments from your local MAC. The remaining 20% should ideally be collected from the patient at the time of services, unless they have a supplemental or secondary policy.

   Note: If the patient has supplemental or secondary coverage which covers the deductible/or patient co-insurance, in most cases you will not charge the patient these amounts.

8. **Collect the Patient Portion of the Fee**
   - When collecting the patient portion, if there is an unmet deductible, this amount would be more than the unadjusted amount of $9.50*.
   - Once the deductible is met, the local MAC will pay 80% of the Non-PAR allowed amount directly to you. The patient portion/responsibility is the remainder of the cost of that service, up to the Medicare Limiting Charge.

   Note: If the patient has supplemental or secondary coverage which covers the deductible and/or patient co-insurance, in most cases, you will not charge the patient these amounts.

9. **Bill Medicare the Limiting Charge**
   - Bill Medicare no more than the Limiting Charge. Your local MAC will adjust and pay you 80% of the Non-PAR allowed amount less any applicable adjustments.

   Note: If the patient has supplemental or secondary coverage which covers the deductible/or patient co-insurance, do not charge the patient these amounts.

10. Collect the Limiting Charge

Collect up to the limiting charge from the patient. You may collect less if you choose. The limiting charge is 115% of the Non-PAR allowed amount. Your local MAC pays 80% of the Non-PAR allowable to the patient.

11. Bill Medicare the Limiting Charge

The limiting charge is 115% of the Non-PAR allowed amount. Your local MAC is billed in order to reimburse the patient.

> **Alert – Limiting Charge Pricing Exception:**
> It is illegal for non-participating providers to bill the patient more than the limiting charge. However, there is one exception to the rule which states that Non-PAR providers may round the Limiting Charge to the nearest dollar without penalty, as long as they round consistently.

Quality Payment Program Adjustments

Once the base Medicare fee has been determined, the base is then adjusted according to the Quality Payment Program (QPP) path the healthcare provider has chosen to participate in. As mandated by MACRA, Eligible Clinicians (ECs), if they are not exempted, may choose to participate in either the Merit-based Incentive Payment System (MIPS) or Advanced Alternative Payment Models (APMs). There are also bonus payments for those participating in advanced APMs (see *Figure 2.4*). Regardless of the program chosen, every healthcare practice needs to take time to focus on quality.

> **Resource:** See Resource 168 for detailed information from innoviHealth and CMS regarding these programs, including information on whether or not your practice needs to participate.

Adjustments to fees will follow a specified timeline over the next several years as these new programs are fully implemented. See *Figure 2.4* to evaluate the different options. As shown, MIPS participants will experience payment adjustments (negative or positive) based on the composite score of four quality categories. APM participants can qualify for a 5% incentive payment.

Figure 2.4 - Fee Schedule Adjustment Timeline

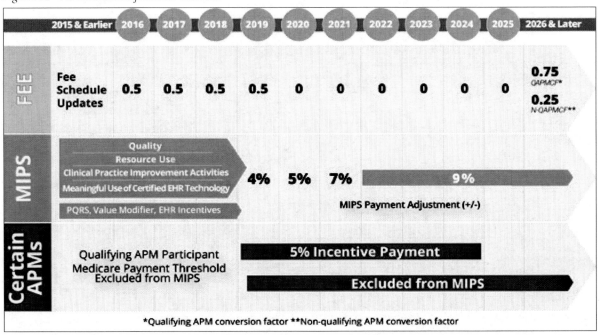

Merit-Based Incentive Payment System (MIPS)

MACRA mandated a new program called the Merit-based Incentive Payment System (MIPS) which replaced EHR, PQRS, and Value Based Payment Modifier (VBM), and added a new quality measure category: Improvement Activities. Data gathering for MIPS calculations began January 2017. As of 2019, either a bonus or penalty will be assessed (see *Figure 2.4*) based on how well a provider meets certain thresholds for the four quality categories: Quality, Resource Use (Cost), Improvement Activities, and Promoting Interoperability. Payments are adjusted based on their composite score.

Resource: See Resource 168 for more information on the MIPS program including how a composite score is calculated.

Payment adjustments are based on the performance of the provider from two years prior. In addition to these payment adjustments, after 2026, the conversion factor will increase at a rate of 0.25% per year.

Note: MIPS does not apply to hospitals or facilities.

Advanced Alternative Payment Models (APMs)

The second payment path (APMs) would exempt the provider from MIPS payment adjustments and would qualify them for a 5 percent Medicare Part B incentive payment. According to CMS, in order to qualify for this incentive, providers "would have to receive enough of their payments or see enough of their patients through Advanced APMs. Advanced APMs are the CMS Innovation Center models, Shared Savings Program tracks, or statutorily-required demonstrations where clinicians accept both risk and reward for providing coordinated, high quality, and efficient care. These models must also meet criteria for payment based on quality measurement and for the use of EHRs." APMs will have have their conversion factor increase by a rate of 0.75% per year after 2026.

Resource: See Resource 150 to learn more about APMs.

Notes:

Notes:

2.3 Medicare Appeals

Medicare Appeals Process

Medicare regulations provide an appeals process for providers and beneficiaries dissatisfied with the initial claim determination made by the Medicare Administrative Contractor (MAC). Because re-submitting a corrected claim that has been denied is not the same thing as the formal Medicare appeals process, it is important to understand the differences between a reopening and an appeal. Appeals can only be filed under the following scenarios:

- PAR: Participating providers (required to accept assignment on all claims)
- NON-PAR:
  - Non-Participating providers who accepted assignment
  - Non-Participating providers who did not accept assignment, but may be responsible for refunding money to the beneficiary
  - Non-Participating providers who otherwise do not have appeal rights may appeal when the beneficiary dies and there is no one else to make the appeal
  - Non-Participating providers, who did not accept assignment may appeal on behalf of a patient, but only when they have valid transfer of appeal rights

Alert: Effective March 20, 2017, new standards for Medicare appeals went into effect. Most of the changes were aimed at the third step: Review by ALJ.

Resource: See Resource 250 for more about these changes.

Before Submitting a Medicare Appeal

There are three situations which should be resolved through a reopening – NOT through the formal appeals process. In the following situations, contact your local MAC by either telephone or letter and request a reopening:

1. Correcting incomplete or invalid claims submission. For example, a missing provider NPI or an incorrect patient ID number.
2. A minor error or omission which caused the claim to be denied. For example, an improper modifier.
3. Failure to respond within 45 days to an Additional Documentation Request (ADR) has resulted in a denial. The reopening must be requested within 120 days from the initial determination to be considered.

The following time frames for a reopening are outlined in the *Medicare Claims Processing Manual*:

- Within one year from the date of the initial determination or redetermination for any reason; or
- Within four years from the date of the initial determination or redetermination for good cause as defined in §10.11; or
- At any time if the initial determination is unfavorable, in whole or in part, to the party thereto, but only for the purpose of correcting a clerical error on which that determination was based. Third party payer error does not constitute clerical error as defined in §10.4.

If the reopening results in an unfavorable determination, then the appeals process may be initiated.

Tip – Unprocessable Claims: Claims that are "unprocessable" should be corrected and re-submitted instead of using the appeals or reopening process. Carefully review the Medicare Summary Notice or the Remittance Advisory for two specific codes: CO16 and MA130. Code CO16 indicates that the claim is unprocessable, while code MA130 means there are no appeal rights. Typically, there is a third code which varies and will be the reason that the claim is unprocessable. If you see these codes simply correct the error and promptly re-submit the claim.

Caution: According to Medicare: "If you submit more than one claim for the same item or service, you can expect your duplicate claims to be denied. In addition, duplicate claims: 1) may delay payment; 2) could cause you to be identified as an abusive biller; or 3) if a pattern of duplicate billing is identified, may generate an investigation for fraud."

Resource: See Resource 285 for more information by CMS regarding duplicate claims.

Medicare Appeals – After the Initial Determination

The Medicare appeals process has five levels. Each level must be completed for each claim before proceeding to the next level. The entire process could take up to 780 days.

1. **Redetermination** – by a different reviewer at the Medicare contractor
2. **Reconsideration** – by a Qualified Independent Contractor (QIC)
3. **Hearing** – by an Administrative Law Judge (ALJ)
4. **Review** – by the Medicare Appeals Council
5. **Review** – by the Federal District Court

On the following pages are instructions for proper Medicare appeals. They are sufficient for most offices. Providers and billers will want to master all components and steps, especially when large dollar amounts are involved.

Tip: Once a claim has been processed as "assigned," it remains that way. If a Non-Par provider mistakenly accepts assignment on a claim, the assignment status cannot be appealed. Other types of appeals, such as denials, may still be pursued.

Alert: In 2016, 65.2% of Part B claim appeals were overturned and ruled to be in the provider's favor and according to a September 2018 OIG report, only 1% of denied Medicare Advantage (Part C) claims were appealed and of those claims, 75% were overturned.

Figure 2.5 summarizes the appeals levels process. Pay close attention to timing deadlines and monetary amounts.

Transfer of Appeal Rights (for non-assigned claims)

The *Transfer of Appeal Rights* form (#CMS-20031) allows you to pursue payment through the appeals process. Keep each completed form on file. The form includes a second page with patient information.

Note: When the provider makes the appeal, they give up the right to bill the patient for that claim if their appeal fails. The patient is still responsible for any deductibles or coinsurance.

Resource: See Resource 240 for a full-size version of this form.

When do payments to providers become non-recoverable?
Medicare uses the same four-year regulation to reopen claims for recovery of overpayments. However, a provision in the American Taxpayer Relief Act of 2012 extends this time frame to five years, after which payments to providers are considered non-recoverable.

Redetermination and Reconsideration

Step 1. Redetermination

After the initial determination and denial, the Redetermination review process is performed by your contractor. Your request must be submitted in written form. Your MAC generally makes a decision within 60 days from the time they receive your request. This decision will be in the form of a letter, *Medicare Summary Notice (MSN)*, or *Remittance Advice (RA)* – also known as an *Explanation of Medicare Benefits (EOMB)*.

File the *Medicare Redetermination Request* form (#CMS-20027) with your Medicare Administrative Contractor (MAC) within 120 days of their initial determination. Be sure to attach all evidence if you check item #14 on the form.

Resource: See Resource 241 for more information.

Troubleshooting by Using the RA/EOMB

One of the most valuable tools available to a practice for the reimbursement process is the *Remittance Advice (RA)/Explanation of Medicare Benefits (EOMB)* or payment report. The effectiveness of the entire billing process can be monitored by carefully reading these forms. If the claims in your practice are consistently being down-coded, bundled, or denied as medically unnecessary or unreasonable, you could be on the road to an audit. Corrective action in the practice can prevent many of these types of denials.

Additionally, contact the patient and ask what reasons were given to him/her for the denial. There are different standards about what information goes to the patient and what goes to the provider. You may find out information that can help you in the appeal process.

Checklist for Submitting a Redetermination

Correspondence should include the items on the following checklist. Keep a checked copy with the *Redetermination Request Form* in the patient record for easy reference.

- A cover letter explaining why the Redetermination is being requested. However, according to *Claims Processing Manual*, "Chapter 29, Section 310.1(B)(2)," you do not need a letter if you use form CMS-20027.
- A copy of the claim and a copy of the *Remittance Advice (RA)*, or *EOMB*, as evidence of prior payment or denial.
- The patient's name and Medicare number.
- The Health Insurance Claim (HIC) or claim control number for the claim in question (circle this number on the remittance number or *EOMB*).
- The date of service for the claim in question.
- The physician provider number (NPI) and that of the organization (if applicable).

Figure 2.5

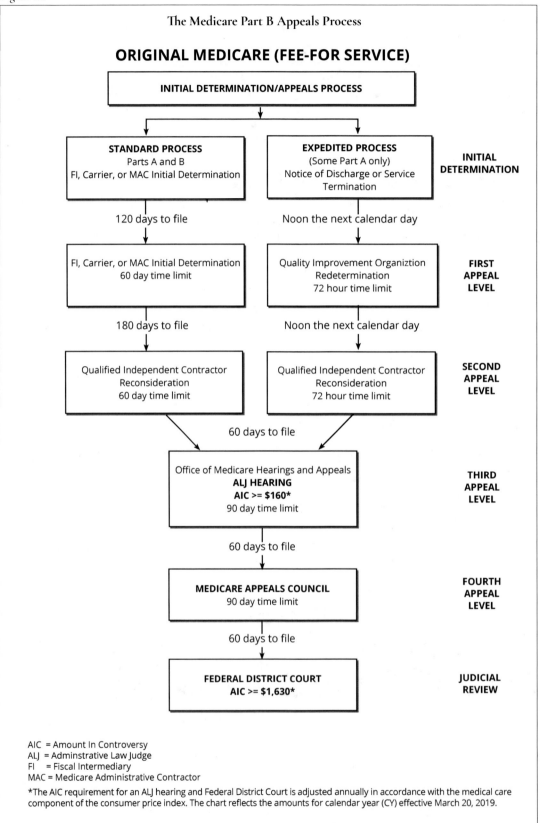

Tip: Frequently, the primary reason for denial is that Medicare does not consider the care to be "medically reasonable or necessary." In this situation, your appeal letter and supporting documents should clearly indicate your rationale for medical necessity.

Supporting Documentation

In addition to the above, include supporting documentation. Highlight information that you want to be considered. The goal is to support your position in reversing the original determination. You will want to enclose the patient's medical history, examination findings, documentation of severity or acute onset, radiology reports, test results, treatment plans, consultation reports, referral requests and reports, and/or copies of communication between provider and patient, as well as the daily notes. The submission of the Electronic Health Record (EHR) can assist in this process if your Medicare Administrative Contractor (MAC) is able to receive it. If you use handwritten notes or use your own style of shorthand or abbreviations, it is appropriate to transcribe and/or translate your notes before submitting them for review. You cannot add information but can interpret the information that is there into a more readable format. Be sure to include copies of the originals along with the transcribed information.

Tip: When making copies of records, if different colored ink is utilized by the provider for documentation and it is necessary for accurate interpretation, you should make color copies.

Book: See Chapter 4 — Documentation for more information on documentation and the EHR.
Resource: See Resource 810 for the latest information.

Signature Requirements

The only acceptable signatures are:
- handwritten (this is defined as a mark or sign by an individual on a document to signify knowledge, approval, acceptance, or obligation),
- electronic,
- digital,
- facsimiles of original written signature, and/or
- digitized.

Do not use "Signature on File" or a stamp signature. If the signatures are not legible, or if you used initials, be sure to include a signature log which could also include an attestation statement. Additionally, if you have not signed your notes, be sure to include an attestation statement. See the *CMS Medicare Program Integrity Manual* "(Pub. 100-08), Chapter 3, Section 3.3.2.4.C" for guidance on attestation statements.

Resource: See Resource 416 for a sample attestation statement and Resource 417 for a signature log.

Step 2. Reconsideration

Reconsiderations are processed by Qualified Independent Contractors (QICs). File the *Medicare Reconsideration Request* form (#CMS-20033) with the QIC within 180 days of your local Medicare Administrative Contractor (MAC)'s Redetermination denial. Use the *Medicare Reconsideration Form* and be sure to review the Checklist for Submitting a Redetermination in Step 1. Evidence submitted should include a clear explanation of why you disagree with the redetermination, a copy of the *Medicare Redetermination Notice (MRN)* and any other useful documentation. This is the last level at which you can submit new evidence to reinforce your case.

Additional documentation submitted at this step could increase the time allotted for the QIC to make a decision. See Resource 242 for more information.

Hearings and Reviews

If there is not satisfaction at levels one and two of your appeals, you can advance through these last three steps. Please note that these reviewers cannot review any new evidence, but only review the evidence which was submitted to the QIC (Level 2). At this level, it may be wise to retain the services of a qualified healthcare attorney to assist with this process.

The number of appeals at the third and fourth levels has been increasing over the years and there is now a backlog of appeals due to insufficient funding.

HHS has developed a three-pronged strategy to address the backlog:

1. Invest in new resources at all levels of appeal to increase adjudication capacity and implement new strategies to alleviate the current backlog.
2. Take administrative actions to reduce the number of pending appeals and encourage resolution of cases earlier in the process.
3. Propose legislative reforms that provide additional funding and new authorities to address the appeals volume.

Resource: See Resource 203 to read more about the backlog and actions being taken by HHS to resolve the problem.

Resource: If you advance to these final levels of appeal, see Resource 243 for additional information.

Clinical Review Judgment

Clinical Review Judgment impacts all physicians, providers, and suppliers who provide services to Medicare beneficiaries and then bill Medicare contractors.

Medicare claim review contractors are required to instruct their clinical review staffs to use clinical review judgment when making complex review determinations about a claim.

According to the Medicare Program Integrity Manual, Clinical Review Judgment involves two steps.

1. "The synthesis of all submitted medical record information (e.g. progress notes, diagnostic findings, medications, nursing notes, etc.) to create a longitudinal clinical picture of the patient; and

2. The application of this clinical picture to the review criteria to determine whether the clinical requirements in the relevant policy have been met."

This is very important to healthcare providers because previously, auditors could demand certain records that had very little to do with the patient's progress. Further, reviewers could choose to ignore submitted records that demonstrated positive outcome. Now, "all submitted medical record information" must be considered in determining if the treatment goals have been met.

Resource: See Resource 454 for more information.

Step 3. Hearing by an Administrative Law Judge (ALJ)

If after Step 2, the disputed amount exceeds the designated amount remaining in controversy (e.g., $180 as of 2021), you may request an ALJ hearing within 60 days of receipt of the reconsideration decision. Please note that this amount changes annually. Use the Request for a Medicare Hearing by an Administrative Law Judge form to submit your request. The ALJ is employed by the Social Security Administration and not CMS/Medicare. Only the documentation from the second level (Reconsideration) and the law is considered. Detailed instructions regarding this step are included in the reconsideration decision letter. See Resource 244 and 245 for more information.

> **Alert:** Effective March 20, 2017, there were significant changes to this step of the appeals process. These changes are intended to streamline this step and reduce the backlog of these cases.
>
> **Resource:** See Resource 250 for more information.

Step 4. Review by the Medicare Appeals Council (MAC)

The Departmental Appeal Board (DAB), also known as the Medicare Appeals Council, provides the final review by the Social Security Administration. The purpose of the DAB review is to correct any errors that might be made by the ALJ in Step 3. Use the Request for Review of Administrative Law Judge (ALJ) Medicare Decision/Dismissal form to submit your request. See Resource 246 for more information.

Step 5. Review by a Federal District Court

This Federal judicial review is the final step in the appeals process. Its mission is to correct any errors by the Social Security Administration's hearing and review. To request a review, follow the instructions in the MAC decision letter from Step 4.

> **Resource:** See Resource 247 to review the official CMS instructions regarding Medicare Appeals.

Medicare "Advantage" Part C Appeals

Medicare Advantage is the beneficiary option for a traditional fee-for-service (FFS) plan. Providers and patients who participate in these entities have the same rights as if they were in the traditional Part B plans. Accordingly, Medicare appeal rights are included in these programs too.

Late Filing Exceptions

As a general rule, providers have one year from the date of service to file a claim. However, it should be noted that there are exceptions to the rule. The *Medicare Claims Processing Manual* (Section 240, Chapter 29) outlines the general procedure for establishing any unusual good cause for late filing.

> **Book:** See Chapter 1.3 — Claims Processing for more information on timely filing.

Notes:

3. Compliance

Chapter Contents

3. Compliance Essentials 123
    About Compliance 123
    The Importance of Having a Compliance Plan 126
    OIG Compliance Programs 127
    Fraud and Abuse 128
    OSHA Compliance 132
    HIPAA Compliance 133
    Other Compliance Concerns 135
    Managing Audits 138

3. Compliance Essentials

About Compliance

A compliance program is a powerful tool for staying abreast of regulations and minimizing your risk of oversight and error, in addition to protecting your practice from implications of insurance abuse or fraud. Developing a compliance program can help every part of your business adhere to best practices, and present opportunities for process improvement which could also lead to increased efficiency, productivity, and profitability. Most importantly, an essential part of your practice's compliance strategy is establishing and maintaining a compliance program which includes regular (at least once per year) refresher training sessions for all healthcare providers and staff. An active, effective, well-documented compliance program can also demonstrate to regulatory agencies or reviewers that there was intent to comply which may, in some cases, mitigate (reduce) penalties assessed. Compliance programs should be a source of **continuous** incremental improvement for your practice.

Continued compliance requires each of the following actions:

1. Pursuing regular education and training to understand which rules and regulations apply to your situation.
2. Creating a documented plan of action regarding these rules. This is the policy and procedure portion of compliance.
3. Reporting your findings to the decision makers and appropriate designated compliance personnel in your practice. If errors are found, corrections need to be made. Policies and procedures should be re-evaluated and updated on a regular basis in order to stay current.

Compliance is about more than just claims and payments. Standards in recordkeeping, business practices, patient privacy, and security also play an important role. The challenge for providers is to not only stay current with correct billing and documentation, but to understand all of the complex legal requirements of practicing medicine.

Note: Some providers are unaware of the reality that a request for records from a payer is a type of compliance audit. When you send your documentation to a payer, it is carefully reviewed (audited), and the results of this review will determine whether or not additional scrutiny and audits will take place.

Alert: Prior to submitting medical records that have been requested by a payer for review, take a moment to verify that the documentation adequately supports the codes submitted and meets the requirements of the payer's policies. **Never** alter documentation previously entered. If additional information is needed or was accidentally left out, follow the proper rules of adding an addendum to the note which includes the pertinent information along with the current date and time. Altering the content of a medical record that has been signed may bring heavy penalties and accusations of fraud.
Book: See "Guidelines for Corrections" in Chapter 4.1 — Documentation Essentials.

Book: See "Managing Audits" on page 137 for more about the role of audits as they relate to compliance.
Resource: See Resource 800 for additional information on compliance, including articles and webinars.

In all fairness, already strained healthcare programs lose billions of dollars due to fraud and abuse. These offenders must be found and held accountable. Many organizations have been found guilty of not adequately protecting their patient's privacy or following other laws. Organizations who are guilty of misappropriating patient information or improper coding and billing practices place increased scrutiny on ethical providers who are trying to follow the laws and provide excellent patient care.

Steeper fines and ever-increasing audits have caused a financial strain on many providers. Some have gone out of business or even declared bankruptcy as a direct result of compliance audits resulting in exorbitant fines and refund demands. It has been said that the best defense is a good offense and this adage holds true when it comes to compliance. Be proactive in identifying and resolving potential compliance shortcomings instead of waiting to see what happens when an outside party finds a problem.

The weakest defense against expanding regulations and inspections is to resist, deny, postpone learning about them, and hope that nothing happens. The strongest defense is to create a proactive, comprehensive compliance system, as described in this chapter.

Compliance Is Inescapable

There is no "one size fits all" compliance program. Learn the components of compliance and implement a program that best suits your practice. Having a compliance program that is ill defined, not applicable to the practice, or not followed may result in worse consequences than not having one in place at all.

This new climate of compliance inspection, in which agencies pay more attention to your documented procedures than to your claims, changes the game. This process can be highly invasive, but it can also be advantageous.

> **Warning:** Healthcare providers should be aware that some practice management companies teach tactics that could be considered fraudulent. Before implementing a new policy, verify that it doesn't violate any rules. Consider consulting a qualified healthcare attorney or a certified compliance specialist to review and qualify the plan/policy before implementing it.
>
> For example, do not "tweak" your documentation in order to justify billing bundled services separately. Healthcare providers should be sure that their documentation supports and justifies the services rendered.

Who Demands Compliance?

Compliance is a requirement for:

- **Government Payers:** Government agencies have significant funding for data analysis, education outreach, and policy research. Be sure to apply the appropriate policies and compliance program requirements to the applicable government program to reduce denials and possible negative audit findings. Many private payers copy the actions of CMS and the OIG, although they often do not provide as many safeguards for providers. With the federal government focusing on inspecting offices for compliance, it is likely that non-government insurance companies will do the same.

- **ERISA:** It may be good to consider compliance as it relates to both ERISA and non-ERISA actions. ERISA cases follow federal laws while non-ERISA cases are adjudicated on the state level. Be prepared for any differences this may cause when you set up your compliance program. Common denials that should be investigated for ERISA plans include timely filing deadlines and the application of third-party administrator (TPA) internal policies instead of the ERISA home plan policies. See Resource 804 for additional information about ERISA.

- **Commercial Plans:** It has become common for commercial payers to incorporate compliance policies in their provider contracts. Be sure to review any compliance policies, including specific items such as timely filing deadlines for a clean claim, appeal deadlines, EDI submission errors, and coverage policies. As payers often will update policies online and expect providers to adhere to them, their online changes and notifications should be regularly reviewed. Signing up for their newsletters is one good way of knowing if there have been changes made.

- **State Departments of Labor and Industries:** Healthcare providers may also have to defend their practice against the Department of Labor (DOL) and Industries if they provide services in workers compensation cases. Workers compensation laws are governed by each individual state and thus vary from state to state.

- **States:** In addition to DOL requirements, some states also have other compliance program requirements. They may have different privacy rules, identify certain providers who can or cannot provide specific types of service, or include laws surrounding how telemedicine services are provided. These variations from federal rules must be part of your Compliance Program. State support for compliance programs can be extremely beneficial when the state has passed laws on the lookback period for payers. While federal programs (e.g., Medicare, Medicaid) may audit several years of data, commercial payers must adhere to the state laws for how far back they can review claims data. For example, Arizona law permits only a one-year lookback period. See Resource 31A for more information on lookback periods.

- **U.S. Department of Justice:** The U.S. Department of Justice, headed by the Attorney General, is responsible for federal law enforcement. As such, federal crimes, such as false claims, are often prosecuted by this department. Many of these cases are forwarded by investigators (and whistleblowers) to the HHS Office of the Inspector General (OIG). From there, the cases may be forwarded to the Justice Department. See Resource 265 for more about this federal department

Tip: Watch out for payer compliance programs which may waive your appeal rights. For example, Medicare started a pilot program called PSAVE back in 2018 which did just that. Although the PSAVE program is no longer active (See Resource 314 for more information about that program) self-audits continue to be encouraged.

Who is Being Targeted?

Any provider type may be targeted for a compliance audit, from the rural sole proprietor to the very large corporation. Federal, state, and commercial payers have been busy creating and implementing a myriad of tools to help them identify providers with questionable billing practices. Additionally, the loss of a computer or flash drive initiates a HIPAA breach investigation which can also lead to an investigation of a healthcare provider's billing practices.

A common tool being used by payers to examine billing practices is "data mining," which is the process by which submitted claims are aggregated and statistically analyzed in order to identify potential areas of fraud or abuse. Payers are using analytic software programs to find ways to increase revenues, cut costs, identify provider outliers who may be over or under reporting services, and discover potentially fraudulent, abusive, or wasteful billing activities. If your billing patterns fall outside their established statistical pattern for similar healthcare providers of your specialty in your geographic area, you may be flagged for an audit. Proper documentation should support the medical necessity for cases that do not conform to typical patterns.

Small healthcare practices tend to be targeted for the following reasons:

- Limited resources for keeping up to date on policies and procedures as well as changes in laws and regulations. Small practices sometimes employ only a few people (e.g., the doctor and a receptionist or assistant). Every activity that is not related to patient care is time spent away from earning, and patient care often becomes a priority over paperwork. It can be difficult to keep up with ever-changing legislation. OIG audit reports show that the vast majority of providers have not kept current with compliance requirements.

- Skewed statistical analysis results. Statistical analysis of all submitted claims includes data from large organizations. Often large medical practices have different billing patterns than smaller practices. Due to the larger number of claims submitted by large groups, the billing trends and data analysis are skewed towards their billing patterns. If only claims from small or solo practices were analyzed, then the trend would likely be very different. As such, it may *appear* that a provider is not within statistical norms when in reality, they would be considered normal if only small providers were included in the data analysis.

- Specialty-oriented, solo practitioners limiting the number of codes reported. Commonly, the vast majority of their claims only utilize a handful of diagnosis and procedure codes, which can make the provider look like they are reporting more of those codes than other providers in multi-specialty or solo practices of another specialty.

Note: Individuals may be held accountable for corporate wrongdoing. The Yates Memo issued in 2015 has enabled prosecutors to pursue criminal charges against an individual. Not only is the business fined, but individuals have also experienced prosecution for their role in the situation.

Resource: See Resource 379 to be linked to an article with more information about the impact of the Yates Memo.

The Importance of Having a Compliance Plan

A compliance plan allows a practice to maintain consistency in the delivery of healthcare services and provides a written outline of the appropriate actions for a practice. It also assures continuity of actions by employees during staff turnover. In the circumstance of an audit with subsequent fines, a viable compliance plan may be used as a mitigating factor to avert or decrease fines and jail time. To realize the importance of having a viable compliance plan, consider the following averages of recoupment from an audit. Over the last several years, the government recovered over $8.00 for every dollar spent on fraud and abuse investigations. With such a substantial return on their investment, they are serious about these programs and providers should be too.

Although compliance plans overseen by certified compliance officers have been implemented in hospitals, medical clinics, nursing homes, and other health facilities, it has been largely ignored by small provider offices. Certified compliance officers can effectively implement a compliance plan that will meet the OIG guidelines.

When considering hiring a compliance officer or consultant, keep in mind that many know general compliance topics while others may be more well versed in your particular specialty. It is imperative that you hire a certified compliance specialist who knows the operation, documentation, and coding requirements for your specialty. The compliance officer will aid in identifying and rectifying problems prior to an external audit as well as implementing a plan of action for handling any other compliance issues.

Alert — Compliance Diminishes Fines: Industry consultants have confirmed with top officials that even an appearance of active, ongoing efforts towards maintaining a compliance program can demonstrate intent and can be successful in reducing penalties. In the words of one consultant, "Virtually every federal agency and the federal sentencing guidelines consider the existence of an effective compliance program as a mitigating factor in the imposition of fines and civil monetary penalties."

Benefits of a Compliance Program

An active compliance program is essential for healthcare practices of all sizes and does not have to be costly or resource-intensive. With the development of a formal program, a healthcare practice may find it easier to comply with its affirmative duty to ensure they are following the law and the accuracy of claims submitted to payers for reimbursement. Numerous benefits can be gained by implementing an effective compliance program. These benefits may include:

- Development of effective internal procedures to ensure compliance with regulations, payment policies, and coding rules
- Improved medical record documentation
- Improved education for practice employees

- Lowering the probability of the occurrence of a HIPAA breach
- A reduction in the number of claim denials
- More streamlined practice operations through better communication and more comprehensive policies
- Avoidance of potential liability arising from noncompliance
- Reduced exposure to audits, investigations, and penalties
- Improved patient care resulting from an increased focus on safety, security, and quality

The OIG will consider the existence of an active, effective compliance program that predates any governmental investigation when addressing the appropriateness of administrative sanctions; however, the burden is on the practice to demonstrate the operational effectiveness of their compliance program. It is widely held that if you hope for leniency during an audit or investigation, then you must follow these guidelines as closely as possible. Importantly, penalties may potentially be reduced if the organization can demonstrate their good faith efforts by implementing and adhering to compliance related guidelines on an ongoing basis.

Alert: A formal compliance program that is not enforced in your practice may create greater liability. Do not purchase a compliance product and then allow it to collect dust on the bookshelf and then hope it will save you during a compliance audit.

Tip — Marketing Warning: Be careful that advertisements and social media posts do not violate any compliance rules (e.g., waiving deductibles). Always state your usual fee on the ad. Also, be sure that the advertisement does not violate any state laws about deceptive and misleading advertising.

Summary

A successful compliance program must consider a variety of regulations which include HIPAA, OIG, OSHA, and other risk management and operational safety measures that must be evaluated regularly by practices in order to properly plan, train, and maintain that program. Every practice, including small offices, should be concerned about compliance.

Implementing a compliance program is preventive. An effective compliance program also sends an important message to a practice's employees that while the practice recognizes that mistakes can occur, employees have an affirmative, ethical duty to come forward and report fraudulent or erroneous conduct so it may be corrected.

OIG Compliance Programs

The Office of Inspector General (OIG) is the enforcement division of the Department of Health and Human Services (HHS) and their mission is to fight waste, fraud, and abuse in Medicare, Medicaid, and more than 300 other HHS programs. They do this through a nationwide network of audits, investigations, and evaluations which result in cost-saving or policy recommendations for decision-makers and the public. That network also assists in the development of cases for criminal, civil, and administrative enforcement.

Each year, the OIG conducts statistical analysis on claims received. They report on their findings and develop an official Work Plan which is the basis for RAC and many MAC reviews. In addition to the Work Plan, they also monitor the Affordable Care Act's "Ethics and Compliance Program."

Another responsibility of the OIG is the creation of compliance program guidance in an effort to involve healthcare providers in preventing the submission of erroneous claims and combating fraud. Be aware that as of June 2017, the OIG updates their Work Plans as often as monthly on their website.

OIG Compliance Program Guidance

In 2000, the OIG published guidance on a voluntary compliance program for individuals and small group physician practices. The Patient Protection and Affordable Care Act of 2010 (PPACA) mandated that a compliance program become compulsory as of a future date to be determined by the Secretary of HHS. As of the date of this publication, final compliance program guidelines have **not** been released **for healthcare providers**. The information included in this segment is from the Final Compliance Program Guidelines currently in place for other Medicare programs. It is highly likely that any final compliance guidelines for providers will closely mirror these guidelines.

Once the final compliance dates and details have been set, this program will be **required** for all providers who bill federal healthcare programs (e.g., Medicare, Medicaid, etc.) If you do not participate in federal healthcare programs, this plan is not required. However, every office should carefully review the components of the OIG compliance program guidance and voluntarily implement steps to further ensure the safety and protection of their patients. It is likely that other payers will eventually require a formal compliance program in the future.

Creating an OIG compliance program is similar to creating a HIPAA compliance plan in that organizations need to appoint a compliance officer and create a working notebook or manual which contains the currently recommended components. Highly sensitive information, such as contracts, should be kept in a separate, secure place and only be referenced in the Compliance Manual.

Tip: Many offices find it easier to engage a professional compliance auditor to visit the practice, investigate and document the workflow, look for weak spots and suggest remediations, and to create the ongoing processes by which the office can continue with the compliance program thereafter.

Fraud and Abuse

Fraud and abuse is considered to be a huge and costly problem for Medicare, Medicaid, and other government and private health care programs. For example, in 2020, 8.4% of the billions the federal government paid for healthcare Part B reimbursements were for fraudulent bills or non-compliant billing practices. Error rates are published annually in the CERT Annual Improper Payment Reports.

Resource: See Resource 420 to review the most current report.

According to CMS, the primary difference between fraud and abuse is intention. They are defined as follows:

"Fraud: When someone intentionally executes or attempts to execute a scheme to obtain money or property of any healthcare benefit program."

"Abuse: When healthcare providers or suppliers perform actions that directly or indirectly result in unnecessary costs to any healthcare benefit program."

What used to be referred to as abuse is now categorized as fraud because even if a provider did not know a certain practice was improper, they "should have known." The responsibility is now placed on providers to understand and follow all laws that affect their practice.

Be aware though, that during an investigation, it can be extremely difficult or even impossible to determine whether an incident is fraud or abuse because the presence or absence of knowledge is subjective. For this reason, it is critical for practices to implement appropriate policies, procedures, training, and other checks and balances to best minimize the risk of an investigation.

Erroneous or Fraudulent?

According to the OIG, there is a distinction between mistakes and intentional deception or fraud. Their Program Integrity Reviews have identified various causes of improper payments ranging from innocent errors to intentional deception. The following list shows these different levels of improper payments as they increase in severity. Level 1 problems can often be resolved through the payer's "corrected claim" process. However, higher levels can have penalties associated with them.

1. Mistakes/errors
2. Inefficiency/waste
3. Bending the rules/abuse
4. Intentional deception/fraud

Monitoring

The government has an ongoing program to monitor settlement agreements with providers who have had previous compliance problems. It is important to note that:

- Under the False Claims Act,
  - A whistleblower ("relator") can be rewarded up to 25%-30% of the recovered fraudulent amount.
  - The government does not need to prove that the provider intended to commit fraud. They only need to have reasonable suspicion.
  - The definition of "knowingly" means: 1) actual knowledge; 2) reckless disregard for the truth; or 3) deliberate ignorance.
  - More than 60% of the whistleblower cases involve healthcare fraud.

- The OIG encourages beneficiaries to be involved in the identification of fraudulent activities, which results in their hotline receiving a very high volume of calls. Hotline information is included in the OIG's semi-annual report to Congress.

- Millions are allocated annually to both the FBI and the Health Care Fraud and Abuse Programs for healthcare investigations. Consequently, special units are well funded for aggressive investigations.

Tip: Medicare does not and will not negotiate settlement amounts. However, according to one healthcare attorney, some Medicaid auditors have been more willing to work out a settlement agreement, but that varies by state.

Important Fraud and Abuse Laws

The following federal fraud and abuse laws are very important to healthcare providers: the False Claims Act (FCA), the Anti-Kickback Statute (AKS), the Physician Self-Referral Law (Stark law), the Eliminating Kickbacks in Recovery Act (EKRA), the Exclusion Authorities, the Civil Monetary Penalties Law (CMPL), and the Health Care Fraud statute.

Understanding these laws can help your organization avoid potential problems.

1. *False Claims Act [31 U.S.C. §§ 3729–3733]* It is illegal to submit claims for payment to Medicare or Medicaid that you know or should know are false or fraudulent. No INTENT to defraud is required, reckless disregard or "deliberate ignorance" are also considered fraudulent.

   Penalty: Fines up to three times the programs' loss plus a specified amount per claim filed. The specified amount is adjusted annually for inflation. For 2021, this was $11,803 to $23,607 per claim filed. Additionally, criminal charges and prison time are a possibility.

Tip: If the provider does not repay an overpayment within 60 days from the date that the incident was confirmed as being owed, they may be liable under the False Claims Act. Note that the 60 day clock begins after confirmation, NOT when it is suspected but not investigated.

Book: See "Handling Overpayments" in Chapter 1.4 — Claims Management for more information.

2. *Anti-Kickback Statute [42 U.S.C. § 1320a-7b(b)]* Federal healthcare programs specifically prohibit any type of "remuneration" for patient referrals. You cannot receive any type of gift or anything of nominal value for referring a patient to another provider. It is illegal. As of December 2016, nominal value is defined as "having a retail value of no more than $15 per item or $75 in the aggregate per patient on an annual basis." However, it should be noted that in December 2020, the OIG made some changes to safe harbors wherein that amount increases to $500, but only in certain situations (e.g., value based arrangements). See Resource 32A for more information.

   The Affordable Care Act changed the burden of proof standard. Now, providers can be held liable **without** specific knowledge of or specific intent to violate the law.

   Under this law, routinely waiving the patient co-pay, coinsurance and/or deductible is illegal.

   Book: See the "Discounts" segment in Chapter 1.5 — Establishing Fees for more about compliantly discounting fee schedules.

   Penalty: Criminal and administrative penalties apply to both parties. The Bipartisan Budget Act of 2018 significantly increased fines and penalties. Fines are up to $100,000 per kickback plus three times the amount of the actual kickback value. Jail time of up to 10 years and exclusion from participation in federal healthcare programs can also be applied.

   Kickbacks are also pursued under the "False Claims Act" which carries a heftier penalty.

3. *Physician Self-Referral Law [42 U.S.C. § 1395nn]* Known as the Stark law, this law prohibits providers from referring patients for "designated health services" payable by Medicare or Medicaid to a business where the provider or an immediate family member has a financial relationship. Specific intent to violate the law is not required.

   Penalty: Fines and exclusion from participation in federal healthcare programs.

   The simplest way to avoid violation of the Stark Law, or a state's version, called a mini-Stark Law, is to always pay attention when referring patients to other practitioners or service providers.

   Be especially cautious when referring to:
   - Clinical laboratory services
   - Physical therapy services
   - Mobile diagnostic units
   - Occupational therapy services
   - Radiology services, including magnetic resonance imaging (MRI)
   - Computerized axial tomography scans and ultrasound services
   - Radiation therapy services
   - Durable medical equipment
   - Parenteral and enteral nutrients, equipment, and supplies
   - Prosthetics, orthotics, and prosthetic devices
   - Home health services
   - Outpatient prescription drugs
   - Inpatient and outpatient hospital services

Some of these situations may not apply to your specialty, but it is wise to be aware of where potential Stark Law violations often occur. In order to maintain a safe harbor, some organizations have advised their doctors never to refer to just one entity, but to the three closest entities. Also, working within a bona fide "physician group" can help you avoid possible violations of this law. Know the laws in your state before making referrals, and consult your attorney before entering into any practice agreements.

It is important to document your financial relationships with referring physicians in your Compliance Manual. Be careful about productivity bonuses and gifts as they could fall under Stark laws too. Avoid things that sound too good to be true because it could likely get you in trouble with this law.

Resource: See Resource 328 for more information.

Resource: See Resource 32A for more information on the changes to Stark Law and the Anti-Kickback Statute aimed at better enabling coordination of care.

4. *Eliminating Kickbacks in Recovery Act (EKRA) [18 U.S.C. 220]* EKRA is an anti-kickback statute signed into law in October 2018 which applies to services covered by a "healthcare benefit program." This law includes federal programs like Medicare as well as private payers. It specifically addresses patient brokering and due to the broad nature of the definition of laboratory, it thus is applicable to all healthcare providers who request any laboratory testing. There are seven 'exceptions' which are similar to the Anti-Kickback Statue, but there are some differences:

- EKRA applies to both employees and independent contractors.
- EKRA only protects payments made by an employer to an employee or independent contractor if the payment is NOT determined by or DOES NOT vary by certain factors (e.g., number of tests performed).

Penalty: For each violation, there may be up to a $200,000 fine, 10 years of imprisonment, or both.

5. *Exclusion Statute [42 U.S.C. § 1320a-7]* Individuals who are specifically excluded from participation in federal healthcare programs because of a felony charge, patient abuse, and/or neglect, cannot participate in any federal (e.g., Medicare, TRICARE) or state (e.g., Medicaid) healthcare program — either directly or indirectly (through an employer or group practice). Exclusions extend beyond those providing direct patient care services. It can include those in executive positions (e.g., director, office manager) as well as volunteer or administrative positions (e.g., accounting, information technology services).

Penalty: Organizations who employ an individual listed in an Exclusions Database can be assessed Civil Monetary Penalties (CMP) of up to $10,000 for each item or service provided by the excluded individual and an assessment of up to three times the amount claimed for such items or services. Additional fines may also be pursued (e.g., $10,000 per day for each day an excluded party retains ownership or control). It could also trigger False Claims Act penalties. Criminal penalties may also be pursued.

Alert: Healthcare providers are required to verify that none of their employees, contractors, and vendors are on *any* exclusion database. This verification must take place every 30 days! At the time of publication, there were over 40 exclusion databases that need to be checked.

Document your searches and if you discover that you have unknowingly employed or worked with an excluded individual, you must notify the OIG. It would be wise to contact a healthcare attorney prior to notifying the OIG.

Resource: See Resource 268 for more information.

6. **Civil Monetary Penalties (CMP) Law [42 U.S.C. § 1320a-7a]** This law, enforced by the OIG, applies to a broad range of activities such as violating Medicare assignment provisions or the Medicare physician agreement.

    Penalty: Penalties can be adjusted annually. For 2018, the CMP ranged from $20,000 to $100,000 **per violation** plus damages up to three times the amount of the improper claim. Depending on the type and number of violations, penalties have been reported that are well over a million dollars.

    Resource: See Resource 269 to read more about this law.

7. **Health Care Fraud Statute [18 U.S.C. § 1347]** This federal law is part of HIPAA. The following is the official definition:

    > **TITLE 18 - CRIMES AND CRIMINAL PROCEDURE**
    > **PART I - CRIMES**
    > **CHAPTER 63 - MAIL FRAUD**
    > **§ 1347. Health care fraud**
    > Whoever knowingly and willfully executes, or attempts to execute, a scheme or artifice—
    > (1) to defraud any health care benefit program; or
    > (2) to obtain, by means of false or fraudulent pretenses, representations, or promises, any of the money or property owned by, or under the custody or control of, any health care benefit program, in connection with the delivery of or payment for health care benefits, items, or services, shall be fined under this title or imprisoned not more than 10 years, or both. If the violation results in serious bodily injury (as defined in section 1365 of this title), such person shall be fined under this title or imprisoned not more than 20 years, or both; and if the violation results in death, such person shall be fined under this title, or imprisoned for any term of years or for life, or both.

    Penalty: Up to 10 years in prison for just one count of fraud, 20 years if a patient is injured, and life in prison if the patient dies as a result of the fraud committed.

OSHA Compliance

The Occupational Safety and Health Administration (OSHA) was created to assure safe and healthful working conditions for working men and women by setting and enforcing standards and by providing training, outreach, education, and assistance.

While generally associated with industrial facilities or construction sites, OSHA rules apply in healthcare practices as well. If you have one employee, then you must have an OSHA plan in place. Some have tried to skirt the law by saying that independent contractors are not employees. As far as OSHA is concerned, if they work in your office, they are considered an employee, no matter what title they are given.

Like HIPAA rules, OSHA federal requirements are the minimum standard. At the time of publication, there were 26 states (and 2 territories) which have their own OSHA plans which may be different than federal rules. Be aware of your individual state requirements.

As with all other compliance related investigation and enforcement organizations, OSHA has also increased the ease for workforce members to file complaints. Every OSHA complaint filed is required to be investigated. Quite often, an OSHA inspection begins with a complaint from either an employee or a patient. Your office will then be given an on-site visit. To help you avoid being blindsided by these on-site visits, it is important to understand these requirements.

Tip: Be sure that employees are properly trained in all areas of OSHA compliance, as well as the reporting procedures for injuries and other safety related occurrences. Make sure all training is thoroughly documented in your Compliance Manual.

Fines and penalties for OSHA violations are adjusted for inflation. As of 2021, they ranged from $13,653 to $136,532 per violation, depending on several factors, including the severity of the incident, the type and size of the business entity and the provider's willingness to comply with the law. Penalties for small offices with up to 25 employees may be reduced. Providers who have not had any previous violations and who can demonstrate a good faith effort may be able to significantly reduce those fines. For this reason, it is wise to implement an OSHA Compliance Program in your office in order to demonstrate a "good faith" effort.

Resource: See Resource 812 for more information about OSHA including tips, a quick start guide, forms, and other resources.

Resource: See Resource 270 for the list of states with their own OSHA requirements.

HIPAA Compliance

The legislation known as "HIPAA" stands for the Health Insurance Portability and Accountability Act of 1996. The intent of the Administrative Simplification, or Accountability portion, of this law was to establish standards and requirements to improve the efficiency and effectiveness of the healthcare industry and safeguard health information. Legislation enacted over the last few years has expanded and, in some cases, changed the responsibilities of providers. Even though no major legislative changes have occurred recently, official guidance has been periodically issued on various topics such as texting and how much you can charge a patient for their medical records.

HIPAA is too comprehensive a subject to be covered in this publication and it directly impacts almost all healthcare providers as well as their business associates. innoviHealth recommends that providers carefully review HIPAA guidelines to ensure compliance. It is prudent to seek the counsel of a qualified healthcare law attorney licensed in your state for additional guidance.

Another important thing to keep in mind is that HIPAA is only the federal minimum standard when it comes to privacy and security. Healthcare practices must also abide by any state regulations applicable to healthcare providers and all healthcare matters, including confidentiality of patient information. It is good business practice to always maintain policies and procedures aimed at protecting patient information.

Alert: HIPAA Compliance plans need to be regularly revised and reviewed. If you have not performed a Risk Analysis, be sure to complete one this year.

Resource: See Resource 24A for more information about a free Security Risk Assessment (SRA) Tool from HealthIT.gov which helps providers conduct an annual SRA. There are other more robust SRA products available in the market which offer additional features beyond the free tool offered by the government.

Resource: See Resource 814 for more resources including links, articles, and webinars.

Store: See the *Complete & Easy HIPAA Compliance* publication (Resource 116) for a more comprehensive review of HIPAA. It is a do-it-yourself guide which includes customizable policies, compliance plans, and required forms.

Tip: All providers need to be concerned about protecting patient information. Most states have laws regarding privacy of medical records which may be different than the federally mandated HIPAA standards. It is important to be aware of individual state requirements.

HIPAA Components

There are five HIPAA components for covered entities: Electronic Transactions, Privacy, Security, Identifiers, and Enforcement. Each has its own rules. If you are a "covered entity," you are held accountable and must comply with all laws, standards, rules, and regulations related to HIPAA. If you have state laws which exceed these HIPAA standards, they prevail (override). The following is an overview of the requirements for each of the **five** basic HIPAA areas:

1. **Electronic Transaction and Code Set Standards Requirements**

    The Transaction and Code Set rules provide national standards for the electronic exchange of health care information including formats and data content. HIPAA requires every provider who does business electronically to use the same health care transactions and code sets. It is important for you to know about these requirements and how they impact your office. Transaction and code set requirements were created to give the healthcare industry a common language to make it easier to transmit information electronically (e.g., a physician's office inquires about a patient's insurance eligibility, or submits a bill to a health plan for payment).

2. **Privacy Requirements**

    The privacy requirements limit how patient Protected Health Information (PHI) may be used and/or disclosed. Patients are provided with basic rights related to the use and disclosure of information related to their past, present and future health. Confidential data must be securely guarded and carefully handled when conducting the business of health care.

    It is critical for practices to have a solid understanding of HIPAA privacy requirements and patient rights in order to avoid costly mistakes. Proper staff training is essential to maintain compliance.

3. **Security Requirements**

    The security requirements outline the minimum administrative, technical, and physical systems required to protect the availability, integrity, and confidentiality of Electronic Protected Health Information (EPHI). Security procedures must be put in place to prevent unauthorized access to ePHI. The requirements include both required and addressable activities that must take place.

    Alert — Mobile Devices & Breaches: Mobile devices such as cell phones, tablets, and laptops have been linked to a significant number of HIPAA breaches. The problem is so widespread that the OIG has included this on their Work Plan and the Department of Health and Human Services (HHS) has created a special resource page for all healthcare professionals which includes web training. Be sure to document all training in your Compliance Manual.
    Resource: See Resource 280 for additional information and training by HHS.

    Note: The presence of ransomware or malware) is considered a security incident under HIPAA that may **also** result in an impermissible disclosure of PHI (a Privacy Rule violation) and possibly also a breach, depending on the circumstances of the attack. See Resource 32C for more information about protecting your practice against ransomware.

4. **HITECH Enforcement Rule**

    The enforcement rule contains the regulations governing the investigation of probable violations and their associated penalties. The HITECH Act of 2009 expanded this rule by making penalties for violations more strict, creating tiered violation levels, and splitting the responsibility of HIPAA enforcement between the Department of Health and Human Services (HHS) and the Federal Trade Commission (FTC).

5. **National Identifier Requirements**

    HIPAA requires all healthcare providers, health plans, and employers to have a national number that will identify them on standard transactions. Providers are required to use the their National Provider Identifier (NPI) which is a unique 10-digit number that is required on electronic transactions.

Alert — Overseas Billing Caution: Many companies have outsourced their billing overseas in order to cut costs. Keep in mind that there could be some costly side effects. As an example, a provider had PHI stolen by someone employed by an overseas billing company. The provider, who had a properly executed *Business Associate Agreement*, is suing the billing company, but there is a significant problem—the backlog of lawsuits in that country can take up to 24 years. Fines imposed by the U.S. Government are payable immediately. Most businesses would find it difficult to wait 24 years to recoup their money.

Note: At the time of publication, CMS was considering revisions to simplify some of the HIPAA requirements. We will publish information in our newsletter when it becomes available. Go to FindACode.com/newsletter to sign up for our newsletter.

Other Compliance Concerns

This chapter is not all-inclusive when it comes to possible compliance pitfalls. This segment includes a few more things to pay attention to; however, it is not a comprehensive list. If you have any questions or concerns, we recommend contacting a healthcare attorney to ensure that you are following the rules.

Discrimination

There are several different types of discrimination that all healthcare organizations need to be concerned about. The following are federal regulations. Be aware of state-specific rules that may also apply. Section 1557 of the Patient Protection and Affordable Care Act (PPACA, also known as the ACA) includes a nondiscrimination provision. The law expands previous federal civil rights laws which prohibit discrimination on the basis of race, color, national origin, sex (including sexual orientation and gender identity), age, or disability. These protections extend to individuals who participate in health programs or activities HHS provides or funds, including health plans offered in Health Insurance Marketplaces.

Note — Notice Requirement: Healthcare providers are required to post nondiscrimination notices in "conspicuous physical locations where the entity interacts with the public." These notices alert individuals of their compliance with federal law. They must also be posted on the company website, if one exists.
Resource: See Resource 375 to download required notices directly from HHS.

Language Discrimination

Prior to the ACA, language interpreters were only required to be "competent." The new rules require healthcare providers to offer "qualified interpreters" to patients and their caregivers with limited English proficiency (including those who are deaf or hard of hearing) patients and their caregivers. They must interpret both oral and written information. The interpreter does not need to be on-site to provide these services (i.e., remote interpretation is permitted); however, they must meet all of the following requirements:

- Adhere to generally accepted interpreter ethics principles, including client confidentiality
- Has demonstrated proficiency in speaking and understanding both spoken English and at least one other spoken language
- Is able to interpret effectively, accurately, and impartially, both receptively and expressly, to and from such language(s) and English, using any necessary specialized vocabulary and phraseology
- Is NOT a minor child, adult family member, or friend of the patient unless the situation is "an emergency involving an imminent threat to the safety or welfare of an individual or the public where no qualified interpreter is immediately available"

- Is an adult family member or friend specifically requested by the patient to act as their interpreter; however, it is still recommended that another interpreter also be used to legally protect the healthcare provider/organization

- Has formal training as a medical interpreter and has demonstrated that they are a qualified medical interpreter — it's not enough just to have the training.

Alert: It is illegal for providers to "coerce individuals to decline language assistance services."

Your Compliance Plan needs to include a written "language access plan" which is appropriate to your location. The law states that this plan will "vary depending on the entity's particular health programs and activities, its size, its geographic location, and other factors." For example, if you are a small provider and there is no Vietnamese population in your area, then there is not a legal need to provide a Vietnamese interpreter.

Code of Conduct

As part of a preventive compliance program, one way to encourage ethical actions of employees is through the use of a *Code of Conduct* form. Code of Conduct standards should be included in your organization's Policies and Procedures Manual to identify your expectations and guiding principles for appropriate workplace behaviors. One of the first compliance tasks for a new employee is to review the Code of Conduct policy and sign the *Code of Conduct* form acknowledging that they understand your organization's standard of compliance and will make every attempt to act accordingly. All employees need to have a signed form in their personnel file. If you have any employees who have not already signed this form, now would be a good time to update their files.

Harassment

Be sure that your *Code of Conduct* form and Policy includes comprehensive information on harassment. Even though there are federal anti-harassment laws, every state has rules which need to be incorporated into your policy. Be sure your policy addresses the following questions:

- What are the parameters regarding violations for sexual misconduct by a doctor of a patient, within the office between staff members, and between other staff in the office and a patient?

- What risk management steps are you taking to prevent this in your practice? For example, do you have mandatory training?

Resource: See Resource 327 to download a sample *Code of Conduct* form.

Privacy

Many providers mistakenly think that if they follow HIPAA's Privacy Rule that they are "covered" when it comes to privacy compliance. In addition to HIPAA, there are also federal and state privacy laws that require healthcare providers to obtain a patient's written consent before disclosing health information to other people and organizations, even for treatment. This publication only includes some general information about privacy regulations. Healthcare organizations need to obtain training about all applicable laws.

Privacy laws often protect regulations related to health conditions or situations considered "sensitive" by most people (e.g., criminal background). Federal laws related to sensitive health information include:

- Mental Health and Substance Use Disorders: Mental Health Parity and Addiction Equity Act (42 CFR Part 2)

- Student Health Records: Family Educational Rights and Privacy Act (FERPA) and HIPAA

- Family Planning: Title 42 – Public Health – 42 CFR 59.11

Resource: See Resource 336 to access the Legal Action Center's website which includes publications, webinars, videos, training materials, and sample forms regarding the rights of individuals with "sensitive" information.

Because privacy laws vary between states, we recommend contacting your state professional association or a qualified healthcare attorney to ensure that you are meeting applicable state privacy regulations.

Alert: There have been lawsuits where an individual claimed their privacy was violated when a healthcare provider asked about a history of either substance abuse or HIV status. Healthcare providers DO have the right to **ask** about these conditions because it can impact the treatment of the patient. It is NOT a violation of their privacy to ask these questions. Do **NOT** settle out of court in frivolous cases such as these. Contact your state professional association or a qualified healthcare attorney for assistance.

Music Copyright Violations

It is illegal to use a personal music account like Spotify or Pandora in a place of business (e.g., medical office). If you look at the agreement you signed, it specifically states that you may listen to the music for personal, not business use. A place of business could be considered a "public performance" and thus a violation of law. Even though this particular violation sounds like a small infringement, if you have an on-site audit, this is one area that they can find fault. Lately, the music business has begun to crack down on this customer agreement violation which carries penalties that can exceed $60,000.

Cannabis Products

There are some states with medical marijuana laws which allow healthcare providers to prescribe cannabis products; however, according to federal law, cannabis is classified as a Schedule I substance under the Controlled Substances Act, making it illegal at the federal level. Under federal law, as of January 2018, according to a Marijuana Enforcement Memorandum, federal prosecutors are instructed to "weigh all relevant considerations, including federal law enforcement priorities set by the Attorney General, the seriousness of the crime, the deterrent effect of criminal prosecution, and the cumulative impact of particular crimes on the community."

Be sure you understand your state-specific requirements and ensure that you are following them carefully. For example, be sure you know what percentage of THC your state allows in order for a product to be considered "THC free." Some providers have discovered that even when a product was labeled THC free, the percentage of THC in a particular product violated their state laws.

Contracts

There are quite a few things that need to be considered when it comes to contracts — too many to be included in this publication. A good healthcare attorney can help ensure that your contracts are proper. The following are a few things to watch out for:

- Third-party billing contract: Be sure you have a written contract which meets HIPAA provisions. An oral contract is not sufficient. Also, do not include "percentage-based" fees if not allowed by either the state of the billing company or the location of the practice.

Note: Some states and Medicaid programs require healthcare billing companies to be registered. If this applies to you, make sure the billing company is properly registered.

- Provider contract: Be sure there is NOT any provision which might violate self-referral laws (e.g., reward/bonus for bringing in additional clients).

Managing Audits

It used to be that when you submitted a claim it was simply processed and either paid or denied; however, it is no longer that straightforward. Data analytic software has greatly increased the odds of postpayment audits and overpayment refund demands. Providers who repeatedly fail to pass a payer-initiated audit may be required to comply with a prepayment review process in order to continue as a contracted provider that payer (see "Prepayment Review" on page 163). It should be noted that the Department of Health and Human Services (HHS) recovers billions annually through their fraud prevention and enforcement efforts. Since 2012, the federal government, state officials, several leading private health insurance organizations, and other healthcare anti-fraud groups have been working together and sharing data in order to prevent fraud. The need for provider compliance has never been greater.

Resource: See Resource 31A for vital information about how far back (look-back period) a payer may review claims on postpayment audits.

Technological advances in data analysis allows payers to more quickly and easily identify providers whose reporting habits (billing patterns) are outside the norm (i.e., outliers) for providers of the same specialty, subspecialty, and geographic location. Now that these data analytic systems are readily available, the result is that all providers in any geographic locale, regardless of practice size, can easily be reviewed so there is no way to fly "under the radar." Keep in mind that there may be valid reasons for being an outlier, but if the provider stands out in a crowd of their peers, they are likely to be audited.

When a provider is flagged as an outlier, they often receive medical record requests for claims they have submitted prior to payment determination. The payer will review the records to see if they support the services reported, accurately reflect the diagnosis, and meet the requirements of any published payer policies. If not, and it is determined the provider has repeatedly misrepresented the services, diagnosis, or medical necessity of the claims submitted, an audit of those services often ensues.

With this increased scrutiny on provider documentation, coding, and billing practices, there is also an increased risk of losing revenue due to errors in these areas. Once a provider has been flagged as an outlier or has failed an audit, resulting in a repayment demand for the unsupported services, they are at greater risk of subsequent audits by other payers and a continuing cycle of review and overpayment demand.

Audits are a reality for all healthcare practices; therefore, significant attention should be focused on managing them. It has been said that a good offense is a good defense, and that certainly applies in this situation. You need to be prepared to defend your standards. This requires an understanding of state and federal laws/regulations (i.e., fraud, waste, and abuse laws and compliance regulations).

Resource: See Resource 815 for the latest information, articles, and webinars on protecting your practice from audits

Book: See Chapter 4 — Documentation for guidelines about using documentation as a preventative measure against an audit.

Alert — Piggy-back Audits: If you have been audited by a government entity and the outcome is not favorable, it becomes public record. The special investigation units of private payers review those public records and often will follow with their own audit. In some states they actually work with the government audit agencies.

While compliance is a broad term that includes all regulatory aspects of health care, this chapter is focused on claims and reimbursement related issues.

Prepayment Review

When a provider consistently demonstrates incorrect coding and billing practices with a contracted payer, they may be placed on a prepayment review. This is a common practice with CMS contractors (e.g., Noridian, Novitas) and many commercial payers as well. A prepayment review status means all claims for the specified payer must be submitted along with supporting documentation to determine if there was correct code reporting. Once the claims are approved, they are typically returned to the provider to submit for processing, which may take an additional 30-90 days. The entire process from claim submission, review, and then finally to payment may take up to 120 days to complete. Depending on the size of the practice, this kind of delay can be devastating.

If your organization begins to notice an abnormal amount of medical record requests, it may be a sign that a payer is reviewing services to determine if their medical necessity requirements are being met. Prior to submitting requested records, it is recommended that the services and their supporting documentation be audited internally for medical necessity and coding compliance. If a large number of record requests are coming in, especially if they are for the same type of procedure or service, it may be an indicator of a full-scale audit taking place. In this situation it is **strongly** recommended that the practice contact a healthcare attorney in order to engage the services of an experienced, certified medical coding auditor to perform an internal audit of the services for which medical records were requested. This does not mean you withhold the requested records from the payer, but rather that an internal audit of those same services be performed to determine if there are any outstanding issues regarding code assignment, documentation, or specific payer policies that could put the practice at risk.

Tip: Do not alter medical records or change the original documentation. If the provider feels strongly that information vital to the service was not included or incorrectly added, it should be handled through an addendum or provider attestation.

Book: See "Guidelines for Corrections" in Chapter 4.1 — Documentation Essentials.

Once a payer has placed a provider under a prepayment review it is vital for the provider to demonstrate that their coding and billing practices are compliant in order to return to normal billing without a prepayment review process as quickly as possible. The provider must consistently prove the documentation, diagnosis, and codes selected support the service performed. Medical necessity, while always a requirement, becomes front and center for every claim where previously it was typically only occasionally scrutinized on a postpayment review. Engaging an auditor to review the records and ensure the provider can pass a prepayment review is an important first step. Once the provider has demonstrated compliance by successfully passing review on several sets of claims, they should begin negotiating the end of their prepayment review status.

Why Be Concerned?

A seemingly innocent mistake can lead to thousands of dollars in payment demands that are difficult to fight. It begins innocently enough; for example, your office receives a "Preliminary Audit Report" which states that a random sampling of claims over a specified time period (usually several years) indicated an error rate of $1.81 per claim (as an example). That may not sound so bad.

The next part of the letter is where math and random sampling become troublesome. They apply that calculated error rate to **every** single **claim** filed during that time period, use a statistical formula for cluster sampling, and that $1.81 turns into more than $20,000 due in 15 days. This "repayment" amount does not include investigative, legal, or expert witness fees that are incurred by the auditing entity during this process. Additionally, there could be fines up to $23,607 (for 2021) for each claim determined to be a "false claim." The bottom line is that medical practices are increasingly vulnerable to the risk of audits and associated penalties assessed for noncompliance. A monetary penalty may not always be the end of the problem. Depending upon audit findings, other complications are possible such as payment suspension, license suspension, license revocation, criminal type investigations, etc. The best protection for a healthcare practice is to adhere to a well documented and effective compliance plan.

Note: We have heard of cases where attorneys have been able to successfully challenge the extrapolation formulas applied to random sampling. Therefore, if your organization receives a letter like this, we recommend hiring a healthcare attorney familiar with this situation.

Internal and External Audits

There are two types of audits: those initiated by the practice and those initiated by an outside party. *For the purposes of this book*, an audit **initiated by the practice** is considered internal, whether performed by an employee of the practice or done by an outside consultant brought in to do the audit for the practice. An external audit is **initiated by an outside party** such as a payer reviewing claims.

One highly effective way to manage audits is to utilize the same methodologies as a compliance program. Perform a risk assessment (self-audit), identify problem areas, and then make a plan to reduce the likelihood of fines and/or penalties as a result of an external audit. This can be accomplished through ongoing, internal training, and monitoring.

Implement a Compliance Program

Part of any audit management plan is to implement a compliance program. This includes monitoring billing, documentation, and other procedures as they relate to all compliance programs, such as HIPAA. Having this information documented is very helpful in an audit to demonstrate compliance.

 Alert — Your Best Defense is An Effective, Current Compliance Plan:
Carefully constructing and following a compliance plan is the best thing you can do. This plan includes an annual internal audit (it is even better if that audit is done by a Certified Compliance Specialist.) The OIG stated that, among other things, an effective, documented compliance plan can be used as a mitigating factor against fines and jail time.
Remember, a compliance plan is only effective if it is appropriately being adhered to.
Resource: See Resource 303 for more about mitigating factors used by the federal government in determining penalties.

Internal/Self-Auditing

It may seem counterintuitive in a chapter on audit management to discuss a self-audit, but it is a critical component of any effective compliance program. A self audit helps identify current and potential problems and gives the practice an opportunity to address and fix them before they are discovered by an outside auditor. Additionally, self-audits demonstrate your compliance efforts should you be required to defend the practice against allegations of fraud or abuse. Some states, like New Mexico, require providers to conduct routine self-audits.

Since 1998, the Office of Inspector General (HHS-OIG) has been promoting implementation of active compliance plans for all healthcare organizations and in 2000 published recommended guidance in the Federal Register. Since that time, multiple government agencies and acts have pushed to make compliance plans mandatory. Currently, there is a provision of the Affordable Care Act (ACA) requiring providers to have a compliance program but they have not yet issued regulations or enforced it. It is important to know that provider contracts often require a compliance program, or at least the elements of one, so providers should be aware of these guidelines or requirements to remain compliant with contract requirements.

Whether mandated by government programs or by individual payer contracts or not, self-audits help demonstrate compliance and reduce the risk of failing a payer audit or accusations that your billing patterns are inappropriate. For comparison purposes, payers gather data identifying the billing patterns of contracted providers who are of the same specialty, subspecialty, and geographic location. This data allows payers to identify providers billing outside of the average data patterns of their peers (payer benchmarks) and flag them for medical record reviews to investigate whether or not the services provided are legitimate. While it can be helpful to review a payer's benchmark information for comparison purposes, the primary concern of the provider should be to ensure that they are treating the patient according to medical necessity, fully documenting the need for the level(s) of treatment or service rendered, and submitting claims according to the appropriate coding and billing guidelines noted in the applicable official codesets.

Tip: A Comparative Billing Report (CBR) from Medicare can provide helpful benchmarking information. They are sent to providers whose billing patterns are different from their peers. Although providers cannot request a CBR, the website does have sample CBRs and training available for review.

Resource: See Resource 323 to be linked to the CBR website.

Self-audits can be quick or more complex and in-depth. Quick audits of common services or at-risk high-value services should be performed daily. This could entail a senior coder or auditor reviewing claims that have been approved and are ready for submission to ensure guidelines are adhered to and the documentation supports the services being reported on the claim. Additional audits that are helpful to perform include:

- Individual provider audits to determine if proper E/M code selection has been done based on new E/M guidelines and documentation
- New technology procedures or services
- High-value services or those that may be of less value but are frequently performed
- Services that have updated or new guidelines
- Services that have had payer medical record requests

If a self-audit indicates that there is a need for provider or staff education, updates, or changes to coding protocols or guidance, these activities should be noted in the Policies and Procedures Manual to demonstrate active, ongoing compliance efforts to:

In summary, according to a CMS e-Bulletin, self-audits can help:

- Reduce fraud and improper payments
- Improve patient care
- Lower the chances of an external audit
- Create a robust culture of compliance

Resource: See Resource 302 for information by CMS about self-audits.

Quick Audits

A quick audit should be done often, if not daily. There are many different ways to accomplish this, but for the most part, having checklists for common tasks such as documentation or billing can ensure compliance on a daily basis. Sometimes small issues can be eliminated by just creating a standard process in your office. Once you have a repeatable system in place, steps in the process should be completed correctly every time. As problems are revealed by an internal baseline audit, improvements or changes should be made to your current process to avoid making these same errors in the future.

Medical Record Self-Audit Form

Some practices use a *Medical Record Self-Audit* form on every chart before it is filed. It is a quick check for some of the necessary components of documentation. Be sure that the form you use includes any additional requirements needed for your state. An added benefit to doing this type of quick audit is that when it comes time for an Internal Baseline Audit, there is less to review because you have already done part of the audit during this step.

Resource: See Resource 295 for a sample *Medical Record Self-Audit* form.

Don't Forget to Check

Although not an exhaustive list, the following are some suggested items to include in your quick audit. They are known problems that should be considered as part of your medical record self-audit or as part of your internal baseline audit:

1. **Abbreviations.** Some auditors are not medically trained. Of those that are medically trained, there is a high probability that the auditor reviewing your claim is not trained in your specialty. As such, they may be unfamiliar with some of the acronyms specific to your practice. Therefore, if you use abbreviations, it is important to provide a legend to avoid potential misunderstandings. See Chapter 4.1 — Documentation Essentials for a sample of commonly accepted medical abbreviations.

2. **E/M Component Scoring.** The level of E/M reported must be supported by the documentation. As of 2021, E/M guidelines and scoring requirements for certain categories of E/M changed while others remained the same. Be sure to verify the category of E/M services being reported and whether or not the new guidelines or old guidelines apply to scoring the level of service. Then, verify the documentation supports the level of service reported based on the applicable guidelines. The new E/M guidelines applicable to 99202-99215 require the medical record to support the code selection through scoring of time or medical decision making (MDM), which includes a medically appropriate history/examination and MDM, which should be clearly documented. Other E/M services require documentation to support individual components of history (i.e., CC, HPI, ROS, PFSH), history, and elements of MDM (i.e., diagnosis, data, risk).

    If patient questionnaires are used and scanned into the health record, be sure they are included with any notes sent to the payer to validate portions of the history that may have referred to the questionnaire in the documentaion.

    Note: Auditors often closely examine the Review of Systems (ROS) to ensure it correlates with the chief complaint and the rest of the encounter note.

    Book: See Chapter 5.3 — Evaluation & Management Coding for more about E/M required components for documenting both the History and Review of Systems.

3. **Scheduling.** When services are selected based on time (e.g., E/M services) and there is a question as to the number of hours a provider would have had to work in any given day to meet those time requirements, auditors will often review a provider's schedule, provider check-in and check-out times, and even review parking lot camera recordings to investigate possible fraud. Because physicians typically spend 45 minutes or more of face-to-face time on higher levels of Evaluation and Management services, one great self-audit to perform is to add up the total time documented on a given day for each provider to determine if time was accurately documented.

    With the 2021 changes to E/M coding, time may become a highly scrutinized item in an audit, especially considering E/M service changes. Consider the following as you conduct your self-audits:

    - Changes to the actual service times for 99202-99215 but not the other E/M codes

    - Time or MDM may be used to determine the level of E/M and a time statement is not required (although we strongly recommend you include a brief statement about what was done during the time spent with the patient)

    - Prolonged services codes, guidelines, and times have undergone significant changes, including the time at which point these codes are applicable, based on Medicare or commercial payer policies

- Provider documentation habits are difficult to change, which may make it easy for auditors to identify discrepancies or documentation failures

The Medicine Services and Procedures category of the CPT codebook also contains many time-based codes that are commonly miscalculated and thus often scrutinized in an audit. Understanding the specific payer policies surrounding how to properly calculate units based on total time or surpassing the midpoint of the total time is vital to ensuring correct coding and avoiding audit failures and refund demands.

Book: See "Timed Codes" in Chapter 5.3 — Common Procedure Codes & Tips for more information.

If a provider consistently reports time-based services that, when added together, equal a total number of hours that would be considered impossible to sustain, time is likely not being properly calculated or documented. For example, a provider whose time-based services consistently indicate they spend more than 10 hours a day caring for patients based on reporting time-based services would be a provider whose documentation habits and coding processes should be reviewed. To have a payer discover this type of reporting problem could be devastating, but to identify it internally, correct it, and document that correction can help to demonstrate that an active compliance program is in place.

4. **Allergies.** Be sure to clearly document relevant allergies if you prescribe any medications or supplements.

5. **Diagnoses.** For E/M services, be sure to list diagnoses that were monitored, evaluated, assessed, or treated during the encounter and those that had to be considered in the decision-making process or treatment options for prescription options or risk factors. Do not give credit for conditions being treated by another provider unless required to evaluate and treat that condition or discuss it with the provider because its presence or current treatment may affect the condition(s) being treated at the current encounter. Status conditions (e.g., amputations, transplants) may be reported annually as long as a status for them is documented in the record, but unless these are monitored, evaluated, treated, or affect treatment decisions at the current encounter, they should not be considered for E/M scoring purposes. While providing the correct ICD-10-CM codes for the diagnoses is very helpful, be sure to write out the patient's diagnosis for accuracy in reporting and clarification

General Tips

The following are some additional quick tips to be prepared for an audit:

- **Claim scrubbing.** Using claim scrubbing software helps detect claim errors before they are submitted. Many billing systems and electronic clearinghouses offer this type of feature. Even though this type of software can help to detect some errors, it is not a substitute for proper coding. Healthcare providers and coding personnel must understand applicable coding and billing guidelines before utilizing claim scrubbing software.

Resource: See Resource 462 for a claim scrubbing tool.

- **Current code book.** Using outdated codes or unofficial terminology can be confusing to someone reviewing your records, including auditors. It can also indicate that you are not up-to-date with other things like documentation, making your office appear less than fully compliant.

Audit Risk Management

Managing risk in the following areas will yield the most effective results. Some of these problems overlap. For example, much of the Evaluation and Management down-coding occurs because of documentation problems. A payer may use any one of the following areas to initiate an audit. Keep in mind that once they have the records, they will likely review other aspects of the practice. Begin by focusing on coding and billing patterns (see the "Provider Profiling" segment that follows), which are the most likely audit triggers; then evaluate the other risk management areas on the following list of common reasons for an audit:

1. Provider profiling
2. Disgruntled people
3. Excessive or improper modifier use
4. Documentation
5. E/M billing
6. Lack of medical necessity
7. Behavioral Health-Specific Services

1. Provider Profiling

Provider profiling is probably the most common cause for an audit. Most insurance payers (if not all) track billing statistics on all providers and use them to compare a provider's billing patterns to those of his/her peers. Billing pattern reviews assess how, when, and what is billed. In addition to the information that follows, it is important to carefully review the OIG Work Plan for additional triggers. Below are *some* known billing pattern issues:

- **Diagnosis determines treatment.** Whatever diagnosis is chosen, it should be fully supported by appropriate documentation. Using the same diagnosis code on every claim or using diagnoses that do not correlate to the procedures performed could indicate careless diagnostic skills or lack of appropriate care. Diagnoses need to support the services rendered.

- **Clustering.** This is the practice of coding/charging one or two middle levels of service codes exclusively, under the philosophy that some will be higher, some lower, and the charges will average out over an extended period (in reality, this overcharges some patients while undercharging others).

- **Upcoding by a staff member or a billing company.** A staff member may do this to help you make more money. A billing company could do this to help increase their own commissions. Either scenario can easily trigger an audit.

- **Double billing.** Although duplicate billing can occur due to simple error, knowingly submitting duplicate claims – which is sometimes evidenced by systematic or repeated double billing – can create liability under criminal, civil, and/or administrative law.

- **Misuse of provider identification numbers.** The healthcare provider ID associated with the service must be the ID of the individual who rendered that service.

- **Unbundling.** This is billing for each component of the service instead of using an all-inclusive code.

- **Improper ICD-10-CM coding.** On submitted claims, any of the following could be considered improper: 1) high usage of general, non-specific codes, 2) not using highest level of specificity, and 3) selecting a diagnosis that is not supported by the documentation.

- **Inconsistent coding among partners in a practice.** When different partners in a practice code and treat for varying levels of care for the same conditions or patients, it sends up red flags.

- **Coding patterns.** Many payers utilize data mining programs which mathematically estimate coding norms based on claims billed. When a provider falls outside what the payer considers their normal coding pattern, the provider may be considered an 'outlier' and thus be flagged for an audit.

- **Frequency of services.** Review the following:
  - How often are laboratory tests referred to the same lab? This can raise concerns about who owns the lab. Is this a self-referral violation?
  - Timed codes are frequently over-reported. See Chapter 5.2 — Procedure Codes & Tips for more information about correctly reporting timed codes.

- **Licensing/Certifications.** There are several licensing/certification issues to consider:
  - Some services may only be provided by a licensed healthcare provider
  - Some locations may also need to be certified (e.g., substance abuse facilities)
  - Non-physician providers, such as an assistant, may only render services they are legally able to provide in accordance with state law as well as payer contracts
- **Physician orders.** Some services require referrals (e.g., x-ray consultation) and an audit of those services will require the provider referral order to be on file.

2. Disgruntled People

This is one of the biggest triggers because all it takes is a phone call. It doesn't matter where the complaint comes from, if there is a complaint, it is quickly investigated to determine whether or not it is true. Complaints usually are initiated by one of the following:

- **Disgruntled employees.** A disgruntled employee is more likely to turn in a healthcare provider than anyone else. If you have an employee who thinks you are not doing something right, it is very important to get it cleared up with them. Sit down and make sure that everyone understands. Get a second opinion if necessary. It is NOT worth having a disgruntled employee lodge a complaint. Document all complaints and resolutions.
- **Disgruntled patients.** Sometimes a patient becomes disgruntled, often due to the receipt of an unexpected bill. To mitigate this risk, it is important to clearly emphasize patient financial responsibilities with all the necessary paperwork. Be sure that you have good policies and procedures in place in your compliance plan so that everyone understands and follows through to ensure compliance. You can reduce the likelihood of a disgruntled patient filing a complaint by doing all you can to establish good communication between employees and patients.

> **Book:** See the "Establish Patient Financial Responsibility" segment in Chapter 1.1 — Insurance & Reimbursement Essentials for more information.

- **Disgruntled competitors.** It is becoming increasingly common to have a competitor lodge a complaint in order to "even the score." There is not much that you can do about this problem. Your documented compliance efforts will show auditors the real story.
- **Healthcare Providers.** Many of the qui tam (whistleblower) lawsuits against large healthcare organizations have been initiated by healthcare providers who work for the organization itself. Many have been put in management or positions as compliance regulators to ensure the organization is doing things correctly. Some organizations make a significant amount of money by doing things wrong, or purposefully looking for ways to work around the rules. When honest providers bring poorly executed practices to the attention of management, they may be told it will be looked into, investigated, or changed, but this often does not happen. The responsibility of a compliance officer is not to appease management or improve the bottom line, but rather to enforce compliance policies, government regulations, and laws (e.g, federal and state). They are to listen to and act upon the information provided to them and ensure it is handled properly.

3. Excessive or Improper Modifier Use

- **Separating the professional component (modifier 26) from the technical component (modifier TC).** Separating the global fee into technical (TC) and professional (26) could allow for a higher reimbursement. Remember that any time something is done for financial intent, rather than out of clinical necessity, it could be construed as abuse or fraud.
- **Improper use of modifiers.** A review can be triggered if you use the wrong modifiers, use a modifier too much, or use certain ones more frequently than other healthcare providers of your specialty in your area. Overutilization of modifier 59 is a common audit target. In some cases, providers add it when it is not necessary, and in other instances an outside billing company may add the modifier without the provider's knowledge.

Tip: Modifiers 25 and 59 are commonly reported inaccurately and are often not supported by the documentation. Excessive reporting of these modifiers may quickly lead to an audit. If properly reported and supported by the documentation and NCCI edit policies, these modifiers should be reported and reimbursed appropriately.

Book: See Appendix B — Modifiers for more information on CPT and HCPCS modifiers.

4. Documentation

Documentation problems such as missing treatment plans, poorly documented visits, cloned records, and other such issues tend to be the biggest problem facing providers when it comes to audits. Properly documented visits help you avoid audits and defend against them as well.

Tip: Remember that documentation drives the coding, not the other way around.

Book: See Chapter 4 — Documentation for additional information about quality documentation standards.

5. Evaluation and Management Billing

A common mistake is the improper reporting and documenting of Evaluation and Management services. See innoviHealth's *Comprehensive Guide to Evaluation & Management* for more information on how to properly document these types of services to ensure proper code selection.

Note: Beware of inappropriately billing new patient codes for established patients. Existing patients who have a new payer due to a new injury, such as an accident, should still be billed as an established patient.

Alert: Never attempt to 'fly under the radar' of the auditors by coding an inappropriate level of service. Always bill and properly document every visit with supportive notes. Then, if your practice is ever identified as an 'outlier,' your records will support your claims.

Downcoding has the potential to negatively alter any future payer calculations of coding patterns based on submitted claims. More importantly, undercoding could be considered fraud because it is making a false statement about the treatment provided. Instead of downcoding as a defensive tactic, use proper documentation.

Store: Significant changes became effective January 1, 2021 affecting E/M services in the Office or Other Outpatient setting (99201-99215). Avoid mixing and matching documentation and scoring requirements by reviewing the new guidelines and coding scenarios available in innoviHealth's Comprehensive Guide to Evaluation & Management available in the online store.

6. Lack of Medical Necessity

One of biggest problems providers face when audited is that many services are deemed not medically necessary and are routinely denied. Much of the proof falls back on the medical record. Here are some specific situations as they relate to audits.

- **Irrelevant/Missing History and/or Physical Examination.** New guidelines affecting the Office or Other Outpatient E/M codes (99202-99215) allow the provider to determine the extent of the patient's history or physical exam. However, an appropriately documented history and physical exam can provide additional support for medically necessary decision making, testing, and treatment. Performing a higher level of history or examination (other than for codes 99202-99215) for the purpose of billing a level of E/M service with a higher reimbursement rate puts a provider at risk of accusations of upcoding or fraud.

- **Unnecessary Durable Medical Equipment (DME).** There must be clinical rationale for the DME and proof that it supports the healing process.

- **Unsupported diagnostic testing.** The need for any diagnostic testing must be substantiated in the documentation. The rationale for ordering the test should be based on the provider's inability to establish a diagnosis to a reasonable degree of clinical certainty without the test results and/or to rule out pathologies, etc.

Individual payer policies often require conservative treatment options to have been performed prior to ordering specific and/or more expensive testing (e.g., imaging, lab work). Proper medical record documentation can support a physician's orders for internal testing performed in the office setting. In fact, unless specifically required by the payer, it is not necessarily required to have a separate physician's order filled out and filed with the payer. In order for the order within a medical record to be valid, it must include the patient's name, date of birth, diagnosis, and intent to order the service, along with the provider's signature and date signed. If laboratory or imaging services are being ordered to be performed at an independent lab or hospital facility, a written physician's order with a supporting diagnosis should be provided to that entity and documented/maintained within the patient's medical record.

- **Unnecessary services.** It is inappropriate to bill for procedures for parts of the body that are not associated with the patient complaint, presenting problem, or those found through objective measures. Be aware of individual payer policies of what they consider medically necessary.

- **Unjustified frequency of re-examinations and/or re-x-rays.** This is an issue when there is little or no documented clinical assessment of the patient's progress that would require the billing for such services. Essential and required information should be in the daily notes. If progress has not been noticed, there should be a referral for further testing and evaluation.

- **Experimental/unproven services.** Performing and billing for services deemed "experimental or unproven" by payers is potentially problematic. For this reason, many payer policies include lists of services that are specifically excluded from coverage.

- **Routine Services.** Another issue is billing for services which are performed on a routine basis as opposed to clearly establishing and supporting medical necessity per third-party billing requirements. When these types of services do not meet coverage guidelines, they are easily identified when evaluating provider claims.

- **Static treatment plans.** This occurs when every patient gets the same treatment plan with the same duration and frequency, regardless of the diagnosis. Patient care should always be individualized and treatment plans should be regularly re-evaluated.

7. Behavioral Health-Specific Services

- **Coding patterns.** Many payers utilize data mining programs which mathematically estimate coding norms based on claims billed. When a provider falls outside what the payer considers their normal coding distribution, the provider may be considered an 'outlier' and thus be flagged for an audit. Keep in mind that patterns can vary based on the severity and chronicity of your patient pool. Documenting all diagnoses relevant to your treatment plan helps to justify the need for services.

As an example of a coding pattern, according to the American Psychological Association Practice Directorate, psychotherapy frequency in 2013 was 90832 (30.6%), 90834 (46.4%), and 90837 (22.9%).

Warning: Do not attempt to make your practice fit these numbers, just understand that the further you are from a payer's established patterns, the more likely it is that you will need to prove that your services were medically necessary.

Note: Percentages can change annually and vary by payer. The numbers shown here are just a reference.

- **Failure to identify type of provider.** Many payers require the use of specific modifiers to identify the type of provider rendering the service (e.g., AH for psychologist). Using the wrong modifier in order to increase payment is considered fraud.

- **Static treatment plans.** Treatment plans are carefully monitored by payers. A static plan is one that is the same for every patient, regardless of the diagnosis. Not only should care be individualized, it should also be revised and updated frequently as care progresses. According to Medicare's CBR201808 report, the treatment plan should be updated/addressed at each visit.

- **Incorrect code selection based on time.** Many services (e.g., psychotherapy, test administration and scoring) are time based services. You must meet the mid-point to be able to report the service. If your patient ends a service before reaching that mid-point, it is NOT reportable — even with a modifier.

> **Book:** See "Timed Codes" in Chapter 5.3 — Common Procedure Codes & Tips for additional information.

- **Auxiliary personnel billing.** Payers have strict rules regarding which services may be performed by nonphysician healthcare providers (e.g., assistant, student). Be sure you understand the rules for each payer as well as the rules for your state. In some cases, auxiliary personnel services might fall under 'incident to' rules.

> **Book:** See "Incident To Services" in Chapter 2.1 — Medicare Essentials for additional information.

- **Routine Services.** Another issue is billing for services which are performed on a routine basis as opposed to clearly establishing and supporting medical necessity per third-party billing requirements. When these types of services do not meet coverage guidelines, they are easily identified when evaluating provider claims.

- **Static treatment plans.** This occurs when every patient gets the same treatment plan with the same duration and frequency, regardless of the diagnosis. Patient care should always be individualized and treatment plans should be regularly re-evaluated.

What to Do When You Are Audited

Does your staff know what to do when they receive a request for medical records from a payer? The following steps may assist you in processing and dealing with a payer's request for medical records that may or may not be related to a specific audit

- If the records request is specific to a payer audit, immediately notify administration of the audit and request for medical records.

- If the request is for a single claim, it is recommended that a review be performed of the services and the documentation to ensure proper code assignment and supporting information with the medical record.

- Determine when to involve an experienced healthcare attorney. A healthcare attorney who is well versed on Medicare, Medicaid, ERISA, commercial payer contracts, and auditing is strongly recommended. Those without this experience and knowledge will spend a lot of time (and provider money) learning how to handle these audits while one experienced in them will know how to immediately respond, saving the practice money in the long run. Be aware that communications regarding auditing information and how the records are handled may only fall under attorney client privilege if handled correctly. Be certain to follow any attorney instructions to the letter to protect this privilege while investigating the audit-related documents.

- Identify the information requested. Under the HIPAA minimum necessary standard, covered entities must ensure access to PHI is limited to the minimum amount of information necessary to fulfill/satisfy the intended purpose of a particular disclosure, request, or use so do not send more than what meets that requirement.

Store: See innoviHealth's *Complete & Easy HIPAA Compliance* publication (Resource 116) for a more comprehensive review of HIPAA including the minimum necessary standard

- Have a certified medical coding auditor or certified coder review the claims and supporting documentation to ensure the records exist, are correctly documented, signed, dated, and support the services billed. Failing to provide a physician's order to support performance of a diagnostic service or procedure can lead to audit failure.

- DO NOT alter or add to your **original** notes or records in any way. You may add an addendum along with the current date and time or the provider of record may provide a signed attestation to clarify any documentation errors or missing information. Ideally, this is done with the assistance of the provider's healthcare attorney.

Book: See "Guidelines for Corrections" in Chapter 4.1 — Documentation Essentials.

- Using a spreadsheet can help keep record requests and audit findings organized. For each claim for which information is being requested, include the patient's name, date of service, payer, codes reported, modifiers, and paid/denial information. Include a column for notes and another to identify whether or not your independent claim review indicates it is supported by the medical record. Be sure to check for content, signatures, orders, etc. See also "Implement a Tracking and Review System" on page 175.

- Review pertinent findings with the healthcare attorney and provider being audited. Be sure that all spreadsheets, correspondence, and emails regarding the audit are marked as directed by the attorney for maximum attorney-client privilege.

- Be sure to submit the requested documents within the timeframe noted in the request to avoid an automatic audit failure and send them certified mail or through the attorney's HIPAA-compliant software sharing program.

  a. **Paper Records:** Send copies only (not the originals) and send them certified return receipt since this information is very important in an audit.

  b. **Electronic Records:** Work with the attorney and payer to determine an electronic format in which the records may be submitted. **Never** provide a username and password to the payer which allows them general access to your internal files. Remember, HIPAA only allows them limited access to those documents needed to satisfy the specific review.

Implement a Tracking and Review System

Every practice should have a tracking system which actively monitors 1) records requests, 2) claim denials 3) underpayments, and 4) appeals. This system should include an official policy and procedure for each situation. Clearly define requirements to quickly respond to requests for records and where that information is logged, i.e., when the request was received, who received it, and when the records were submitted. To minimize future problems, your tracking system should also analyze data obtained and use it to train all staff on resolutions.

Book: See Chapter 1.4 — Claims Management for more about monitoring unpaid claims.

Notes:

4. Documentation

Chapter Contents

4.1 Documentation Essentials 153
    Introduction 153
    The Role of Medical Necessity 155
    Documentation and Recordkeeping Standards 156
    Transitioning from Active Care 167
    The Treatment Plan 168

4.2 Provider Documentation Training 173
    Provider Documentation Guides (PDGs) 174
    Diagnostic Statement 186
    Lessons from the Clinical Example 194

4.3 Documentation Tips 197
    Tips 200

4.1 Documentation Essentials

Introduction

Years ago, documentation was not submitted to Medicare or other payers. The chances of a medical record becoming a legal document in a malpractice case were minimal. Since most patient records were only seen by the doctor and staff, documentation was done with the assumption that no one else needed to understand the patient chart. No standards existed for recording/documenting patient information.

Times have changed dramatically. Documentation is now a critical component in both the Reimbursement Life Cycle (see Chapter 1.1 — Insurance & Reimbursement Essentials) and as evidence of care for reviews, audits, or medical malpractice cases. This is because documentation:

- provides clear evidence of continuity of care to communicate with other providers.
- outlines a clear course of care and the patient's response to treatment.
- acts as a legal record of the care given.
- allows comparisons between differing patient episodes, as well as other patients with similar conditions.
- supports the billing for services rendered.

Figure 4.1

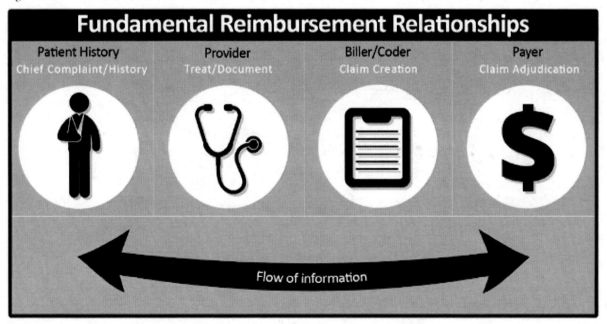

Figure 4.1 shows the fundamental relationships between the different entities involved in the Reimbursement Life Cycle. Information flows frequently between each of these entities. For example, the patient needs to ensure that all essential information is communicated to the provider who then has the responsibility to not only examine, diagnose, and treat the condition(s), but also the responsibility to ensure that the encounter is properly documented. If the patient encounter is thoroughly documented, it becomes possible for both the biller and the payer to efficiently and correctly perform their responsibilities.

When considering these Fundamental Reimbursement Relationships, documentation is the recording of pertinent facts and observations about a patient's health history and physical examination of the system(s) applicable to the current encounter. It may include testing, decision making, treatment planning, treatment, and outcomes assessment.

In cases where third-party reimbursement is needed, as shown in *Figure 4.1*, the biller/coder then uses the information contained in the documentation created by the provider to submit a claim for each patient encounter. Thus we see that without appropriate documentation, there is insufficient information to make correct coding and claims adjudication decisions. Claims cannot and do not stand alone – they rely on the provider's record of the patient encounter. The entire third party insurance payer industry, including government and private enterprises, are increasingly using the health care record to determine whether they consider the services on the submitted claims to be both reasonable and medically necessary. In some cases, they may even interview the patient to determine if the documentation matches the patient encounter.

When a patient encounter is documented properly, another healthcare provider or reviewer can read the notes and know exactly what happened during that encounter and why. The notes should be readable and the most recent patient record should not read like the first patient record. Good documentation will concisely record the patient's condition, both subjectively from the patient's point of view and objectively from the healthcare provider's point of view, what treatment was performed, why the treatment was performed, and how well the patient is progressing toward the treatment goals.

It should be noted that all patient encounters should be recorded in the patient's file. This includes telephone calls and encounters with staff members as they relate to patient care.

Like treatment plans, progress notes document a client's progression on the specified treatment plan. Progress notes can help assist in the justification of continued treatment beyond the original treatment plan. It is a common practice for third party payers to grant a set number of visits based on a diagnosis. When requesting further covered visits in behalf of the client, progress notes can help to establish medical necessity.

Any successful implementation of documentation protocols will depend largely on the willing participation of the entire staff from the front desk to the clinician.

To summarize, the medical record performs several functions. Not only does it support medical necessity, justify submitted claims and reduce your exposure to audits, it also reduces medical errors and professional liability exposure, facilitates claims review, provides clinical data for both education and research, promotes continuity of care among providers, serves as a measure of patient safety, and demonstrates quality of care. The medical record, with all these functions, facilitates the smooth flow of information necessary for a successful and thriving practice.

Resource: See Resource 816 for the latest information, webinars and articles.

Book: See Chapter 1.3 — Claims Processing for more about claims submission requirements.

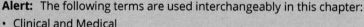

Alert: The following terms are used interchangeably in this chapter:
- Clinical and Medical
- Clinical Chart and Medical Record
- Medically Necessity and Clinical Necessity
- Electronic Health Record (EHR) and Electronic Medical Record (EMR)
- Treatment Plans and Care Plans

Tip – Did It Really Happen?

The phrase, "If it is not documented it did not happen" has been used for years by payers for denial purposes. However, from a legal perspective it could have happened. Even if there is no legal action (including malpractice cases), insufficient documentation can cause a myriad of problems.

Conclusion: If in doubt, document it. It is better to correctly document in the first place than to deal with the potential repercussions of insufficient record-keeping.

The Role of Medical Necessity

Medicare defines **medical necessity** as services or items reasonable and necessary for the diagnosis or treatment of illness or injury, or to improve the functioning of a malformed body member. Consequently, the medical record has become the vital determining factor when assessing what is medically reasonable and necessary. Although this definition from Medicare sounds like a hard and fast rule, keep in mind that there are almost as many versions of "medical necessity" as there are payers, laws, and courts to interpret them.

Tip: Generally speaking, most definitions of medical necessity incorporate the principle of providing services which are "reasonable and necessary" or "appropriate" in light of clinical standards of practice in one's medical community.

The lack of objectivity inherent in these terms often leads to widely varying interpretations by healthcare providers and payers, which in turn can result in the care provided not meeting the payer definition of necessity. Last, but not least, the decision as to whether the services were medically necessary is often made by a payer's reviewer, who has never seen the patient, and may not even have medical training.

CMS/Medicare has long been determining medical necessity, and correct billing practices of providers, by requiring its Medicare Administrative Contractors (MACs) to perform current and postpayment reviews. These types of reviews check claims against chart documentation to ensure that dollars spent were administered appropriately. Third party payers also commonly perform the same types of claim and documentation reviews. Reviews are now simply a fact of life for all payers, not just Medicare.

Book: See Chapter 2 — Medicare for more about Medicare reviews.

Book: See Chapter 3 — Compliance Essentials for information about other fraud concerns.

If a payer determines that services were medically unreasonable or unnecessary after payment has been made, it is treated as an overpayment. Generally, payers demand overpayments to be refunded immediately, often with penalties and/or interest. Moreover, if a pattern of claims appears to demonstrate that the healthcare provider knows, or should have known, that the services were not medically necessary, they may also face allegations of fraud which can include large monetary penalties and/or exclusion from government programs such as Medicare. Additionally, criminal prosecution could be considered.

Alert: Many payers include coverage policies which list diagnosis codes that support medical necessity. While it is appropriate to review this information, choosing a diagnosis code only because it is on a "covered" list is fraud. Your diagnosis should always be based on sound clinical judgment.

Medical Necessity Quick-Check

The following criteria may be considered when determining if a particular service is medically necessary.

1. Does the record show a patient complaint that is consistent with an injury or condition? Does the clinical documentation clearly identify the chief complaint (the reason for the encounter)? Does the record establish the medical necessity of the care provided?
2. Do the exam findings confirm the existence of a condition that is consistent with the complaint? If the area is not examined and consequently, there are no exam findings, treatment is not justified. When there is a patient complaint or pain in the absence of positive exam findings, it can be difficult to explain and usually requires further investigation. It is necessary to document a causal chain from the mechanism of injury or disease process to the patient complaint, to the exam findings, to the diagnosis, and ultimately to the treatment.

3. Is the selected case management and treatment appropriate for the diagnosis and phase of the condition? For example, care for the same diagnosis might vary between two patients based on gender, age, comorbidities, etc. Also, as patients heal, certain treatments may need to be discontinued and replaced by other types of treatment.

4. Is there documented progress based on a care plan? The plan should include specific and measurable goals. Medical necessity is not present if patient complaints and objective findings remain the same over long periods. Improvement must be noted over time.

Book: See "The Treatment Plan" on page 168 for additional information on measurable progress.

Tip: The four elements of medical necessity are:
1. Complaint
2. Explanation
3. Appropriate treatment
4. Progress

This quick test can be applied to each and every procedure code billed on a claim. If all four criteria are met, the service is likely to be deemed medically necessary.

Documentation and Recordkeeping Standards

How Much Documentation?

Documenting every detail of a service is not necessary, reasonable or practical. The degree of documentation required depends on many factors such as level of service or provider specialty. The higher the level of service billed, the more detailed the documentation should be. A claim may be denied, downcoded, or undergo further scrutinization if the documentation is borderline. It is just as important to document routine medical services as it is to document unusual medical services. Even the specialty of the physician providing the services has an effect. A normal "head and neck exam" means different things to an orthopedic surgeon, an otolaryngologist (ear, nose, and throat specialist), and a chiropractor.

Figure 4.1 shows that proper record keeping begins with the patient who provides the history and chief complaint which the provider then uses to create a record with an initial diagnosis and treatment plan. This record needs to be an accurate representation of what happened in the patient encounter with sufficient information to enable the biller/coder to create an accurate claim. This will ensure that the payer receives everything they need to process the claim correctly.

Tip: It is not appropriate to keep more than one chart for each patient. Separate charts for private pay, auto accident insurance, and workers' compensation can appear very suspicious to payers, once discovered, because they can give the appearance that the provider is attempting to hide important patient information.

The objective in chart organization is to create a picture of the care the patient has received, beginning with the presentation of their initial problem, continuing through every patient encounter and treatment session, and concluding with a discharge and/or referral. Anyone reviewing the chart should be able to quickly understand the logic of the chosen course of treatment(s). It it important to note that a chart's organization is primarily dependent on the type of chart used, i.e., EHR versus paper. In an EHR, chart organization is largely determined by the software. In contrast, a paper chart requires more methodical methods of organization.

For either type, the following are all important elements of a chart:

- patient-completed intake forms
- patient demographics
- patient-completed outcomes assessment forms
- prior medical records
- medical records obtained from referrals (e.g., imaging studies, specialty consultations)
- correspondence with patient, payers, and other providers, and
- the provider's own chart notes, which may also be further subcategorized

Reports should be filed in chronological order and linked to the appropriate diagnosis from the problem list. When outside reports are received, acknowledge that you have reviewed them by creating a chart memo which includes a summary of the findings and a statement of how it may or may not affect your diagnosis and/or treatment plan. In addition to maintaining all pertinent clinical data, the patient's chart should also have associated financial and other supporting data (e.g., forms for patient registration, assignment, authorizations, releases, consent to treat, HIPAA privacy, etc.)

Tip — Do it Once, But Do it Correctly: It is preferable to complete your daily chart for each patient while in the treatment room because that is the best time to accurately recall pertinent case information. Some states or payers may require that records be complete within 24 hours of a rendered service.

Try to avoid doing only partial charting during the patient encounter and then waiting until the end of the day to finish. It is like waiting for a root canal. You know that if you get five more patients, your root canal is just that much longer at the end of the day. Stalling the documentation diminishes your incentive to grow your practice and the accuracy of your records.

SOAP Notes

SOAP is an abbreviation for the Subjective data, Objective data, Assessment, and Plan. It is the heart and body of the chart. Its format encourages comprehensive records and organization of the notes, with rapid and easy retrieval of information. Keep in mind that when documenting for evaluations, innoviHealth suggests a format that more closely resembles the requirements for an E/M code, as outlined in either the 1995 or 1997 Documentation Guidelines.

Store: See innoviHealth's *Comprehensive Guide to Evaluation & Management* for information regarding E/M requirements.

Subjective Data

This is the patient's point of view which includes their pain level, perception of function level, etc.

- Presenting complaint, including the severity and duration of the symptoms
- Whether this is a new concern or an ongoing / recurring problem
- Changes in the patient's progress or health status since the last visit
- Family and patient's past medical history when relevant (i.e., initial exam)
- Aggravating and/or relieving factors
- Patient statement of functional limitations and/or challenges
- Context of the condition (how, when, and where)

Objective Data

These are factors which the healthcare provider can measure, as objectively as possible, such as:

- Relevant vital signs
- Physical examination, with emphasis on the chief complaint
- Positive exam findings with any specific details
- Pertinent negative exam findings

Assessment

With subjective and objective data, a provider can express a sound opinion of what's going on. The assessment, which is based on the S and O components of SOAP, should consider a review of medications, diagnostic results, and consultation reports. These elements are the basis for arriving at a clinical impression/diagnostic statement. ICD-10-CM codes should be listed in this part of a SOAP note. Note that the ICD-10-CM codes are listed in the assessment, but they may also contain information from the Plan, or "P," in SOAP. For example, seventh character extensions often specify the episode of care. External cause codes, if used, are often based on information reported in the "Subjective" portion of the note.

The assessment is a short discussion which should include the following:

- Patient risk factors (as appropriate)
- Ongoing/recurring health concerns (as appropriate)
- Diagnostic problem statement or clinical impression, including a differential diagnosis (as appropriate)
- Patient response to treatment

Book: See Chapter 4.2 — Provider Documentation Training to learn more about a proper Diagnostic Statement.

Plan

According to Medicare, a plan is "an ordered assembly of expected or planned activities, including observation goals, services, appointments and procedures, usually organized in phases or sessions, which have an objective of organizing and managing health care activity for the patient." To summarize, it's a plan to address the patient condition based upon specific clinical endpoint(s), e.g., resolution, referral, and re-evaluation. The plan should document (where applicable) the:

- recommended therapeutic procedures, modalities, and other treatments.
- rationale for treatment linked to a diagnosis or patient complaint.
- tests or procedures to be performed.
- consultation requests including the reason for the referral.
- self and/or home care recommendations (e.g., home exercise plan).
- frequency of visits.
- estimate of total number of visits recommended or length of care.
- specific and measurable goals, correlated with the services provided.
- anticipated date of re-evaluation/re-assessment.
- specific patient instructions as it pertains to function — what to do/what not to do.
- specific concerns regarding the patient, including the patient's refusal to comply with your recommendations.

When a diagnosis is inconclusive or yet to be determined, the plan describes the steps necessary to reach a diagnostic conclusion such as orders for imaging, labs, or referral for specialty consultation.

Tip – The Perfect SOAP Note:
There is no such thing as a perfect SOAP note that meets medical necessity requirements. This is because one purpose of a SOAP note (or any documentation) is to communicate what is going on with your patient to someone who is not there.

While there are certain elements that should be part of every good SOAP note, it also should be flexible enough to change with the patient. For example, you have three patients who have the same chief complaint. Even though their presenting problem is the same, they range from 5 to 85 years of age. Therefore, their documentation should look different.

Simplification can be good, but there is a danger in too much simplification. As such, is it unwise to utilize a single 'perfect' SOAP note as a template for all your patients.

Alert: For behavioral health services, due to HIPAA requirements, keep Psychotherapy Notes in a separate section of the chart or in another location, such as a separate filing cabinet.
Book: See Resource 505 for more about Psychotherapy Notes.

Tip: When evaluating a SOAP note to identify the key components for an Evaluation and Management encounter, remember that the "subjective" portion will contain the patient's history, the "objective" will contain the physical examination, and the "assessment" and "plan" will contain the medical decision making.

Quality Patient Records

Here are points to ponder for better records:

- Maintain one separate chart with a unique medical record number for each patient. Do not use the same record for other family members and do not use more than one active chart for the same patient.

- The patient's identifying information, including full name and date of birth (requirements may differ from state to state) must be on each page or both sides of the page as applicable. Pages should be numbered when there is more than one page for a specific date's chart entry. Chart entries should be ordered in chronological or reverse chronological order.

- Anything that relates to the patient encounter should be in the patient record. Remember that from the reviewer's perspective: "If it's not documented, it didn't happen."

- Non-compliance with doctor recommendations, missed appointments, displeasure, negative events, and reactions must be documented.

- Patient records should tell the complete story of the patient. Can the patient's past and current health concerns be understood by a person seeing the record for the very first time?

- Patient records may provide significant evidence in lawsuits, hearings, or inquests when the care provided is in question. Regardless of the type of assessment or investigation, a good or bad patient record may have a significant positive or negative impact on the outcome of the process.

- Recommendations for home care, exercises, and referrals (to and from other providers) must be documented.

- All recommended tests must have a report in the file. Be sure to include the rationale for ordering diagnostic and other ancillary services if it is not easily inferred.

- If records are handwritten, they must be legible. However, it is recommended that chart records are NOT handwritten. This is due to the fact that even legible records are difficult to read when copied. Compounding the problem, those records become increasingly more difficult to read when third party record reviewers make additional copies. Records that cannot be read, especially handwritten ones, may be treated similarly to undocumented services. "If it isn't documented it didn't happen" becomes "If it isn't legible then it may as well not have been written down." If you, your staff, or colleagues are having difficulty with the legibility of your records, you should consider alternate means of note-taking such as transcription and/or EHRs. If you have not yet transitioned to EHR and are using a paper documentation system, be sure to document using dark blue or black ink.

- Only standard abbreviations should be used. If you have developed an individualized style of reporting and documenting using acronyms, you should ensure that a key with your full meaning is readily available (see "Abbreviations" on page 166).

- Blank spaces on an exam form or chart note may not be used to imply that a test result was normal. Consider using acronyms such as "WNL" for "within normal limits" or "NAD" for "no abnormality detected."

- Entries should be written or dictated and signed within 24 hours of the patient encounter. Timeliness is essential for accuracy.

- All entries **must** be dated and signed by the healthcare provider. Patient documentation is a legal document!

- An addendum to a medical record should be dated the day the information is added to the medical record rather than the date the service was provided.

Electronic Health Record (EHR) Considerations

An EHR refers to storing patient information in an electronic format that keeps it private and allows the information to be shared easily with others who may need it to perform their duties, such as third party payers or consulting providers.

These systems often help providers create more thorough documentation; however, with this benefit comes an increased caution about "canned" or "cloned" records. Clinical documentation should reflect each patient encounter independently, and no two encounters are exactly alike. Thus, the notes for two separate visits may be similar; but as long as they are completely and accurately describing the encounter, there is little likelihood of them being exactly the same. Claims reviewers believe that copied and pasted notes usually do not accurately reflect the encounter, or that they indicate a lack of progress. Avoid the appearance of cloned records by recording information specific to a particular patient, such as their actual pain rating on the Verbal Numeric Rating Scale instead of "decreased pain." Customize care plans based on age, co-morbidities, severity of the complaint, and other factors that differ from patient to patient. For a single patient, emphasize the changes since the last visit rather than restating the initial findings.

Although many providers have desired to "keep things simple" by avoiding the implementation of EHR, the option to do so may be expiring. Some states already require EHR and, with the Quality Payment Program, providers who bill Medicare will be subject to payment adjustments based in part on EHR use. According to the Quality Payment Program fact sheet published by CMS, "Clinicians would choose to report customizable measures that reflect how they use electronic health record (EHR) technology in their day-to-day practice, with a particular emphasis on interoperability and information exchange. Unlike the Meaningful Use program, the "Promoting Interoperability" category would not require all-or-nothing EHR measurement or quarterly reporting." Please note that the QPP still requires providers to demonstrate that EHR is being used in a meaningful way to qualify for those incentive payments.

Resource: See Resource 398 for more about Medicaid's EHR program.

EHR use continues to be one of the most frustrating aspects of practicing medicine in today's healthcare climate. A July 2016 Mayo Clinic survey found that 44% of physicians were dissatisfied with the EHR technology, compared to only 36% who were satisfied. In addition, an overwhelming 63% don't believe EHR use improves efficiency. Compounding this frustration, a 2014 study from Northwestern Medicine showed that physicians who used an EHR spent three times longer looking at a computer screen during patient encounters than their counterparts who did not. Given these findings, it is not surprising that providers who simply want to practice medicine have resorted to shortcuts in their EHR documentation. Using templates and copy/paste features may save time in the short run, but without proper care to ensure that the documentation matches exactly what happened in the patient encounter, these features could potentially leave a provider more vulnerable to negative outcomes in the current environment of increasing audits. These helpful shortcuts don't have to be removed from the documentation process entirely, but it is incredibly important to be aware of the risk they present.

Alert: When using some shortcut features in EHR software, use caution and be sure to properly edit and review before finalizing the record. Failure to take these steps can yield a record which does not accurately reflect the patient encounter, leaving you vulnerable to the possibility of having payments recouped or facing allegations of fraud in the event of an audit.

Common Errors

Providers need to be aware of the most common documentation errors. Establish procedures to ensure that common errors are avoided. Although not a comprehensive list, here are some common errors to be aware of:

- Illegible records
- Missing dates
- Missing signature
- Missing informed consent
- Missing re-assessment
- Missing patient identifiers
- Missing metrics/objective
- Blanks used to indicate "Within Normal Limits" (WNL)
- Missing legend for abbreviations
- Missing care plan
- Diagnoses that do not support the service(s) rendered or vague symptom diagnoses that do not justify the type or level of care
- Using unedited pre-populated templates (i.e., cloning records)

Other Important Considerations

Detailed and thorough documentation should be kept for all patient case types. It is also essential to be aware of and adhere to specific payer guidelines or documentation requirements. Remember that even for non-insurance (cash) patients, your records might be requested for review or reference in certain situations, such as malpractice claims or complaints to regulatory agencies like state boards.

Alert: HIPAA rules mandate that providers must comply with the rules regarding the proper uses and disclosures of Protected Health Information (PHI). For example, if a payer wishes to review records for a patient who is not their client, they must have the required releases in order to view them.

Store: See *Complete & Easy HIPAA Compliance* (Resource 116) in the online store for more information about PHI.

Date and Time

Since the medical record is a legal document, a patient encounter is invalid without a date. Signatures, even those that are electronic, should include a time and date stamp. See "Signatures" on page 163 for more on signatures. Time could also be important when reconstructing services provided to a patient on the same date. When recording services in which a time element is in the code description, be sure to record the amount of time spent with the patient for those particular procedures. It is most accurate to record actual start and end times, but, depending on payer policies, it may be sufficient to document the total time for each procedure instead.

Resource: See Resource 616 for the Medicare definition of timed codes with examples.

Also, keep in mind that payers often have established timelines for episodes for care for certain conditions which makes it essential to fully document dates of all of the following that apply:

- exacerbation
- regression
- re-injury
- new injuries which support a continuation of service as active care rather than maintenance care
- end of active care
- beginning or resumption of maintenance care

Do not leave blank spaces in the chart because this encourages entering information out of order. Information should always be entered in the patient chart chronologically. Results of x-rays or other tests should be entered when received rather than on blank lines left by the date of service information. This method could give the impression that the physician saw the information at the time of service which creates an inaccurate picture of the patient encounter. If data is pending, make a note in the chart stating that results are expected.

Tip: When additional chart information, such as results of x-rays, tests, or reports from other providers is received, make a separate chart entry or memo on that date. Include a brief notation or summary including comments on how the results may influence the diagnosis or treatment plan.

X-Ray Reports

A written x-ray report is necessary when the x-ray study was performed in your office. If the films are sent out for radiological review, a chart notation is appropriate. However, it is not ideal or recommended to use a checklist for the report. Imaging reports should be distinct from, rather than embedded within, the daily encounters so that it can be sent out if requested by another provider.

The following list of recommended documentation is based on information from the American College of Radiology:

1. Demographics including:
   - The facility or location where the study was performed
   - Name of patient and another identifier such as date of birth or record number (this is a HIPAA standard)
   - Name or type of examination
   - Date of the examination
   - Inclusion of the following additional items is encouraged:
     - Date of dictation
     - Date and time of transcription
     - Patient's date of birth or age
     - Patient's gender

2. Relevant clinical information such as patient history or exam findings that elicited the need for the imaging
3. Body of the report
   - Findings: use appropriate anatomic, pathologic, and radiologic terminology
   - Potential limitations that may affect the quality of the films, such as patient habitus or expected artifacts
   - Comparison studies and reports if available
4. Impression (conclusion or diagnosis)
   - A specific diagnosis should be given when possible
   - A differential diagnosis should be rendered when appropriate
   - Follow-up or additional diagnostic studies to clarify or confirm the impression should be suggested when appropriate
   - Any significant patient reaction should be reported

Signatures

The individual who ordered/provided services must be clearly identified in the medical records. Each chart entry must be legible and should include the practitioner's first and last name. For clarification purposes, Medicare recommends you include your applicable credentials (e.g., MD). The purpose of a provider signature in the medical record is to demonstrate the services have been accurately and fully documented, reviewed and authenticated. Furthermore, it confirms the provider has certified the medical necessity and reasonableness for the service(s) submitted for payment consideration.

The healthcare provider's name and signature are different. Both are required. Furthermore, in an electronic record, the provider's signature "locks" the record, preventing it from being modified after the entry has been signed. This is vital to the authenticity of the record.

Tip: All documents in the chart, including chart notes, patient-completed forms, records received from other offices, and entries by staff should be signed. Once a note is signed, it is closed and any additions would need to be added as an addendum with a new signature and date.

Medicare Requirements for Valid Signatures

Acceptable methods of signing records/test orders and findings include:
- Handwritten signatures (legible)
- Electronic signatures may be acceptable in several forms:
  - Digitized signature – an electronic image of an individual's handwritten signature reproduced in its identical form using a pen tablet
  - Electronic signature – a method which contains date and timestamps and includes printed statements, (e.g., 'electronically signed by,' or 'verified/reviewed by,') followed by the practitioner's name and preferably a professional designation
  - Digital signature – an electronic method of a written signature that is typically generated by special encrypted software that allows for sole usage

Resource: See Resource 371 for more on Medicare signature requirements.

Unacceptable Signatures

The following have been declared unacceptable by Medicare and most third party payers:

- Signature 'stamps' alone in medical records are NO LONGER recognized by Medicare as valid authentication
- Reports or any records that are dictated and/or transcribed, but do not include valid signatures 'finalizing and approving' the documents are not acceptable
- Initials may not be used
- Indications that a document has been 'Signed but not read' or "dictated but not read" are not acceptable as part of the medical record. Lack of time is not an acceptable reason to use this approach.

Signature Log and Attestation

A signature log is a typed listing of the provider(s) name(s), including credentials, with corresponding handwritten signature(s) and initials. This may be an individual log or a group log. A signature log may be used to establish signature identity, particularly when the signature could be considered illegible or initials are used. Medicare also requires a signature attestation if a signature is missing or illegible. This attestation is a statement that must be signed and dated by the author of the medical record entry and must contain sufficient information to identify the beneficiary. Be aware of individual payer requirements.

Resource: See Resource 416 for a sample attestation statement and Resource 417 for a signature log.

Electronic Signatures

While EHR may simplify and automate the signature process, be aware that electronic and digital signatures are not the same as "auto-authentication" or "auto-signature" systems, some of which do not mandate or permit the provider to review an entry before signing or do not meet the requirements noted above.

CMS has cautioned that both computer systems and software products (e.g., EHR software) must include protections against modification. Be sure to implement appropriate administrative safeguards which meet state and federal laws. Finally, check with your malpractice insurance regarding their requirements for electronic signatures.

Resource: See Resource 819 and search on "electronic signatures" for more information.

Evaluation and Management Requirements

When documenting Evaluation and Management (E/M) services, there are distinct requirements that must be met in order to qualify for a specific level of service. It is essential to fully document all requirements as outlined by official CPT and payer guidelines. While SOAP notes may outline the clinical information necessary for a patient encounter, E/M requirements are more thorough and must satisfy all three key components in order to be billed.

Store: See innoviHealth's *Comprehensive Guide to Evaluation & Management* for more information

Dictation/Voice Recognition

The growth of EHRs and voice recognition technology (considered a form of dictation) are permitting healthcare providers to have instant documentation. As such, analog/manual dictation is not as common as it used to be. Regardless of the technology used, it is easy for errors to slip into the record, therefore it must be carefully reviewed for accuracy before signing (whether electronically or manually). The provider is ultimately responsible for the content of dictated records.

Computer Generated Notes

There has been a great deal of abuse and misuse of software generated notes and their randomization function. When documentation is worded exactly like, or similar to, previous entries from visit to visit on a single patient or from patient to patient, it is referred to as cloned documentation. Even though it appears to be related to patient cases, in reality it does not have an accurate story to tell to allied professionals, or to those who may take over a case.

Computer generated notes must be specific to the particular patient on each day of service. Cloned records could lead to claim denials because the notes are not specific enough. They do not demonstrate why services were necessary on each day of service or why they were required by an individual patient. Regional contractors such as Palmetto GBA have warned that if cloned records are detected, it could result in denial of services for lack of medical necessity and recoupment of all overpayments made.

Alternatively, there is the problem of using "spinner" or "random text generator" software to produce "cloned records with a difference." With a spinner, the order of the words is switched around and synonyms are commonly substituted. In many healthcare fields, where patients often receive similar treatments, spinners save time but could create documentation problems.

Notes should be patient specific for each date of service, and as detailed as possible. Factors that should be taken into account should be:

- Age
- Severity of condition
- Past response to treatment
- Frequency of treatment
- Complicating factors

Again, it is important to demonstrate why the service was necessary on that particular day.

The Department of Health and Human Services (HHS) previously issued a letter condemning "cloning" software and EHR software which inappropriately up-code documentation. They said, "False documentation of care is not just bad patient care; it is illegal." As a result, they are now more closely scrutinizing medical records.

 Resource: See Resource 374 to read this letter in its entirety.

Guidelines for Corrections

Sometimes the patient record needs to be corrected. This is acceptable as long as the change is clearly indicated as such. Paper records will need to include the date of the change along with your initials. EHR software has a different process for corrections depending on the program being used. A medical record should not be changed if it is subpoenaed for possible legal action. Any alterations at this time could damage the physician's credibility in court. Most attorneys would rather defend a physician with no medical record than defend a physician with an inappropriately altered record.

- It is important that corrections only be in the form of additions.
- There must be no erasures, white-out or overwriting on the record, such that the original entry is lost.
- To make additions or corrections to a paper record, draw a single line through inaccurate or incorrect information to make sure a reviewer can still read it, write in the correction, and then date and initial [or sign] it.
- Add omitted information chronologically by the date the information is actually entered in the chart.
- When necessary, attach an addendum with additional information, such as accidentally left out documentation of a procedures step. These chart entries should include a separate signature with a time and date stamp.

Illustrations

Drawings, illustrations, and pictures may be used when appropriate. These are effective methods of medical shorthand which can quickly and clearly demonstrate the location of a symptom or verify a completed service. Illustrations may be hand-drawn or be commercially purchased illustrations. The chart should include the patient's name, date of birth, medical record number, and date. The physician's signature is an appropriate confirmation. Utilizing initials may be insufficient, especially if there is more than one provider in the clinic with the same initials.

Subjective Judgments and Statements

Patient medical information should be entered in an objective manner. Personal opinion and subjective judgment about the patient or the patient's behavior have no place in the medical record. A patient who is slurring, staggering, and smells of alcohol should not be labeled as intoxicated unless a blood test establishes this fact. As an alternative, describe the patient with objective statements about the way the person speaks, walks, and smells. Some medical conditions are misleading. For example, ketoacidosis, which can occur in patients with diabetes, can cause symptoms similar to intoxication.

Avoid any written or verbal statements which could be interpreted as a guarantee. Rather than stating that the "patient will recover 100%," or "60% of patients see improvement," it is more appropriate to state that "improvement is anticipated with the recommended treatment plan."

Communications and Unusual Circumstances

All interactions between a patient and staff members (physician, receptionist, other staff) that could potentially affect the patient's care should be recorded in the patient chart. This includes not only patient/staff conversations, but also less obvious interactions such as a staff member overhearing a patient express unwillingness to follow the physician's treatment plan. What may seem like an offhand comment should be recorded because the patient's intent not to follow the physician's instructions has the potential to impact future care. In addition, any unusual circumstance, such as a patient who does not speak English, uses a wheelchair, or is uncooperative, may influence the patient's medical care and therefore should be documented.

Telephone calls between the patient and staff, cancellations, and no shows should also be documented. If there should be a legal action for a bad outcome, the healthcare provider will be in a much better position when it can be shown that the patient did not show up for appointments or follow the recommended course of treatment.

Abbreviations

Utilizing standardized abbreviations can help to lessen the time required to write daily visit notes. The notes need to be readable to any medical professional that should need to review them, so it is wise to limit your abbreviations to those that are common in the health care professions. If you do develop our own set of abbreviations, you need to provide a key.

Common acronyms and abbreviations are listed below:

symbol	meaning
A	assessment
@	at
a. c.	before eating
c̄	with
CC	chief complaint
cm	centimeter
D	day

symbol	meaning
NKMA	no known medical allergies
p̄	after
P	plan
p. c.	after eating
PE	physical examination
PMH	past medical history
PMI	point of maximum intensity

symbol	meaning
Disp	disposition
DOB	date of birth
Dx	diagnosis
E/M	evaluation and management
Fx	fracture
HPI	history of present illness
ht	height
HTN	hypertension
Hx	history
Ⓛ	left
LE	lower extremity
MCL	midclavicular line

symbol	meaning
PRN	as needed for
Pt	patient
Ⓡ	right
R/O	rule out
ROS	review of systems
s̄	without
SOB	shortness of breath
Sx	sign/symptom
Tx	treatment
WNL	within normal limits
Wt	weight
x̄	except

Transitioning from Active Care

At some point during the subsequent treatment visits, the patient will no longer require active or continuing care. For example, they may have reached their optimum level of improvement or they may need to be referred to another provider.

Most third party payers do not cover situations where the patient is not progressing. At each visit, progress should be assessed. If there is no improvement over a reasonable period of time, or no further improvement could be reasonably anticipated, then the patient either discontinues care, moves into a maintenance care situation, or they need to be referred to another provider.

Referrals

There are many different types of referrals. When making or receiving referrals, carefully follow payer specific provider referral requirements. The following are some situations in which the patient may be referred:

- Second opinions (e.g., specialty consultations) to obtain assistance in properly diagnosing a patient whose clinical presentation is unclear
- Concurrent care for the condition being treated (e.g., physical therapy, massage therapy)
- Recommendations to seek concurrent care for unrelated conditions (e.g., primary care provider, mental health counseling)
- Transferring care to another provider

Maintenance Care

When the patient's chief complaint has been addressed, he/she may want to continue treatment to maintain their current state. These types of visits should not be confused with annual wellness visits, rather, they are for the purpose of avoiding regression or deterioration of a condition. These maintenance visits may be clinically indicated for certain illnesses; however, coverage for these types of visits depends on the payer and/or the diagnosis so be aware of differences in payer policies.

The documentation for these visits needs to clearly identify the type of care being provided. For Medicare patients, when the provider knows that the care is likely to be non-covered, it is important to include a signed *ABN* in the patient chart.

Book: See the segment "Medicare Coverage" in Chapter 2.1 — Medicare Essentials for more about the *ABN*.

Tip: If maintenance care is recommended, it may be necessary to update your diagnosis as you begin a new treatment plan. Please note that most payers do not cover maintenance treatment/visits unless certain limited conditions are met. Unless there is a supplemental policy that requires a denial, do NOT bill the third party for non-covered maintenance services.

The Treatment Plan

After the healthcare provider has conducted a thorough history and physical examination, and ordered the relevant studies (such as lab testing or x-rays), the next step is to create a treatment plan. It is very difficult to defend treatment denials from third party payers when there are no plans or goals for the outcome of care. If you needed to build a house, you would have to select a blueprint, order materials, hire a contractor, etc. The house would never come together if you just started pounding nails into boards haphazardly. Likewise, third-party payers want to see that there is a plan for patient improvement, and perhaps even more importantly, a way to measure that improvement. Treatment plans and outcomes assessments are integral components of both the initial evaluation and subsequent re-evaluations.

The proper documentation of a treatment plan cannot be overemphasized. Claims reviewers are looking for a treatment plan when they request records. Without a viable treatment plan, the care provided may be considered medically unnecessary and will likely result in a denial. Another important reason for a well-documented treatment plan is to help establish the clinical reasoning or thought process behind the care given. If the healthcare provider does not include the treatment plan in the clinical record, he/she cannot say that the plan is being followed. Keep in mind that a treatment plan should never be set in stone. Rather, it is a dynamic program that should frequently change based on the patient's progress. Because of its dynamic nature, medical reviewers look negatively on static, non-customized treatment plans.

This plan need not be lengthy, however, it needs to be relevant, timely, and thorough. Thorough does not mean all of your time is spent doing treatment plans. There are many treatment planners and treatment plan software programs on the market. Choose the one(s) which best fits the needs of your practice.

> **Alert — Software Caution**
> In some cases, lawyers have successfully argued in court that not much time or thought went into the treatment plan if the same plan is used for every patient with the same diagnosis. Their argument is that this demonstrates the provider was not giving the best treatment possible. Software programs should be able to let you customize a treatment plan. Customize any provided templates to reflect the patient's unique clinical needs.
>
> **Tip:** Some payers may require the use of their own special form for treatment plans. Verify individual payer requirements before submitting plans.

Effective Treatment Plan Components

Different payers may have different requirements or policies related to treatment plans which may vary depending on the condition(s) being treated. innoviHealth recommends including each of the following elements for an effective plan:

- Treatments selected – Which treatment options were discussed and why they were selected?
- Recommended level of care (duration and frequency of visits) – How long and how often are you going to see the patient?
- Specific treatment goals – What are you trying to accomplish?

- Objective measures to evaluate treatment effectiveness – How do you know when you have accomplished the goal(s)?
- Patient tasks – What tasks or activities is the patient responsible to complete?

 Tip: Don't forget to document that the patient has signed an informed consent document regarding the treatment plan prior to the initiation of treatment. See Chapter 1.1 — Insurance & Reimbursement Essentials for more information.

Prognosis

A prognosis is an important component of treatment goals. This is a forecast of the probable result of treatment for a patient's condition. Be sure to include specific concerns regarding the patient, including non-compliance. A prognosis may be classified into the following types.

1. Excellent – Full symptomatic and functional recovery is expected.
2. Good – Symptomatic and functional recovery is expected.
3. Fair – The patient can expect to have a reduction of their symptom(s), although complete recovery is not necessarily indicated.
4. Guarded – The patient's prognosis is unknown due to extenuating factors, including potential inability to follow treatment protocol.
5. Poor – The nature of the patient's condition(s) (e.g., severity, etc.) bring into doubt the likelihood of full recovery.

The prognosis may be updated at each re-evaluation as the provider's assessment changes, based on the information gathered. This may lead to a revised treatment plan.

Evidence Based Treatment Planning

Payers are increasingly requiring providers to create care plans using the best available evidence. When providers and payers rely on the same evidence, reviews should become more impartial. When following evidence-based treatment planning standards, once an initial diagnostic assessment has been established, a care plan must be formulated for every condition. It should include the estimated duration and frequency of care, indicated modalities and procedures, exercise/rehabilitation recommendations, instructions regarding activities of daily living, prognosis, and the establishment of any total or partial disability period.

Assessment of the patient will become more refined and streamlined to reflect clinical changes in response to care which can be measured (e.g., patient questionnaire). This is the language that payers expect when assessing medical necessity. Providers who understand and communicate clearly in this language will minimize claims delays and denials.

The benefits of this approach transcends mere cost savings, as the ultimate benefactor to the public and patient through the delivery of high quality value-based care that is provided in a clinically efficient and effective manner.

Outcomes Assessment Tools (OATs)

An important key element to an effective treatment plan is the proper use of outcomes assessment tools (or questionnaires) to measure functional loss and gains. This is because they help to establish reliable, objective measures which make them effective communication methods for the patient record.

There are many outcomes assessment tools and systems available (e.g., disorder specific severity measures, disability measures, personality inventories, etc.) These patient assessment measures were developed to be administered at the initial patient interview and to monitor treatment progress, which helps the provider to determine:

- initial symptomatic status,
- patient reported outcome (PRO) information, and
- severity.

Be aware of individual payer requirements. For example, some government programs have compiled their own lists of recommended OATs for specific conditions and the reporting of these OATs are required for quality based reimbursement.

Notes:

Notes:

4.2 Provider Documentation Training

Codes provide valuable information which claims reviewers can use to determine if the care provided is medically necessary. However, code selection can only be as good as the medical record which was used to select them. Documentation has many functions, but, for the provider, one of the most significant roles may be its relationship to reimbursement. This chapter is limited to discussing diagnosis code documentation standards.

Store: For information on properly documenting Evaluation and Management visits, see innoviHealth's *Comprehensive Guide to Evaluation & Management*.

Book: See Chapter 4.1 — Documentation Essentials for a more complete discussion on how to properly document the patient encounter in order to establish medical necessity.

Figure 4.2

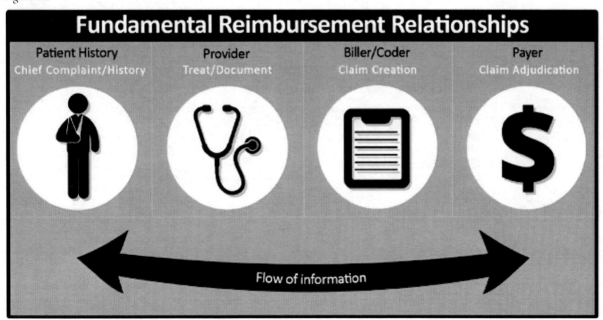

Figure 4.2 depicts the relationship between the parties involved in the healthcare reimbursement process. It all begins with an encounter, initiated by a patient who seeks care. The patient presents with a chief complaint and provides a health history. This information then becomes part of the healthcare record and the provider begins to document all relevant information regarding the patient and provide care. If someone were to review the record created by the provider, and interview the patient, the information should match.

Next, it is the responsibility of a biller and/or coder to translate the information from the medical record into a claim (paper or electronic). Ideally, the codes chosen will match exactly what was documented, which in turn matches what actually happened to the patient during the encounter. In order for this to happen, and the entire process to flow smoothly, both the provider and the biller must understand coding rules, descriptions, and documentation requirements. This publication was designed with that goal in mind. "*Provider Documentation Guides™*" which are explained in this chapter, help to accomplish that goal. Finally, the claim form with all the right codes goes to the payer. The payer then applies their payment policies, which ideally, are satisfied by the information found on the submitted claim. In some cases, the payer might request additional information from either the provider or the patient. With proper communication between all of these groups, additional requests for information should be minimal.

Provider Documentation Guides (PDGs)

innoviHealth formulated a method for helping providers become proficient with the ICD-10-CM documentation and coding requirements for the conditions they encounter most often. The process, which we call a *Provider Documentation Guide (PDG)*, is explained here and can be used with any ICD-10-CM code. It is a one to two page summary of all the components a provider and coder need to know to properly document and code a condition. Each *PDG* is like a ready-made ten minute training session, which could be used in weekly office meetings to improve both ICD-10-CM documentation and code selection.

The following items are all included in each *Provider Documentation Guide*:

1. The condition (i.e., diagnosis), including the ICD-10-CM code or code range
2. Helpful information (e.g., terminology, what to document, list for the provider, and notes for the coder)
3. Applicable instructional notes/guidelines and indicator(s) at the chapter and block levels
4. Information conveyed by each character level with instructional notes, guidelines, and indicators applicable at the category and subcategory levels

The above information is presented in each *PDG* in order to facilitate correct documentation to support the diagnoses reported. When a patient presents with the condition, the *PDG* acts as a tool to help the provider ensure that all the necessary information is documented. It also serves as a guide to coders/billers by providing the correct codes for the diagnosis, as well as all of the relevant guidelines and terminology associated with the code description. Without a *PDG*, it would be necessary to thoroughly review multiple pages of the Tabular List and guidelines to locate all of the pertinent information. As an example, the following segment explains two complete *PDGs* in detail.

 Alert: The two examples presented here are for training purposes. While they may not be relevant to your practice, they cover the information contained in innoviHealth's Provider Documentation Guides. See Appendix C — Provider Documentation Guides for specialty-specific guides.

Item 1: Condition and Codes

The first item to identify is the condition, which serves as the title. The terms within the title can be based on common names for the condition, the exact medical term, or most often, the coategory of the codes this *PDG's* range covers.

Also included in the first item is the ICD-10-CM code or code range. Most *PDGs* cover several diagnoses, often grouping together laterality and anatomic site codes for more convenient access.

Diabetes Mellitus Type 1 with Neurologic Complications

ICD-10-CM: E10.40 - E10.49

Atypical Femoral Fracture

ICD-10-CM: M84.750A - M84.759S

Item 2: Helpful Information

This section of the *PDG* compiles helpful information for both the provider and the coder. It can include a documentation checklist for the provider, relevant terminology now required in ICD-10-CM, a brief description of what needs to be documented in order to support a code fully, and any critical guidelines. This section is designed to clarify information regarding the documentation of the codes in the range.

Atypical Femoral Fracture	Diabetes Mellitus Type 1 with Neurologic Complications
What to Document	**What to Document**
4th Character: Type of nontraumatic fracture 6th Character: Complete/incomplete, type of fracture, and laterality 7th Character: Episode of care and healing status **Document:** -External cause, if any **Terminology:** **Atypical fracture:** A type of fracture that has specific radiological features and could potentially be associated with long-term use of bisphosphonates in patients with osteoporosis. Sometimes referred to as "Fossamax fractures." **Complete fractures:** A complete break, one that goes completely across the bone, causing it to be separated into two or more fragments. **Incomplete fracture:** A partial fracture of a bone, where the bone is broken but still connected as in Greenstick, torus, or buckle fractures. **Transverse fracture:** A fracture that extends across the bone in a horizontal fashion. **Oblique fracture:** A fracture that extends across the bone diagonally.	3rd Character: Type and etiology of diabetes 4th Character: Organ system affected, if any 5th Character: Complications affecting the organ system **Document:** -Functional activity, if any **Terminology:** **Mononeuropathy:** Damage to a nerve outside of the brain and spinal cord, usually caused by an injury. **Polyneuropathy:** Degeneration of general peripheral nerves spreading toward the center of the body. **Autonomic polyneuropathy:** Damage to nerves that causes disruption in areas of the autonomic nervous system that manage daily body functions, such as blood vessels, heart, sweat glands, blood pressure, intestines, pupils, bladder, etc. **Amyotrophy:** Breakdown of muscle tissues.

For some conditions, this summary may be all that is needed. Others may require using more of the information contained in later sections of the *PDG* in order to create a record that completely supports the diagnosis. Tips and definitions can be especially helpful for beginners or coders who lack sufficient training in anatomy or pathology.

Item 3: Applicable Guidelines at the Chapter and Block Levels

The next piece of a *PDG* summarizes the relevant instructional notes/guidelines at the chapter and block levels.

Atypical Femoral Fracture

Chapter Guidelines

13. Diseases of the musculoskeletal system and connective tissue (M00-M99)

Notes:
  Use an external cause code following the code for the musculoskeletal condition, if applicable, to identify the cause of the musculoskeletal condition

Excludes2:
  arthropathic psoriasis (L40.5-)
  certain conditions originating in the perinatal period (P04-P96)
  certain infectious and parasitic diseases (A00-B99)
  compartment syndrome (traumatic) (T79.A-)
  complications of pregnancy, childbirth and the puerperium (O00-O9A)
  congenital malformations, deformations, and chromosomal abnormalities (Q00-Q99)
  endocrine, nutritional and metabolic diseases (E00-E88)
  injury, poisoning and certain other consequences of external causes (S00-T88)
  neoplasms (C00-D49)
  symptoms, signs and abnormal clinical and laboratory findings, not elsewhere classified (R00-R94)

OSTEOPATHIES & CHONDROPATHIES (M80-M94)

DISORDERS OF BONE DENSITY & STRUCTURE (M80-M85)

For the Atypical Femoral Fracture *PDG*, there are no instructional notes/guidelines at the block levels. However, there are instructional notes/guidelines that apply to any code in Chapter 13. The "Notes" specify how to report an external cause code in more detail than is provided in Item 2 above. The Excludes2 notes also apply to any Chapter 13 code.

Diabetes Mellitus Type 1 with Neurologic Complications

Chapter Guidelines

4. Endocrine, nutritional and metabolic diseases (E00-E89)

Notes:
  All neoplasms, whether functionally active or not, are classified in Chapter 2. Appropriate codes in this chapter (i.e. E05.8, E07.0, E16-E31, E34.-) may be used as additional codes to indicate either functional activity by neoplasms and ectopic endocrine tissue or hyperfunction and hypofunction of endocrine glands associated with neoplasms and other conditions classified elsewhere.

Excludes1:
  transitory endocrine and metabolic disorders specific to newborn (P70-P74)

DIABETES MELLITUS (E08-E13)

See Guidelines: 1;C.15.g

For the Diabetes Mellitus Type 1 with Neurological Complications *PDG*, the "Note" and Excludes1 note applies to codes in Chapter 4. The "Notes" provide more detail on the meaning of "Functional activity, if any" in Item 2.

The "See Guidelines" is applicable to the block of codes from E08-E13. To ensure proper reporting, the cited guidelines may need to be referenced.

Store: See innoviHealth's *ICD-10-CM Coding* books for easy to read Official ICD-10-CM guidelines.

Items 4–8: Third, Fourth, Fifth, Sixth, and Seventh Character Information

These remaining sections go into detail about each character in the code. Each of these sections will contain:

- A restatement of what needs to be documented.

- Any applicable instructional notes/guidelines. Remember that instructional notes/guidelines showing up at one level (e.g., category, subcategory) apply to all downstream codes. In other words, an instructional note/guideline appearing at the category level applies at the subcategory and code levels as well.

- A list of all the possible categories, subcategories, or codes for a given character; the one that narrows the code choices toward the ICD-10-CM code for the condition will be highlighted.

If a seventh character exists for a given code or group of codes, highlighting may only occur to the fifth or sixth character, followed by a list of character options to choose from. This allows the provider or individual using the *PDG* to see all the codes affected on one *PDG*, rather than spread across multiple *PDGs*.

Each *PDG* will have a section for all seven characters, even if they are not used, as a way to standardize the look of *PDGs* and help the provider ensure that all necessary information has been documented.

Third Character Information
Atypical Femoral Fracture

3rd Character

Document: Type and etiology of diabetes

E08-	Diabetes mellitus due to underlying condition
E09-	Drug or chemical induced diabetes mellitus
E10-	Type 1 diabetes mellitus
E11-	Type 2 diabetes mellitus
E13-	Other specified diabetes mellitus

Diabetes Mellitus Type 1 with Neurologic Complications

3rd Character

M80-	Osteoporosis with current pathological fracture
M81-	Osteoporosis without current pathological fracture
M83-	Adult osteomalacia
M84-	Disorder of continuity of bone
M85-	Other disorders of bone density and structure

Neither *PDG* contains any additional instructional notes at the category level. The highlighting directs to the fourth character options. Whenever there is a hyphen, it means that more characters are required to form a complete code.

Fourth Character Information

Atypical Femoral Fracture

4th Character

Document: Type of nontraumatic fracture

Excludes2:
traumatic fracture of bone-see fracture, by site

M84.3- Stress fracture
M84.4- Pathological fracture, not elsewhere classified
M84.5- Pathological fracture in neoplastic disease
M84.6- Pathological fracture in other disease
M84.7- Nontraumatic fracture, not elsewhere classified
M84.8- Other disorders of continuity of bone
M84.9 Disorder of continuity of bone, unspecified

For the Atypical Femoral Fracture *PDG*, we have another Excludes2 note that applies to any code beginning with M84-.

The highlighted subcategory, M84.7-, directs to the fifth character options for the diagnosis.

M84.9 "Disorder of continuity of bone, unspecified" is a complete code, indicated by the bold font. *PDGs* are, in part, designed to avoid selecting unspecified codes so don't simply choose the first bold code in the *PDG* if the documentation points to a more specific code.

Diabetes Mellitus Type 1 with Neurologic Complications

4th Character

Document: Organ system affected, if any

Includes:
brittle diabetes (mellitus)
diabetes (mellitus) due to autoimmune process
diabetes (mellitus) due to immune mediated pancreatic islet beta-cell destruction
idiopathic diabetes (mellitus)
juvenile onset diabetes (mellitus)
ketosis-prone diabetes (mellitus)
Excludes1:
diabetes mellitus due to underlying condition (E08.-)
drug or chemical induced diabetes mellitus (E09.-)
gestational diabetes (O24.4-)
hyperglycemia NOS (R73.9)
neonatal diabetes mellitus (P70.2)
postpancreatectomy diabetes mellitus (E13.-)
postprocedural diabetes mellitus (E13.-)
secondary diabetes mellitus NEC (E13.-)
type 2 diabetes mellitus (E11.-)

E10.1- Type 1 diabetes mellitus with ketoacidosis
E10.2- Type 1 diabetes mellitus with kidney complications
E10.3- Type 1 diabetes mellitus with ophthalmic complications
E10.4- Type 1 diabetes mellitus with neurological complications
E10.5- Type 1 diabetes mellitus with circulatory complications
E10.6- Type 1 diabetes mellitus with other specified complications
E10.8 Type 1 diabetes mellitus with unspecified complications
E10.9 Type 1 diabetes mellitus without complications

For the Diabetes Mellitus Type 1 with Neurological Complications *PDG*, the Includes and Excludes1 notes apply to the codes beginning with E10-.

E10.4- is highlighted, so the fifth characters shown in the next box apply to codes beginning with E10.4-.

E10.8 and **E10.9** are complete codes, indicated by the bold font. Again, avoid using unspecified codes when possible.

Fifth Character Information

Atypical Femoral Fracture

5th Character

Indicator(s): CC (7th A/K/P), POAEx (7th D/G/K/P/S)

M84.75- Atypical femoral fracture

For the Atypical Femoral Fracture *PDG*, there is only one option for the fifth character.

Note the indicators, as they point to the correct seventh character extension to use in different situations.

Book: See *Figure F.1* in Appendix F — Coding Reference Tables for a table of all the indicators that can be seen in a *PDG*.

Diabetes Mellitus Type 1 with Neurologic Complications

5th Character

Document: Complications affecting the organ system

Indicator(s): CMS22: 18 | CMS23: 18 | CMS24: 18 | RxØ5: 3Ø | HHSØ4: 2Ø | HHSØ5: 2Ø

0   diabetic neuropathy, unspecified
1   diabetic mononeuropathy
2   diabetic polyneuropathy
      Including: neuralgia
3   diabetic autonomic (poly)neuropathy
      Including: gastroparesis
4   diabetic amyotrophy
9   other complication

For the Diabetes Mellitus Type 1 with Neurological Complications *PDG*, the fifth character is the final character for E10.4- codes. Just take the correct fifth character and add it on to E10.4-. For example, if the documentation indicated the patient had diabetic neuralgia, the final code would be **E10.42** "Type 1 diabetes mellitus with diabetic polyneuropathy."

The indicator conveys the various HCC categories in the different HCC models the code belongs to.

Book: See *Figure F.3* in Appendix F — Coding Reference Tables for a list of HCC codes and descriptions.

Store: See innoviHealth's *ICD-10-CM Coding for Risk Adjustment/HCC* for more information on Hierarchical Condition Category coding.

Sixth Character Information

Atypical Femoral Fracture

6th Character

Document: Complete/incomplete, type of fracture, and laterality

> *The appropriate 7th character is to be added to each code from M84.75:*
> *A - initial encounter for fracture*
> *D - subsequent encounter for fracture with routine healing*
> *G - subsequent encounter for fracture with delayed healing*
> *K - subsequent encounter for fracture with nonunion*
> *P - subsequent encounter for fracture with malunion*
> *S - sequela*

0   unspecified
1- Incomplete right leg
2- Incomplete left leg
3- Incomplete unspecified leg
4- Complete transverse right leg
5- Complete transverse left leg
6- Complete transverse unspecified leg
7- Complete oblique right leg
8- Complete oblique left leg
9- Complete oblique unspecified leg

For the Atypical Femoral Fracture *PDG*, the gray box provides the list of seventh character extensions, which will also be shown under "7th Character" below.

The sixth character options will follow M84.75-, and all of these sixth characters will be followed by one of the seventh characters in the gray box

Tip: When a *PDG* stops highlighting characters, it means that the characters in the next section apply to any of the character options. So, in the case to the left, whether selecting 0, 1, 2, etc. as the sixth character, the seventh character options remain the same. This can occur for up to 4 character sections at a time.

Diabetes Mellitus Type 1 with Neurologic Complications

6th Character

N/A

The diabetes *PDG* ends at the fifth character, there are no sixth (or seventh) character options.

Seventh Character Information

Atypical Femoral Fracture

7th Character

Document: Episode of care and healing status

A initial encounter
D subsequent encounter with routine healing
G subsequent encounter with delayed healing
K subsequent encounter with nonunion
P subsequent encounter with malunion
S sequela

The Atypical Femoral Fracture *PDG* has six options for the seventh character extension. Select the one that applies.

Diabetes Mellitus Type 1 with Neurologic Complications

7th Character

N/A

The diabetes *PDG* ends at the fifth character, there are no seventh (or sixth) character options.

Diabetes Mellitus Type 1 with Neurologic Complications

ICD-10-CM: E10.40 – E10.49

What to Document

3rd Character: Type and etiology of diabetes
4th Character: Organ system affected, if any
5th Character: Complications affecting the organ system

Document:
-Functional activity, if any

Terminology:
Mononeuropathy: Damage to a nerve outside of the brain and spinal cord, usually caused by an injury.
Polyneuropathy: Degeneration of general peripheral nerves spreading toward the center of the body.
Autonomic polyneuropathy: Damage to nerves that causes disruption in areas of the autonomic nervous system that manage daily body functions, such as blood vessels, heart, sweat glands, blood pressure, intestines, pupils, bladder, etc.
Amyotrophy: Breakdown of muscle tissues.

Chapter Guidelines

4. Endocrine, nutritional and metabolic diseases (E00-E89)

Notes:
All neoplasms, whether functionally active or not, are classified in Chapter 2. Appropriate codes in this chapter (i.e. E05.8, E07.0, E16-E31, E34.-) may be used as additional codes to indicate either functional activity by neoplasms and ectopic endocrine tissue or hyperfunction and hypofunction of endocrine glands associated with neoplasms and other conditions classified elsewhere.

Excludes1:
transitory endocrine and metabolic disorders specific to newborn (P70-P74)

DIABETES MELLITUS (E08-E13)

See Guidelines: 1;C.15.g

3rd Character

Document: Type and etiology of diabetes

- E08- Diabetes mellitus due to underlying condition
- E09- Drug or chemical induced diabetes mellitus
- **E10- Type 1 diabetes mellitus**
- E11- Type 2 diabetes mellitus
- E13- Other specified diabetes mellitus

4th Character

Document: Organ system affected, if any

Includes:
brittle diabetes (mellitus)
diabetes (mellitus) due to autoimmune process
diabetes (mellitus) due to immune mediated pancreatic islet beta-cell destruction
idiopathic diabetes (mellitus)
juvenile onset diabetes (mellitus)
ketosis-prone diabetes (mellitus)

Excludes1:
diabetes mellitus due to underlying condition (E08.-)
drug or chemical induced diabetes mellitus (E09.-)
gestational diabetes (O24.4-)
hyperglycemia NOS (R73.9)
neonatal diabetes mellitus (P70.2)
postpancreatectomy diabetes mellitus (E13.-)
postprocedural diabetes mellitus (E13.-)
secondary diabetes mellitus NEC (E13.-)
type 2 diabetes mellitus (E11.-)

- E10.1- Type 1 diabetes mellitus with ketoacidosis
- E10.2- Type 1 diabetes mellitus with kidney complications
- E10.3- Type 1 diabetes mellitus with ophthalmic complications
- **E10.4- Type 1 diabetes mellitus with neurological complications**
- E10.5- Type 1 diabetes mellitus with circulatory complications
- E10.6- Type 1 diabetes mellitus with other specified complications
- E10.8 Type 1 diabetes mellitus with unspecified complications
- E10.9 Type 1 diabetes mellitus without complications

5th Character

Document: Complications affecting the organ system

Indicator(s): CMS22: 18 | CMS23: 18 | CMS24: 18 | RxO5: 30 | HHS04: 20 | HHS05: 20

- 0 diabetic neuropathy, unspecified
- 1 diabetic mononeuropathy
- 2 diabetic polyneuropathy
    Including: neuralgia
- 3 diabetic autonomic (poly)neuropathy
    Including: gastroparesis
- 4 diabetic amyotrophy
- 9 other complication

Diabetes Mellitus Type 1 with Neurologic Complications (continued)

6th Character
N/A

7th Character
N/A

Notes

Atypical Femoral Fracture

ICD-10-CM: M84.750A - M84.759S

What to Document

4th Character: Type of nontraumatic fracture
6th Character: Complete/incomplete, type of fracture, and laterality
7th Character: Episode of care and healing status

Document:
-External cause, if any

Terminology:
Atypical fracture: A type of fracture that has specific radiological features and could potentially be associated with long-term use of bisphosphonates in patients with osteoporosis. Sometimes referred to as "Fossamax fractures."
Complete fractures: A complete break, one that goes completely across the bone, causing it to be separated into two or more fragments.
Incomplete fracture: A partial fracture of a bone, where the bone is broken but still connected as in Greenstick, torus, or buckle fractures.
Transverse fracture: A fracture that extends across the bone in a horizontal fashion.
Oblique fracture: A fracture that extends across the bone diagonally.

Chapter Guidelines

13. Diseases of the musculoskeletal system and connective tissue (M00-M99)

Notes:
Use an external cause code following the code for the musculoskeletal condition, if applicable, to identify the cause of the musculoskeletal condition

Excludes2:
arthropathic psoriasis (L40.5-)
certain conditions originating in the perinatal period (P04-P96)
certain infectious and parasitic diseases (A00-B99)
compartment syndrome (traumatic) (T79.A-)
complications of pregnancy, childbirth and the puerperium (O00-O9A)
congenital malformations, deformations, and chromosomal abnormalities (Q00-Q99)
endocrine, nutritional and metabolic diseases (E00-E88)
injury, poisoning and certain other consequences of external causes (S00-T88)
neoplasms (C00-D49)
symptoms, signs and abnormal clinical and laboratory findings, not elsewhere classified (R00-R94)

OSTEOPATHIES AND CHONDROPATHIES (M80-M94)

DISORDERS OF BONE DENSITY AND STRUCTURE (M80-M85)

3rd Character

M80- Osteoporosis with current pathological fracture
M81- Osteoporosis without current pathological fracture
M83- Adult osteomalacia
M84- Disorder of continuity of bone
M85- Other disorders of bone density and structure

4th Character

Document: Type of nontraumatic fracture

Excludes2:
traumatic fracture of bone-see fracture, by site

M84.3- Stress fracture
M84.4- Pathological fracture, not elsewhere classified
M84.5- Pathological fracture in neoplastic disease
M84.6- Pathological fracture in other disease
M84.7- Nontraumatic fracture, not elsewhere classified
M84.8- Other disorders of continuity of bone
M84.9 Disorder of continuity of bone, unspecified

5th Character

Indicator(s): CC (7th A/K/P), POAEx (7th D/G/K/P/S)

M84.75- Atypical femoral fracture

6th Character

Document: Complete/incomplete, type of fracture, and laterality

> *The appropriate 7th character is to be added to each code from M84.75:*
> *A - initial encounter for fracture*
> *D - subsequent encounter for fracture with routine healing*
> *G - subsequent encounter for fracture with delayed healing*
> *K - subsequent encounter for fracture with nonunion*
> *P - subsequent encounter for fracture with malunion*
> *S - sequela*

0- unspecified
1- Incomplete right leg
2- Incomplete left leg

Atypical Femoral Fracture (continued)

6th Character (continued)
3- Incomplete unspecified leg
4- Complete transverse right leg
5- Complete transverse left leg
6- Complete transverse unspecified leg
7- Complete oblique right leg
8- Complete oblique left leg
9- Complete oblique unspecified leg

7th Character

Document: Episode of care and healing status

A   initial encounter
D   subsequent encounter with routine healing
G   subsequent encounter with delayed healing
K   subsequent encounter with nonunion
P   subsequent encounter with malunion
S   sequela

Diagnostic Statement

As indicated at the beginning of this chapter, using a Diagnostic Statement (sometimes called a Problem Statement, or Clinical Impression as part of an assessment) is another way to ensure a smooth flow of information between all parties involved in the Fundamental Reimbursement Relationships (*see Figure 4.2*).

Essentially, a Diagnostic Statement is a summary of the healthcare provider's impression of the patient history and exam findings, worded in a manner that anyone with an understanding of ICD-10-CM can easily find what they are looking for when auditing a record, regardless of their level of familiarity of terms and phrases used within your specialty. The Diagnostic Statement, included in an initial report, clearly identifies which codes apply to the case.

A current issue arising from the use of electronic health records (EHRs) and electronic medical records (EMRs) is the replacement of the diagnostic statement with a bulleted diagnosis list and accompanying codes. The details of diagnosing the patient's condition and all the treatment options available to them is discussed in detail with the patient, but often, this information is not included in the documentation. The functionality of current EHR/EMR systems indirectly encourages the reporting of only a code and a diagnosis. The detail needed to show medical necessity and the provider's train of thought are lost in this process. The diagnostic statement (or clinical impression) identifies medical necessity and the provider's thought process in developing a diagnosis and treating it.

Note: It is a mistake to assume that a Diagnostic Statement includes *only* objective information. Many ICD-10-CM codes, such as symptom codes or external cause codes, are based on the patient history and other subjective information. The purpose of the Diagnostic Statement is to make the diagnosis code documentation easy to find and evaluate while still accurately representing the patient's condition.

The following Clinical Example provides a framework for understanding why a Diagnostic Statement is helpful. It is not intended to be a complete record, rather it only includes relevant information for the purpose of demonstrating the ICD-10-CM diagnosis code selection process and the creation of a Diagnostic Statement. It begins with "Relevant History" and "Relevant Exam Findings" for the codes selected.

Figure 4.3

Clinical Example

CC: Patient brought in by parents because of increased irritability, agitation and aggression in their 10 year old child.

Relevant History: Patient has been this way since a young age. Previously diagnosed with depression and ADHD and is currently being treated with 20 mg Prozac. Things have been getting worse over last couple of months, particularly the last couple of weeks since learning that his Grandma has cancer. These symptoms are impacting peer interactions as patient is becoming more withdrawn and easily agitated when peers want to do something different than his desires. He has become more controlling in his peer relationships. Academically, his grades have dropped and he is struggling with schoolwork.

Relevant Exam Findings: Patient's appearance is adequately groomed and dressed. He appeared his stated age and there were no signs of sensory or motor problems. He describes his mood as anxious and denies any suicidal or homicidal ideation. His thought process is linear. He denies experiencing any auditory, visual or tactile hallucinations. He reports no delusions, paranoia or other perceptual disturbances. His sleep patterns are disrupted due to difficulty falling asleep for fears of being alone in the dark. His appetite is appropriate. His memory appears to be intact. Insight and judgment are considered fair.

> **Clinical Example (continued)**
>
> Codes that might be assigned to this case:
>
> F41.1   *Generalized anxiety disorder*
> F34.1   *Dysthymic disorder*
> Z63.79   *Other stressful life events affecting family and household*
> Z55.4   *Educational maladjustment and discord with teachers and classmates*
> Z86.59   *Personal history of other mental and behavioral disorders*
> F40.298 *Other specified phobia*

Though the documentation provided in *Figure 4.3* is sufficient to support the selected codes, it does not necessarily use the same vocabulary as the ICD-10-CM code set. Consequently, if an auditor were reviewing this documentation, it would be an arduous task for them to sift through the history and the exam findings and then compare it to the codes selected. This might require someone with clinical expertise in order to correctly correlate the sample documentation with the codes assigned.

To avoid potential misunderstandings and a breakdown in the flow of information, the provider can make it easier for others to review his or her notes by creating a Diagnostic Statement that specifically states which codes the healthcare provider deems appropriate to the case. *Figure 4.4* is an example of a Diagnostic Statement for this clinical example:

Figure 4.4

> **Diagnostic Statement:** Patient has a history of ADHD and suffers from generalized anxiety disorder and dysthymic disorder, complicated by a stressful life event. He has sleep disturbance due to phobia (fear of the dark) and is experiencing educational maladjustment

If the diagnosis information in a record is audited, the last thing a provider wants to do is explain themselves to the reviewer. If the provider can give the auditor exactly what they want, as long as it is an accurate reflection of the patient encounter, there will be no need for clarification and denials will be far less likely. That is the purpose of a well designed Diagnostic Statement.

> **Alert:** It is inappropriate to select diagnosis codes based solely on what will get the claim reimbursed. First and foremost, the diagnosis must be an accurate reflection of the patient's presentation, as depicted by *Figure 4.2 - Fundamental Reimbursement Relationships*. Medical necessity is the overarching criteria for claim payment. The Diagnostic Statement should accurately reflect the patient's condition and medical necessity for the treatment plan.

On the following pages, each code for this case will be reviewed one at a time. Compare the highlighted phrases from the History and Exam Findings to the highlighted phrases in the Diagnostic Statement. Note how they are converted into words that better match the code, but still reflect the patient presentation.

> **Store:** See innoviHealth's *Comprehensive Guide to Evaluation & Management* for more about the required elements of a psychiatric exam.

F34.1 "Dysthymic Disorder"

The Diagnostic Statement specifically mentions dysthymic disorder, whereas the history and exam provide the findings, but do not make the diagnosis obvious. The Relevant Exam Findings mention "previously diagnosed with depression," but they do not offer up any key terms to aid in code selection. Technically, a phrase such as "depression" is insufficient because the code does not identify the type or duration of the depression. This Diagnostic Statement identifies the type of depression. A competent audit or might be able to infer that information from the record, but the provider can make the note easier for a coder/auditor to approve if the provider simply aligns his or her documentation with the terms that the coder/auditor expects to see.

Clinical Example

Relevant History:

Patient has been this way since a young age. Previously diagnosed with depression and ADHD and is currently being treated with 20 mg Prozac. Things have been getting worse over last couple of months, particularly the last couple of weeks since learning that his Grandma has cancer. These symptoms are impacting peer interactions as patient is becoming more withdrawn and easily agitated when peers want to do something different than his desires. He has become more controlling in his peer relationships. Academically, his grades have dropped and he is struggling with schoolwork.

Relevant Exam Findings:

Patient's appearance is adequately groomed and dressed. He appeared his stated age and there were no signs of sensory or motor problems. He describes his mood as anxious and denies any suicidal or homicidal ideation. His thought process is linear. He denies experiencing any auditory, visual or tactile hallucinations. He reports no delusions, paranoia or other perceptual disturbances. His sleep patterns are disrupted due to difficulty falling asleep for fears of being alone in the dark. His appetite is appropriate. His memory appears to be intact. Insight and judgment are considered fair.

Codes that might be assigned to this case:

F34.1	Dysthymic disorder
F41.1	Generalized anxiety disorder
Z63.79	Other stressful life events affecting family and household
Z55.4	Educational maladjustment and discord with teachers and classmates
Z86.59	Personal history of other mental and behavioral disorders
F40.298	Other specified phobia

versus

Diagnostic Statement:

Patient has a history of ADHD and suffers from generalized anxiety disorder and dysthymic disorder, complicated by a stressful life event. He has sleep disturbance due to phobia (fear of the dark) and is experiencing educational maladjustment

F41.1 "Generalized Anxiety Disorder (GAD)"

The statement "Patient suffers from generalized anxiety and dysthymic disorder" is used in the Diagnostic Statement because those are the words associated with **F41.1** and **F34.1**. The Relevant History and Exam Findings support a diagnosis of "GAD," but they do not offer up any key terms to aid in code selection.

According to the diagnostic criteria of DSM-5, all of the following symptoms must be present:

- "Excessive anxiety and worry, occurring more days than not for at least 6 months, concerning a number of events;
- The individual finds it difficult to control the worry;
- The anxiety and worry are associated with at least three of the following six symptoms (only one item required in children):
  - Restlessness, feeling keyed up or on edge.
  - Being easily fatigued
  - Difficulty concentrating
  - Irritability
  - Muscle tension
  - Sleep disturbance
- The anxiety, worry or physical symptoms cause clinically significant distress or impairment in important areas of functioning;
- The disturbance is not due to the physiological effects of a substance or medical condition;
- The disturbance is not better explained by another medical disorder" (American Psychiatric Association).

(example on next page)

Clinical Example

Relevant History:

Patient has been this way since a young age. Previously diagnosed with depression and ADHD and is currently being treated with 20 mg Prozac. Things have been getting worse over last couple of months, particularly the last couple of weeks since learning that his Grandma has cancer. These symptoms are impacting peer interactions as patient is becoming more withdrawn and easily agitated when peers want to do something different than his desires. He has become more controlling in his peer relationships. Academically, his grades have dropped and he is struggling with schoolwork.

Relevant Exam Findings:

Patient's appearance is adequately groomed and dressed. He appeared his stated age and there were no signs of sensory or motor problems. He describes his mood as anxious and denies any suicidal or homicidal ideation. His thought process is linear. He denies experiencing any auditory, visual or tactile hallucinations. He reports no delusions, paranoia or other perceptual disturbances. His sleep patterns are disrupted due to difficulty falling asleep for fears of being alone in the dark. His appetite is appropriate. His memory appears to be intact. Insight and judgment are considered fair.

Codes that might be assigned to this case:

F34.1	*Dysthymic disorder*
F41.1	*Generalized anxiety disorder*
Z63.79	*Other stressful life events affecting family and household*
Z55.4	*Educational maladjustment and discord with teachers and classmates*
Z86.59	*Personal history of other mental and behavioral disorders*
F40.298	*Other specified phobia*

versus

Diagnostic Statement:

Patient has a history of ADHD and suffers from generalized anxiety disorder and dysthymic disorder, complicated by a stressful life event. He has sleep disturbance due to phobia (fear of the dark) and is experiencing educational maladjustment.

Z63.79 "Other stressful life events affecting family and household"

The History specifically mentions a significant life event "Grandma has cancer." In this case, this could be a contributing cause which may be exacerbating the other symptoms which are causing the patient to seek treatment. However, that particular piece of information is not included in ICD-10-CM terminology. As such, by adding the phrase "stressful life event," it makes it clear to the reviewer that this particular factor is influencing the status of the patient.

Clinical Example

Relevant History:

Patient has been this way since a young age. Previously diagnosed with depression and ADHD and is currently being treated with 20 mg Prozac. Things have been getting worse over last couple of months, particularly the last couple of weeks since learning that his Grandma has cancer. These symptoms are impacting peer interactions as patient is becoming more withdrawn and easily agitated when peers want to do something different than his desires. He has become more controlling in his peer relationships. Academically, his grades have dropped and he is struggling with schoolwork.

Relevant Exam Findings:

Patient's appearance is adequately groomed and dressed. He appeared his stated age and there were no signs of sensory or motor problems. He describes his mood as anxious and denies any suicidal or homicidal ideation. His thought process is linear. He denies experiencing any auditory, visual or tactile hallucinations. He reports no delusions, paranoia or other perceptual disturbances. His sleep patterns are disrupted due to difficulty falling asleep for fears of being alone in the dark. His appetite is appropriate. His memory appears to be intact. Insight and judgment are considered fair.

Codes that might be assigned to this case:

- F34.1 *Dysthymic disorder*
- F41.1 *Generalized anxiety disorder*
- Z63.79 *Other stressful life events affecting family and household*
- Z55.4 *Educational maladjustment and discord with teachers and classmates*
- Z86.59 *Personal history of other mental and behavioral disorders*
- F40.298 *Other specified phobia*

versus

Diagnostic Statement:

Patient has a history of ADHD and suffers from generalized anxiety disorder and dysthymic disorder, complicated by a stressful life event. He has sleep disturbance due to phobia (fear of the dark) and is experiencing educational maladjustment.

Z55.4 "Educational maladjustment and discord with teachers and classmates"

The History reports several indications that the patient is having trouble with school. It should be noted that the diagnostic criteria for General Anxiety Disorder states "The anxiety, worry or physical symptoms cause clinically significant distress or impairment in important areas of functioning" however, the problems with school are not completely tied to the anxiety disorder. If, as part of the treatment plan, the provider wishes to also address the academic problems, then the additional diagnosis supports the treatment plan.

Clinical Example

Relevant History:

Patient has been this way since a young age. Previously diagnosed with depression and ADHD and is currently being treated with 20 mg Prozac. Things have been getting worse over last couple of months, particularly the last couple of weeks since learning that his Grandma has cancer. These symptoms are impacting peer interactions as patient is becoming more withdrawn and easily agitated when peers want to do something different than his desires. He has become more controlling in his peer relationships. Academically, his grades have dropped and he is struggling with schoolwork.

Relevant Exam Findings:

Patient's appearance is adequately groomed and dressed. He appeared his stated age and there were no signs of sensory or motor problems. He describes his mood as anxious and denies any suicidal or homicidal ideation. His thought process is linear. He denies experiencing any auditory, visual or tactile hallucinations. He reports no delusions, paranoia or other perceptual disturbances. His sleep patterns are disrupted due to difficulty falling asleep for fears of being alone in the dark. His appetite is appropriate. His memory appears to be intact. Insight and judgment are considered fair.

Codes that might be assigned to this case:

- F34.1   *Dysthymic disorder*
- F41.1   *Generalized anxiety disorder*
- Z63.79 *Other stressful life events affecting family and household*
- Z55.4   *Educational maladjustment and discord with teachers and classmates*
- Z86.59 *Personal history of other mental and behavioral disorders*
- F40.298 *Other specified phobia*

versus

Diagnostic Statement:

Patient has a history of ADHD and suffers from generalized anxiety disorder and dysthymic disorder, complicated by a stressful life event. He has sleep disturbance due to phobia (fear of the dark) and is experiencing educational maladjustment.

Z86.59 "Personal history of other mental and behavioral disorders"

Personal history codes are used to document conditions that are not currently being treated, but which may require continued monitoring. The History states that the patient is being treated with medication more indicative of depressive than ADHD symptoms. Additionally, the documented symptoms in the Clinical Example do not appear to meet the criteria for ADHD. The provider is clearly not managing the ADHD at this encounter, however, it still needs to be monitored. The personal history code **Z86.59** is included here to indicate that information.

Clinical Example

Relevant History:

Patient has been this way since a young age. Previously diagnosed with depression and ADHD and is currently being treated with 20 mg Prozac. Things have been getting worse over last couple of months, particularly the last couple of weeks since learning that his Grandma has cancer. These symptoms are impacting peer interactions as patient is becoming more withdrawn and easily agitated when peers want to do something different than his desires. He has become more controlling in his peer relationships. Academically, his grades have dropped and he is struggling with schoolwork.

Relevant Exam Findings:

Patient's appearance is adequately groomed and dressed. He appeared his stated age and there were no signs of sensory or motor problems. He describes his mood as anxious and denies any suicidal or homicidal ideation. His thought process is linear. He denies experiencing any auditory, visual or tactile hallucinations. He reports no delusions, paranoia or other perceptual disturbances. His sleep patterns are disrupted due to difficulty falling asleep for fears of being alone in the dark. His appetite is appropriate. His memory appears to be intact. Insight and judgment are considered fair.

Codes that might be assigned to this case:

- F34.1 *Dysthymic disorder*
- F41.1 *Generalized anxiety disorder*
- Z63.79 *Other stressful life events affecting family and household*
- Z55.4 *Educational maladjustment and discord with teachers and classmates*
- Z86.59 *Personal history of other mental and behavioral disorders*
- F40.298 *Other specified phobia*

versus

Diagnostic Statement:

Patient has a history of ADHD and suffers from generalized anxiety disorder and dysthymic disorder, complicated by a stressful life event. He has sleep disturbance due to phobia (fear of the dark) and is experiencing educational maladjustment.

Website: FindACode.com offers a tool (available by subscription) called Code-A-Note™. Simply copy and paste the body of a note into this tool which then scans the note for potential code options in the ICD-10-CM, CPT, and HCPCS code sets. No Protected Health Information (PHI) is required or retained. It is a great tool when working with an unfamiliar specialty, or when trying to locate difficult codes.

Lessons from the Clinical Example

Provider Documentation Guides *(PDGs)*

The *Provider Documentation Guides* (*PDGs*) for the codes chosen for the Clinical Example can be helpful in determining if the codes are properly documented. For example, the *PDG* for Other Anxiety Disorders makes it easy to see that the fourth character for F41.- codes indicate the type of anxiety disorder. The words in the documentation should match up with the diagnosis code.

Symptom Codes

Guideline *1.B.5* states that "symptoms that are associated routinely with a disease process should not be assigned as additional codes." DSM-5 guidelines state that the insomnia should be clinically significant on its own to warrant a diagnosis. Since insomnia is routinely associated with many psychiatric conditions, it would be unnecessary and even incorrect to report insomnia in addition to conditions in which insomnia is a symptom of that condition, unless it is clinically significant on its own. It could be argued that insomnia is significant since it is affecting educational or academic functioning, but it should be noted that one of the DSM-5 diagnostic criteria points for insomnia is "The insomnia is not explained by coexisting mental disorders or medical conditions". If however, after several months of treatment, the provider may determine that the insomnia is unresolved, despite the fact that generalized anxiety disorder and dysthymic disorder have been alleviated. It may then be appropriate to report **F51.09** "Other insomnia not due to a substance or known physiological condition" in place of **F34.1** and **F41.1** to indicate the need for ongoing care.

Personal History Codes

Guideline *1;C.21.c.4* states that "Personal history codes explain a patient's past medical condition that no longer exists and is not receiving any treatment, but that has the potential for recurrence, and therefore may require continued monitoring." The documentation did state that **F90.1** "Attention-deficit hyperactivity disorder, predominantly hyperactive type" was a previous diagnosis. However, this diagnosis code is not reported even though it is clearly documented in the history.

Other Codes

Guideline *1;A.9.a* states that "Codes titled "other" or "other specified" are for use when the information in the medical record provides detail for which a specific code does not exist." In our clinical example, we included the **F40.298** to describe the fear of the dark since there is no official ICD-10-CM diagnosis code for fear of the dark. Although technically this code may not be required since sufficient information is in the clinical record, it was provided here for instructional purposes to demonstrate the use of "other" codes.

Excludes2

The *PDGs* for behavioral disorders have many great tips. For example, at the 3rd character level, there is an Excludes2 note for **F34.1** "Dysthymic disorder." According to Guideline *1.A.12.b*, "Excludes2 indicates that the condition excluded is not part of the condition represented by the code, but a patient may have both conditions at the same time." Therefore, anxiety should be added to the depressive disorder since it was also documented. In this clinical example, the anxiety met the criteria for Generalized anxiety disorder. Therefore, the addition of an anxiety code is appropriate. It could be argued that anxiety can be a symptom of depression, but the ICD-10-CM guidelines make it clear that two codes are now required to describe both conditions. As a result, the provider should document them distinctly.

Use of the Word "and"

The official description for code **Z55.4** says "Educational maladjustment and discord with teachers and classmates." In the Clinical Example, only the decline in grades and struggling with schoolwork were mentioned. Even though nothing about trouble with the teacher was documented, use of this code is acceptable because Guideline *1.A.14* states that "the word 'and' should be interpreted to mean either 'and' or 'or' when it appears in a title." Therefore, one or the other must be present, *but not necessarily both*. The Diagnostic Statement was designed with this guideline in mind.

Factors Influencing Health Status

The external cause codes included in the Clinical Example specify events or conditions which may influence the patient prognosis and treatment plan. Therefore all of that information must be clearly documented. These codes are subjective; that is, they are typically reported by the patient or caregiver, rather than observed by the clinician as with most other diagnosis codes.

The instructions for Factors influencing health status and contact with health services (Z00-Z99) at the beginning of Chapter 21 in the Tabular List have the following guidelines:

> *Note:*
> *Z codes represent reasons for encounters. A corresponding procedure code must accompany a Z code if a procedure is performed. Categories Z00-Z99 are provided for occasions when circumstances other than a disease, injury or external cause classifiable to categories A00-Y89 are recorded as 'diagnoses' or 'problems'. This can arise in two main ways:*
> *(a) When a person who may or may not be sick encounters the health services for some specific purpose, such as to receive limited care or service for a current condition, to donate an organ or tissue, to receive prophylactic vaccination (immunization), or to discuss a problem which is in itself not a disease or injury.*
> *(b) When some circumstance or problem is present which influences the person's health status but is not in itself a current illness or injury.*

In our Clinical Example, these additional factors support the diagnoses selected. Even though payers may not require all of these additional codes for claims adjudication, during a claim review, they help to establish clinical need and support the diagnosis chosen.

Code Sequencing

Section IV, paragraph G of the Official Guidelines says "List first the ICD-10-CM code for the diagnosis, condition, problem, or other reason for the encounter/visit shown in the medical record to be chiefly responsible for the services provided." In this scenario the anxiety was deemed to be the most serious, followed by the depression and insomnia. The "Z" codes and phobias were only contributing factors in this clinical example.

Notes:

4.3 Documentation Tips

As discussed in Chapter 4.1, documentation plays a crucial role in clearly establishing medical necessity and communicating with payers. Proper documentation can yield significant savings in the form of reduced payer takebacks and helps to defend against allegations of fraud or abuse. The information presented in this chapter is based on information compiled from a variety of resources including Medicare. Considering that many other payers follow or adopt Medicare guidelines, this information is relevant to both Medicare participating and non-participating providers. See Chapter 2.1 — Medicare Essentials for more information about becoming a Medicare participating provider.

Does Your Documentation Protect You From Accusations of False Claims?

To answer this question, first consider how a false claim is explained by CMS:

> While the False Claims Act imposes liability only when the claimant acts "knowingly," it does not require that the person submitting the claim have actual knowledge that the claim is false. A person who acts in reckless disregard or in deliberate ignorance of the truth or falsity of the information, also can be found liable under the Act. 31 U.S.C. 3729(b).

What do they mean by "reckless disregard" or "deliberate ignorance?" Could "reckless disregard" include doing nothing to correct poorly constructed EHR templates that lead to "note bloat" resulting in incorrect coding? Could not taking time to become better educated on the coding, billing, and documentation guidelines, regardless of your reasons for not doing so, be considered "deliberate ignorance?" Asking these questions now and addressing them as part of a formal compliance plan will help to prevent accusations of false claims and protect your organization.

As of January 2020, the penalties for the submission of a single false claim were $11,665 to $23,331. Although it is less likely the government will come after you for a single false claim, even a single false claim can be very costly. The example that follows demonstrates how expensive coding one level higher than the note allows could be (using the lowest penalty rate and the Medicare allowed amount for a participating provider). See how much it could cost if a claim was submitted for Evaluation and Management service 99214 (the most commonly reported with the highest percentage of error) and the documentation only supported 99213.

Example:
E/M Established patient 99214	$131.20
E/M Established patient 99213	− $ 92.47
Overpayment	$ 38.73
Multiplied by 3 for damages	$116.19
Plus one false claim penalty	$11,803.00 (the lowest penalty amount)
Grand Total	**$11,919.19**

As shown in the grand total, this adds up to a whopping minimum fine of $11,919.19 for a single false claim that only had an overpayment of $38.73.

The best way to avoid the risk of penalties (as shown in the previous example), which would be assessed over multiple claims, is to improve documentation by doing the following:

- review coding rules and guidelines for the codes most commonly reported by your specialty
- conduct internal auditing protocols for your practice

- provide ongoing provider education and training on important documentation issues and document that training (including logs of attendees) in your Compliance Manual

Book: See Chapter 3 — Compliance Essentials for more about false claims, internal audits, and Compliance Manuals.

Remember, everything begins with the documentation found in the medical record, so the most important thing providers can do after providing excellent care to their patients is to know what needs to be documented and then document it well.

Clear Documentation Facilitates Correct Code Selection

There are quite a few electronic health record (EHR) systems that also provide some degree of code selection; however, the code options presented from a quick main term entry are seldom the correct code and almost always are missing key instructional notations such as "code first," "excludes1," and "excludes2," which are key pieces of information for proper coding and reimbursement. Documentation tips for providers, which will help facilitate accurate coding include:

1. Have the provider document the patient's history of present illness (HPI), using complete sentences that tell the patient's story. Be sure to include information like:

   - context
   - duration
   - location
   - timing
   - modifying factors
   - quality
   - severity
   - associated signs and symptoms.

Store: See innoviHealth's *Comprehensive Guide to Evaluation & Management* (available in the online store) for more information about properly documenting E/M visits.

2. Create a diagnostic statement identifying the diagnoses, symptoms, or working diagnosis the patient may have, starting with the most serious. This should be a provider's impression that summarizes the subjective and objective findings that resulted in the diagnoses listed, not a bulleted list of codes.

Book: See Chapter 4.2 — Provider Documentation Training for more about diagnostic statements.

3. Document details such as:

   - laterality (e.g., right, left, bilateral)
   - anatomic location and episode of care for injuries (e.g., torus fracture of the upper end of the left radius, subsequent encounter)
   - circumstances surrounding an injury or accident (e.g., fell off a trampoline in neighbor's yard)

- stage or type of illness/condition (e.g., diabetes type 1, insulin dependent)
- status of condition (e.g., essential hypertension, stable on furosemide).

4. Using proper wording, identify any connection of the condition being treated to existing co-morbid conditions (e.g., ulcer of the left great toe secondary to uncontrolled insulin dependent diabetes mellitus type 2).

Know What Documentation is Required by your MAC

CMS contracts with private companies, referred to as Medicare Administrative Contractors (MACs), to manage Medicare claims. There are several MACs and each is contracted to provide guidance, claims processing, and review for specific assigned geographic locations. While CMS may create National Coverage Determinations (NCDs) which provide national level coverage guidance on documenting and reporting specific codes, the MACs have the ability to create Local Coverage Determinations (LCDs) for a geographic region, which provide coverage guidance details and other criteria required to support medical necessity.

Note: If the LCD contradicts the NCD, the guidelines of the NCD take precedence over the LCD and should be followed.

These documents often contain terminology, definitions, and documentation criteria that aid providers in creating medical records that will support medical necessity. Guidance may include instructions to document conservative therapies tried and failed (failed as in the therapy didn't work or the patient couldn't tolerate it), the use of any durable medical equipment (e.g., braces, TENs) that was tried and failed, a trial of over-the-counter or prescription medications, physical therapy(ies), and more. If this required information is not documented adequately in the medical record, the MAC may deny the claim. Because MACs don't usually request medical records for every service provided, claims with insufficient documentation may still be paid; however, if the MAC later decides to audit these services and requests the medical records, claims lacking required documentation will be denied and monies recouped. If the activity appears abusive or suspicious, the case may be turned over to a Recovery Audit Contractor (RAC) for potential fines and penalties, which could lead to discovery of additional problems such as other claim problems, allegations of false claims, or even fraud.

Website: FindACode.com has a direct link to any CPT/HCPCS code with applicable NCDs, as well as LCDs and Articles, based on the user's geographic location. These documents are updated throughout the year and users are able to have multiple locations set up in their profile to facilitate coding and auditing across multiple states and MACs. Identify the CPT and HCPCS codes billed most frequently in your practice and search for any NCDs, LCDs, and Articles linked to them to identify documentation requirements which support medical necessity and reimbursement.

Insufficient Documentation Errors

Claims are determined to have insufficient documentation errors when the medical documentation submitted is either nonexistent or inadequate to support reimbursement for the service. Poor documentation makes it difficult for the reviewer to determine if the services were actually provided, provided at the level billed, and/or medically necessary.

Claims are also placed into this category when a specific documentation element that is required as a condition of payment is missing, such as a physician signature on an order, or a form that is required to be completed in its entirety.

The following are some insufficient documentation errors identified by CMS's Comprehensive Error Rate Testing (CERT) program:

- Incomplete progress notes (e.g., unsigned, undated, insufficient detail)

- Unauthenticated medical records (e.g., no provider signature, no supervising signature, illegible signatures without a signature log or attestation to identify the signer, an electronic signature without the electronic record protocol or policy that documents the process for electronic signature)
- No documentation of intent to order services and procedures (e.g., incomplete or missing signed order or progress note describing intent for services to be provided)

Book: See "Common Errors" in Chapter 4.1 — Documentation Essentials for a list of common documentation errors.

Tips

Disclaimer: The information in this chapter contains general information and is the opinion of the authors. It should not be interpreted by providers/payers as official guidance. As such, this information should not be used for claim adjudication. Third party payers should utilize their own payment policies based on clinically sound guidelines.

Index

Developmental Testing/Screening (96110-96113, G0451)	201
Diagnostic Evaluation (90791, 90792)	202
External Cause Codes	203
Health Behavior Assessment/Intervention	204
Neurobehavioral Status Examination (96116, 96121)	206
Other Psychotherapy Procedures (90845-90880)	207
Pharmacologic Management (90863)	208
Psychological & Neuropsychological Testing (96130-96139)	209
Psychotherapy for Crisis (90839-90840)	211
Psychotherapy Services (90832-90838)	211

Format Conventions

MEDICAL NECESSITY: describes conditions where services are considered medically necessary.

PERFORMED BY: describes which provider types are allowed to perform these procedures. The definitions for each provider type are found in Resource 470. The following acronyms are used throughout this chapter:

MD/DO - Physician (MD/DO)	CP - Clinical Psychologist
CSW - Clinical Social Worker	NP - Nurse Practitioner
CNS - Clinical Nurse Specialist	PA - Physician Assistant
IPP - Independently Practicing Psychologist	PNP - Psychiatric Nurse Practitioner

COVERAGE: means what is payable or meets the payer requirements for reimbursement

NONCOVERAGE: situations where it is known that the service will not be paid by Medicare

Alert: The information in this chapter is adapted primarily from published Medicare guidelines and regulations. Be aware of state laws which could supersede the information included here. Also, there could be variations between different payer plans.

Alert: For the purposes of this "Tips" section, when there is a significant and separately identifiable service which should be reported with an E/M code, documentation requirements are different than what is included here.

Book: See Chapter 5.3 — Evaluation & Management Coding for more information on E/M requirements.

NonCovered Services

The following are Medicare noncovered services:

- Geriatric day care programs
- Environmental intervention
- Marriage counseling
- Biofeedback training

Alert: It is fraud to modify a record in order to make one of these noncovered services appear to be a covered service. For example, if marriage counseling is being performed, DO NOT submit a bill or falsify a Medicare record so that it appears that individual psychotherapy was performed.

Developmental Testing/Screening (96110-96113, G0451)

Documentation should include ALL of the following:

- Time involved, preferably with start and stop times, including time for interpretation and report

Note: When services span more than one day, documentation should clearly indicate the time spent on each day. However, payers may have different requirements for the reporting of dates when submitting a claim. Be aware of these differences.

- Tests administered and scored
- Interpretation of findings and written report
- Present evaluation
- Diagnosis (if no mental/neurocognitive disorder/condition was found during the screen, report the diagnosis that was the basis for the testing)
- Recommendations for interventions, if necessary
- Name and credentials of provider performing the service
- Referral – if these services are being requested by another healthcare professional, include the reason for the referral and the name of the referring provider

Tip: Please be aware of the differences between these codes. See Chapter 5.2 — Common Procedure Codes & Tips for more information.

PERFORMED BY:
- MD, DO CP, NP, CNS, PA, IPP – to the extent authorized under state scope of practice.
- Always verify your state scope of practice to ensure coverage. Students/trainees performing tests are NOT covered.

Additional IPP Guidelines:

When diagnostic psychological tests are performed by a psychologist who is not practicing independently, but is on the staff of an institution, agency, or clinic, that entity bills for the psychological tests.

The A/B MAC (B) considers psychologists as practicing independently when:
- They render services on their own responsibility, free of the administrative and professional control of an employer such as a physician, institution or agency;
- The persons they treat are their own patients; and
- They have the right to bill directly, collect and retain the fee for their services."

– *Medicare Benefit Policy Manual, Chapter 15, Section 80.2*

Diagnostic Evaluation (90791, 90792)

Documentation must include ALL of the following components:

- Date, name, age, sex, date of birth (DOB), date of service (DOS), chief complaint
- Referral source, including name and credentials of the referring provider, where applicable
- Time involved, preferably with start and stop times, including time for interpretation and report

Note: When services span more than one day, documentation should clearly indicate the time spent on each day. However, payers may have different requirements for the reporting of dates when submitting a claim. Be aware of these differences.

- Pertinent history of present illness (including current medications)
- Pertinent past psychiatric history
- Pertinent medical history (including past, family, social)
- Pertinent mental status examination and symptoms (e.g., ADL, posture/gait, eye contact, motor activity [increased/decreased], affect, memory, rate/volume of speech, mood, associations, general knowledge, concentration, orientation, abstraction, paranoid ideation, hallucinations, idea of reference, appetite, sleep disturbance, etc.)
- Appropriate high risk factors (e.g., suicidal/homicidal ideation)
- All relevant diagnoses in the following order:
  - chief complaint, or reason for the visit
  - other clinical or personality disorders contributing to the chief complaint
  - general medical conditions contributing to the chief complaint, and
  - psychosocial and environmental problems
- Functional assessments including severity and/or disability where indicated
- Initial treatment plan (including diagnostic test results, medications)

- Where psychotherapy is planned and there is a diagnosis of dementia, confusion, or any type of impaired cognition, the documentation should indicate that the patient consents to, and is able to, participate in and benefit from the psychotherapy
- Long term goals and prognosis when possible
- Anticipated treatment duration (interval) where applicable
- Therapeutic techniques and approaches

Note: When the patient is unable to interact through normal verbal communicative channels such as: age (<17 years old), organic mental deficits, or catatonic or mute, be sure to also document interactive complexity. See "Interactive Complexity (90785)" in Chapter 5.2 — Common Procedure Codes & Tips for more information.

Additional 90792 Requirements: Documentation must also indicate the additional 'medical' components, such as the following, when clinically indicated:

- Physical examination elements
- Review of prescription of medications
- Review and ordering of laboratory or other diagnostic studies
- Non-mental health diagnosis, as applicable (e.g., Parkinson's)

Performed by: MD, CP, CSW, NP, CNS – to the extent authorized under state scope of practice.

Coverage: Generally covered once, per provider/discipline, at the onset of an illness/condition or suspected illness/condition. However, it may be utilized again, for the same patient, if a new episode of illness/condition occurs after a respite, or an admission, or readmission, to an inpatient status due to complications of the underlying condition.

External Cause Codes

Although there is no HIPAA mandate for reporting external cause codes, some payers may require them. Reporting external cause codes on submitted claims may also reduce the amount of records requests for patients involved in accidents and injuries. This information helps payers verify who is responsible for claims due to injuries (e.g., automobile, workers compensation, home).

There is important information that must be included when documenting injuries and external cause codes in ICD-10-CM. There are expanded sections on poisonings and toxins making it more convenient to code, as ICD-10-CM is very specific.

When documenting injuries, include the following:

- Episode of care (e.g., initial, subsequent, sequela)
- Injury site (Be as specific as possible)
- Etiology (How was the injury sustained, e.g., sports, motor vehicle crash, pedestrian, slip and fall, environmental exposure, etc.)
- Place of occurrence (e.g., school, work, etc.) Initial encounters may also require, where appropriate:
- Intent (e.g., unintentional or accidental, self-harm, etc.)
- Status (e.g., civilian, military, etc.)

Book: See "External Causes and Encounters" in Appendix E — Common Diagnosis Code Tips for coding options.

Health Behavior Assessment/Intervention

Note: Codes 96156-96171 were new in 2020. See Chapter 5.2 — Common Procedure Codes & Tips for more information about these codes.

Documentation for all health behavior services (96156-96171) should include the following:

- **Diagnosis:** Report a covered non-psychiatric diagnosis code. Behavioral health diagnosis codes F01-F99 should not be used to report these services. See "Health Behavior Assessment and Intervention" in Chapter 5.2 — Common Procedure Codes & Tips for additional information about covered diagnosis codes for these services.

- **Patient status:** The patient must be alert, oriented, and have the ability to understand and respond meaningfully during the encounter. Be sure to include how these services impact the management of their condition(s) and activities of daily living.

- **Barriers:** Services must focus on the following areas:
  - Cognitive
  - Emotional
  - Social
  - Behavioral functioning

- **Provider type:** CPT and Medicare guidelines state that those who are allowed to use E/M and/or Preventive Medicine services codes should not use these codes. Therefore, the documentation needs to clearly identify the type of provider rendering these services. According to one MAC, only a clinical psychologist may perform these services. Review payer policies to determine provider type requirements.

- **Reasonable and necessary:** Payer policies will generally outline what they consider to be reasonable and necessary. Where possible, be sure that documentation addresses why it meets their criteria.

- **Patient compliance:** How well is the patient complying with their medical treatment plan? How well do they adhere to the plan? What obstacles are preventing them from complying? Do they understand their treatment plan, as well as the benefits and risks of procedures being performed?

Resource: See Resource 485 for information by the American Psychological Association about these services.

NonCoverage: If documentation includes any of the following it may indicate that either different codes should be reported (e.g., psychotherapy, behavioral health integration) or they are not covered services (e.g., recreational services):

- Update/educate family on patient's condition
- Educate staff on patient's care plan or treatment planning
- Provide family psychotherapy or mediation
- Educate diabetic patients or family
- Deliver medical nutrition therapy

- Personal, social, recreational, and general support services
- Maintain the patient's or family's existing health and overall well-being

ASSESSMENT/RE-ASSESSMENT (96156)

Documentation for both the assessment and re-assessment should include, but are not limited to, the following:

- **Time:** Even though code 96156 does not have a time component, from an audit perspective, it is recommended that this information be included in the documentation.
- **Referral:** Many other payers require a referral from another healthcare provider (e.g., physician, nurse practitioner, physician assistant) requesting these services to address patient barriers.
- **Care coordination:** There should be evidence of care coordination with the referring provider, primary care provider, and/or other agencies involved in the patient's care.
- **Evaluation:** This face-to-face, health-focused clinical interview is an evaluation of the patient's response(s) to their condition(s) with a focus on the referral question. According to CPT guidelines, this includes their "outlook, coping strategies, motivation, and adherence to medical treatment." Where possible, document psychological and environmental factors which may be significantly affecting either the treatment or medical management of their condition(s).
- **Behavioral Observations:** Both direct and indirect observations of the QHP are employed to assess how the patient responds during the interview process.
- **Clinical Decision Making:** All portions of the evaluation, including information obtained prior to the patient evaluation, are utilized to formulate the clinical impressions and diagnoses (or suspected diagnoses) including treatment recommendations.
- **Measurable Goals:** The initial assessment will set individualized patient goals which will be evaluated and revised as needed during the re-assessment.

Initial Assessment

In addition to the previously discussed items, documentation should include ALL of the following components:

- Onset and history of diagnosis of medical condition(s)
- Rationale for assessment
- Assessment outcome
- Recommendations including goals and anticipated duration (including frequency) of interventions, where applicable

Re-assessment

Some payer policies indicate that ALL of the following documentation components were required:

- Date of change in psychological or medical status which justifies the need for re-evaluation of the patient's capacity to understand and cooperate with the medical interventions necessary to their health and well being
- Rationale for reassessment
- Indication of precipitating event
- Changes in goals, duration and/or frequency of services

HEALTH BEHAVIOR INTERVENTION (96158-96171)

Documentation of intervention services needs to include the following, where applicable:

- **Time:** These are timed services so start and stop times need to be part of the medical record. See "Timed Codes" in Chapter 5.2 — Common Procedure Codes & Tips for a helpful table.
- **Type of encounter:** Was this an individual, group, or family encounter? Identify all individuals present.
- **Compliance:** Is there evidence of improved patient compliance with the treatment plan?
- **Capacity:** The patient has a capacity to understand and respond meaningfully.
- **Responses:** What are their responses to clinical intervention?
- **Plan:** Evidence of clearly addressing the patient's intervention plan.
- **Frequency:** Rationale provided for frequency and duration of service.

Tips

- Be sure that is it clear that these services could not be reported with another type of service (e.g., medical nutrition therapy).
- Payers may have limitations on frequency of services (e.g., 12 hours regardless of the number of sessions) so be sure cumulative time is carefully monitored and documented.

Neurobehavioral Status Examination (96116, 96121)

Documentation should include the following:

- Time involved, preferably with start and stop times, including time for interpretation and report

Note: When services span more than one day, documentation should clearly indicate the time spent on each day. However, payers may have different requirements for the reporting of dates when submitting a claim. Be aware of these differences.

- Why testing is needed
- Type
  - Initial: suspected diagnosis, neuropsychological abnormality, and/or central nervous system dysfunction
  - Follow-up: assessment of changes in disease/condition, progression over time, and/or comparison to previous testing, whether by this provider or another provider
- Test(s) administered and scored
- Interpretation of findings/results and written report
- Clinical assessment of thinking, reasoning, and judgment (e.g., acquired knowledge, attention, language, memory, planning and problem solving, visual spatial abilities)
- Treatment recommendations
- Support the fact that the procedure meets the payer's statutory and benefit category requirements
- Be legible, maintained in the patient's medical record, and made available upon request
- Referral – if these services are being requested by another healthcare professional, include the reason for the referral and the name of the referring provider

MEDICAL NECESSITY:

The following information from a retired LCD provides some guidance on what that MAC considered medically necessary:

1. Detection of neurologic diseases based on quantitative assessment of neurocognitive abilities (e.g., mild head injury, anoxic injuries, AIDS dementia);
2. Differential diagnosis between psychogenic and neurogenic syndromes;
3. Delineation of the neurocognitive effects of CNS disorders;
4. Neurocognitive monitoring of recovery or progression of CNS disorders; and/or
5. Assessment of neurocognitive functions for the formulation of rehabilitation and/or management strategies among individuals with neuropsychiatric disorders.
6. Where it will impact the management of the patient by confirmation or delineation of diagnosis.

– WPS LCD L30489

PERFORMED BY: MD, DO CP, IPP, NP, CNS, PA – to the extent authorized under state scope of practice

Other Psychotherapy Procedures (90845-90880)

Family Psychotherapy (90846, 90847, 90849)

MEDICAL NECESSITY: Documentation should support the rationale for the necessity of these services, such as:

- Identifying maladaptive behavior(s) of family members that are exacerbating the beneficiary's mental health condition(s) and hindering the patient's treatment progress
- Contacting family members in order to obtain information necessary for diagnosis and treatment planning because the patient is comatose, withdrawn, and/or uncommunicative

PERFORMED BY: MD, DO, CP, CSW, PA, CNP, CNS or others authorized by state. RNs with special training may also be considered.

Group Psychotherapy (90853)

Documentation must include ALL of the following components:

- The number of actual participants - group size typically cannot be more than 12 people
- The name and credentials of the qualified professional leading the group
- Interactive methods used, where applicable
- Individual treatment plan must support the necessity of group therapy

PERFORMED BY: MD, DO, CP, CSW, PA, CNP, PNP, CNS or others authorized by state. RNs with special training may also be considered.

NONCOVERAGE:

- Socialization, music therapy, recreational activities, art classes, excursions, sensory stimulation or eating together, cognitive stimulation, motion therapy, etc.
- Self-help groups or support groups without a qualified professional present

Psychoanalysis (90845)

This is not a time based code and may only be billed once per daily session, regardless of the time. To determine a fee, the RVU is based on a 45-60 minute face-to-face session.

The medical record must clearly document the indications for psychoanalysis, description of the transference, and the psychoanalytic techniques used.

Performed by: Only providers trained by an accredited program of psychoanalysis

Hypnotherapy (90880)

If these services are being requested by another healthcare professional, be sure the documentation includes the reason for the referral and the name of the referring provider.

Narcosynthesis (90865)

Documentation should include ALL of the following:

- Rationale for this procedure (e.g., the patient had difficulty verbalizing his/her psychiatric problems without the aid of the drug)
- Pharmacological agent name and the dosage administered
- Results (i.e., whether the technique was effective or noneffective)
- Therapy notes

Performed by: MD, DO only

Pharmacologic Management (90863)

These guidelines only apply to management by a healthcare provider (e.g., prescribing psychologist) who is not authorized to perform Evaluation and Management Services.

Book: See Chapter 5.3 — Evaluation & Management Coding for more information on physicians and other qualified healthcare professionals (e.g., psychiatric nurse practitioners) who are required to report medication management as part of an Evaluation and Management visit.

Documentation should include ALL of the following components:

- Relevant history (including diagnosis)
- Pertinent signs and symptoms
- Mental status exam results
- Medical decision making components (i.e., assessment of treatment response and ongoing treatment formulation)
- Medication(s) prescribed
- Medication(s) problems, reactions, side effects (if any)

Where applicable, the following should be included:

- Psychopharmacologic agents initiated or adjusted
- Referral – if psychotherapy services are being provided by another healthcare professional, include reason for the referral and the name of the referring provider

Performed by: Healthcare providers who are authorized to prescribe medication in their state, but are not eligible to report Evaluation and Management codes. Physicians should NEVER use code 90863.

NonCoverage:

- Actual medication administration
- Observation of patient taking an oral medication
- Administration and supply of oral medication

 Alert: 90863 is not covered by Medicare. Be aware of individual payer policies and documentation requirements for this code.

Psychological & Neuropsychological Testing (96130-96139)

As of 2019, both psychological and neuropsychological testing services must report the administration and scoring (96136-96139) separately from the evaluation (96130-96133) portion of the testing service.

The following information from one payer provides guidance on what needs to be included in the documentation to differentiate between psychological and neuropsychological testing:

> Examples of problems that might lead to neuropsychological testing are:
> - Detection of neurologic diseases based on quantitative assessment of neurocognitive abilities (e.g., mild head injury, anoxic injuries, AIDS dementia)
> - Differential diagnosis between psychogenic and neurogenic syndromes
> - Delineation of the neurocognitive effects of central nervous system disorders
> - Neurocognitive monitoring of recovery or progression of central nervous system disorders; or
> - Assessment of neurocognitive functions for the formulation of rehabilitation and/or management strategies among individuals with neuropsychiatric disorders.
>
> The content of neuropsychological testing procedures differs from that of psychological testing in that neuropsychological testing consists primarily of individually administered ability tests that comprehensively sample cognitive and performance domains that are known to be sensitive to the functional integrity of the brain (e.g., abstraction, memory and learning, attention, language, problem solving, sensorimotor functions, constructional praxis, etc.). These procedures are objective and quantitative in nature and require the patient to directly demonstrate his/her level of competence in a particular cognitive domain. Neuropsychological testing does not rely on self-report questionnaires such as the Minnesota Multiphasic Personality Inventory 2 (MMPI-2), rating scales such as the Hamilton Depression Rating Scale, or projective techniques such as the Rorschach or Thematic Apperception Test (TAT) when questions of how brain damage or degenerative disease processes (e.g. right hemisphere CVA) may be affecting emotional expression or how significant emotional distress or mood impairment might be affecting cognitive function (e.g. question of presence of "pseudodementia") arise.
>
> Typically, psychological testing will require from four (4) to six (6) hours to perform, including administration, scoring and interpretation. Supporting documentation in the medical record must be present to justify greater than 8 hours per patient per evaluation. If the testing is done over several days, the testing time should be combined and reported all on the last date of service. If the testing time exceeds eight (8) hours, medical necessity for extended time should be documented. Medical records may be requested.
>
> *– Psychiatry and Psychology Services (L33632)*

Tips

- Timed services must meet the minimum thresholds. See "Timed Codes" in Chapter 5.2 — Common Procedure Codes & Tips for a helpful table.
- When services span more than one day, documentation should clearly indicate the time spent on each day. However, payers may have different requirements for the reporting of dates when submitting a claim. Be aware of these differences.

- To meet Medicare medical necessity requirements, documentation must indicate that the patient has a suspected mental health disorder, neuropsychological abnormality, or central nervous system dysfunction.

- Be aware of payer definitions or state scope of practice laws regarding technicians and which test(s) they are authorized to perform. For example, for codes 96138 and 96139, one Medicare Administrative Contractor (MAC) allows the reporting of these services by a technician who is supervised by the primary or qualified healthcare professional who interprets the tests.

- Scope of practice for 96130-96133, 96136, 96137 is generally limited to an MD, DO, CP, IPP, NP, CNS, or PA – to the extent authorized under state scope of practice as a qualified healthcare provider (QHP).

- Typically, one initial testing and a follow up re-testing evaluation within a 12-month period by the same provider or group is allowed. If there is a need for further testing, the medical necessity of those services must be documented.

- The following situations may be considered noncovered for testing services:
  - Patient not cognitively able to meaningfully participate
  - General screening tests
  - Educational or vocational purposes
  - Self-administered or self-scored screening/inventories (e.g., AIMS, Folstein Mini-Mental Status Exam)
  - Non medical decision making situations
  - Patient is on medications which may invalidate the results
  - When patient has substance abuse history and any of these situations apply:
    ◊ ongoing substance abuse would render inaccurate test results
    ◊ currently under the influence or intoxicated
    ◊ patient is less than 10 days post-detox
  - Neuropsychological assessment could have been obtained through regular clinical evaluation
  - History of brain dysfunction where testing would have no impact on treatment plan
  - Adjustment disorder or dysphoria is associated with moving to skilled nursing facility or nursing home
  - Using a standard battery of tests instead of customized to the individual case when only a few tests would have been adequate

Testing Administration and Scoring (96136-96139)

Documentation must include ALL of the following components:

- Total time involved, with beginning and ending times, for all tests performed, including the scoring of individual tests, as well as the actual testing time(s)

- Names of tests administered and scored

- Date(s) of testing participation

- Name and credentials of individual(s) administering the test(s)

- Referral – if services are being requested by another healthcare professional, include the reason for the referral and the name of the referring provider

Testing Evaluation Services (96130-96133)

Documentation must include ALL of the following components:

- Time involved, preferably with start and stop times, including time for interpretation and report
- Why testing is needed
- Type
    - Initial: suspected diagnosis, neuropsychological abnormality, and/or central nervous system dysfunction
    - Follow-up: assessment of changes in disease/condition, progression over time, and/or comparison to previous testing, whether by this provider or another provider
- Interpretation of test(s) previously administered
- References to previous evaluation(s) and testing services, including the rationale for testing services
- Communication with others (e.g., referring provider, caregiver(s), other sources)
- Treatment recommendations
- Recommendations for interventions, if necessary
- Presence of physical and/or mental health disorder or signs/symptoms of psychiatric disorder for which testing is indicated (rationale and medically necessary reason for testing)

Psychotherapy for Crisis (90839-90840)

Documentation should include ALL of the following components:

- History of the crisis state
- Mental status exam results
- Disposition of the patient
- Level of psychotherapy services provided
- Description of mobilization of resources to defuse the crisis and restore safety
- Description of the psychotherapeutic interventions implemented to minimize the potential for psychological trauma
- Total duration of time face-to-face with the patient and/or family, preferably with start and stop times

Psychotherapy Services (90832-90838)

A Noridian Medicare review demonstrated that 46.25 percent of the individual psychotherapy sessions were denied due to poor documentation. Furthermore, 16.75 percent were reduced in payment because the medical record either did not indicate the service time or the documentation did not meet the level of service billed. To avoid denials or payment reductions, be sure documentation meets payer and code description requirements.

Note: These are time-specific codes. A recent OIG report on one provider group stated that their documentation did NOT meet requirements because it lacked start and stop times. As such, it is recommended that providers include both start and stop times.

Psychotherapy times are for face-to-face services with the patient and/or family member. The patient must be present for all or some of the service. Choose the code closest to the actual time (i.e., 16-37 minutes for 90832 and 90833, 38-52 minutes for 90834 and 90836, and 53 or more minutes for 90837 and 90838). Do not report psychotherapy of less than 16 minutes duration.

Book: See Chapter 5.3 — Evaluation & Management Coding for details about when it is appropriate to bill an E/M visit at the same encounter as psychotherapy services.

Documentation should include ALL of the following components:

- Date of service, patient name, and age
- Face-to-face time with the patient
- Reason for the encounter and pertinent interval history - clearly explained
- Medication prescription and monitoring — Note that this is not the same as managing medication. See also "Pharmacologic Management (90863)" on page 208.
- Appropriate high risk factors (S/I, H/I) where applicable
- Interventions used including psychotherapeutic, medications, diagnostic test(s), consults, family, other
- Clinical test results where applicable
- Summary of diagnosis, functional status, treatment plan, symptoms
- Patient assessment (prognosis, progress to date or regression, concerns of client/provider)
- Status of the following: mental and physical function, cognitive
- Interactive complexity specifics, where applicable. See Chapter 5.2 — Common Procedure Codes & Tips for additional information
- For E/M services (Evaluation and Management) include evidence of medical decision making. See Chapter 5.3 — Evaluation & Management Coding for additional information
- Evidence of patient's ability to participate and permission to treat must include:
    1. Evidence of their capacity to participate and benefit from psychotherapy, and
    2. A signed agreement to treat by the patient or responsible party (if involuntary treatment is authorized for state welfare and institute, include appropriate documentation (e.g., 5150 or 5250 form for California)
- Treatment obstacles
- Summary of the following: diagnosis, functional status, treatment plan, symptoms, prognosis, progress and progress to date
- Legible name and professional degree of practitioner and 'incident to' practitioner where applicable

Book: See the "Signatures" segment in Chapter 4.1 — Documentation Essentials for information regarding acceptable signatures.

Alert: Psychotherapy services over 90 minutes (with no E/M involvement) may report an appropriate prolonged services code (99354-99357). However, the documentation MUST clearly support the necessity of this extended, unusual circumstance.

Tip — Psychotherapy Notes

The following items are protected under the HIPAA Psychotherapy Notes provision:
- Information which documents or analyzes the counseling session, or
- Information which does not integrate with non-protected aspects (see below).

The following items are **NOT** protected and must be included in the general medical record:
- Medication prescription and monitoring
- Session start and stop times
- Modalities and frequencies of treatment
- Clinical test results

Resource: See Resource 505 for more about Psychotherapy Notes and HIPAA.

Tips

- Coverage may be limited to a set number of visits (e.g., 26 per year). However, documentation clearly establishing the medical necessity of additional services can help with seeking coverage of additional services.

- The following are not psychotherapy services and should not be billed as such:
  - Viewing films or other activities that are not face-to-face psychotherapy
  - Teaching grooming skills, monitoring activities of daily living (ADL), recreational therapy (dance, art, play) or social interaction
  - Oversight activities such as housing, financial management, etc.
  - Provider travel time

- In situations where the patient has a severe enough cognitive defect (e.g., dementia) that psychotherapy would be ineffective, it is typically not a covered benefit

Note: Psychotherapy is typically not covered for a patient with either severe or profound intellectual disabilities (F72, F73). However, other services (e.g., E/M, rehabilitative services) might be covered depending on payer policy.

- Scope of practice: Be aware of payer limitations on who can provide these services. Medicare requirements are:
  - Codes 90832, 90834, 90837: MD, DO, NP, PNP, CP, PA, CSW, or CNS
  - Codes 90833, 90836, 90838: MD, DO (Also NP, PNP, and CNS when performed in collaboration with a physician and within state scope of practice laws). This is because these codes are for Evaluation and Management services.

Notes:

5. Procedure Coding

Chapter Contents

5.1 Procedure Coding Essentials 217
    Introduction 217
    Getting Started with CPT 219
    NCCI Coding Edits 222
    Evaluation and Management (E/M) Services 223

5.2 Procedure Codes & Tips 225
    Procedure Code Tips 225
    Common Procedure Codes 273

5.3 Evaluation & Management Coding 311
    The Basics 311
    Office/Other Outpatient E/M Services 316
    Coding Scenario 1: 2020 E/M Guidelines 324
    Code Selection by Counseling Time (2020 Version) 341
    Coding Scenario 2: Current Office E/M Guidelines 343
    Evaluation and Management Codes 346

5.1 Procedure Coding Essentials

Introduction

The information in this chapter is specific to the basic reporting of services and procedures using the Healthcare Common Procedural Coding System (HCPCS), which includes both Current Procedural Terminology (CPT) codes and HCPCS codes. Services performed by healthcare providers may be reported as either Professional or Institutional as explained below:

Professional Services/Procedures: These are performed by physicians or other healthcare providers in the office or other types of facility settings. These services, regardless of where they are provided, are reported on the *1500 Claim Form* (or electronic equivalent) with the two HIPAA-compliant code sets: the American Medical Association's Current Procedural Terminology, Fourth Edition, (CPT®) and the Healthcare Common Procedure Coding System (HCPCS).

Institutional Services/Procedures: These are performed in hospitals, ambulatory surgery centers, and other facilities where rooms (e.g., operating, ICU, neonatal unit), staff, equipment, and supplies are provided for patient care occurring in the facility. These services/procedures are reported on the *UB-04 Claim Form*. When professional services are rendered in a facility or institutional setting, they are typically reported on the *1500 Claim Form* (or electronic equivalent) as a professional service. Nevertheless, different payers could have varying policies for reporting those services. See the segment "Procedure Coding for Facilities" on page 315 for more information.

Note: Codes are used to describe service(s) rendered, but their existence does not ensure coverage by third party payers. Individual payer policies govern how services are reported so each provider should be sure to review payer contracts and payer-published policies carefully to ensure accurate reporting.

Only HIPAA-approved codes are included in this publication. See "ABC Codes" on 218 for information on Advanced Billing Concepts (ABC) codes, which may be valuable for internal record keeping, but not for HIPAA-approved transactions.

Current Procedural Terminology (CPT) Fourth Edition

Current Procedural Terminology (CPT®), Fourth Edition is maintained and published by the American Medical Association (AMA) who owns the copyright to the codes and their associated descriptions. Medicare also refers to these codes as the *Healthcare Common Procedure Coding System (HCPCS)* Level I code set. This set of codes, descriptions, and guidelines are intended to describe professional procedures and services performed by physicians and other healthcare professionals. For the most part, CPT codes are updated annually on January 1st; however, there can be some codes released early. For example, vaccine codes, Molecular Pathology Tier 2 codes, Administrative MAAA codes, and Category III codes are released in January or July, therefore, they are typically not found in the current year printed codebook. Each procedure or service is identified with a five-character code. The use of CPT codes simplifies the reporting of services. The CPT codes are not all inclusive, meaning there are many new technologies or services that may be considered common, but the AMA has not created codes to describe them in the CPT code set.

> "Inclusion of a descriptor and its associated five-digit code number in the *CPT codebook* is based on whether the procedure is consistent with contemporary medical practice and is performed by many practitioners in clinical practice in multiple locations. Inclusion in the *CPT* codebook does not represent endorsement by the American Medical Association (AMA) of any particular diagnostic or therapeutic procedure. Inclusion or exclusion of a procedure does not imply any health insurance coverage or reimbursement policy." –*CPT*, by the AMA

The CPT codes in this chapter are selected because of their relevance to this specialty-specific publication.

Resource: See Resource 817 for additional information, articles and webinars about procedure coding.
Website: See FindACode.com for access to electronic searching for CPT codes, descriptions and related information (available by subscription).

Healthcare Common Procedure Coding System (HCPCS)

The Healthcare Common Procedure Coding System (HCPCS) is divided into two principal subsystems, referred to as Level I and Level II of the HCPCS (pronounced "hick-picks"). As discussed previously, HCPCS Level II codes are a five-character alphanumeric code set created and maintained by the Centers for Medicare and Medicaid Services (CMS). The Level II HCPCS codes describe a variety of healthcare services and supplies. This code set also includes some quality data codes such as those used to report performance in the Quality Category of the Quality Payment Program (QPP). QPP codes are not included in this publication (see Resource 168).

One benefit of this code set is the increased specificity for services and supplies that may be unavailable, ill-defined, or defined differently by payers than they are within the CPT code set. Providers should be aware of individual payer preferences regarding the use of HCPCS to avoid claims processing errors (e.g., Medicare often requires the provider report a HCPCS G-code in place of a CPT published code for certain services).

Book: See Chapter 6.2 — Common Supply Codes & Tips for HCPCS supply codes.

Tip: New, revised, and deleted codes are implemented quarterly. Depending on the quarter, your specialty may or may not be impacted. FindACode.com always has the most up-to-date codes and also has a list of these updates.

ABC Codes

ABC codes, created and maintained by Alternative Link, use a five-character alphabetic system with a two-digit identifier based on provider type. They do not use modifiers. ABC codes fill in the gaps or replace general (unspecific) codes for procedures in the CPT and HCPCS code sets, allowing for the recording of services at a higher level of specificity for practitioners, patients, payers, and researchers. **Currently, these codes may only be used for recording procedures internally and not for HIPAA-regulated transactions.**

ABC codes may be particularly beneficial for practices that offer alternative services where there is no insurance coverage or billing involved. ABC codes provide a standardized method of recording treatment details, which is necessary to keep an office running efficiently. For example, alternative services such as footbaths, Class IV laser, PEMF, and many others can be coded using ABC codes. This provides for not only improved and compliant communications for healthcare providers, but also an efficient method of tracking service details and statistics for the practice.

Resource: See Resource 346 to search for and learn more about ABC codes.
Book: See Chapter 4 — Documentation for more about proper documentation.

Procedure Coding for Facilities

Reporting facility services is not the same as reporting professional services. Typically, facility services are room and board rates, supplies, equipment, and technical services; however, some facilities have all-inclusive rates. To report these types of services, Diagnostic Related Group (DRG) codes or revenue codes are utilized on the *UB-04 Claim Form* or its electronic equivalent. When professional services are rendered in an institution (hospital, facility), such as Evaluation and Management services, operations, or procedures, they are reported separately as a professional service on a *1500 Claim Form* using the appropriate CPT/HCPCS code(s). Whether to use the *UB-04* or the *1500 Claim Form* depends on the type of service, location where it was rendered, and specific payer policies (e.g., some payers prefer revenue codes over CPT codes for partial hospitalization services).

Resource: See Resource 473 for information on billing facility services.

Instructions for Procedural Coding for Professional Services

The instructions from CPT state: *"Select the name of a procedure that accurately identifies the service performed. Do not select a CPT code that merely approximates the service provided."* There are a few remedies for reporting services when there is not a CPT code that "accurately identifies" the service performed. These include:

- **Modifiers:** Application of a CPT or HCPCS modifier that, when applied to the code that most closely represents what was performed, accurately identifies the service.

- **HCPCS Level II:** Search for a HCPCS Level II code (if one exists) that accurately describes the service and is accepted by the payer.

- **Unlisted Code:** Report an unlisted code specific to the category of codes the service belongs to. Unlisted codes always end in '99' (e.g., 64999 "Unlisted procedure, nervous system"). Be sure to enter a brief description of the service in either Item Number 19 or the shaded area of Item Number 24 on the *1500 Claim Form* (or Form Locator 80 on the *UB-04* as required by the payer) and send with a copy of the medical report.

- **CPT Category III:** Check to see if there is a CPT Category III code available to report the service. These are temporary codes for emerging technologies, services, procedures, and paradigms. Individual payer policies vary regarding reimbursement of these codes.

- **Payer Guidelines:** Check with individual payers for any additional guidelines they may require.

Resource: See Resource 178 for detailed CMS and NUCC claim form instructions.

Specific guidelines for each section are available from the original source documents, as published by the AMA and the Centers for Medicare and Medicaid Services (CMS). General coding guidance to assist you in understanding and using each of these code sets is included in this book.

Getting Started with CPT

In general, CPT codes are not restricted to any specialty or group, and may be used by any qualified healthcare practitioner. However, certain CPT codes may only be used by a "physician" or other Qualified Healthcare Professional (QHP) and the definition of which practitioners are "physicians" or QHPs may vary by state (as specified by statutes) and sometimes by payer policies (e.g., Medicare publishes a list of who they consider to be a physician and nonphysician practitioner).

Resource: See Resource 402 for more about who is considered an `other qualified healthcare professional.'

Format of the Terminology

In order to save space and improve readability, codes have been formatted with the main information on the first line; code differentiation is included below and is indented. The primary component of the text is placed before the semicolon, and is part of the code.

For example:

	Work hardening/conditioning;
97545	initial 2 hours
97546	each additional hour

Therefore, the full descriptions for these codes would be:

97545	Work hardening/conditioning; initial 2 hours
97546	Work hardening/conditioning; each additional hour

Modifiers

Modifiers should be used to "accurately identify" a procedure or service that does not meet the exact description of a CPT code. In other words, the service or procedure is slightly different from what is described by the code, but is accurately described with the application of a modifier.

Determining the correct modifier to report often depends on specific payer policies. For example, Medicare policies require bilateral procedures to be reported with modifier 50 on a single claim line (e.g., 69436-50), while many other payers accept either a single claim line (e.g., 69436-50) OR two claim lines (e.g., 69436-RT and 69436-LT).

As noted in the previous paragraph, the appropriate application of a modifier to the most accurate CPT code description allowed the service to be reported correctly. When application of a modifier still does not accurately reflect the service described in the medical record, it may require reporting an unlisted code. Unlisted codes may also require application of a modifier.

Book: See Appendix B — Modifiers for more comprehensive information about modifiers and a listing of both CPT and HCPCS modifiers.

Add-on Codes

Add-on codes mean exactly what the name implies. They never stand alone in the CPT codebook and are always placed on the second line after the primary code associated with it. For easy identification, in both the CPT codebook and in the tips portion of this publication, these codes are identified with a plus symbol "**+**" (see example that follows). In the code listing portion of Chapter 5.2 — Procedure Codes & Tips they are identified with the indicator "Add On."

Example:

Prolonged service(s) in the outpatient setting requiring direct patient contact beyond the time of the usual service;

★+99354   first hour (List separately in addition to code for outpatient **Evaluation and Management** or psychotherapy service, except with office or other outpatient services [99202-99215])

★+99355   each additional 30 minutes (List separately in addition to the code for prolonged services)

Code 99354 for prolonged treatment for an unusual circumstance is shown with the description (List separately in addition to code...) Use this code in addition to the standard office or outpatient evaluation and management codes, when services exceed the usual and customary services.

Resource: See Resource 53A for more information about the proper usage of these codes.

Unlisted Codes

An unlisted code is reported when there is not a CPT or HCPCS code available that accurately describes the service or procedure performed and application of a modifier or multiple modifiers is not sufficient to accurately describe it (as previously stated). Each section of the CPT codebook contains unlisted service codes for reporting these services within the specific service categories such as 60699 "Unlisted procedure, endocrine system" or 76496 "Unlisted fluoroscopic procedure (eg, diagnostic, interventional)." There are also unlisted HCPCS codes such as L8499 "Unlisted procedure for miscellaneous prosthetic services."

Store: FindACode.com subscribers can search the word "unlisted" to see unlisted code options.

When reporting an unlisted code, ensure the patient documentation clearly describes the components of the procedure or service performed. When submitting the claim, enter the name of the service and/or a brief description of it in Item Number 19 of the *1500 Claim Form*. This allows the payer to review the information provided and if sufficient, authorize payment. However, if additional information is still needed, they may request documentation (e.g., operative report).

Tip: To facilitate faster payment, it is recommended that the unlisted service or procedure be compared (by the provider of the service) to another procedure that has similar work, practice expense, and malpractice expense RVUs. This enables the payer to more easily identify and compare the unlisted procedure or service to one that they know the provider has evaluated as similar and thus determine a fair reimbursement amount.

Special Reports

A special report is used to code services that are new, variable, unusual, or rarely provided. These special reports are used to determine medical necessity or medical appropriateness of the service, and are used to justify payment.

Special reports should document the need and extent of the service, including duration of treatment and equipment needed. Special reports can also include treatment plans, therapeutic findings, and exacerbating or other conditions that arise during treatment.

The CPT codebook lists the following as reasons to create a special report: "complexity of symptoms, final diagnosis, diagnostic and therapeutic procedures, concurrent problems, and follow-up care."

Examples:

- 99080 Special reports such as insurance forms, more than the information conveyed in the usual medical communications or standard reporting form
- 99199 Unlisted special service, procedure or report

Alert — Results/Testing/Reports:
These three terms are not interchangeable and providers need to understand their differences to ensure proper communication. According to the CPT Editorial Panel, "Results are the technical component of a service. Testing leads to results and those results lead to interpretation. Reports are the work product of the interpretation of numerous test results."

NCCI Coding Edits

As part of their ongoing efforts to reduce inappropriate payments of Part B claims, the Centers for Medicare & Medicaid Services (CMS) developed the National Correct Coding Initiative (NCCI) edits which are tools used to determine the appropriate reporting of CPT and HCPCS codes. In an effort to promote correct coding nationwide and assist healthcare providers to correctly code and report their services, the policies developed are based on:

- Coding conventions in the American Medical Association's CPT codebook
- National and local policies and edits
- Coding guidelines developed by national societies
- Analysis of medical and surgical practices and current coding practices

NCCI is a system of preventing overpayments by identifying and bundling code pairs that have overlapping or integrative components when performed together in addition to identifying the number of units that would be considered reasonable, likely, or probable for each code. There are three types of NCCI edits:

- **Medically Unlikely Edits (MUEs):** Prevents payment for an inappropriate quantity of the same service performed in a single day.

- **Procedure-to-Procedure (PTP) edits:** Prevents inappropriate payment of services that should not be reported together unless a clinically appropriate PTP-associated modifier is also reported.

- **Add-on Code (AOC) edits:** A listing of CPT/HCPCS add-on codes with their respective primary codes. An add-on code may only be paid if the respective primary code has also been reported and is eligible for payment. See Resource 53A for more information about add-on codes.

NCCI edits are maintained and updated by CMS on a quarterly basis and their Policy Manual is updated annually. A change in an edit is not retroactive and has no bearing on prior services **unless** it has been specifically updated with a retroactive effective date. The NCCI Policy Manual is published with the edits and identifies general guidelines to explain the reason(s) for specific edits. Red text noted throughout the manual indicates changes for the current year. When reviewing a claim and comparing them to the edits for compliance purposes, it is important to apply the edits that were effective as of the date of service being reviewed.

Website: NCCI edits are updated quarterly and Find-A-Code links each edit and table of edits to each individual code to improve efficiency. Subscribers also have access to a simple way of verifying current NCCI PTP edits and MUEs using the National CCI Edits Validator™ tool. For a tutorial on how to use this tool, sign into FindACode.com, click on "Tools", then "Scrubbing & Validation", and then CCI Validator™ (non-facility or facility) and then click on the "Demo Video" button in the upper right corner of the screen.

Who Uses NCCI Edits?

NCCI is not applicable to all medical claims. Review your third-party payer contracts and their published policies to determine if they use them or a version of them. Medicare requires contracted providers to adhere to the NCCI edits, NCCI Policy Manual guidance, and MUEs while other payer types have the option to decide whether or not to adopt them into their policies. Payers who adopt NCCI edits must publish that they have done so in their policies and procedures, and in their provider contracts identify which parts (i.e., NCCI Policy Manual, NCCI PTP Edits, MUEs) they are adopting/using. When these policies are not published or made part of a provider's contract, the payer may not hold the provider accountable to follow them.

An example of this is liability payers (e.g., workers compensation, auto) who are not held to the same standards for coding and billing as Medicare, Medicaid, and commercial payers. As such, providers are not required to follow NCCI unless agreed upon through a provider contract. If these payers deny insurance claims based on NCCI edits and policies, and there is no agreement requiring the use of NCCI edits included in the contract, the claim may be appealed for proper payment.

Book: See Appendix A — NCCI Edits for a list of commonly used specialty-specific NCCI edits.

Resource: See Resource 53B for detailed information on NCCI, PTP edits, MUEs, and using the NCCI Policy Manual.

Evaluation and Management (E/M) Services

Evaluation and Management (E/M) services are a type of patient encounter between a physician or other qualified healthcare professional (QHP) and a patient seeking medical advice and care for symptoms, conditions, illnesses, or injuries. Commonly, E/M services are face-to-face encounters between the provider and patient, but there are several E/M encounter types that may transpire over the phone, online, or through telehealth/telemedicine (real-time audiovisual) or another form of telecommunication.

Book: See Chapter 5.3 — Evaluation & Management Coding for more information about these services.

Store: See innoviHealth's *Comprehensive Guide to Evaluation & Management* (available in the online store) for more information about properly documenting E/M visits.

Who May Use E/M Codes? Evaluation and Managements codes can only be used by a physician or 'other qualified healthcare professional.' See Resource 402 for more about who is an 'other qualified healthcare professional.'

Notes:

5.2 Procedure Codes & Tips

The codes included in this chapter are a selection of codes for behavioral health. They are selected from both the official Current Procedural Terminology (CPT) code book and the Healthcare Common Procedure Coding System (HCPCS) code set. The complete listing of both code sets can be found at FindACode.com.

Procedure Code Tips

The following tips for procedure codes are derived from a variety of sources, including Medicare. It is designed to be a quick reference to assist in the code selection process. Only some commonly billed procedure codes are included in the "Procedure Code Tips" segment. A more comprehensive, specialty-specific list is found in the "Common Procedure Codes" section which begins on page 273.

Book: See Chapter 4.3 — Documentation Tips for information regarding requirements for proper documentation.
Website: Go to FindACode.com for additional procedure code information including fees and third party payer information.

Disclaimer: The information in this chapter contains general information and is the opinion of the authors. It should not be interpreted by providers/payers as official guidance. As such, this information should not be used for claim adjudication. Third party payers should utilize their own payment policies based on clinically sound guidelines.

Code Tip Index

2022 — New/Revised Codes	227
Adaptive Behavior Services	228
Alcohol/Substance Use Screening and Counseling	231
Assessment and Testing Services	240
Cognitive Impairment Services	248
Diagnostic Evaluations	252
Evaluation & Management	253
Health Behavior Assessment and Intervention	255
Intensive Outpatient Program (IOP)	256
Interactive Complexity (90785)	257
Partial Hospitalization Program (PHP)	258
Pharmacologic Management	258
Preventive Services	259
Psychiatric Collaborative Care (99492-99494, G2214)	259
Psychotherapy	262
Remote Monitoring	268
Telehealth Services	269
Timed Codes	270
Transcranial Magnetic Stimulation (TMS)	270
Veteran's Affairs Services	271

Important Notes About This Chapter

The codes in this chapter are grouped together by service types and include segments such as, "Diagnoses," "Coding Tips," etc. As stated in the disclaimer, these segments are general in nature.

Diagnoses

The "Diagnoses" segments include possible ICD-10-CM code categories for each procedure. They are not complete lists of all possible diagnoses for the associated procedure. Providers should always use sound clinical judgment when determining the appropriate diagnosis for a case. Do not use the "Diagnoses" listings as a substitute for proper diagnosis code selection.

Medicare has stated that "it is the responsibility of the provider to code to the highest level specified in the ICD-10-CM. The correct use of an ICD-10-CM code does not assure coverage of a service. The service must be reasonable and necessary in the specific case and must meet the criteria specified in this determination."

Unless otherwise noted in the sections that follow, generally most codes in Chapter 5 "Mental, Behavioral and Neurodevelopmental Disorders (F01-F99)" of ICD-10-CM are appropriate as long as they meet medical necessity criteria and individual payer policy requirements.

Additionally, the following may likely be covered, given medical necessity criteria are met:

A50.4-	E66-	G21-	**G24.02**	**G24.4**	G25.7-	**G26**	G30-	G31-	G47-	**H93.25**
R37	**R40.0**	**R40.1**	R41-	**R45.7**	R45.85-	**R47-**	**R48.0**	**R49.1**	T74.02-	T76-

Book: See Appendix E — Common Diagnosis Code Tips for additional information on coding common diagnosis codes.

Store: For codes not included in Appendix E — Common Diagnosis Code Tips, see innoviHealth's *ICD-10-CM Coding for Behavioral Health* book or the *ICD-10-CM Comprehensive CodeBook* (available in the online store).

All Criteria Must Be Met for CPT and HCPCS Codes

Each CPT and HCPCS code has an assigned description identifying the work that must be done and documented in order to bill for the service. When the required elements are not documented in the medical record but the service is still billed, the claim submitted may be denied. However, when the claim is paid, it could be audited at a future date to verify proper documentation. Constant requests for medical records to support services billed may be an indicator of an upcoming audit or investigation into the documentation, coding, and billing habits of your organization.

As CPT and HCPCS codes are updated annually, it is important for your organization to maintain the current manuals or have access to an online code information database like the one at FindACode.com where current updates are strictly maintained. Vital information regarding codes, description, NCCI edits, modifiers, and more are easily obtained online with one of our subscription options.

Website: Contact FindACode.com for a free demo to see how our many tools and features can benefit your organization.

Conventions

The following conventions are used in this chapter:

Type Styles

Excerpts from the AMA's CPT codebook are in a type style like this.

Explanations added by innoviHealth are in a type style like this. Tables are the exception. All text in tables, including codes, notations or explanations by innoviHealth, will be in **a type style like this.**

Tables like this include official instructions or quotes from payers.

Revision Identifiers

N Signifies a code added this year.

R Signifies a code revised this year. Revised codes may have had a change to their description, inclusion terms, and/or instructional notes.

2022 — New/Revised Codes

During 2021, new codes were added which should be noted by a behavioral health practice. There are also changes which are effective January 1, 2022.

Care Management Services

Care management services have expanded. There are four new codes for Principal Care Management to report the management of a patient with a single complex chronic condition which is expected to last at least 3 months. See the "Principal Care Management" segment in Chapter 5.3 — Evaluation & Management Coding for additional information.

COVID PHE Additional Supplies & Work

On September 8, 2020, code 99072 was added to report the additional supplies, materials, and clinical staff time over and above what is typically included for an office visit in consequence of the COVID PHE. Even though the RVS Update Committee recommended an approved amount of $6.57, CMS has denied payment for this code and so have many other payers. At the time of publication, the 2022 Final Rule stated that CMS was still considering comments so there will be no Medicare coverage in 2022.

Evaluation and Management Office Visits

The big changes to E/M services for Office or Other Outpatient Visits took place in 2021. For 2022, there is one small change; the phrase "usually the presenting problems are minimal" was removed from code 99211. See Chapter 5.3 — Evaluation & Management Coding for additional information.

Remote Patient Monitoring

Digital medicine also continues to expand. Over the last few years, new codes have been added and this pattern continues with the addition of several codes. In fact, the CPT codebook includes a new appendix devoted entirely to digital medicine. See "Remote Monitoring" on page 268 for more information.

Veteran's Affairs

Last year new codes were added for chaplain services and this year another new code has been added. See "Veteran's Affairs Services" on page 271 for more information.

Adaptive Behavior Services

Explanation

A new section was added to the CPT codebook along with additional guidelines and definitions in 2019. These codes may be used for patients of any age who have any of the following:

- Deficient adaptive behaviors (e.g., impaired social skills)
- Maladaptive behaviors (e.g., repetitive behaviors or those causing harm to others or property)
- Impaired functioning secondary to deficient or maladaptive behaviors (e.g., instruction-following, self-care)

They are not limited to just individuals with autism spectrum disorders (ASDs). They are also appropriate for other diagnoses or conditions such as developmental disabilities or head trauma. Reimbursement and medical necessity requirements vary by payer, although most will require a reasonable expectation of improvement where ongoing therapy is not necessary to maintain or prevent deterioration of a certain level of functioning.

Codes 0362T "Behavior identification supporting assessment" and 0373T "Adaptive behavior treatment with protocol modification" require a physician or other qualified health care professional (QHP) to be "on-site," which means that they are close and immediately available should the technician require assistance. They do not necessarily need to be in the same room while the service is being performed.

According to the Behavior Analyst Certification Board (BACB), a technician is someone who has received formal training (e.g., Registered Behavior Technician) and a QHP can be a Licensed Behavior Analyst, Licensed Assistant Behavior Analyst, Board Certified Behavior Analyst-Doctoral, Board Certified Behavior Analyst, Board Certified Assistant Behavior Analyst, or other credentialed professional whose scope of practice, training, and competence includes applied behavior analysis.

Note: All adaptive behavior services are reported in 15 minute increments. As of 2019, add-on codes are not used to report additional time.

Resource: See Resource 412 for more information about these codes.

ASSESSMENTS

Adaptive behavior assessments are either conducted and administered by a physician or QHP or administered by one or more technician(s) under the direction of the physician/QHP. They are divided into behavior identification and supporting assessments, both of which may include functional analysis and/or behavior assessments.

Adaptive Behavior Assessments Coding Table			
Code	Description	By	Notes
Assessment, Face-to-face, each 15 min, with patient and guardian(s)/caregiver(s)			
97151	Behavior identification assessment	Physician/QHP	May include any or all of the following: • non-face-to-face time analyzing data • score, interpretation, and report • develop plan of care which may include supportive assessments • discuss results/options w/patient/caregiver(s)

Supporting Assessment, Face-to-face, each 15 min, with one patient			
97152	Supporting assessment • **deficient** adaptive/maladaptive/impaired	1 tech	• No "on-site" requirement for phys/QHP, but done under their direction • Includes phys/QHP interpretation of results
0362T	Supporting assessment with required components including: • patient with **destructive** behavior(s) • customized patient environment	Phys/QHP with 2+ techs	• "On-site" requirement for phys/QHP • Time reporting is a single tech's time • Environment customized to patient's behavior

Notes:
- All assessments may include functional analysis and/or behavior assessment
- Deficient adaptive/maladaptive/impaired = Patient has deficient adaptive/maladaptive behavior(s), or other impaired functioning secondary to deficient adaptive/maladaptive behavior
- Codes 97152 and 0362T may be used with 97151

Coding Tips

- These assessments do not describe diagnostic (90791, 90792), speech (92521-92524) or occupational therapy evaluations (97165-97168), health/behavior assessment/interventions (96156-96171), or neuropsychological testing (96132-96146)

- Adaptive behavior assessments may include any or all of the following (see FindACode.com or a CPT codebook for more comprehensive definitions):

  - **Functional behavior assessment:** identify behaviors and/or triggering events by utilizing caregiver interviews, questionnaires, and/or observation

  - **Functional analysis:** evaluate effects of environmental events on potential target behavior by observing and measuring occurrences of the behavior in response to those events

  - **Other structured observations**

  - **Instruments and procedures**

    - *Standardized:* administered and scored in the same way for all patients (e.g., Pervasive Developmental Disabilities Behavior Inventory)

    - *Nonstandardized:* Used to assess behaviors and associated environmental events specific to an individual patient and their behaviors

- Code 97152 also includes the physician's or QHP's interpretation of assessment results to determine the levels of adaptive and maladaptive behavior

- Supporting assessments (97152, 0362T) may be:

  - reported in conjunction with 97151

  - repeated on different days until the behavior identification assessment (97151) is complete

  - reported based on the type of behavior being addressed — use 97152 for deficient and 0362T for destructive

- For code 0362T, only the face-to-face time of one technician may be reported so one hour with 3 techs is reported as 1 unit, not 3 units

- Destructive behavior (0362T) is defined by the CPT codebook as one or more "maladaptive behaviors associated with high risk of medical consequences or property damage (e.g., elopement, pica, or self-injury requiring medical attention, aggression with injury to other(s), or breaking furniture, walls, or windows)"

TREATMENT

Adaptive behavior treatment (ABT) focuses on goals and targets established by previous assessments (97151, 97152, 0362T). Treatment protocols are established by a physician or QHP and then administered by either a physician/QHP or technician. These services may include ongoing assessments and/or modifications to the treatment protocol by the physician/QHP when there is a problem(s) with the current protocol. Code selection is based on the type of behavior addressed (e.g., deficient, destructive), who performs the service (e.g., QHP, technician[s]), and to whom (e.g., patient, group).

Adaptive Behavior Treatment (ABT) Coding Table

Code	Description	By	Notes
Treatment — One Patient, Face-to-face, each 15 minutes			
97153	ABT by protocol	1 tech	• No "on-site" requirement for phys/QHP • **Deficient** adaptive/maladaptive/impaired • Do not report with 92507
97155	ABT w/protocol modification, by physician/QHP, may include simultaneous direction of tech	Phys/QHP with 0-1 tech	• "On-site" requirement for phys/QHP • **Deficient** adaptive/maladaptive/impaired • **Destructive** behavior(s) • Do not report phys/QHP instruction of tech w/o patient present • Do not report with 92507
0373T	ABT w/protocol modification, with required components including: • patient with **destructive** behavior(s) • customized patient environment	Phys/QHP with 2+ techs	• "On-site" requirement for phys/QHP • Time reporting is a single tech's time • Environment customized to patient's behavior
Notes: • Deficient adaptive/maladaptive/impaired = Patient has deficient adaptive/maladaptive behavior(s), or other impaired functioning secondary to deficient adaptive/maladaptive behavior • Do not report any of these codes with 90785-90899, 96105-96155			
Treatment — Group (2-8; patient or family) All Face-to-face			
97154	Group ABT by protocol; 2-8 patients	1 tech	• Do not report with 92508, 97150
97158	Group ABT w/protocol modification; 2-8 patients	Phys/QHP	• Do not report with 92508, 97150 • Protocol modifications made during session
97156	Family ABT guidance; one family; w/wo patient	Phys/QHP	
97157	Multi-family ABT guidance; w/o patient	Phys/QHP	
Notes: • Do not report these codes if more than 8 patients or families are present • Do not report any of these codes with 90785-90899, 96105-96155			

Coding Tips

- For code 0373T, only the face-to-face time of one technician may be reported so one hour with 3 techs is reported as 1 unit, not 3 units

- Destructive behavior (97155, 0373T) is defined by the CPT codebook as one or more "maladaptive behaviors associated with high risk of medical consequences or property damage (e.g., elopement, pica, or self-injury requiring medical attention, aggression with injury to other(s), or breaking furniture, walls, or windows)"

- Treatment guidance (97156, 97157) includes identifying potential treatment targets and training parent(s)/guardian(s) on how to implement the patient's protocols at home. The patient may or may not be present for these sessions depending on code selection.

- Pay attention to payer-specific requirements such as clinical rationale for the length and frequency of treatment.

Alcohol/Substance Use Screening and Counseling

Explanation

There are a variety of code options for substance use disorder (SUD) screenings and subsequent treatment. Most commonly, SUD treatment services (with the exception of the items discussed in this segment) are reported with psychotherapy codes 90832-90838, intensive outpatient, or partial hospitalization services. This segment discusses the following:

- Drug testing
- Medication assisted treatment (MAT)
- Opioid use disorder treatment
- Screening and brief intervention services (SBIRT)

 Book: See also "Intensive Outpatient Program (IOP)" on page 256 and "Partial Hospitalization Program (PHP)" on page 258.

DRUG TESTING

Drug testing may be either presumptive or definitive and is used to monitor chronic pain management as well as compliance with substance use disorder treatment. Bundled services may include drug testing, depending on payer policy (see "Bundled Services" on page 233). Where allowed, the following are some commonly used codes for drug testing.

Drug test(s), **presumptive**, any number of drug classes; any number of devices or procedures, (eg, immunoassay), includes sample validation when performed, per date of service;

80305	capable of being read by direct optical observation only (eg, dipsticks, cups, cards, cartridges)
80306	read by instrument-assisted direct optical observation (eg, dipsticks, cups, cards, cartridges)
80307	by instrumented chemistry analyzers (eg, immunoassay, enzyme assay, TOF, MALDI, LDTD, DESI, DART, GHPC, GC mass spectrometry)

Alcohol (ethanol);

82075	breath
82077	any specimen except urine and breath, immunoassay (eg, IA, EIA, ELISA, RIA, EMIT, FPIA) and enzymatic methods (eg, alcohol dehydrogenase)

Drug test(s), **definitive**, utilizing drug identification methods able to identify individual drugs and distinguish between structural isomers (but not necessarily stereoisomers), including, but not limited to GC/MS (any type, single or tandem) and LC/MS (any type, single or tandem and excluding immunoassays (eg, IA, ELISA, EMIT, FPIA) and enzymatic methods (eg, alcohol dehydrogenase));

qualitative and quantitative, all sources, includes specimen validity testing, per day, per # of drug classes as listed below. Includes metabolite(s) if performed;

- G0480   1-7 drug class(es)
- G0481   8-14 drug class(es)
- G0482   15-21 drug class(es)
- G0483   22 or more drug class(es)
- G0659   performed without method or drug-specific calibration, without matrix-matched quality control material, or without use of stable isotope or other universally recognized internal standard(s) for each drug, drug metabolite or drug class per specimen

Note: Tests using codes 80307, G0482, G0483 can be expensive, so verify coverage prior to ordering.

Resource: See Resource 541 for more comprehensive information.

Alert: Drug testing may only be performed with the patient's consent and must comply with applicable state laws.

MEDICATION-ASSISTED TREATMENT/MANAGEMENT (MAT)

Explanation

Pharmacotherapeutic agents can play a critical role in treating substance use disorders (SUDs) and vary depending on the disorder being treated. They serve several purposes: reducing acute withdrawal symptoms, detoxifying, curtailing cravings, and preventing relapses. For tobacco cessation, nicotine replacement therapies are typically utilized. For alcohol SUDs, naltrexone, acamprosate, and disulfiram are utilized. Opiate SUDs (OUDs) employ agonist therapies such as methadone and buprenorphine.

Note: CMS recently expanded MAT by exempting physicians from certain certification requirements needed to prescribe buprenorphine for opioid use disorder (OUD) treatment. See Resource 52B for more information.

Some payers bundle all substance use disorder treatment services together under one payment rate while others allow breaking out services and reporting them separately. Many payers consider weekly per diem rates to include several types of services (e.g., medication management). It is up to the provider to understand what the payer considers bundled and not bill these services separately. For example, one state's Medicaid weekly "bundled rate" for methadone maintenance services included the following:

- Intake evaluation
- Initial physical examination
- On-site drug abuse testing and monitoring
- Individual, group, and family counseling services

>
> **Alert:** One large organization was fined a significant amount of money because they billed psychotherapy separately for Medicaid patients undergoing SUD treatment. You must know the individual payer policies and ONLY bill according to those policies.
>
> Also, be sure to verify which medications are covered by each payer as well as the level of education or licensing they require for the healthcare provider who is performing counseling services.
>
> **Book:** See Appendix B — Modifiers for a list of modifiers (e.g., HO "Masters Degree Level") which may be used to identify the level of education or licensing of the treating provider.

MAT in the ED Setting

OUD services in the emergency department (ED) setting can be different than other settings. According to CMS, "the term MAT generally refers to treatment of OUD that includes both an FDA-approved medication for the treatment of OUD and behavioral/psychosocial treatment, but that care provided in the ED typically would include medication for the treatment of OUD and referral or linkage to primary care or a hospital-based bridge clinic for continuation of medication and potentially other services, including counseling and other psychosocial services." To more accurately describe the services provided in an ED, the following new code was created:

G2213   Initiation of medication for the treatment of opioid use disorder in the emergency department setting, including assessment, referral to ongoing care, and arranging access to supportive services (List separately in addition to code for primary procedure)

This new code includes payment for assessment, referral to ongoing care, follow-up after treatment begins, and arranging access to supportive services, but it should be noted that the drug itself will be paid separately. See Chapter 6.2 — Supply Codes & Tips for information about the drugs used for MAT.

Bundled Services

Some payers bundle payments for substance use disorders since medication assisted treatment (MAT) should be combined with other behavioral modification techniques (e.g., psychotherapy) for optimal treatment outcomes. Federal guidelines (42 CFR 8.12) require opioid treatment programs (OTP) to include MAT along with psychosocial and support services including the following:

- physical exam and assessment
- psychosocial assessment
- treatment planning
- counseling
- medication management
- drug administration, where applicable
- comprehensive care management and supportive services
- care coordination
- management of care transitions
- individual and family support services
- health promotion
- overdose education furnished in conjunction with providing an opioid antagonist medication (new for 2021)

Medicare-Enrolled Opioid Treatment Program

Medicare's opioid treatment program (OTP), which began in January of 2020, includes a number of bundled codes for the weekly treatment of opioid use disorders. These bundled codes include the following services:

- dispensing and/or administration of medication
- substance use counseling
- individual and/or group therapy
- and toxicology testing (if performed)

There are codes that include medication and those that do not. These codes may *only* be used by a Medicare-enrolled Opioid Treatment Program and the facility must have a current, valid certification from the Substance Abuse and Mental Health Services Administration (SAMHSA) since these medications are controlled substances.

Note: As of January 1, 2021, CMS expanded the definition of OUD treatment services to include opioid antagonist medications (e.g., naloxone) which have been approved by the FDA for emergency treatment of known or suspected opioid overdose.

Intakes for new patients and periodic assessments for established patients are additional necessary services which may be separately billed with the following codes:

G2076 **Intake activities**, including initial medical examination that is a complete, fully documented physical evaluation and initial assessment conducted by a program physician or a primary care physician, or an authorized healthcare professional under the supervision of a program physician or qualified personnel that includes preparation of a treatment plan that includes the patient's short-term goals and the tasks the patient must perform to complete the short-term goals; the patient's requirements for education, vocational rehabilitation, and employment; and the medical, psychosocial, economic, legal, or other supportive services that a patient needs, conducted by qualified personnel; List separately in addition to code for primary procedure

G2077 **Periodic assessment**; assessing periodically by qualified personnel to determine the most appropriate combination of services and treatment; List separately in addition to code for primary procedure

Resource: These codes are only for services rendered in a Medicare-enrolled OTP. See Resource 643 to go to the CMS website which has more information about this program including enrollment information.

Medicare-Enrolled OTP MAT Coding Table

Drug	Oral	Take Home	Implant Insert	Implant Remove	Implant Insert & Remove	Injectable
buprenorphine	G2068	G2079	G2070	G2071	G2072	G2069
	All	Take Home				
methadone	G2067	G2078				
naltrexone	G2073	--				
drug NOS	G2075	--				
Take Home	Nasal	Injectable				
naloxone	N G1028 R G2215	G2216				

Notes:
- **All** = All modes of administration (i.e., oral, implant, injectable)
- **Add-on:** Code G2080 may be added to any of these codes (except "Take Home") for each additional 30 minutes of non-routine group or individual counseling
- **Take Home** = *Add-on* for codes when up to 7 days worth of medication is sent home with the patient, except for naloxone which may only be prescribed once every 30 days
- Naloxone prescription requires patient education about the proper use of this drug

Note: Medicare's OUD treatment codes G2086-G2088 do NOT include MAT. See "Opioid Use Disorder (OUD) Treatment" on page 236 for information about those services.

Coding Tips

- If a medication is NOT dispensed/administered, use code G2074 to report that the other expected services were provided.

- Therapy and counseling services may be provided via telehealth. See also "Telehealth Services" on page 269.

  As of January 1, 2022, when two-way audio/video communication technology is not available to the beneficiary and all other applicable requirements are met, these services may be provided using audio-only telephone calls. In this situation, it is required to document why two-way audio/video was not available to the patient. It should also be noted that when using the add-on code for additional counseling and therapy, the practitioner is "...required to certify, in a form and manner specified by CMS, that they had the capacity to furnish the services using two-way, audio/video communication technology, but used audio-only technology because the beneficiary did not have access to two-way audio/video communication technology."

  CMS has stated that it is up to the clinician's "...judgment to determine whether in-person counseling or therapy, rather than the use of audio-only telephone calls, would be most appropriate in certain circumstances, such as for patients who are considered to be high risk."

Note: After the COVID-19 PHE is over, when therapy and counseling bundled services are provided via audio-only communication, submitted claims must add modifer FQ.

- Unlike other Medicare services, beneficiaries have a flat copayment of $0.

- There is no limit on how long the patient may undergo OUD treatment.

- Intakes and periodic assessments (G2076, G2077) may be furnished by a program physician, a primary care physician, or an authorized healthcare professional under the supervision of a program physician or qualified personnel such as nurse practitioners (NPs) and physician assistants (PAs).

- At a minimum, the patient must receive at least one of the five services included in these bundled codes.

- There must be at least eight random drug abuse tests per year.

- Naloxone is only to be provided on an as-needed basis.

- Before billing the bundled OTP codes (e.g., G1028, G2215, G2216), check to see if the patient already has received a prescription paid under either Part B or Part D. CMS has stated that this would be considered duplicative if a claim for the same medication is separately paid for the same beneficiary on the same date of service, and CMS would recoup any duplicative payment made to an OTP for medication included in the bundled rate or paid for under the take-home add-on option.

Book: See Resource 644 for more comprehensive information about these services including billing requirements for institutional claims. Note that with recent changes to guidelines, this resource might not be immediately updated by CMS.

Non-Bundled Services

Some commonly used procedure codes are:

	Drug Delivery Implant;		
	Insertion	Removal	Removal w/Reinsertion
bioresorbable, biodegradable, non-biodegradable	11981	—	—
non-biodegradable	—	11982	11983
4 or more (services for subdermal rod implant)	G0516	G0517	G0518
biodegradable or bioresorable	—	—	17999

Other Medication Services

96372	Therapeutic, prophylactic, or diagnostic injection (specify substance or drug); subcutaneous or intramuscular
H0020	Alcohol and/or drug services; methadone administration and/or service (provision of the drug by a licensed program)
H0033	Oral medication administration, direct observation
S0109	Methadone, oral, 5 mg

 Note: H0020, H0033, and S0109 are not payable by Medicare. Also, some payers bundle services for code H0020. Review payer policies to determine their preferred code options and what services they include with these codes.

Alert: When using code H0020, pay close attention to what the payer defines as a unit and what they consider bundled into that code. Keep in mind that requirements may vary by both the payer and the state. Using Medicaid as an example in California the unit is daily, in Maryland it is weekly, and in Vermont it is monthly. So if you were billing Medicaid in California, you would bill one unit of code H0020 for every day of service, but if you were in Vermont, you would bill one unit of H0020 for the entire month of service.

Coding Tips

- Methadone maintenance services are being closely monitored by the OIG.
- When providers administer prepurchased medications, they may bill them separately if not billing bundled payment codes.
- Do not use J codes if the medication is just being prescribed and not administered.

 Alert: For pregnant women with an opioid use disorder, the American College of Obstetricians and Gynecologists recommends opioid agonist pharmacotherapy (methadone).

OPIOID USE DISORDER (OUD) TREATMENT

CMS-created OUD bundled payment codes are billed monthly and include management, care coordination, psychotherapy, and counseling activities. Even though they represent bundled services, they do not include Medication-Assisted Treatment (MAT) or drug testing so those services may be billed separately. The first code is for the initial month of treatment as it also includes an intake assessment and the development of the treatment plan.

Alert: The 2021 Medicare Physician Fee Schedule Final Rule indicated that these codes would be changed by replacing "opioid use disorder" with "a substance use disorder." However, the official code set release at the time of publication did not include that change. Watch for announcements of any updates to Medicare policies or code descriptions.

Office-based treatment for opioid use disorder, including care coordination, individual therapy and group therapy and counseling;

G2086   including development of the treatment plan; at least 70 minutes in the first calendar month

G2087   at least 60 minutes in a subsequent calendar month

G2088   each additional 30 minutes beyond the first 120 minutes (List separately in addition to code for primary procedure)

CMS payment is based on the assumption that there will be an average of two individual psychotherapy sessions and four group psychotherapy sessions per month; however, the frequency of services will vary based on the patient and their progress. The 2021 Final Rule said "For example, the needs of a particular patient in a month may be unusually acute, well beyond the needs of the typical patient; or there may be some months when psychosocial stressors arise that were unforeseen at the time the treatment plan was developed, but warrant additional or more intensive therapy services for the patient." Add-on code G2088 may be billed in cases of extraordinarily high usage of services.

 Note: When additional services are needed, be sure to document why they were needed (medical necessity) and report with add-on code G2088. This code can only be used with G2086 or G2087.

Treatment services are not limited to any particular physician or nonphysician practitioner specialty and may be provided by professionals "who are qualified to provide the services under state law and within their scope of practice 'incident to' the services of the billing physician or other practitioner."

Coding Tips

- All three of these codes may be rendered via telehealth.
- These codes were created by Medicare so be aware of different coding requirements from other payers such as Medicaid or commercial plans.
- Codes 90832, 90834, 90837, and 90853 may not be reported by the *same* practitioner for OUD treatment for the same beneficiary in the same month as these services. However, these services may be separately billed for treating co-occurring diagnoses.
- At least one psychotherapy service must be furnished in order to bill these services.
- These codes should not be billed more than once per month per beneficiary according to Medicare guidelines.
- According to Medicare, these codes are not limited to any particular physician or nonphysician provider (NPP) specialty.
- **New patient rules:** Prior to reporting these codes, there must be an initiating visit which evaluates the patient's needs. According to the proposed rule, the initiating visit could be an E/M visit (levels 2 through 5), annual wellness visit (AWV), initial preventive physical exam (IPPE), or transitional care management (TCM) services (99495 and 99496).
- **Emergency department:** These codes do not apply for this setting. See "MAT in the ED Setting" on page 233 for care initiated in this setting.

Book: Report the applicable opioid use disorder code from category F11- found in Appendix E — Common Diagnosis Codes & Tips.

SCREENING AND BRIEF INTERVENTION SERVICES (SBIRT)

Explanation

Screenings and counseling, also known as screening and brief intervention services (SBIRT), for Substance Use Disorders (SUDs) are typically a covered preventive service for most payers. As a preventive service, copayment/coinsurance and deductibles are typically waived. An SBIRT includes three components: a screening/assessment using a standardized tool, a brief intervention, and a referral for treatment when indicated.

Note: These are NOT considered SUD treatment services. For treatment, see psychotherapy codes (90832-90838), G2067-G2080, G2086-G2088, and "Intensive Outpatient," and "Partial Hospitalization."

SBIRT Coding Table

Description	Payer	Code
Assessment/Screening		
Alcohol and/or substance (other than tobacco) use/misuse structured screening (eg, AUDIT, DAST), and brief intervention (SBI) services;		
5-14 min	Commercial, Medicaid, Medicare	★G2011
15 to 30 min	Commercial, Medicaid	★99408
	Medicare	★G0396
greater than 30 min	Commercial, Medicaid	★99409
	Medicare	★G0397
Alcohol and/or drug assessment	Medicaid, Workers Comp	H0001
Annual alcohol misuse screening, 15 minutes	Medicare	★G0442
Alcohol and/or drug screening	Medicaid	H0049
Intervention Services		
Alcohol and/or drug services, brief intervention, per 15 minutes	Medicaid	H0050
Alcohol and/or drug intervention service (planned facilitation)	Medicaid, Workers Comp	H0022
Brief face-to-face behavioral counseling for alcohol misuse, 15 minutes	Medicare	★G0443

Notes:
- Medicaid and Workers Compensation plans are state-specific and may or may not use these codes.
- Codes with a star "★" symbol may be rendered via telehealth. See "Telehealth Services" on page 269 for more information.
- Other commercial payers might have other codes. Consider the following and verify with the payer:
  - H2012   Behavioral health day treatment, per hour
  - T1007   Alcohol and/or substance abuse services, treatment plan development and/or modification
  - T1015   Clinic visit/encounter, all-inclusive
  - T1023   Screening to determine the appropriateness of consideration of an individual for participation in a specified program, project or treatment protocol, per encounter

According to Medicare, dependence is defined as meeting at least 3 of the following:

- Tolerance
- Withdrawal symptoms
- Impaired control
- Preoccupations with acquisition and/or use
- Persistent desire or unsuccessful efforts to quit
- Sustains social, occupational, or recreational disability
- Use continues despite adverse consequences

Book: See "Substance Use Disorders" in Appendix E — Common Diagnosis Codes & Tips for more about selecting an appropriate diagnosis code(s).
Resource: As a reminder, PHI relating to substance abuse has greater confidentiality requirements than other medical records. See Resource 623 for more information.

Coding Tips

- Some of these services are timed codes, so be sure to document start and stop times and follow payer guidelines regarding the reporting of time. See "Timed Codes" on page 270 for more information.
- Screenings often use a short pre-screen (e.g., the National Institute on Alcohol Abuse and Alcoholism's [NIAAA] 3 Question Screen) to identify individuals who need a more comprehensive screening. Pre-screenings are not reported separately. To report these services, you must administer a standardized tool such as the Alcohol Use Disorders Identification Tool (AUDIT) or The Drug Abuse Screening Test (DAST).
- Document the following five components:

    1. **Assess:** Ask about/assess behavioral health risk(s) and factors affecting choice of behavior change goals/methods.
    2. **Advise:** Give clear, specific, and personalized behavior change advice, including information about personal health harms and benefits.
    3. **Agree:** Collaboratively select appropriate treatment goals and methods based on the patient's interest in and willingness to change the behavior.
    4. **Assist:** Using behavior change techniques (self-help and/or counseling) to aid the patient in achieving agreed-upon goals by acquiring the skills, confidence, and social/environmental supports for behavior change, supplemented with adjunctive medical treatments when appropriate.
    5. **Arrange:** Schedule follow-up contacts (in person or by telephone) to provide ongoing assistance/support and to adjust the treatment plan as needed, including referral to more intensive or specialized treatment.

    – NCD 210.8

- Medicare coverage information:
    - Four counseling sessions (G0443) are covered
    - The patient must be competent and alert when face-to-face (or telehealth where applicable) counseling is provided
    - Counseling provided by a primary care provider (e.g., doctor or nurse practitioner) in a primary care setting (e.g., doctor's office or clinic)
    - Screenings provided in any of the following settings are not covered:
        - Ambulatory surgical center
        - Emergency department

- Hospice
- Independent diagnostic testing facility
- Inpatient hospital setting (outpatient may be covered if other criteria are met)
- Inpatient rehabilitation facility
- Skilled nursing facility

Alert: As of January 1, 2021, CMS includes SUD screenings as part of the Initial Preventive Physical Examination (IPPE) or the Annual Wellness Visit (AWV) so it may not be separately reported.

Resource: See Resource 612 for more information.

Resource: See Resource 624 to review the Department of Veterans Affairs and Department of Defense's "Clinical Practice Guideline for the Management of Substance Use Disorders" for additional helpful information.

Assessment and Testing Services

Explanation

The CPT codebook section on developmental, psychological, and neuropsychological assessment and testing services was significantly modified in 2019 to more closely align with other procedure code descriptions which have a primary base code describing the main service and add-on code(s) to report additional work performed beyond the base service. The technical component (performing the test) is separated from the professional component (interpretation and report). Time spent scoring tests by a physician, QHP, or technician is now considered to be billable time.

These central nervous system services are organized into the following:

- Assessment of Aphasia and Cognitive Performance Testing (96105, 96125)
- Developmental/Behavioral Screening and Testing (96110-96113 [page 243], 96127 [page 245])
- Psychological/Neuropsychological Testing
  - Neurobehavioral Status Examination (96116, 96121), see page 245
  - Testing Evaluation Services (96130-96133), see page 247
  - Test Administration and Scoring (96136-96139), see page 246
  - Automated Testing and Result (96146) describes computerized or electronic testing wherein a test is administered and scored automatically without the assistance or direction of a technician or healthcare provider. Report one unit for every automated, standardized test taken by the patient. The results may be incorporated into the medical decision making portion of other evaluation services (e.g., 96130, 90791).

Book:
- For adaptive behavior assessment or testing, see page 228.
- For alcohol or substance use assessments, see page 238.
- For health behavior assessments, see page 255.

Alert: The following assessment and testing codes have been deleted: 96101, 96102, 96103, 96111, 96118, 96119, 96120. See the tables that follow for the appropriate codes for services.

The following table outlines the different testing services and what is included when they are rendered by a physician or other qualified healthcare professional (QHP). For other provider types, see the "Services Performed by Others" table that follows.

Services Performed by Physician/QHP

Code	Add-on	Unit	Description	Page	Test	E/F	I/R	Face
96105	n/a	Hour	Aphasia assessment		X		X	
96125	n/a	Hour	Cognitive performance testing		X		X	X
96110	n/a	Instrument	Developmental screening	243				
96112	96113	Hour/30 min	Developmental testing	243	X		X	
★96116	96121	Hour	Neurobehavioral status examination	245	X		X	X
96136	96137	30 min	Test administration and scoring (2+ tests), psychological or neuropsychological	246	X			X
96132	96133	Hour	Testing evaluation, neuropsychological	247		X	X	X
96130	96131	Hour	Testing evaluation, psychological	247		X	X	X

Table Key:
- ★   Telehealth code
- Add-on   The code to add to the primary procedure for additional intra-service work
- E/F   Evaluation and Interactive Feedback
- Face   Includes a face-to-face service, if applicable
- I/R   Interpretation and Report
- Page   See this page for more information about these services
- Test   Test administration/scoring
- Unit   The reporting unit. Developmental testing is unique in that the first unit is an hour and each additional 30 minutes is reported with the add-on code of 96113.

Resource: See Resource 402 for additional information on qualified healthcare professionals (QHPs).

The "Services Performed by Others" table that follows outlines services that may be reported when rendered by an automated, computerized program or by someone other than a physician or QHP. According to the CPT codebook, clinical staff is defined as "a person who works under the supervision of a physician or other qualified health care professional and who is allowed by law, regulation and facility policy to perform or assist in the performance of a specified professional service, but who does not individually report that professional service. Other policies may also affect who may report specific services."

The CPT codebook does not define a technician. Generally speaking, a technician is someone performing technical work of a service under the direction of a professional. The services that may be delegated largely depends on state law and/or payer policies. There may also be information from professional organizations that provide guidance. For example, the American Academy of Clinical Neuropsychology, and the National Academy of Neuropsychology both have policies on the use and training of technicians.

Services Performed by Others							
Code	Add-on	Unit	Description	Page	Tech	Staff	Auto
96110	n/a	Instrument	Developmental screening	243	X	X	
96127	n/a	Instrument	Emotional/behavioral assessment, brief	245		X	
96138	96139	30 min	Test administration and scoring (2+ tests), psychological or neuropsychological	246	X		
96146	n/a	Instrument	Automated test administration and scoring, single, psychological or neuropsychological				X

Table Key:
Add-on The code to add to the primary procedure for additional intra-service work
Auto   Automated, computerized test administration with an automated result
Page   See this page for more information about these services
Tech   Technician
Staff   Staff member qualified/trained to perform the service
Unit   The reporting unit

Coding Tips

- Do not report (bill) if time is less than 31 minutes for hour-based codes (e.g., 96130). For codes with a unit of 30 minutes, do not report if time is less than 16 minutes.

  Book: See "Timed Codes" on page 270.

- Be aware of payer policies which may require the use of an applicable modifier to identify the level of training of the individual performing the testing services (e.g., HN "Bachelors degree level").

  Book: See Appendix B — Modifiers for a comprehensive listing of modifiers to report the applicable provider type.

- Assessments performed by a chaplain may be reported with new code Q9001. See "Veteran's Affairs Services" on page 271 for more information.

- Providing interactive feedback to patient or caregiver(s) has been added to psychological and neuropsychological testing evaluation services. See page 259.

- Typically, routine re-evaluation of chronically disabled patients is not considered medically necessary by payers

- Do not report these services at the same time as Adaptive Behavior Services (97151-97158, 0362T, 0373T)

- Dementia screenings by a physician or QHP should be reported with E/M codes

- Testing services (96105, 96112, 96113, 96125, 96130-96133) must include an interpretation and report

- Automated testing (96146) must include an automated result

- Be aware of payer policies regarding the reporting of services covering multiple days. Some may want only the last day reported while others may want the date range.

- When documenting complex patient encounters where multiple services are rendered, it becomes very important to have the patient record clearly state the beginning and ending times for **each type of service** provided.

Audit Alert: Testing more than 8 hours per patient, per evaluation typically requires a copy of the report to support medical necessity.

Reminder: Technicians and trainees (e.g., students, interns, post-doctoral fellows) are not the same thing. Individual payers determine whether supervised, unlicensed trainees may bill services.

Coding Example

The following example and table outline codes that might be billed for a complex patient encounter where services cover multiple days with varying types of testing.

> **Example**
> Jane Feelsbad is a 16 year old female who, according to her parents, is currently experiencing symptoms of anxiety, depression, and erratic behavior. Her therapist requests testing to better assess her symptoms and formulate a treatment plan. She comes to the clinic and spends 175 minutes taking a computerized MMPI-A, MACI, and the Beck Depression Inventory. She later returns to meet with the psychologist who spends 2 hours and 20 minutes administering and scoring the WISC-V. He talks on the phone with the school counselor for 20 minutes. He spends 145 minutes reviewing and interpreting all gathered information, including the previously administered tests, the WISC which he performed, and writing a report. When the report is complete, Jane and her parents come in together for 50 minutes to discuss the results and decide on treatment options.

Codes to Report for the Example					
Code	Description	Time	Units	Explanation/Notes	
96146	MMPI-A, MACI, and the Beck depression inventory	n/a	2	Time is not counted. Use 1 unit for each computerized test. Only 2 units are counted because the Beck Depression Inventory is a self-reported, non-automated/computerized test so it cannot be reported separately.	
	Psych testing by QHP			2 hours 20 minutes (140 minutes) total includes both administering and scoring the tests, but NOT the interpretation and report	
96136	first 30 minutes	30	1		
96137	each addt'l 30 min	110	4	If this had been 76-105 minutes, then 3 units would have been billed.	
	Psych testing evaluation services			215 minutes total includes • 20 minute phone call with school counselor • 145 minutes interpretation and report • 50 minutes interactive feedback with family	
96130	first hour	60	1		
96131	each addt'l hour	155	3	Subtracting the first unit (60 minutes) from the total (215) leaves 155 minutes (2 hours and 35 minutes). Since 35 minutes is past the midpoint (31 minutes) an additional unit may be reported.	

DEVELOPMENTAL TESTING/SCREENING (96110-96113, G0451)

Explanation

These codes identify developmental testing or developmental screenings performed to identify or rule-out developmental delays using standardized tools. Areas of development evaluated include fine motor, gross motor, visual motor/adaptive, language, and personal and social skills.

96110   Developmental **screening** (eg, developmental milestone survey, speech and language delay screen), with scoring and documentation, per standardized instrument

G0451   Development testing, with interpretation and report, per standardized instrument form

Developmental **test administration** (including assessment of fine and/or gross motor, language, cognitive level, social, memory and/or executive functions by standardized developmental instruments when performed), by physician or other qualified health care professional, with interpretation and report

96112   first hour

+ 96113   each additional 30 minutes (List separately in addition to code for primary procedure)

Coding Tips

- Code 96110 is described as a screening, whereas 96112, 96113, and G0451 are described as testing. Please be aware of the differences. Even though the description for code G0451 uses the word 'testing,' its RVU is the same as 96110, so it is priced as a screening and intended to be less comprehensive than testing services.

- Medicare covers G0451 but not 96110.

- For developmental testing services, the individual administering the test interprets the results and provides a written report of findings.

- Students/trainees performing tests are generally NOT covered.

- A United coverage policy regarding 96110 states: "Because a physician obtains developmental information as an intrinsic part of a Preventive Medicine service (99381-99397, G0402) for an infant or child and because this information is sometimes obtained in the form of a questionnaire completed by the parents, it is expected that this code will be reported in addition to the Preventive Medicine visit only if the screening meets the code description. Physicians should report the specific CPT code, for developmental screening or other similar screening or testing, separate and distinct from the Preventive Medicine service only when the testing or screening results in an interpretation and report by the physician being entered into the medical record."

- For an emotional/behavioral assessment, use 96127 (see page 245).

- For Early Periodic Screening Diagnosis and Treatment (EPSDT) services, some payers may require the use of code S0302. This code may be reported with E/M services.

Diagnoses

96110/G0451: Consider ICD-10-CM codes from the following:

B20	F01- to F09	F10.11	F10.120 to F48.9	F50- to F82	F84-	F88
F89	F90- to F98.9	F99	G13-	G20	G21-	G24- to G25-
G26	G30- to G31-	G35	G40-	G44.209	G47.52	G47.53
G80.3	G91-	G93.1	G94	H91.3	H93.25	I60-
I69-	R37	R40.0	R40.1	R41.0 - R41.3	R41.8-	R45.1
R45.2	R45.5 to R45.83	R47.02	R47.1	R47.8-	R47.9	R48-
S06-	T50.9-	T74-	T76-	Z00.12-	Z87.890	

96112/96113: Consider ICD-10-CM codes from the following:

F80-	F81-	F82	F84-	F88	F89	F90-	F94-	F98.9	H93.25	R62.0
R62.5-	Z00.121	Z13.4 -								

Note: Routine developmental screenings of children are coded with Z00.12- instead of Z13- codes.

EMOTIONAL/BEHAVIORAL ASSESSMENT, BRIEF (96127)

Explanation

Use this code to report a brief assessment for a variety of conditions including ADHD, depression, suicidal risk, anxiety, substance abuse, eating disorders, etc. Because no professional involvement is required for the administration, scoring, and documentation of this assessment, it may be performed by administrative staff.

This service is not used to diagnose a specific condition or disorder. It is used to indicate a possible need for in-depth assessment or further intervention.

Coding Tips

- These assessments are typically performed for a variety of diagnoses.

- See also G0444 "Annual depression screening, 15 minutes."

- This code may be reported multiple times since multiple different instruments may be administered in an individual patient encounter. For example, one or more instruments could be administered to the same informant or the same instrument could be administered to one or more informants (e.g., same instrument used to assess attention-deficit/hyperactivity disorder (ADHD) is administered to a teacher and a parent in order to evaluate two different situations the child may be in).

- Some payer policies state that this code may be billed on the same date of service as other common psychiatric services such as psychotherapy. However, according to NCCI edits, 96127 will not be paid if billed with codes 90832-90853 and many E/M codes. This may be an NCCI edit error as some payer policies specifically state the opposite.

- Do not bill separately when these test(s) are included as part of a battery of tests for a more comprehensive evaluation. For example, do not report 96127 in conjunction with a diagnostic evaluation (90791, 90792).

- Commonly covered tests. The following list is not exhaustive. Please check with individual payer policies for coverage:

    - *Child/adolescent:* Ages and Stages Questionnaire: Social-Emotional, Australian Scale for Asperger's Syndrome, Beck Youth Inventories - 2nd Edition, Behavior Assessment Scale for Children - 2nd Edition, Behavioral Rating Inventory of Executive Function, Briggance Screens, Brief Infant and Toddler Social Emotional Assessment, Connor's Rating Scale, Kutcher Adolescent Depression Scale, Patient Health Questionnaire, Pediatric Symptom Checklist, Screen for Child Anxiety Related Disorders, Strength and Difficulties Questionnaire, Substance Abuse and Alcohol Abuse Screening, Vanderbilt Rating Scales

    - *Adult:* Alcohol Use Disorders Identification Test, Beck Depression Inventory, Columbia-Suicide Severity Rating Scale, Drug Abuse Screening Test, Generalized Anxiety Disorder, Geriatric Depression Scale, Life Event Checklist, Patient Health Questionnaire

Diagnoses

- There are no commonly associated diagnosis codes since this type of testing is utilized in a variety of situations to determine if further diagnostic testing or treatment is warranted.

NEUROBEHAVIORAL STATUS EXAMINATION (96116, 96121)

Explanation

A neurobehavioral status exam consists primarily of individually administered ability tests that comprehensively sample cognitive and performance domains that are known to be sensitive to the functional integrity of the brain (e.g., abstraction, memory and learning, attention, language, problem solving, sensorimotor functions, constructional praxis, etc.) These tests are objective and quantitative and require the patient to directly demonstrate his or her level of competence in the cognitive domain(s) being evaluated.

Use code 96116 for the first hour and 96121 for each additional hour.

Coding Tips

- Do not use automated or computerized questionnaires such as the *Minnesota Multiphasic Personality Inventory 2 (MMPI-2)*, rating scales such as the *Hamilton Depression Rating Scale*, or projective techniques such as the *Rorschach* or *Thematic Apperception Test (TAT)*. Use 96146 "Psychological/neuropsychological test administration and scoring, single automated" instead.

- These codes may NOT be used to report the administration of a *Mini Mental Status Exam (MMSE)*. The OIG recently prosecuted a provider for billing 96116 when they performed a MMSE. CPT guidelines state "For mini mental status examination performed by a physician, see evaluation and management services codes." Assessing a patient's memory, orientation, and arithmetic calculation skills are part of an E/M service.

- Be aware of payer policies which may limit testing to those for whom there is an expectation that neuropsychological testing would impact the individual's medical, functional, or behavioral management. For example, this may exclude a patient previously diagnosed with certain brain dysfunctions such as stable Alzheimer's disease wherein testing would NOT help with medical decision making.

TEST ADMINISTRATION AND SCORING (96136-96139)

Explanation

These codes describe only the administration and scoring of two or more psychological and neuropsychological tests when provided by a physician, qualified healthcare professional, or technician. Select the code based on the type of provider. The interpretation and report is billed separately with codes 96130-96133.

> Psychological tests are used to address a variety of questions about people's functioning, diagnostic classification, co-morbidity, and choice of treatment approach. For example, personality tests and inventories evaluate the thoughts, emotions, attitudes, and behavioral traits that contribute to an individual's interpersonal functioning. The results of these tests determine an individual's personality strengths and weaknesses and may identify certain disturbances in personality or psychopathology. One type of personality test is the projective personality assessment, which asks a subject to interpret some ambiguous stimuli, such as a series of inkblots. The subject's responses can provide insight into his or her thought processes and personality traits.
>
> *- First Coast Service Options Medicare LCD L34520*

Psychological or neuropsychological test administration and scoring **by physician or other qualified health care professional**, two or more tests, any method;

- 96136 first 30 minutes
- + 96137 each additional 30 minutes (List separately in addition to code for primary procedure)

Psychological or neuropsychological test administration and scoring by **technician**, two or more tests, any method

- 96138 first 30 minutes
- + 96139 each additional 30 minutes (List separately in addition to code for primary procedure)

Resource: See Resource 402 for additional information on qualified healthcare professionals (QHPs).

Coding Tips

- Each individual psychological/neuropsychological test administered must be medically necessary. A standard battery of tests is only medically necessary if each individual test in the battery is medically necessary.

- Psychological and neuropsychological testing codes should be reported by the performing provider (i.e., clinical psychologist, neuropsychologist, physician, or technician) who administered the test.

- These codes are typically reported in conjunction with test evaluation services (96130-96133)
- The following example demonstrates how these codes may be reported together:

Example:
A technician spends 2 hours administering and manually scoring two tests and then a psychiatrist spends an additional 3 hours interpreting those results, gathering additional information, reporting their findings, and talking to the patient about the results.

Code	Units	Explanation
96138	1	Technician time, first 30 minutes
96139	3	additional tech time
96130	1	Psychologist time interpreting and reporting
96131	2	additional psychologist time

Diagnoses

Some commonly used codes are listed here. See also the listing at the beginning of this segment.

Consider ICD-10-CM codes from the following:

F01.5- to **F09**	**F10.120** to **F39**	F40- to **F48.9**	F50- to **F59**	F60- to **F79**	F80- to **F82**
F84-	**F88-F99**	H90-	H91-	I60- to I66-	**R07.0**
R41.0 to **R41.3**	R47-	**R49.1**	Z71.0		

Other ICD-10-CM codes to consider:

G13-	G21-	G24-	G25-	**G26**	G30-	G31-	**G44.209**	**G47.52**	**G47.53**	**G80.3**
G91-	**G93.1**	**G94**	**H93.25**	I69-	**R37**	**R40.0**	**R40.1**	R41.8-	R45-	R47-
R48-	S06-	T50.905-	T74-	T76-	**Z87.890**					

TESTING EVALUATION SERVICES (96130-96133)

Explanation

These services include the professional work of integrating patient data and interpreting test results and clinical data to facilitate clinical decision making, treatment planning as required for psychological (96130, 96131) and neuropsychological (96132, 96133) testing services. It can also include face-to-face, interactive feedback with the patient, family member(s), or caregiver(s). Psychological and neuropsychological evaluations focus on different areas of functioning.

- **Neuropsychological:** intellectual function, attention, executive functioning, language and communication, memory, visual-spatial function, sensorimotor function, emotional and personality features, adaptive behavior
- **Psychological:** emotional and interpersonal functioning, intellectual function, thought processes, personality, psychopathology

Coding Tips

- An interpretation and report is required
- These are hour based codes. Do not report services less than 31 minutes.

Book: See "Timed Codes" on page 270.

- Do not use codes 96130-96133 if only reading the testing report or explaining the results to the patient or family. In that circumstance, it would be more appropriate to use other codes such as those for evaluation and management services.

Alert: Be aware that diagnostic evaluations (90791, 90792) and testing evaluation services (96130-96133) have overlapping required components (i.e., recommendations, communication/feedback with family, and review of diagnostic studies). Even though at the time of publication there were no NCCI edits to address this issue, we feel that this is a potential audit concern. Be careful; do NOT double-report your time.

Cognitive Impairment Services

Explanation

Due to the increasing needs of Medicare beneficiaries, CMS has expanded the services available for treating cognitive impairments. Additionally, screenings for cognitive impairment (e.g., 3755F, 3720F) are on the list of quality measures for Medicare (See Resource 168 for more about the Quality Payment Program). This section discusses services which could be rendered after a screening or cognitive performance testing (96125) has been completed. They are:

- Assessment of and care planning for a patient with cognitive impairment (99483)
- Cognitive therapeutic interventions (97129, 97130 — new codes for 2020)

Book: See also "Psychiatric Collaborative Care (99492-99494, G2214)" on page 259.

ASSESSMENT/CARE PLANNING (99483)

Explanation

These services are rendered to a patient (new or established) exhibiting signs and/or symptoms of cognitive impairment in order to support the diagnosis, its etiology, and the level of severity. It includes a comprehensive assessment with many required components (see the "Coding Tips").

Note: 99483 may be used for either a new or existing patient who exhibits signs or symptoms of cognitive impairment. Like other E/M codes, it may only be reported by a physician or QHP and "incident to" rules apply (see "Incident To Services" in Chapter 2.1 — Medicare Essentials).

Store: See innoviHealth's *Comprehensive Guide to Evaluation & Management* (available in the online store) for additional information about reporting these E/M services.

Coding Tips

- May only be reported once every 180 days
- Consider using chronic care management codes (99439, 99487, 99489, 99490-99494) for patients with greater complexity
- If any of the required elements (see next bullet) are missing, use an appropriate E/M code instead of code 99483

- Assessment (typically 50 minutes face-to-face with patient and/or family or caregiver) must include ALL of the following:
  - Cognition-focused evaluation including a pertinent history and examination
  - Current and likely progression of the disease
  - Medical decision making of moderate or high complexity (see "Medical Decision Making" in Chapter 5.3— Evaluation & Management Coding for more information)
  - Functional assessment (e.g., basic and instrumental activities of daily living), including decision-making capacity
  - Use of standardized instruments for staging of dementia (e.g., functional assessment staging test [FAST], clinical dementia rating [CDR])
  - Contributing factors (e.g., medication, chronic pain syndrome, infection, depression, tumor, stroke, normal pressure hydrocephalus)
  - Medication reconciliation and review for high-risk medications
  - Evaluation for neuropsychiatric and behavioral symptoms (e.g., depression) which can include the use of standardized screening instrument(s)
  - Evaluation of safety (e.g., home, operating a motor vehicle)
  - Identification of caregiver(s), caregiver knowledge, caregiver needs, social supports, and the willingness of caregiver to take on caregiving tasks
  - Develop, update/revise, or review an Advance Care Plan
  - Creation of a written care plan, including initial plans to address:
    - any neuropsychiatric symptoms, neuro-cognitive symptoms
    - functional limitations
    - referrals of the patient and/or caregiver to community resources as needed (e.g., rehabilitation services, adult day programs, support groups) and provide initial education and support
- May NOT be reported with many other E/M services (e.g., office visits, chronic care management services) or psychiatric services (e.g., testing, behavioral assessments).

Book: See Appendix A — NCCI Edits for a more comprehensive list of excluded codes.

- Chronic Care Management (99490) is an appropriate code to use for monthly care management with dementia, where there is at least one other chronic condition, but only AFTER a cognitive impairment care plan has been developed and documented.

The following list of suggested measurements is from the Alzheimer's Association:

Suggested Measures to Support the Care-Planning Process		
Domain	**Suggested Measures**	**Comments**
Cognition	Mini-Cog GPCOG Short MoCA	≤ 3 min, validated in primary care Patient/informant components ~ 5 min, needs testing in primary care
Function	FAQ (IADL), Katz (ADL), Lawton-Brody (IADL)	Caregiver rated

Suggested Measures to Support the Care-Planning Process		
Domain	**Suggested Measures**	**Comments**
Stage of cognitive impairment	Mini-Cog + FAQ	Brief, better in milder stages: see Steenland et al, 2008 for interpretation of combined tools.
	Dementia Severity Rating Scale	Caregiver rated, correlates with Clinical Dementia Rating
Decision-making	3-level rating: able to make own decisions, not able, uncertain/needs more evaluation	Global clinician judgment
Neuropsychiatric symptoms Depression	NPI-Q BEHAVE 5+ PHQ-2	10 items 6 high-impact items Depression identification
Medication review and reconciliation	Med list + name of person overseeing home meds	Identify/reconsider high risk meds; assess for reliable administration by self or other
Safety	Safety Assessment Guide	7 questions (patient/caregiver)
Caregiver identification and needs assessment	Caregiver Profile Checklist Single-Item Stress Thermometer PHQ-2	Ability/willingness to care, needs for information, education, and support Rapid identification of stress Depression
Advance care planning	End-of-Life Checklist	Screen for preferences and legal needs

Diagnoses

G30.0 G30.1 G30.9 F01.50 F01.51 F02.80 F02.81 F03.90 F03.91 G31.01 G31.09
G31.83 G31.84 G31.85

COGNITIVE THERAPEUTIC INTERVENTIONS (97129, 97130)

Explanation

Cognitive rehabilitation describes the therapeutic processes utilized by a healthcare professional to restore or enhance a patient's cognitive functioning level when deficits are due to brain or neurologic dysfunction (e.g., traumatic brain injuries, cerebral vascular accidents). The goal is to improve (or attempt to improve), manage, or cope with these deficits, through retraining the ability to think, problem solve, use reasoning (good judgment), and make decisions. The focus is on correcting deficits in memory, reasoning, concentration (attention), visual processing, perception, learning, planning, sequencing, and judgment.

Treatment typically involves a structured set of activities or tasks which can include computer-assisted training aimed at reinforcing or reestablishing previously learned patterns of behavior or to establish new compensatory mechanisms for neurologic deficits. According to a National Institutes of Health panel, these interventions "are structured, systematic, goal-directed, and individualized and they involve learning, practice, social contact, and a relevant context."

> Therapeutic interventions that focus on cognitive function (eg, attention, memory, reasoning, executive function, problem solving, and/or pragmatic functioning) and compensatory strategies to manage the performance of an activity (eg, managing time or schedules, initiating, organizing, and sequencing tasks), direct (one-on-one) patient contact;
>
> 97129   initial 15 minutes
>
> 97130   each additional 15 minutes (List separately in addition to code for primary procedure)

Alert: Failure to document face-to-face time with the patient on ANY time-based code often results in an adverse audit determination.

Note: As of 2020, code G0515 was deleted.

Further guidance can be found in the following Medicare LCD:

> Cognitive skill training should be aimed towards improving, restoring, maintaining or preventing further deterioration of specific functions which were impaired by an identified illness or injury, and expected outcomes should be reasonably attainable by the patient as specified by the plan of care. Therefore, cognitive skills training that do not require skilled services to improve, restore, maintain or prevent deterioration would not be appropriate. Evidence-based reviews indicate that cognitive rehabilitation (and specifically memory rehabilitation) is not recommended for patients with severe cognitive dysfunction.
>
> Cognitive skills are an important component of many tasks, and the techniques used to improve cognitive functioning are integral to the broader impairment being addressed. Cognitive therapy techniques are most often covered as components of other therapeutic procedures, and typically would not be separately reported.
>
> Cognitive skills activities include only those that require the skills of a therapist and must be provided with direct (one-on-one) contact between the patient and the qualified professional/auxiliary personnel. These services are also reimbursable when billed by clinical psychologists; please refer to LCD, L35070, Speech-Language Pathology (SLP) Communication Disorders. Those services that a patient may engage in without a skilled therapist qualified professional/auxiliary personnel are not covered under the Medicare benefit.
>
> *– LCD L35036*

Aetna policy number 0214 includes the following guidance (emphasis added):

> The plan of care should be ongoing, (i.e., updated as the patient's condition changes), and treatment should demonstrate reasonable expectation of improvement. Cognitive therapy is considered medically necessary only if there is a **reasonable expectation** that cognitive therapy will achieve **measurable improvement** in the patient's condition in a reasonable and predictable period of time.
>
> The therapist should re-evaluate the patient regularly (this is typically done on a monthly basis) and document the progress toward the goals of cognitive therapy in the patient's clinical record. The treatment goals and subsequent documentation of treatment results should specifically demonstrate that cognitive therapy services are contributing to such improvement.

Coding Tips

- These are time based codes so follow each payer's time reporting standards. See "Timed Codes" on page 270.
- Code 97130 is an add-on code for 97129.
- There must be direct (one-on-one) patient contact aimed at improving Activities of Daily Living (ADL).
- May be performed by a physician, psychologist, physical, occupational, or speech therapist, or a therapist/therapy assistant under the direct or general supervision, as applicable, of a therapist. Keep in mind that this is not considered a skilled therapy service.
- Some payers require neuropsychological testing prior to performing these services so that testing results are used as the guide for rehabilitation goals when creating an appropriate, patient-specific treatment plan.
- May be performed in either an inpatient or outpatient setting. When performed in the inpatient setting, it is subject to meeting acute inpatient rehabilitation criteria. When performed in the outpatient setting, it is subject to contract limitations for physical therapy (PT) and/or occupational therapy (OT).
- These services are typically considered medically **unnecessary** when there is a diagnosis of any of the following: cerebral palsy, Down syndrome, Parkinson's or Alzheimer's disease, attention deficit hyperactivity disorder, or a developmental disorder (e.g., autism, schizophrenia).
- Community/work reintegration training should be billed with code 97537.

- There must be a reasonable expectation of improvement, which also explains why certain diagnoses (e.g., Parkinson's, dementia, Down syndrome) may not qualify for coverage because there is a low probability of lasting improvement.

 Book: See Appendix A — NCCI Edits for a list of codes which may not be billed at the same time as these services.

Diagnoses

Most payers consider these services investigational for certain diagnoses (e.g., ADHD, autism spectrum disorder), so verify coverage prior to treatment. See the list that follows for some possible coding options.

Consider ICD-10-CM codes from the following:

| C09- to C14- | **F07.81** | G04- to G05- | I60- to **I62.9** | I63- | I67.8- | I69- | S06- | S09.90- |
| Z87.820 | | | | | | | | |

Modifiers

- **Medicare:** Modifier GN, GO, or GP (whichever is applicable) must be used when reporting these services under a therapy Plan of Care (POC). However, when rendered **outside** a POC by a physician, Nonphysician Practitioner (NPP), or psychologist, do NOT use these modifiers.

Diagnostic Evaluations

90791 PSYCHIATRIC DIAGNOSTIC EVALUATION, 90792 (WITH MEDICAL SERVICE)

Explanation

A psychiatric diagnostic evaluation is an integrated assessment that includes history, mental status, and recommendations. It may include communicating with the family and ordering further diagnostic studies. A psychiatric diagnostic evaluation with medical services includes a psychiatric diagnostic evaluation and a medical assessment. It may require a physical exam, communication with the family, prescription medications, and ordering laboratory or other diagnostic studies. A psychiatric diagnostic evaluation with medical services also includes a relevant physical examination.

Coding Tips

- The provider rendering the evaluation may not report a separate E/M encounter code on the same day. If E/M services are provided, use 90792.
- Psychotherapy may not be billed the same day as a diagnostic evaluation.
- According to *CPT Assistant December 2013*, family psychotherapy services may not be billed on the same day as 90791 or 90792 because family interviews at that time would be considered part of the diagnostic evaluation process.
- This service may only be reported once per day.
- May be reported more than once for a patient when separate evaluations are conducted with the patient and other informants (i.e., family members, guardians, significant others) on different days.
- In certain circumstances family members, guardians, or significant others may be seen in lieu of the patient.

- Medicare contractors generally state that this service is only covered once at the beginning of the illness or suspected illness. However, there are some exceptions which often vary from payer to payer and may include any of the following:
  - There is a "treatment hiatus" where the patient has not been seen for the previously evaluated condition for at least 6 months.
  - The patient is experiencing an acute and/or marked mental status change which requires further assessment.
  - There is an admission to an inpatient facility for a psychiatric condition.
  - A second opinion or diagnostic clarification is necessary to rule out additional treatable psychiatric or neurological conditions.

Alert: Be aware that diagnostic evaluations (90791, 90792) and testing evaluation services (96130-96133) have overlapping required components (i.e., recommendations, communication/feedback with family, and review of diagnostic studies). Even though at the time of publication there were no NCCI edits to address this issue, we feel that this is a potential audit concern. Be careful. Do NOT double-report your time.

What is One Hour? 31-60 minutes of time spent performing the evaluation, interpretation, and report equals one unit of time. If less than 31 minutes, then the definition of the CPT code has not been met and the testing may not be billed.

Book: See also Chapter 4.3 — Documentation Tips for more information about documenting these services.
Book: See also "Timed Codes" on page 270.

Evaluation & Management

Explanation

Evaluation and Management (E/M) codes are used to report professional services rendered by a physician/qualified healthcare professional (usually face-to-face). These services have extensive special guidelines that are essential to understand. For quick reference, a few codes and tips are listed here.

Other Qualified Healthcare Professionals (QHPs): According to the CPT codebook guidelines, certain procedures may be performed by either a physician or an other qualified healthcare professional. A QHP is a licensed healthcare provider who performs professional services within their state scope of practice and independently reports those services. This does not include clinical staff, such as physician assistants, who perform services under the supervision of a physician or other qualified healthcare professional. Physicians also meet this general definition; however, they must also satisfy additional requirements as outlined by state, federal, or private payer rules and regulations.

Resource: See Resource 402 for additional information on QHPs.
Book: See also Chapter 5.3 — Evaluation & Management Coding for a listing of these codes.
Book: See "Coding Tips for E/M Involvement" on page 267 for additional information on coding E/M services with psychotherapy.

Reminder: It is important to remember that medical necessity is the overarching criteria for E/M service level selection and if a higher level of service is justified in component scoring, but the medical necessity indicates a lower level of service, the E/M level selected should be the one that matches the level of medical necessity.

Book: See also "Evaluation and Management (E/M) Services" in Chapter 5.1 — Procedure Coding Essentials for more information about medical necessity.

Store: See innoviHealth's *Comprehensive Guide to Evaluation & Management* (available in the online store) for detailed information about reporting E/M services, including E/M code level selection.

OFFICE VISITS (99202-99205, 99211-99215)

Coding Tips

- When the patient has two or more services (one of them being an E/M) performed on the same day for which there is either an NCCI or CPT edit disallowing them to be reported together, modifier 25 may be used to override the edit IF the E/M service qualifies as a significant and separately identifiable service.

- Do NOT report modifier 25 when only an E/M service is performed or when there is NOT an existing NCCI or CPT edit which indicates that one of the services is bundled into the other.

Book: See Appendix A — NCCI Edits for a more information about these edits and a listing of services considered bundled with E/M services.

- If an existing patient has not received services from any healthcare provider in your practice within the past 3 years, they are considered a new patient.

- The highest levels of service (99205 and 99215) require documentation that supports a high-level of risk to the patient (e.g., suicidal ideation, attempted suicide).

- Although 99211 is referred to as a "nurse's visit," it is considered an incident-to service which requires a supervising physician/QHP to be on site (not in the room) when the service is performed. Documentation must support the service provided and include the proper signatures.

- As of January 1, 2022, the phrase "usually the presenting problems are minimal" was removed from code 99211.

SKILLED NURSING FACILITY VISITS (99307-99310)

These services are subsequent visits in a Skilled Nursing Facility (SNF). Initial SNF care codes (99304, 99305, and 99306) are found in Chapter 5.3 — Evaluation & Management Coding.

Coding Tips

- In this type of setting, frequent visits by the healthcare provider are unnecessary since the patient is already under medical care of the facility itself. However, several visits may be necessary when there is a new episode of illness or an acute exacerbation of a chronic illness (e.g., an acute behavioral cognitive and/or functional change).

- There must be face-to-face interaction with the patient.

- These services may only be reported once per day, so if the physician/QHP performs multiple E/M services in the same day, they may be combined to calculate an overall component score for that day.

Health Behavior Assessment and Intervention

Explanation

Health behavior assessment services are performed to identify biopsychosocial factors (e.g., psychological, behavioral, emotional, cognitive) that may impact the patient's response(s) to disease-related problems. Unlike psychiatric services, which focus on mental health, these services aim to improve the patient's overall well-being through a health-focused clinical interview, behavioral observation, and/or psychophysiological monitoring. Standardized health-oriented questionnaires may be used to evaluate anxiety, pain, coping strategies, and other contributing factors.

The health behavior intervention typically includes cognitive, behavioral, social, and psychophysiological services designed to improve the patient's functioning, minimize their psychological/psychosocial impediments, and help them better cope with their medical condition(s).

Health Behavior Services and Psychotherapy Comparison

	Psychotherapy	Health Behavior Services
Diagnosis	Chapter 5. Mental, Behavioral and Neurodevelopmental disorders (F01-F99)	Medical condition(s) not listed in Chapter 5.
Primary focus	Insight, decision making, alleviate emotional concerns	Psychosocial and psychological factors that hinder improvement in physical functioning, wellness, or recovery
Goal	Change behavior to improve emotional well-being	Improve patient's health through better disease management
Team approach	Typically private	Work closely with referring provider in care management approach

Examples:
- 8-year-old with cancer experiencing extreme anxiety regarding treatment and pain management
- 15-year-old insulin-dependent diabetic who is non-compliant with disease management
- Family of 59-year-old with end-stage renal disease to assess pain management and death/dying concerns
- 8-year-old with coronary artery disease experiencing difficulty managing his treatment plan

Health Behavior Coding Table

Code	Add-on	Unit	Description
96156	n/a	n/a	Assessment
96158	96159	30 min/15 min	Intervention, individual
96164	96165	30 min/15 min	Intervention, group (2+ patients)
96167	96168	30 min/15 min	Intervention, family (with patient)
96170	96171	30 min/15 min	Intervention, family (without patient)

Table Key:
- Add-on   The code to add to the primary procedure for additional intra-service work
- Unit   The reporting unit. The first amount is the amount of time for the primary code and the second amount is for each additional 15 minutes of service.

Coding Tips

- These are time-based codes which include face-to-face time with the family and/or patient(s), as such, documentation must clearly indicate the total amount of time spent providing these services.

- Per Medicare guidelines, 8-22 minutes is counted as one fifteen minute unit, 23-38 minutes is counted as two fifteen minute units. Even if multiple and different time-based services are performed at a single encounter, only one may be billed if the total time does not exceed 22 minutes.

Book: See "Timed Codes" on page 270 for more information.

- Only a qualified, nonphysician healthcare professional may use these codes. Physicians, clinical nurse specialists, or nurse practitioners should use E/M or Preventive Medicine codes instead of these codes. For Medicare, the provider must be registered as CP-Specialty Code 68.

- Medicare did not cover deleted code 96155, so it is likely that they will also not cover the replacement codes (96170, 96171).

- These codes may NOT be billed on same date of service as: Adaptive Behavior Services (97151-97158, 0362T, 0373T), or Psychiatric Services (90785-90899). However, if adaptive behavior services are performed on the same day as these services, just bill the predominant service.

- E/M services, including Preventive Medicine Counseling (99401-99404, 99411-99412) and/or Behavior Change Intervention services (99406-99412), may be reported on the same day if rendered by a different provider.

- These are **not** preventive medicine counseling and risk factor reduction interventions.

- Generally, it is best to bill the diagnosis code obtained from the referring healthcare provider.

Diagnoses

DO NOT use any of the following diagnosis codes:

F01 - F99   G30-   G31.0-   **G31.1**   **G31.83**   **G31.84**

Website: Go to FindACode.com for complete diagnosis code lists and information.

Intensive Outpatient Program (IOP)

Explanation

An Intensive Outpatient Program (IOP) is an intermediate level of care which is commonly considered after the patient has been discharged from inpatient care when the patient still requires more care than is typically available in an outpatient setting. It may also be indicated when the patient requires more than outpatient care, but not enough for an inpatient program (e.g., hospitalization, partial hospitalization). Typically the facility/agency must be licensed by the state to provide these services and the program is generally provided under the supervision of a psychiatrist.

It is essential to understand the billing rules which can vary by payer. For example, some payers consider psychotherapy sessions included (bundled) when you bill a per diem rate, while others do not. Failure to follow payer guidelines often results in denials, post-payment reviews, refund demands, and possibly even allegations of fraud. In August of 2018, the OIG ordered a facility to pay a $1.1 million fine for claims billed to Medicare over the course of seven years for what Medicare considered to be medically unnecessary psychotherapy services rendered in an IOP facility.

There are no CPT codes to describe these services. The two most commonly used codes for non-Medicare payers are:

H0015   Alcohol and/or drug services; intensive outpatient (treatment program that operates at least 3 hours/day and at least 3 days/week and is based on an individualized treatment plan), including assessment, counseling; crisis intervention, and activity therapies or education

S9480   Intensive outpatient psychiatric services, per diem

Note: Both codes may not be billed together. Use one or the other depending on payer preferences.

Resource: See Resource 621 for a comprehensive article on billing IOP services.

Interactive Complexity (90785)

Explanation

Interactive complexity refers to very specific situations where significant communication difficulties encountered during a psychiatric procedure hinders the service/treatment plan. Typically, this occurs when third parties are involved in the psychiatric care of the patient. This could include parents, guardians, other family members, interpreters, agencies, parole officers, or even schools.

At least one of the following must be present in order to report code 90785:

1. Use of play equipment or other physical devices in order to overcome barriers to therapeutic or diagnostic interaction between the provider and a patient who has
   - lost or not developed either expressive language skills to explain symptoms and/or respond to treatment or
   - the receptive communication skills to understand the provider
2. There is a need to manage maladaptive communication, such as high anxiety or reactivity, disagreement between participating individuals, or even repeatedly asking questions.
3. Caregiver emotions or uncooperative behavior interferes with either the understanding of or the implementation of the treatment plan.
4. A 'sentinel event' is reported/disclosed which is mandated to be reported to a third party (e.g., abuse/neglect). This event is then discussed/reported with the patient and any others also present during the encounter.

Note: As of 2022, language translation or fluency in typical language is no longer applicable. Also, some "typical" patient descriptions were removed from the CPT codebook. Be aware of these differences and ensure that policies and procedures are updated.

Coding Tips

- Interactive complexity is an 'add-on' code which may be billed with the following psychiatric services: diagnostic psychiatric evaluation (90791, 90792), psychotherapy (90832-90834, 90836-90838), and group psychotherapy (90853).
- The 2022 CPT codebook removed some outdated language regarding E/M level selection and added language to clarify that 90785 may only be reported in conjunction with a psychiatric diagnostic evaluation or psychotherapy service and is not applicable to performing just an E/M service, but an E/M service COULD be provided with the other psychiatric services.
- When performed with psychotherapy, the interactive complexity component relates only to the increased work intensity of the psychotherapy service, but does not change the time for the psychotherapy service.

- Do not bill with E/M codes when there are no psychotherapy services provided at the same encounter.
- Documentation must clearly indicate ALL of the following:
  - the person does not have the ability to interact through normal verbal communicative channels,
  - which methods or adaptations were utilized in the session and the rationale for employing these interactive techniques, and
  - recommendations for future care.

Diagnoses

Consider ICD-10-CM codes from the following:

| F20.2 | F80- | F84.3 | F84.5 | F84.8 | H90- | H91- | R07.0 | R47- | R49.1 | Z71.0 |

Partial Hospitalization Program (PHP)

Explanation

Psychiatric Partial Hospitalization Programs (PHPs) are a more comprehensive level of care than Intensive Outpatient Programs (IOPs). When the patient requires a minimum of 20 hours per week and hospitalization is not clinically indicated, a PHP can be the most effective type of care. Typically, the patient is either being discharged from an inpatient program or they are at risk of requiring hospitalization without proper intervention.

It should be noted that there are different guidelines and requirements for psychiatric PHPs, substance abuse PHPs, and eating disorder PHPs. Also, like IOPs, billing requirements can vary by payer, so be sure to review individual payer policies to ensure compliance.

Resource: See Resource 622 for a comprehensive article on billing PHP services, including Medicare's admission criteria and services that may be included in the per diem rate.

Pharmacologic Management

Code 90863 is for non-qualified healthcare providers who are licensed to prescribe medication. All others (e.g., physician, NPs, etc.) use E/M codes.

Coding Tips

- Includes prescription and review of medication when performed with psychotherapy services. Psychotherapy services (90832, 90834, 90837) should be reported in addition to this code.
- Pharmacologic management time MAY NOT be included in psychotherapy time.
- According to the CPT guidelines for this code, "for pharmacologic management with psychotherapy services performed by a physician or other qualified health care professional who may report evaluation and management codes, use the appropriate evaluation and management codes 99202-99255, 99281-99285, 99304-99337, 99341-99350 and the appropriate psychotherapy with evaluation and management service 90833, 90836, 90838."

Resource: See Resource 402 for more information about qualified healthcare professionals (QHPs).
Book: For medication management of substance use disorders, see page 232.

Preventive Services

The following are preventive services which are typically covered under the essential health benefits provision of the Affordable Care Act. Certain services can be done for preventive or diagnostic reasons. Only some of the assessments and screenings shown below are included in this chapter.

- Alcohol Use/Misuse Screening and Counseling for Adults: 99385-99387, 99395-99397, 99408, 99409, G0396, G0442, G0443
- Counseling Services: 0403T, 99401, 99402, 99403, 99404, 99406, 99407, 99408, 99409, 99411, 99412, G0296, G0396, G0397, G0443, G0445, G0446, G0447, G0473, H0005, S0257, S0265, S9470, T1006, T1027
- Depression Screening for Adults and Adolescents Ages 12-18: 99384-99387, 99394-99397, G0444
- Developmental & Behavioral Assessments for Children and Adolescents: 96110, 99381-99384, 99391-99394
- Developmental/Behavioral Screening: G0451 (with select diagnosis), 96110, 96127, S0302 (allowed with any diagnosis)
- Preventive Medicine Service (99381-99397, G0402, G0513, G0514) Note: codes 99381-99397 are E/M codes
- Screening Services: G0101, G0102, Q0091, G0442, G0444
- Tobacco Use & Cessation Counseling for Adults: 99406, 99407, G9016, S9453

Note: As of October 1, 2018 additional diagnosis codes were added for screening encounters. See subcategories Z13.3- and Z13.4- to review applicable codes.

Book: See also the "Common Procedure Codes" section which begins on page 273.

Psychiatric Collaborative Care (99492-99494, G2214)

Note: As of January 1, 2021, code G2214 was added to report the first 30 minutes of this service. CPT time rules apply and the service elements for 99493 must be met.

Explanation

According to CMS, the Psychiatric Collaborative Care Model (CoCM) is described as follows:

> A specific model for BHI, psychiatric CoCM typically is provided by a primary care team consisting of a primary care provider and a [behavioral health] care manager who works in collaboration with a psychiatric consultant, such as a psychiatrist. Care is directed by the primary care team and includes structured care management with regular assessments of clinical status using validated tools and modification of treatment as appropriate. The psychiatric consultant provides regular consultations to the primary care team to review the clinical status and care of patients and to make recommendations.

Patients are typically those who may be dealing with a newly diagnosed condition, need help with treatment options, are not responding or engaging sufficiently in a treatment plan, or require further assessment. The CPT codebook refers to an "episode of care" as:

> ...beginning when the patient is directed by the treating physician or other qualified health care professional to the behavioral health care manager and ending with:
> - the attainment of targeted treatment goals, which typically results in the discontinuation of care management services and continuation of usual follow-up with the treating physician or other qualified healthcare professional; or
> - failure to attain targeted treatment goals culminating in referral to a psychiatric care provider for ongoing treatment; or
> - lack of continued engagement with no psychiatric collaborative care management services provided over a consecutive six month calendar period (break in episode).

Resource: See Resource 647 for more information about these services, including the roles of the behavioral healthcare manager and psychiatric consultant.

Resource: See Resource 646 for more comprehensive information about these services including Principal Care Management (PCM) services for a single, high-risk disease (99424-99427). Note that prior to 2022, PCM services were reported with codes G2064 and G2065.

Book: These services may not be reported with many other services. See Appendix A — NCCI Edits for a list of codes which may not be reported with 99492-99494, and G2214.

Book: See also Chapter 5.3 — Evaluation & Management Coding for other information.

The following table summarizes coding options:

Psychiatric Collaborative Care Coding Table		
Type	**Time (total during the month)**	**Code(s)**
Initial	<15 min 16-35 min 36-85 min 86-115 min	Do not report G2214* 99492 99492 x 1 AND 99494 x1
Subsequent	<15 min 16-30 min 31-75 min 76-105 min	Do not report G2214* 99493 99493 x1 AND 99494 x1

Note:
* According to the CPT codebook, services less than 36 minutes may NOT be reported. However, as of January 1, 2021, CMS allows code G2214 to report the first 30 minutes of these services. Verify non-government payer polices to see if this code is allowed.

Coding Tips

- These codes are used to report services provided during a single calendar month.
- A new episode of care begins when care is resumed after there has been at least six months since the last episode of care.
- As of January 2020, Medicare began allowing these services to be reported during the same service period as Transitional Care Management services (99495 and 99496) and Chronic Care Management Services (99439, 99490, 99491) as long as all requirements to report each service are met and time and effort are not counted more than once. Please note that patient consent must be obtained separately for each of these services.

- Services can be rendered in both non-facility and facility settings. In fact, even if the services are provided in a non-facility for part of the month and a facility for the other part, the time all counts towards the same code(s). However, be aware of payer policies regarding special types of facilities. For example, Federally Qualified Health Centers (FQHCs) and Rural Health Clinics (RHCs) report CCM/BHI services with codes G0511 and G0512.

- When either E/M or chronic care management (CCM) services are performed by the provider, they may either be reported separately with the appropriate E/M or CCM code, or counted towards CoCM services. It does NOT count towards both. Note the following FAQ by CMS:

  > CCM and BHI are distinct, differing services even though there is some overlap in eligible patient populations. There may be some circumstances in which it is reasonable and necessary to provide both services in a given month. The BHI codes can be billed for the same patient in the same month as CCM if
  >
  > advance consent for both services and all other requirements to report BHI and to report CCM are met and time and effort are not counted more than once. Billing practitioners should keep in mind that cost sharing and advance consent apply to each service independently and there can only be one reporting practitioner for CCM each month. If all requirements to report each service are met, both may be billed.

- CCM codes 99487, 99490 cannot be reported in the same month as BHI codes 99492-99494. CMS has stated that "a single practitioner must choose whether to report the General BHI code or the CoCM codes in a given month (service period) for a given beneficiary. However, in many cases, it may be appropriate for a single practitioner to report the General BHI code or the CoCM codes for the same beneficiary over the course of several months."

- The psychiatric consultant and behavioral health care manager may, but are not required to be, employees in the same practice as the billing practitioner

- Other qualified individuals (clinical staff) may provide certain aspects of care. According to the CPT codebook, this is "... an individual who performs services 'incident to' (as an integral part of) services of the billing practitioner, subject to applicable state law, licensure, scope of practice, and supervision." The clinical staff may, but are not required to, include individuals who meet the qualifications for the CoCM behavioral health are manager or psychiatric consultant.

- Since Medicare makes payment to the participating billing practitioner for the service, the psychiatric consultant and/or behavioral healthcare manager do not necessarily have to be participating with Medicare.

- Medicare requires written consent from the patient.

  > The patient must be informed about the program and provide general consent, which must be documented in the medical record. This includes giving permission to consult with relevant specialists (including the psychiatric consultant) and the acknowledgement that there is beneficiary cost-sharing/co-payment for both non-face-to-face and face-to face services. Consent may be verbal (written consent is not required) but must be documented in the medical record.

Resource: See Resource 603 to review Medicare's FAQ page regarding billing these types of services.

Diagnosis

These services are for patients with any psychiatric condition(s) (including substance abuse) that, in the clinical judgment of the billing provider, would benefit from these services. According to Medicare, this includes pre-existing condition(s) (see 81 FR 80232).

Psychotherapy

The Psychotherapy Coding Flowchart (*Figure 5.2*) helps outline the decision process for psychiatric services codes. This is only a suggested coding flowchart; however, it does help remind the user which questions need to be asked during the code selection process. It begins with a psychotherapy service and ends with the submission of the appropriate code(s) on a claim for reimbursement from a third party payer.

Notes:

- Pharmacologic management is not included on this chart. Physicians and other qualified healthcare professionals should use the appropriate Evaluation and Management (E/M) encounter code to bill this service. Providers who are not authorized to report E/M services, but whose scope of practice allows prescribing privileges, may use code 90863 in addition to psychotherapy codes 90832, 90834, or 90837. See page 258 for more information.

- Counseling services performed by a chaplain are not included here and may be reported with new codes Q9002 and Q9003. See "Veteran's Affairs Services" on page 271 for more information.

Flowchart Notes

1. **Is this a crisis?**
    - This coding option is for services provided when the patient is in high distress with a complex or life threatening situation which requires urgent and immediate attention. It may not be used with any other psychotherapy code. See page 267 for more information.

2. **Is this Psychoanalysis, Family Therapy, or Group Therapy?**
    - These psychiatric services are reported differently than psychotherapy services and are not included here.

3. **Is this Non-Family Group Therapy?**
    - See the procedures section for other therapy options such as psychoanalysis and Family Group Therapy. These therapy options may NOT add the interactive complexity code.
    - Psychoanalysis and family group therapy cannot be used with the interactive complexity add-on code. When interactive complexity is applicable, both 90853 and 90785 should be used on the claim.

4. **Is E/M Involved?**
    - Does this service qualify for Evaluation and Management (E/M) services in addition to the psychotherapy service? Only physicians and other designated qualified healthcare professionals may use these codes. See "Coding Tips for E/M Involvement" on page 267 for an explanation.
    - Report psychotherapy time separately from the E/M portion of the patient encounter. Documentation must fully support the level of E/M services provided in addition to the psychotherapy services.

5. **Is this a Prolonged Service?**
    - Prolonged services are those that extend beyond the time listed for the procedure/service (e.g., more than 74 minutes for 90837). Be sure to review "7. Add Appropriate Prolonged Services Code" for important information about properly reporting prolonged services.

6. **Is Interactive Complexity Present?**
    - One of the four criteria listed on page 256 must be met in order to use this "add-on" code. Add-on means that code 90785 is also included when billing the other service(s) provided to the patient.
    - Please note the expanded definition of "interactive" on page 257.

Figure 5.2

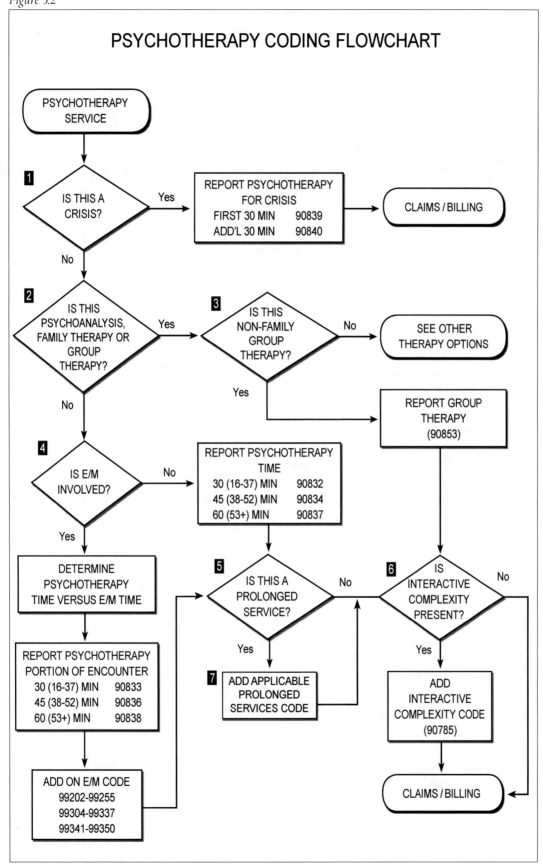

7. **Add Applicable Prolonged Services Code**
   - Correct reporting of prolonged services depends on the type of service that is prolonged (was the psychotherapy prolonged or the E/M service prolonged?), where that prolonged service took place, and the type of patient contact.
   - In a behavioral health setting, prolonged E/M services would not be common. Prolonged psychotherapy would be the most common situation where a prolonged services add-on code would be reported.
   - The following table outlines which prolonged codes may also be reported, as applicable, in conjunction with the primary service:

Prolonged Services Code Options		
Type	**Time**	**Prolonged Code(s)**

Office Visit
    99205
    99215
	
	>73 min
	>54 min
		
		99417*
		99417*

Direct Patient Contact** – Other Outpatient Visit (not office) or Psychotherapy
    90837, 90847 (psychotherapy)
    99241-99245, 99324-99337, 99341-99350, 99483 (E/M)
	30-74 min
	75-104 min
	>104 min
		99354
		99354 x1 AND 99355 x 1
		99354 x1 AND 99355 x 2 or more for each additional 30 min

Direct Patient Contact** – Inpatient, Observation or Psychotherapy
    90837, 90847 (psychotherapy)
    99218-99220, 99221-99223, 99224-99226, 99231-99233, 99234-99236, 99251-99255, 99304-99310 (E/M)
	30-74 min
	75-104 min
	>104 min
		99356
		99356 x1 AND 99357 x 1
		99356 x1 AND 99357 x 2 or more for each additional 30 min

Without direct patient contact – Outpatient, Inpatient, or Observation (NOT office 99205, 99215) See Resource 540 for a detailed explanation and examples.	30-74 min 75-104 min >104 min	99358 99358 x 1 AND 99359 x 1 99358 x 1 AND 99359 x 2 or more for each additional 30 min

Notes:
* Code 99417 includes both face-to-face and non-face-to-face time.

    As of January 1, 2021, CMS created the following shortened prolonged service code which may be reported with 99205, 99215:

    G2212 "Prolonged office or other outpatient evaluation and management service(s) beyond the maximum required time of the primary procedure which has been selected using total time on the date of the primary service; **each additional 15 minutes** by the physician or qualified healthcare professional, with or without direct patient contact (List separately in addition to CPT codes 99205, 99215 for office or other outpatient evaluation and management services)"

** Only face-to-face direct patient contact which includes non-face-to-face services on the patient's floor/unit

   - As of January 1, 2021, CMS created add-on code G2211 to report the additional complexity of treating a patient with a single, serious condition, or a complex condition. However, the implementation of that code has been delayed until 2024.

FAMILY THERAPY (90846-90849)

Explanation

Family therapy is used to describe family participation in the treatment process of the patient. The focus of the psychotherapy is related to the treatment of the patient's condition, and not the treatment of each family member's problems. In situations where the patient is withdrawn and uncommunicative due to a mental disorder, the healthcare provider may contact relatives and close associates to obtain the necessary background information to assist in diagnosis and treatment planning.

Coding Tips

- According to *CPT Assistant December 2013*, family psychotherapy services may not be billed on the same day as 90791 or 90792 because family interviews at that time would be considered part of the diagnostic evaluation process.

- For Medicare, code 90849 is generally noncovered. Family psychotherapy services are covered only where the primary purpose of such psychotherapy is the treatment of the patient's condition. Examples include:
  - When there is a need to observe and correct, through psychotherapeutic techniques, the patient's interaction with family members, and/or
  - Where there is a need to assess the conflicts or impediments within the family, and assist the family members in the management of the patient through psychotherapy.

GROUP THERAPY (90853)

Explanation

Group psychotherapy is administered in a group setting with a trained therapist simultaneously providing therapy to several patients. Personal and group dynamics are discussed and explored in a therapeutic setting allowing emotional catharsis, instruction, insight, and support.

Group therapy, since it involves psychotherapy, must be led by a person who is legally authorized by their state to perform this service. This will usually mean a physician, clinical psychologist, clinical social worker, physician assistant, certified nurse practitioner, clinical nurse specialist, or other person authorized by the state to perform this service.

Coding Tips

- Coverage must meet medical necessity guidelines. For example, Medicare does not cover socialization, music therapy, recreational activities, art classes, excursions, sensory stimulation or eating together, cognitive stimulation, motion therapy, etc.

- Even though there is no time specified in the official CPT definition of this code, individual payers may set their own. For example, Medicaid in California requires a group therapy session to be a minimum of 90 minutes.

- The number of required participants in the group is often established by individual payer policy. For example, the policy may state that "no less than 2 and no more than 8 persons" is reimbursable.

PSYCHOTHERAPY: 90832/3 (30 MIN), 90834/6 (45 MIN), 90837/8 (60 MIN)

Explanation

Psychotherapy is the treatment for mental illness and behavioral disturbances in which the healthcare provider engages the patient in definitive, therapeutic communication with the goal of:

- alleviating emotional disturbances,
- reversing or changing maladaptive behavior patterns,
- encouraging personality growth and development or supporting current evaluation of functioning.

Although maintenance, per se, is not covered; helping a patient maintain his/her highest level of functioning, such as a patient with borderline personality disorder, may be covered on a case-by-case basis. These case-by-case considerations must be supported by the evaluation and a plan with clearly identified goal(s).

Alert: These are time-specific codes. Documentation should include both start and stop times. Previous Medicare inappropriate payment reports indicated a high incidence of downcoded claims because of insufficient documentation of time.

Book: See Chapter 4.3 — Documentation Tips for guidelines regarding documentation and other requirements for using these codes.

Coding Tips

- Psychotherapy time may include face-to-face time with family members (or others involved in the treatment process) as long as the patient is present for the majority of the service.

- Pay particular attention to codes specifying service time and bill appropriately. Do not report services less than 16 minutes.

- To report psychotherapy only, choose the appropriate code based on the following face-to-face times:
  - 16-37 minutes = 90832/90833
  - 38-52 minutes = 90834/90836
  - 53-75 minutes = 90837/90838
  - 75+ minutes = 90837/90838 + (modifier 22 OR prolonged E/M code [see "7. Add Appropriate Prolonged Services Code" on page 264])

Note: Significant changes to prolonged services reporting are now in effect. Be sure to report the applicable prolonged services code as explained on page 264.

Diagnoses

Please note the following limitations:

- Psychotherapy services for patients with severe or profound mental retardation is often not covered. However, rehabilitative, evaluation and management (E/M) codes, or pharmacological management codes are generally covered.

- For patients with dementia, it **must** be mild enough that they have the ability or capacity to retain and recall the therapeutic encounter from one session, individual or group, to another. This capacity to meaningfully benefit from psychotherapy **must** be documented in the medical record. Psychotherapy services are not covered when documentation indicates that dementia has produced a severe enough cognitive defect to prevent psychotherapy from being effective.

Consider ICD-10-CM codes from the following:

F20.2   F80-   **F84.3**   **F84.5**   **F84.8**   H90-   H91-   **R07.0**   R47-   **R49.1**   **Z71.0**

Coding Tips for E/M Involvement

- A separate diagnosis is not required for the reporting of E/M and psychotherapy on the same date of service.

- To report both E/M and psychotherapy, the two services must be significant and separately identifiable.

- If the E/M service is rendered on the same day by a different provider than the one performing the psychotherapy AND they report the services with the same Tax Identification Number (TIN), most payers will consider them to be one entity and therefore a separate E/M service (e.g., 99202-99215) may not be reported.

- Time spent on history, examination, and medical decision making when used for the E/M service is not included in psychotherapy time. However, Prolonged Services may be reported when E/M and psychotherapy are reported together. See "5. Is this a Prolonged Service?" on page 264 for more information.

- When E/M services are included with psychotherapy, select codes by using E/M criteria in addition to the criteria above. Psychotherapy time may not be included in E/M time. Not all practitioners may use E/M codes (see the "Who May Use E/M Codes" note below).

- E/M services performed in addition to psychotherapy may include:
  - Physical examinations, medical diagnostic evaluations, and evaluation of comorbid medical conditions
  - Drug management and evaluation of drug interactions
  - Physician orders, interpretation of laboratory studies, and other medical diagnostic studies and observations

- If E/M services are provided without psychotherapy, select the appropriate code from the E/M section.

 Who May Use E/M Codes? Evaluation and Managements codes can only be used by a physician or 'other qualified healthcare professional.' See Resource 402 for more about who is an 'other qualified healthcare professional.'

PSYCHOTHERAPY FOR CRISIS (90839, 90840)

Explanation

According to the CPT codebook, "Psychotherapy for crisis is an urgent assessment and history of a crisis state, a mental status exam, and a disposition. The treatment includes psychotherapy, mobilization of resources to defuse the crisis and restore safety, and implementation of psychotherapeutic interventions to minimize the potential for psychological trauma. The presenting problem is typically life threatening or complex and requires immediate attention to a patient in high distress."

Coding Tips

- These codes do not include medical services. In a crisis situation, psychiatrists may prefer the appropriate E/M code instead.

- Time includes the total duration of face-to-face time with patient and/or family members, and it does not have to be continuous.

 Alert: The provider's time and attention during a crisis must be completely devoted to the situation. Services cannot be provided to any other patient during that same time period. This requirement will most likely be closely monitored by claims reviewers.

Remote Monitoring

Explanation

As digital medicine continues to expand, new codes are being created to describe the different types of remote care that can be provided to a patient. These services are different from remote clinician-to-patient or clinician-to-clinician interactions which are reported with their own codes (e.g., 99421, 98970, 99451). Generally speaking, the remote services included here can be grouped into two broad categories:

1. Remote Physiologic Monitoring (RPM): 99454, 99457, 99458, 99091

2. Remote Therapeutic Monitoring/Treatment Management (RTM) CPT codes 98975, 98976, 98977, 98980, and 98981)

Note: At the time of publication, additional remote monitoring codes were being considered by the AMA for implementation in 2023.

Note: In 2021, two new codes to report Communication Technology-Based Services (CTBS) by a nonphysician provider were added. See Resource 53D for more information about those services.

Resource: See Resource 64B for a more indepth review of these different types of services.

REMOTE PHYSIOLOGIC MONITORING (RPM)

These services evaluate physiologic data remotely gathered and delivered to a healthcare provider who uses this information to manage patient care. Although the CPT codebook guidelines for 2022 changed, the codes themselves did not. They are:

RPM Services		
Code	Description	Information & Tips
99453 99454	Remote monitoring of physiologic parameter(s) (eg, weight, blood pressure, pulse oximetry, respiratory flow rate), initial; set-up and patient education on use of equipment device(s) supply w/ daily recording(s) or programmed alert(s) transmission, each 30 days	• Use code 99091 for the interpretation of physiologic data submitted by the patient/caregiver.
99457 99458	Remote physiologic monitoring treatment management services, clinical staff/physician/QHP; first 20 minutes each additional 20 minutes	• Requires interactive communication w/patient or caregiver • Services during a single (not calendar) month

Coding Tips

- Clinical staff/physician/QHP evaluate the results of a device defined by the FDA as a "medical device".
- Must be ordered by the physician/QHP.
- Documentation needs to specify how this data is part of the recommended treatment plan.
- Pay attention to CPT guidelines as these codes may NOT be reported with many other services. See Appendix A — NCCI Edits for a list of specialty-specific exclusions or visit FindACode.com for a complete listing.

- Codes 99473 and 99474 are not included here because they are measurements taken by the patient which are later given to a provider, but no active healthcare provider monitoring of these measurements is taking place.

REMOTE THERAPEUTIC MONITORING/TREATMENT MANAGEMENT (RTM)

These services are divided into the work and supplies involved with the monitoring equipment of a device defined as a medical device by the FDA and the work involved by a healthcare provider who evaluates the information from the device in relation to treatment evaluation of the patient. These new codes are:

Remote therapeutic monitoring (eg, respiratory system status, musculoskeletal system status, therapy adherence, therapy response);

98975 initial set-up and patient education on use of equipment

98976 device(s) supply with scheduled (eg, daily) recording(s) and/or programmed alert(s) transmission to monitor respiratory system, each 30 days

Remote therapeutic monitoring treatment management services, physician or other qualified health care professional time in a calendar month requiring at least one interactive communication with the patient or caregiver during the calendar month;

98980 first 20 minutes

98981 each additional 20 minutes (List separately in addition to code for primary procedure)

Coding Tips

- Services must be ordered by a physician or QHP.
- Do NOT report these codes for services less than 20 minutes. The mid-point time rules do not apply.
- Codes 98980 and 98981 have CPT guidelines regarding when these services may be reported along with a caution about overlapping of time of other time-based services including psychotherapy (e.g., 90832, 90838) and adaptive behavior services among others. As such, carefully document remote monitoring time separately from the other services listed in the CPT codebook. See Appendix A — NCCI Edits for a list of specialty-specific exclusions or visit FindACode.com for a complete listing.

Online Digital Cognitive Behavioral Therapy Program

These new codes describe services where a "standardized" prescription digital therapy (PDT) is used which monitors both patient adherence to therapy as well as their responses when using the PDT. Although limited information was available at the time of publication, PDTs may be used to monitor the treatment of conditions such as anxiety, substance use disorder(s), or chronic insomnia. These codes are different from other RTM services in that they are not limited to a medical device as defined by the FDA. These new codes are:

Remote therapeutic monitoring of a standardized online digital cognitive behavioral therapy program **ordered** by a physician or other qualified health care professional;

0702T supply and technical support, per 30 days

0703T management services by physician or other qualified health care professional, per calendar month

Keep in mind that these are Category III codes, which, unlike Category I (CPT) codes, are often not reimbursable by Medicare. Review private or commercial payer policies to determine coverage.

Telehealth Services

Information about telehealth and telemedicine services are not included in this tips chapter.

Book: See Appendix D — Telehealth Codes for more comprehensive information about these services.

Timed Codes

Timed codes are procedure (CPT and HCPCS) codes that identify a specific time that must be met in order to bill for one unit of service. When billing only one timed service, the rules are fairly straightforward — when more than half of a timed code service (e.g, 8 minutes for a 15 minute code) is completed, one unit of service can be billed. However, in order to bill the second unit of service, the full time period (e.g., 15 minutes) of the first code must be completed in addition to the next mid-point (e.g., the first 15 minutes plus an additional 8 minutes [23 min total]) in order to bill for the next unit for a code with a 15 minute time description.

The chart below identifies the amount of minutes required to bill for each unit of service, using the CPT mid-point guidelines.

# of Units	15 min		30 min		60 min	
	Min	Max	Min	Max	Min	Max
0	0	7	0	15	0	30
1	8	22	16	45	31	90
2	23	37	46	75	91	150
3	38	52	76	105	151	210
4	53	67	106	135	211	270
5	68	82	136	165	271	310

This chart only should be used when there is no 'add-on' code to use or there is not a code specifying an additional time (e.g., 90833-90846).

Note: Healthcare providers should base the service provided on the standard of care and not on reimbursement. Service lengths that are outside the normal standard of care *could* identify the provider as an outlier among peers and potentially lead to a medical review or audit.

Resource: See Resource 616 to review Medicare's official guidelines with more coding scenarios.

Book: See Chapter 3 — Compliance Essentials for additional information about medical reviews and audits.

Transcranial Magnetic Stimulation (TMS)

Explanation

Transcranial magnetic stimulation (TMS), also known as repetitive TMS (rTMS), is a noninvasive procedure utilizing magnetic fields to electrically stimulate nerve cells in the brain. A small electromagnetic coil is placed on the scalp near the area to be treated. When turned on, the electromagnetic pulses repeatedly stimulate the brain's nerve cells. It is a painless procedure which is sometimes used for treatment-resistant depression or other psychiatric/neurologic brain disorders (e.g., auditory hallucinations, migraines). It is different from more invasive procedures such as vagus nerve stimulation or electroconvulsive therapy (ECT) which requires anesthesia and, in the case of ECT, produce convulsions. Side effects are generally mild to moderate (e.g., headache, scalp discomfort).

During the initial session, the healthcare provider performs cortical mapping to determine the optimal placement of the electrodes, stimulating pulses, and energy dosage necessary for optimal treatment. Periodically, these settings may be revised (90869) depending on the patient's response to treatment or to manage negative side effects.

Therapeutic repetitive transcranial magnetic stimulation (TMS) treatment;
- 90867   initial, including cortical mapping, motor threshold determination, delivery and management
- 90868   subsequent delivery and management, per session
- 90869   subsequent motor threshold re-determination with delivery and management

Coding Tips

- When reporting a separate Evaluation and Management service on the same day as the TMS service, be sure your documentation supports the individual E/M components for the visit.
- According to AMA guidelines, psychotherapy may be performed on the same day as the TMS service.
- Be aware of individual payer policies which may have differing requirements regarding medications and/or services already tried and failed (e.g., psychotherapy) prior to performing TMS. For example, one payer policy states that psychotherapy must have been conducted for 6 weeks (at least once per week) without significant improvement in depressive symptoms as indicated by a standardized depression assessment tool. Be sure that documentation supports payer requirements.
- Prior to performing TMS, the provider should check for any contraindications (e.g., seizure history, other magnetic sensitive devices) and document these findings in the medical record.

 Book: See Appendix A — NCCI Edits for a list of codes which may not be billed at the same time as these services.

Diagnoses

- Payers are beginning to cover this service for treatment-resistant major depressive disorder (MDD), while other diagnoses are often not covered.

Consider ICD-10-CM codes from the following:

F32.2   F32.3   F33.2   F33.3

Veteran's Affairs Services

In many cases, billing services for veterans simply use the codes listed in other segments of this chapter. However, there are some specialized services which have their own codes. They are chaplain services and whole health partner services.

CHAPLAIN SERVICES

The primary purpose of Chaplain spiritual care is to provide in-depth spiritual and pastoral care and counseling, which is highly integrated into the total care and treatment program. Chaplains provide a full range of spiritual and pastoral care and counseling that is characterized by in-depth assessment, evaluation and treatment of patient's often with many different physical, social, mental and spiritual needs, as part of an integrated and comprehensive bio-psycho-social-spiritual approach, assessing a patient's intrinsic and extrinsic spirituality, ascertaining spiritual preference and practices, exploring and determining patient's spiritual health, coping mechanisms, well-being, and developing goals of spiritual care unique to a patient's needs and family/caregiver support. The chaplain also provides consultation, counseling and support to family members and staff. Professional chaplains are clinically trained to provide this type of spiritual care.

The following codes are used to report these services:

Q9001 Assessment by department of veterans affairs chaplain services

Counseling, by department of veterans affairs chaplain services;
Q9002 individual
Q9003 group

WHOLE HEALTH PARTNER SERVICES

The Veterans Whole Health Program allows the patient and their health team to work together for the overall health of the patient, treating the patient based on their needs and goals. The program involves many resources that can help the patient to live a healthy and happy life.

N Q9004 Department of veterans affairs whole health partner services

Common Procedure Codes

Conventions

The following conventions are used in this segment:

Identifiers/Columns

- **N** Signifies a code added this year.
- **R** Signifies a code revised this year. Revised codes may have had a change to their description, inclusion terms, and/or instructional notes.
- **+** Signifies an add on code which must be used in addition to a primary procedure
- **#** Signifies a resequenced code which had been moved out of numeric order
- **NCCI** Identifies codes to which NCCI edits apply. See Chapter 5.1 — Procedure Coding Essentials for information about NCCI edits. See Appendix A — NCCI Edits for applicable NCCI edits for that code.
- **RVU** This column identifies the total RVU, where applicable, for the code
- **$Fee** This column identifies a Medicare fee for the code. It may be based on the RVU (national, unadjusted amount) or a fee schedule (e.g., laboratory, DME).

Indicators

Special code edits are included in this code list to assist with accurate code selection and reporting. These edits are identified as "indicators." Appropriately employing them may improve coding accuracy and reduce claim denials. Automatic payer edits can identify and deny claims that fail to meet the basic edits identified here. Become familiar with the edits that affect your organization to avoid unnecessary claim denials.

Note: Not every code will have an associated indicator.

Book: See *Figure F.2* in Appendix F — Coding Reference Tables for a list with explanations of the indicators found in this chapter.

CPT Procedure Codes

Disclaimer: The NCCI flags, RVUs and Fees included here are from October 2021 which were the most current edits at the time of publication. NCCI edits for 2022 will be available by January 1st for FindACode.com subscribers.

Code	Description	NCCI	RVU	$Fee

Anesthesia (00100-01999)

ANESTHESIA FOR PROCEDURES ON THE HEAD (00100-00222)

Code	Description	NCCI	RVU	$Fee
00104	Electroconvulsive therapy	NCCI	NE	NE

Surgery (10004-69990)

SURGICAL PROCEDURES ON THE INTEGUMENTARY SYSTEM (10030-19499)

Introduction or Removal Procedures on the Integumentary System (11900-11983)

Code	Description	NCCI	RVU	$Fee
11981	Insertion, non-biodegradable drug delivery implant Indicator(s): AS: 0 | Bilat: 0 | Global: 000 | Mod51: 2 | PC/TC: 0	NCCI	3.05	$106.42
11982	Removal, non-biodegradable drug delivery implant Indicator(s): AS: 0 | Bilat: 0 | Global: 000 | Mod51: 2 | PC/TC: 0	NCCI	3.44	$120.03
11983	Removal with reinsertion, non-biodegradable drug delivery implant Indicator(s): AS: 0 | Bilat: 0 | Global: 000 | Mod51: 2 | PC/TC: 0	NCCI	4.26	$148.64

Surgical Repair (Closure) Procedures on the Integumentary System (12001-16036)

Burns, Local Treatment (16000-16036)

Code	Description	NCCI	RVU	$Fee
16000	Initial treatment, first degree burn, when no more than local treatment is required Indicator(s): AS: 1 | Bilat: 0 | Global: 000 | Mod51: 2 | PC/TC: 0	NCCI	2.18	$76.07

Dressings and/or debridement of partial-thickness burns, initial or subsequent

Code	Description	NCCI	RVU	$Fee
16020	Small (less than 5% total body surface area) Indicator(s): AS: 1 | Bilat: 0 | Global: 000 | Mod51: 2 | PC/TC: 0	NCCI	2.50	$87.23

SURGICAL PROCEDURES ON THE MUSCULOSKELETAL SYSTEM (20100-29999)

Application of Casts and Strapping (29000-29799)

Body and Upper Extremity Application of Casts and Strapping (29000-29280)

Body and Upper Extremity Application of Strapping-Any Age
Strapping

Lower Extremity Application of Casts and Strapping (29305-29584)

Lower Extremity Application of Strapping-Any Age
Strapping

Code	Description	NCCI	RVU	$Fee
29260	Elbow or wrist Indicator(s): AS: 1 | Bilat: 1 | Global: 000 | Mod51: 2 | PC/TC: 0	NCCI	0.88	$30.71
29280	Hand or finger Indicator(s): AS: 1 | Bilat: 1 | Global: 000 | Mod51: 2 | PC/TC: 0	NCCI	0.86	$30.01
29530	Knee Indicator(s): AS: 1 | Bilat: 1 | Global: 000 | Mod51: 2 | PC/TC: 0	NCCI	0.89	$31.05
29540	Ankle and/or foot Indicator(s): AS: 1 | Bilat: 1 | Global: 000 | Mod51: 2 | PC/TC: 0	NCCI	0.82	$28.61

SURGICAL PROCEDURES ON THE RESPIRATORY SYSTEM (30000-32999)

Surgical Procedures on the Nose (30000-30999)

Other Procedures on the Nose (30901-30999)

Code	Description	NCCI	RVU	$Fee
30901	Control nasal hemorrhage, anterior, simple (limited cautery and/or packing) any method Indicator(s): AS: 1 | Bilat: 1 | Global: 000 | Mod51: 2 | PC/TC: 0	NCCI	4.63	$161.56

Code	Description	NCCI	RVU	SFee

SURGICAL PROCEDURES ON THE CARDIOVASCULAR SYSTEM (33016-37799)

Surgical Procedures on Arteries and Veins (34001-37799)

Vascular Injection Procedures (36000-36598)

Venous Procedures

Code	Description	NCCI	RVU	SFee
36410	Venipuncture, age 3 years or older, necessitating the skill of a physician or other qualified health care professional (separate procedure), for diagnostic or therapeutic purposes (not to be used for routine venipuncture) Indicator(s): AS: 1 | Bilat: 0 | Mod51: 2 | PC/TC: 0	NCCI	0.51	$17.80
36415	Collection of venous blood by venipuncture	NCCI	NE	$3.00
36416	Collection of capillary blood specimen (eg, finger, heel, ear stick)	NCCI	NE	NE

SURGICAL PROCEDURES ON THE NERVOUS SYSTEM (61000-64999)

Surgical Procedures on the Extracranial Nerves, Peripheral Nerves, and Autonomic Nervous System (64400-64999)

Neurostimulator Procedures on the Peripheral Nerves (64553-64595)

Percutaneous implantation of neurostimulator electrode array

Code	Description	NCCI	RVU	SFee
64553	Cranial nerve Indicator(s): AS: 0 | Bilat: 0 | Global: 010 | Mod51: 2 | PC/TC: 0	NCCI	71.59	$2,498.00

SURGICAL PROCEDURES ON THE AUDITORY SYSTEM (69000-69979)

Surgical Procedures on the External Ear (69000-69399)

Removal Procedures on the External Ear (69200-69222)

Removal foreign body from external auditory canal

Code	Description	NCCI	RVU	SFee
69200	Without general anesthesia Indicator(s): AS: 1 | Bilat: 1 | Global: 000 | Mod51: 2 | PC/TC: 0	NCCI	2.39	$83.39

Radiology Procedures (70010-79999)

DIAGNOSTIC RADIOLOGY (DIAGNOSTIC IMAGING) PROCEDURES (70010-76499)

Diagnostic Radiology (Diagnostic Imaging) Procedures of the Head and Neck (70010-70559)

Code	Description	NCCI	RVU	SFee
70371	Complex dynamic pharyngeal and speech evaluation by cine or video recording Indicator(s): AS: 0 | Bilat: 0 | Mod51: 0 | PC/TC: 1	NCCI	3.21	$112.01

Magnetic resonance imaging, brain, functional MRI (70554-70555)

Code	Description	NCCI	RVU	SFee
70554	Including test selection and administration of repetitive body part movement and/or visual stimulation, not requiring physician or psychologist administration Indicator(s): AS: 0 | Bilat: 3 | DxImage | PC/TC: 1	NCCI	12.39	$432.33
70555	Requiring physician or psychologist administration of entire neurofunctional testing Indicator(s): AS: 0 | Bilat: 3 | Mod51: 0 | PC/TC: 1	NCCI	NE	NE

Pathology and Laboratory Procedures (0001U-89398)

ORGAN OR DISEASE ORIENTED PANELS (80047-80081)

Code	Description	NCCI	RVU	$Fee
80048	Basic metabolic panel (Calcium, total) This panel must include the following: Calcium, total (82310) Carbon dioxide (bicarbonate) (82374) Chloride (82435) Creatinine (82565) Glucose (82947) Potassium (84132) Sodium (84295) Urea nitrogen (BUN) (84520)	NCCI	NE	$8.46
80050	General health panel This panel must include the following: Comprehensive metabolic panel (80053) Blood count, complete (CBC), automated and automated differential WBC count (85025 or 85027 and 85004) OR Blood count, complete (CBC), automated (85027) and appropriate manual differential WBC count (85007 or 85009) Thyroid stimulating hormone (TSH) (84443)	NCCI	NE	NE
80053	Comprehensive metabolic panel This panel must include the following: Albumin (82040) Bilirubin, total (82247) Calcium, total (82310) Carbon dioxide (bicarbonate) (82374) Chloride (82435) Creatinine (82565) Glucose (82947) Phosphatase, alkaline (84075) Potassium (84132) Protein, total (84155) Sodium (84295) Transferase, alanine amino (ALT) (SGPT) (84460) Transferase, aspartate amino (AST) (SGOT) (84450) Urea nitrogen (BUN) (84520)	NCCI	NE	$10.56
80061	Lipid panel This panel must include the following: Cholesterol, serum, total (82465) Lipoprotein, direct measurement, high density cholesterol (HDL cholesterol) (83718) Triglycerides (84478)	NCCI	NE	$13.39
80076	Hepatic function panel This panel must include the following: Albumin (82040) Bilirubin, total (82247) Bilirubin, direct (82248) Phosphatase, alkaline (84075) Protein, total (84155) Transferase, alanine amino (ALT) (SGPT) (84460) Transferase, aspartate amino (AST) (SGOT) (84450)	NCCI	NE	$8.17

DRUG ASSAY (80305-83992)

Presumptive Drug Class Screening (80305-80307)

	Code	Description	NCCI	RVU	$Fee
#	80305	Capable of being read by direct optical observation only (eg, utilizing immunoassay [eg, dipsticks, cups, cards, or cartridges]), includes sample validation when performed, per date of service	NCCI	NE	$12.60
#	80306	Read by instrument assisted direct optical observation (eg, utilizing immunoassay [eg, dipsticks, cups, cards, or cartridges]), includes sample validation when performed, per date of service	NCCI	NE	$17.14
#	80307	By instrument chemistry analyzers (eg, utilizing immunoassay [eg, EIA, ELISA, EMIT, FPIA, IA, KIMS, RIA]), chromatography (eg, GC, HPLC), and mass spectrometry either with or without chromatography, (eg, DART, DESI, GC-MS, GC-MS/MS, LC-MS, LC-MS/MS, LDTD, MALDI, TOF) includes sample validation when performed, per date of service	NCCI	NE	$62.14

Definitive Drug Testing (80320-83992)

Antidepressants, tricyclic and other cyclicals (80335-80337)

	Code	Description	NCCI	RVU	$Fee
#	80335	1 or 2	NCCI	NE	NE
#	80336	3-5	NCCI	NE	NE
#	80337	6 or more	NCCI	NE	NE

THERAPEUTIC DRUG ASSAYS (80143-80299)

	Code	Description	NCCI	RVU	$Fee
	80173	Haloperidol	NCCI	NE	$15.78
	80178	Lithium	NCCI	NE	$6.61
#	80164	Valproic acid (dipropylacetic acid); total	NCCI	NE	$13.54
#	80165	Valproic acid (dipropylacetic acid); free	NCCI	NE	$13.54

Code	Description	NCCI	RVU	$Fee

URINALYSIS PROCEDURES (81000-81099)

Urinalysis, by dip stick or tablet reagent for bilirubin, glucose, hemoglobin, ketones, leukocytes, nitrite, pH, protein, specific gravity, urobilinogen, any number of these constituents (81000-81003)

Code	Description	NCCI	RVU	$Fee
81000	Non-automated, with microscopy	NCCI	NE	$4.02
81001	Automated, with microscopy	NCCI	NE	$3.17
81002	Non-automated, without microscopy	NCCI	NE	$3.48
81003	Automated, without microscopy	NCCI	NE	$2.25

Urinalysis (81005-81020)

Code	Description	NCCI	RVU	$Fee
81005	Qualitative or semiquantitative, except immunoassays	NCCI	NE	$2.17

CHEMISTRY PROCEDURES (82009-84999)

Code	Description	NCCI	RVU	$Fee
83655	Lead	NCCI	NE	$12.11
84443	Thyroid stimulating hormone (TSH)	NCCI	NE	$16.80
84478	Triglycerides	NCCI	NE	$5.74
84479	Thyroid hormone (T3 or T4) uptake or thyroid hormone binding ratio (THBR)	NCCI	NE	$6.47
84999	Unlisted chemistry procedure	NCCI	NE	NE

Alcohol (ethanol) (82075-82077)

Code	Description	NCCI	RVU	$Fee
82077	Any specimen except urine and breath, immunoassay (eg, IA, EIA, ELISA, RIA, EMIT, FPIA) and enzymatic methods (eg, alcohol dehydrogenase)	NCCI	NE	$17.27

Glucose (82947-82952)

Code	Description	NCCI	RVU	$Fee
82947	Quantitative, blood (except reagent strip)	NCCI	NE	$3.93
82948	Blood, reagent strip	NCCI	NE	$5.04

Hemoglobin (83026-83069)

Code	Description	NCCI	RVU	$Fee
83036	Glycosylated (A1C)	NCCI	NE	$9.71

Thyroxine (84436-84439)

Code	Description	NCCI	RVU	$Fee
84436	Total	NCCI	NE	$6.87

Gonadotropin, chorionic (hCG) (84702-84704)

Code	Description	NCCI	RVU	$Fee
84702	Quantitative *Indicator(s): Female*	NCCI	NE	$15.05
84703	Qualitative *Indicator(s): Female*	NCCI	NE	$7.52

Code	Description	NCCI	RVU	$Fee
HEMATOLOGY AND COAGULATION PROCEDURES (85002-85999)				
85999	Unlisted hematology and coagulation procedure	NCCI	NE	NE

Blood count (85004-85049)

Code	Description	NCCI	RVU	$Fee
85007	Blood smear, microscopic examination with manual differential WBC count	NCCI	NE	$3.80
85008	Blood smear, microscopic examination without manual differential WBC count	NCCI	NE	$3.43
85009	Manual differential WBC count, buffy coat	NCCI	NE	$5.07
85014	Hematocrit (Hct)	NCCI	NE	$2.37
85018	Hemoglobin (Hgb)	NCCI	NE	$2.37
85025	Complete (CBC), automated (Hgb, Hct, RBC, WBC and platelet count) and automated differential WBC count	NCCI	NE	$7.77
85027	Complete (CBC), automated (Hgb, Hct, RBC, WBC and platelet count)	NCCI	NE	$6.47
85032	Manual cell count (erythrocyte, leukocyte, or platelet) each	NCCI	NE	$4.31
85048	Leukocyte (WBC), automated	NCCI	NE	$2.54

Prothrombin time (85610-85611)

Code	Description	NCCI	RVU	$Fee
85610	Prothrombin time	NCCI	NE	$4.29

Sedimentation rate, erythrocyte (85651-85652)

Code	Description	NCCI	RVU	$Fee
85651	Non-automated	NCCI	NE	$4.27

Thromboplastin time, partial (PTT) (85730-85732)

Code	Description	NCCI	RVU	$Fee
85730	Plasma or whole blood	NCCI	NE	$6.01

IMMUNOLOGY PROCEDURES (86000-86849)

Code	Description	NCCI	RVU	$Fee
86376	Microsomal antibodies (eg, thyroid or liver-kidney), each	NCCI	NE	$14.55

Fluorescent noninfectious agent antibody (86255-86256)

Code	Description	NCCI	RVU	$Fee
86256	Titer, each antibody Indicator(s): AS: 0 | Bilat: 0 | Mod51: 0 | PC/TC: 6	NCCI	NE	$12.05

Heterophile antibodies (86308-86310)

Code	Description	NCCI	RVU	$Fee
86308	Screening	NCCI	NE	$5.18

Immunoassay for infectious agent antibody(ies), qualitative or semiquantitative, single-step method (eg, reagent strip) (86317-86328)

Code	Description	NCCI	RVU	$Fee
86317	Quantitative, not otherwise specified	NCCI	NE	$14.99

Immunoelectrophoresis (86320-86327)

Code	Description	NCCI	RVU	$Fee
86320	Serum Indicator(s): AS: 0 | Bilat: 0 | Mod51: 0 | PC/TC: 6	NCCI	NE	$29.92
86325	Other fluids (eg, urine, cerebrospinal fluid) with concentration Indicator(s): AS: 0 | Bilat: 0 | Mod51: 0 | PC/TC: 6	NCCI	NE	$23.13

Code	Description	NCCI	RVU	$Fee

Particle agglutination (86403-86406)

Code	Description	NCCI	RVU	$Fee
86403	Screen, each antibody	NCCI	NE	$11.54

Skin test (86485-86580)

Code	Description	NCCI	RVU	$Fee
86580	Tuberculosis, intradermal Indicator(s): AS: 0 | Bilat: 0 | Mod51: 0 | PC/TC: 3	NCCI	0.29	$10.12

Syphilis test, non-treponemal antibody (86592-86593)

Code	Description	NCCI	RVU	$Fee
86592	Qualitative (eg, VDRL, RPR, ART)	NCCI	NE	$4.27

MICROBIOLOGY PROCEDURES (87003-87999)

Culture, bacterial (87040-87077)

Code	Description	NCCI	RVU	$Fee
87070	Any other source except urine, blood or stool, aerobic, with isolation and presumptive identification of isolates	NCCI	NE	$8.62

Culture, presumptive, pathogenic organisms, screening only (87081-87084)

Code	Description	NCCI	RVU	$Fee
87081	Screening only	NCCI	NE	$6.63
87084	Screening only; with colony estimation from density chart	NCCI	NE	$27.07

Culture, bacterial (87086-87088)

Code	Description	NCCI	RVU	$Fee
87086	Quantitative colony count, urine	NCCI	NE	$8.07
87088	With isolation and presumptive identification of each isolate, urine	NCCI	NE	$8.09

Infectious Agent Antigen Detection (87260-87899)

Infectious agent antigen detection by immunoassay technique, (eg, enzyme immunoassay [EIA], enzyme-linked immunosorbent assay [ELISA], fluorescence immunoassay [FIA], immunochemiluminometric assay [IMCA]) qualitative or semiquantitative; (87301-87451)

Code	Description	NCCI	RVU	$Fee
® 87340	Hepatitis B surface antigen (HBsAg)	NCCI	NE	$10.33
® 87341	Hepatitis B surface antigen (HBsAg) neutralization	NCCI	NE	$10.33

CYTOGENETIC STUDIES (88230-88299)

Chromosome analysis (88261-88264)

Code	Description	NCCI	RVU	$Fee
88262	Count 15-20 cells, 2 karyotypes, with banding	NCCI	NE	$125.49

Molecular cytogenetics (88271-88275)

Code	Description	NCCI	RVU	$Fee
88271	DNA probe, each (eg, FISH)	NCCI	NE	$21.42

Chromosome analysis (88280-88289)

Code	Description	NCCI	RVU	$Fee
88285	Additional cells counted, each study	NCCI	NE	$26.91

Code	Description	NCCI	RVU	SFee

SURGICAL PATHOLOGY PROCEDURES (88300-88399)

Immunofluorescence, per specimen (88346-88350)

Code	Description	NCCI	RVU	SFee
88346	Initial single antibody stain procedure *Indicator(s): AS: 0 | Bilat: 0 | Mod51: 0 | PC/TC: 1*	NCCI	4.18	$145.85

PROPRIETARY LABORATORY ANALYSES (PLA) CODES (0001U-0304U)

Code	Description	NCCI	RVU	SFee
0173U	Psychiatry (ie, depression, anxiety),genomic analysis panel, includes variant analysis of 14 genes	NCCI	NE	NE
0175U	Psychiatry (eg, depression, anxiety), genomic analysis panel, variant analysis of 15 genes	NCCI	NE	NE

Drug assay, definitive (0143U-0150U)

Code	Description	NCCI	RVU	SFee
0143U	120 or more drugs or metabolites, urine, quantitative liquid chromatography with tandem mass spectrometry (LC-MS/MS) using multiple reaction monitoring (MRM), with drug or metabolite description, comments including sample validation, per date of service	NCCI	NE	NE
0144U	160 or more drugs or metabolites, urine, quantitative liquid chromatography with tandem mass spectrometry (LC-MS/MS) using multiple reaction monitoring (MRM), with drug or metabolite description, comments including sample validation, per date of service	NCCI	NE	NE
0145U	65 or more drugs or metabolites, urine, quantitative liquid chromatography with tandem mass spectrometry (LC-MS/MS) using multiple reaction monitoring (MRM), with drug or metabolite description, comments including sample validation, per date of service	NCCI	NE	$114.43
0146U	80 or more drugs or metabolites, urine, by quantitative liquid chromatography with tandem mass spectrometry (LC-MS/MS) using multiple reaction monitoring (MRM), with drug or metabolite description, comments including sample validation, per date of service	NCCI	NE	$114.43
0147U	85 or more drugs or metabolites, urine, quantitative liquid chromatography with tandem mass spectrometry (LC-MS/MS) using multiple reaction monitoring (MRM), with drug or metabolite description, comments including sample validation, per date of service	NCCI	NE	$114.43
0148U	100 or more drugs or metabolites, urine, quantitative liquid chromatography with tandem mass spectrometry (LC-MS/MS) using multiple reaction monitoring (MRM), with drug or metabolite description, comments including sample validation, per date of service	NCCI	NE	$114.43
0149U	60 or more drugs or metabolites, urine, quantitative liquid chromatography with tandem mass spectrometry (LC-MS/MS) using multiple reaction monitoring (MRM), with drug or metabolite description, comments including sample validation, per date of service	NCCI	NE	$114.43
0150U	120 or more drugs or metabolites, urine, quantitative liquid chromatography with tandem mass spectrometry (LC-MS/MS) using multiple reaction monitoring (MRM), with drug or metabolite description, comments including sample validation, per date of service	NCCI	NE	$114.43

Medicine Services and Procedures (0001A-99607)

VACCINES, TOXOIDS (90476-91307)

Code	Description	NCCI	RVU	SFee
90636	Hepatitis A and hepatitis B vaccine (HepA-HepB), adult dosage, for intramuscular use	NCCI	NE	NE

Code	Description	NCCI	RVU	$Fee
Hepatitis A vaccine (90632-90634)				
90632	Adult dosage, for intramuscular use	NCCI	NE	$64.08
90633	Pediatric/adolescent dosage-2 dose schedule, for intramuscular use	NCCI	NE	NE
90634	Pediatric/adolescent dosage-3 dose schedule, for intramuscular use	NCCI	NE	NE

PSYCHIATRY (90785-90899)

Interactive Complexity (90785-90785)

Code	Description	NCCI	RVU	$Fee
+ 90785	Interactive complexity (List separately in addition to the code for primary procedure) Indicator(s): Bilat: 0 | Global: ZZZ | Mod51: 0 | PC/TC: 0 | Telemed	NCCI	0.43	$15.00

Psychiatric Diagnostic Procedures (90791-90899)

Code	Description	NCCI	RVU	$Fee
90791	Evaluation Indicator(s): Bilat: 0 | Mod51: 0 | PC/TC: 0 | Telemed	NCCI	5.18	$180.75
90792	Evaluation with medical services Indicator(s): Bilat: 0 | Mod51: 0 | PC/TC: 0 | Telemed	NCCI	5.78	$201.68

Psychotherapy (90832-90838)

Code	Description	NCCI	RVU	$Fee
90832	30 minutes with patient Indicator(s): Bilat: 0 | Mod51: 0 | PC/TC: 0 | Telemed	NCCI	2.23	$77.81
+ 90833	30 minutes with patient when performed with an evaluation and management service (List separately in addition to the code for primary procedure) Indicator(s): Bilat: 0 | Global: ZZZ | Mod51: 0 | PC/TC: 0 | Telemed	NCCI	2.04	$71.18
90834	45 minutes with patient Indicator(s): Bilat: 0 | Mod51: 0 | PC/TC: 0 | Telemed	NCCI	2.96	$103.28
+ 90836	45 minutes with patient when performed with an evaluation and management service (List separately in addition to the code for primary procedure) Indicator(s): Bilat: 0 | Global: ZZZ | Mod51: 0 | PC/TC: 0 | Telemed	NCCI	2.58	$90.02
90837	60 minutes with patient Indicator(s): Bilat: 0 | Mod51: 0 | PC/TC: 0 | Telemed	NCCI	4.37	$152.48
+ 90838	60 minutes with patient when performed with an evaluation and management service (List separately in addition to the code for primary procedure) Indicator(s): Bilat: 0 | Global: ZZZ | Mod51: 0 | PC/TC: 0 | Telemed	NCCI	3.42	$119.33

Other Psychotherapy (90839-90853)

Code	Description	NCCI	RVU	$Fee
90845	Psychoanalysis Indicator(s): AS: 0 | Bilat: 0 | Mod51: 0 | PC/TC: 0 | Telemed	NCCI	2.81	$98.05
90846	Family psychotherapy (without the patient present), 50 minutes Indicator(s): AS: 0 | Bilat: 0 | Mod51: 0 | PC/TC: 0 | Telemed	NCCI	2.84	$99.10
90847	Family psychotherapy (conjoint psychotherapy) (with patient present), 50 minutes Indicator(s): AS: 0 | Bilat: 0 | Mod51: 0 | PC/TC: 0 | Telemed	NCCI	2.94	$102.59
90849	Multiple-family group psychotherapy Indicator(s): AS: 0 | Bilat: 0 | Mod51: 0 | PC/TC: 0	NCCI	1.01	$35.24
90853	Group psychotherapy (other than of a multiple-family group) Indicator(s): AS: 0 | Bilat: 0 | Mod51: 0 | PC/TC: 0 | Telemed	NCCI	0.79	$27.57

Psychotherapy for Crisis

Code	Description	NCCI	RVU	$Fee
90839	First 60 minutes Indicator(s): AS: 0 | Bilat: 0 | Mod51: 0 | PC/TC: 0 | Telemed	NCCI	4.16	$145.16
+ 90840	Each additional 30 minutes (List separately in addition to code for primary service) Indicator(s): AS: 0 | Bilat: 0 | Global: ZZZ | Mod51: 0 | PC/TC: 0 | Telemed	NCCI	1.97	$68.74

Code	Description	NCCI	RVU	$Fee
Other Psychiatric Services or Procedures (90863-90899)				
+ 90863	Pharmacologic management, including prescription and review of medication, when performed with psychotherapy services (List separately in addition to the code for primary procedure) *Indicator(s): Telemed*	NCCI	0.75	$26.17
90865	Narcosynthesis for psychiatric diagnostic and therapeutic purposes (eg, sodium amobarbital (Amytal) interview) *Indicator(s): AS: 0 | Bilat: 0 | Mod51: 0 | PC/TC: 0*	NCCI	4.86	$169.58
90870	Electroconvulsive therapy (includes necessary monitoring) *Indicator(s): AS: 0 | Bilat: 0 | Global: 000 | Mod51: 0 | PC/TC: 0*	NCCI	5.08	$177.26
90880	Hypnotherapy *Indicator(s): AS: 0 | Bilat: 0 | Mod51: 0 | PC/TC: 0*	NCCI	3.09	$107.82
90882	Environmental intervention for medical management purposes on a psychiatric patient's behalf with agencies, employers, or institutions	NCCI	NE	NE
90885	Psychiatric evaluation of hospital records, other psychiatric reports, psychometric and/or projective tests, and other accumulated data for medical diagnostic purposes	NCCI	1.44	$50.25
90887	Interpretation or explanation of results of psychiatric, other medical examinations and procedures, or other accumulated data to family or other responsible persons, or advising them how to assist patient	NCCI	2.54	$88.63
90889	Preparation of report of patient's psychiatric status, history, treatment, or progress (other than for legal or consultative purposes) for other individuals, agencies, or insurance carriers	NCCI	NE	NE

Therapeutic repetitive transcranial magnetic stimulation (TMS) treatment

Code	Description	NCCI	RVU	$Fee
90867	Initial, including cortical mapping, motor threshold determination, delivery and management *Indicator(s): AS: 1 | Bilat: 0 | Global: 000 | Mod51: 0 | PC/TC: 0*	NCCI	NE	NE
90868	Subsequent delivery and management, per session *Indicator(s): AS: 1 | Bilat: 0 | Global: 000 | Mod51: 0 | PC/TC: 0*	NCCI	NE	NE
90869	Subsequent motor threshold re-determination with delivery and management *Indicator(s): AS: 1 | Bilat: 0 | Global: 000 | Mod51: 0 | PC/TC: 0*	NCCI	NE	NE

Individual psychophysiological therapy incorporating biofeedback training by any modality (face-to-face with the patient), with psychotherapy (eg, insight oriented, behavior modifying or supportive psychotherapy)

Code	Description	NCCI	RVU	$Fee
90875	30 minutes *Indicator(s): Telemed*	NCCI	1.78	$62.11
90876	45 minutes	NCCI	3.09	$107.82

BIOFEEDBACK SERVICES AND PROCEDURES (90901-90913)

Code	Description	NCCI	RVU	$Fee
90901	Biofeedback training by any modality *Indicator(s): AS: 0 | Bilat: 0 | Global: 000 | Mod51: 0 | PC/TC: 0*	NCCI	1.20	$41.87

NEUROLOGY AND NEUROMUSCULAR PROCEDURES (95700-96020)

Sleep Medicine Testing (95782-95811)

Code	Description	NCCI	RVU	$Fee
# 95800	Sleep study, unattended, simultaneous recording; heart rate, oxygen saturation, respiratory analysis (eg, by airflow or peripheral arterial tone), and sleep time *Indicator(s): AS: 0 | Bilat: 0 | Mod51: 0 | PC/TC: 1*	NCCI	4.88	$170.28
# 95801	Sleep study, unattended, simultaneous recording; minimum of heart rate, oxygen saturation, and respiratory analysis (eg, by airflow or peripheral arterial tone) *Indicator(s): AS: 0 | Bilat: 0 | Mod51: 0 | PC/TC: 1*	NCCI	2.62	$91.42

Code	Description	NCCI	RVU	SFee

Routine Electroencephalography (EEG) Procedures (95812-95830)

Electroencephalogram (EEG) extended monitoring (95812-95813)

Code	Description	NCCI	RVU	SFee
95812	41-60 minutes *Indicator(s): AS: 0 | Bilat: 0 | Mod51: 0 | PC/TC: 1*	NCCI	10.13	$353.47
95813	61-119 minutes *Indicator(s): AS: 0 | Bilat: 0 | Mod51: 0 | PC/TC: 1*	NCCI	12.46	$434.77

Electroencephalogram (EEG) (95816-95824)

Code	Description	NCCI	RVU	SFee
95816	Including recording awake and drowsy *Indicator(s): AS: 0 | Bilat: 0 | Mod51: 0 | PC/TC: 1*	NCCI	11.08	$386.62
95819	Including recording awake and asleep *Indicator(s): AS: 0 | Bilat: 0 | Mod51: 0 | PC/TC: 1*	NCCI	13.29	$463.73
95822	Recording in coma or sleep only *Indicator(s): AS: 0 | Bilat: 0 | Mod51: 0 | PC/TC: 1*	NCCI	12.12	$422.90

Evoked Potentials and Reflex Testing Procedures (95925-95939)

Code	Description	NCCI	RVU	SFee
95930	Visual evoked potential (VEP) checkerboard or flash testing, central nervous system except glaucoma, with interpretation and report *Indicator(s): AS: 0 | Bilat: 2 | Mod51: 0 | PC/TC: 1*	NCCI	1.97	$68.74

Short-latency somatosensory evoked potential study, stimulation of any/all peripheral nerves or skin sites, recording from the central nervous system (95925-95938)

Code	Description	NCCI	RVU	SFee
95925	In upper limbs *Indicator(s): AS: 0 | Bilat: 2 | Mod51: 0 | PC/TC: 1*	NCCI	4.62	$161.21
95926	In lower limbs *Indicator(s): AS: 0 | Bilat: 2 | Mod51: 0 | PC/TC: 1*	NCCI	4.26	$148.64
# 95938	Short-latency somatosensory evoked potential study, stimulation of any/all peripheral nerves or skin sites, recording from the central nervous system; in upper and lower limbs *Indicator(s): AS: 0 | Bilat: 2 | Mod51: 0 | PC/TC: 1*	NCCI	10.58	$369.17
95927	In the trunk or head *Indicator(s): AS: 0 | Bilat: 0 | Mod51: 0 | PC/TC: 1*	NCCI	4.18	$145.85

Special EEG Tests (95700-95967)

Functional cortical and subcortical mapping by stimulation and/or recording of electrodes on brain surface, or of depth electrodes, to provoke seizures or identify vital brain structures (95961-95962)

Code	Description	NCCI	RVU	SFee
95961	Initial hour of attendance by a physician or other qualified health care professional *Indicator(s): AS: 0 | Bilat: 0 | Mod51: 0 | PC/TC: 1*	NCCI	9.25	$322.76
+ 95962	Each additional hour of attendance by a physician or other qualified health care professional (List separately in addition to code for primary procedure) *Indicator(s): AS: 0 | Bilat: 0 | Global: ZZZ | Mod51: 0 | PC/TC: 1*	NCCI	7.72	$269.37

Neurostimulators, Analysis-Programming Procedures (95970-95984)

Electronic analysis of implanted neurostimulator pulse generator/transmitter (eg, contact group[s], interleaving, amplitude, pulse width, frequency [Hz], on/off cycling, burst, magnet mode, dose lockout, patient selectable parameters, responsive neurostimulation, detection algorithms, closed loop parameters, and passive parameters) by physician or other qualified health care professional; (95970-95984)

Code	Description	NCCI	RVU	SFee
95970	With brain, cranial nerve, spinal cord, peripheral nerve, or sacral nerve, neurostimulator pulse generator/transmitter, without programming *Indicator(s): AS: 0 | Bilat: 0 | Mod51: 0 | PC/TC: 0 | Telemed*	NCCI	0.56	$19.54

Code	Description	NCCI	RVU	$Fee

Other Neurology and Neuromuscular Procedures (95990-95999)

95999	Unlisted neurological or neuromuscular diagnostic procedure *Indicator(s): AS: 0	Bilat: 0	Mod51: 0	PC/TC: 0*	NCCI	NE	NE

Functional Brain Mapping (96020-96020)

96020	Neurofunctional testing selection and administration during noninvasive imaging functional brain mapping, with test administered entirely by a physician or other qualified health care professional (ie, psychologist), with review of test results and report *Indicator(s): AS: 0	Bilat: 0	Mod51: 0	PC/TC: 1*	NCCI	NE	NE

MEDICAL GENETICS AND GENETIC COUNSELING SERVICES (96040-96040)

96040	Medical genetics and genetic counseling services, each 30 minutes face-to-face with patient/family *Indicator(s): Telemed*	NCCI	1.34	$46.76

ADAPTIVE BEHAVIOR SERVICES (97151-97158)

Adaptive Behavior Assessment (97151-97152)

# 97151	Behavior identification assessment, administered by a physician or other qualified health care professional, each 15 minutes of the physician's or other qualified health care professional's time face-to-face with patient and/or guardian(s)/caregiver(s) administering assessments and discussing findings and recommendations, and non-face-to-face analyzing past data, scoring/interpreting the assessment, and preparing the report/treatment plan *Indicator(s): AS: 0	Bilat: 0	Mod51: 0	PC/TC: 0	Telemed*	NCCI	NE	NE
# 97152	Behavior identification-supporting assessment, administered by one technician under the direction of a physician or other qualified health care professional, face-to-face with the patient, each 15 minutes *Indicator(s): AS: 0	Bilat: 0	Mod51: 0	PC/TC: 0	Telemed*	NCCI	NE	NE

Adaptive Behavior Treatment (97153-97158)

# 97153	Adaptive behavior treatment by protocol, administered by technician under the direction of a physician or other qualified health care professional, face-to-face with one patient, each 15 minutes *Indicator(s): AS: 0	Bilat: 0	Mod51: 0	PC/TC: 0	Telemed*	NCCI	NE	NE
# 97154	Group adaptive behavior treatment by protocol, administered by technician under the direction of a physician or other qualified health care professional, face-to-face with two or more patients, each 15 minutes *Indicator(s): AS: 0	Bilat: 0	Mod51: 0	PC/TC: 0	Telemed*	NCCI	NE	NE
# 97155	Adaptive behavior treatment with protocol modification, administered by physician or other qualified health care professional, which may include simultaneous direction of technician, face-to-face with one patient, each 15 minutes *Indicator(s): AS: 0	Bilat: 0	Mod51: 0	PC/TC: 0	Telemed*	NCCI	NE	NE
# 97156	Family adaptive behavior treatment guidance, administered by physician or other qualified health care professional (with or without the patient present), face-to-face with guardian(s)/caregiver(s), each 15 minutes *Indicator(s): AS: 0	Bilat: 0	Mod51: 0	PC/TC: 0	Telemed*	NCCI	NE	NE
# 97157	Multiple-family group adaptive behavior treatment guidance, administered by physician or other qualified health care professional (without the patient present), face-to-face with multiple sets of guardians/caregivers, each 15 minutes *Indicator(s): AS: 0	Bilat: 0	Mod51: 0	PC/TC: 0	Telemed*	NCCI	NE	NE
# 97158	Group adaptive behavior treatment with protocol modification, administered by physician or other qualified health care professional, face-to-face with multiple patients, each 15 minutes *Indicator(s): AS: 0	Bilat: 0	Mod51: 0	PC/TC: 0	Telemed*	NCCI	NE	NE

Code	Description	NCCI	RVU	$Fee

CENTRAL NERVOUS SYSTEM ASSESSMENTS/TESTS (EG, NEURO-COGNITIVE, MENTAL STATUS, SPEECH TESTING) (96105-96146)

Assessment of Aphasia and Cognitive Performance Testing (96105-96125)

96105	Assessment of aphasia (includes assessment of expressive and receptive speech and language function, language comprehension, speech production ability, reading, spelling, writing, eg, by Boston Diagnostic Aphasia Examination) with interpretation and report, per hour *Indicator(s): AS: 0 | Bilat: 0 | Mod51: 0 | PC/TC: 0 | PS: 04 | Telemed*	NCCI	2.91	$101.54
# 96125	Standardized cognitive performance testing (eg, Ross Information Processing Assessment) per hour of a qualified health care professional's time, both face-to-face time administering tests to the patient and time interpreting these test results and preparing the report *Indicator(s): AS: 0 | Bilat: 0 | Mod51: 5 | PC/TC: 7 | Telemed*	NCCI	3.07	$107.12

Developmental/Behavioral Screening and Testing (96110-96127)

96110	Developmental screening (eg, developmental milestone survey, speech and language delay screen), with scoring and documentation, per standardized instrument *Indicator(s): PS: 04 | Telemed*	NCCI	0.29	$10.12
96112	Developmental test administration (including assessment of fine and/or gross motor, language, cognitive level, social, memory and/or executive functions by standardized developmental instruments when performed), by physician or other qualified health care professional, with interpretation and report; first hour *Indicator(s): AS: 0 | Bilat: 0 | Mod51: 0 | PC/TC: 0 | Telemed*	NCCI	3.77	$131.55
+ 96113	Developmental test administration (including assessment of fine and/or gross motor, language, cognitive level, social, memory and/or executive functions by standardized developmental instruments when performed), by physician or other qualified health care professional, with interpretation and report; each additional 30 minutes (List separately in addition to code for primary procedure) *Indicator(s): AS: 0 | Bilat: 0 | Global: ZZZ | Mod51: 0 | PC/TC: 0 | Telemed*	NCCI	1.68	$58.62
# 96127	Brief emotional/behavioral assessment (eg, depression inventory, attention-deficit/hyperactivity disorder [ADHD] scale), with scoring and documentation, per standardized instrument *Indicator(s): AS: 0 | Bilat: 0 | Mod51: 0 | PC/TC: 3 | Telemed*	NCCI	0.14	$4.89

Psychological/Neuropsychological Testing (96116-96146)

Neurobehavioral Status Examination (96116-96121)

96116	First hour *Indicator(s): AS: 0 | Bilat: 0 | Mod51: 0 | PC/TC: 0 | PS: 04 | Telemed*	NCCI	2.78	$97.00
+ 96121	Each additional hour (List separately in addition to code for primary procedure) *Indicator(s): AS: 0 | Bilat: 0 | Global: ZZZ | Mod51: 0 | PC/TC: 0 | Telemed*	NCCI	2.36	$82.35

Testing Evaluation Services (96130-96133)

96130	Psychological testing; first hour *Indicator(s): AS: 0 | Bilat: 0 | Mod51: 0 | PC/TC: 0 | Telemed*	NCCI	3.46	$120.73
96131	Psychological testing; each additional hour (List separately in addition to code for primary procedure) *Indicator(s): AS: 0 | Bilat: 0 | Global: ZZZ | Mod51: 0 | PC/TC: 0 | Telemed*	NCCI	2.62	$91.42
96132	Neuropsychological testing; first hour *Indicator(s): AS: 0 | Bilat: 0 | Mod51: 0 | PC/TC: 0 | Telemed*	NCCI	3.82	$133.29
96133	Neuropsychological testing; each additional hour (List separately in addition to code for primary procedure) *Indicator(s): AS: 0 | Bilat: 0 | Global: ZZZ | Mod51: 0 | PC/TC: 0 | Telemed*	NCCI	2.98	$103.98

Code	Description	NCCI	RVU	SFee

Test Administration and Scoring (96136-96139)

Code	Description	NCCI	RVU	SFee
96136	By physician or other qualified health care professional, two or more tests, any method; first 30 minutes *Indicator(s): AS: 0 | Bilat: 0 | Mod51: 0 | PC/TC: 0 | Telemed*	NCCI	1.34	$46.76
96137	By physician or other qualified health care professional, two or more tests, any method; each additional 30 minutes (List separately in addition to code for primary procedure) *Indicator(s): AS: 0 | Bilat: 0 | Global: ZZZ | Mod51: 0 | PC/TC: 0 | Telemed*	NCCI	1.20	$41.87
96138	By technician, two or more tests, any method; first 30 minutes *Indicator(s): AS: 0 | Bilat: 0 | Mod51: 0 | PC/TC: 0 | Telemed*	NCCI	1.07	$37.34
96139	By technician, two or more tests, any method; each additional 30 minutes (List separately in addition to code for primary procedure) *Indicator(s): AS: 0 | Bilat: 0 | Global: ZZZ | Mod51: 0 | PC/TC: 0 | Telemed*	NCCI	1.07	$37.34

Automated Testing and Result (96146-96146)

Code	Description	NCCI	RVU	SFee
96146	Psychological or neuropsychological test administration, with single automated, standardized instrument via electronic platform, with automated result only *Indicator(s): AS: 0 | Bilat: 0 | Mod51: 0 | PC/TC: 0*	NCCI	0.06	$2.09

HEALTH BEHAVIOR ASSESSMENT AND INTERVENTION (96156-96171)

Code	Description	NCCI	RVU	SFee
96156	Health behavior assessment, or re-assessment (ie, health-focused clinical interview, behavioral observations, clinical decision making) *Indicator(s): AS: 0 | Bilat: 0 | Mod51: 0 | PC/TC: 0 | Telemed*	NCCI	2.79	$97.35

Health and behavior intervention, individual (96158-96159)

	Code	Description	NCCI	RVU	SFee
	96158	Initial 30 minutes *Indicator(s): AS: 0 | Bilat: 0 | Mod51: 0 | PC/TC: 0 | Telemed*	NCCI	1.91	$66.65
+	96159	Each additional 15 minutes (List separately in addition to code for primary service) *Indicator(s): AS: 0 | Bilat: 0 | Global: ZZZ | Mod51: 0 | PC/TC: 0 | Telemed*	NCCI	0.66	$23.03

Health and behavior intervention, group (96164-96165)

	Code	Description	NCCI	RVU	SFee
#	96164	Initial 30 minutes *Indicator(s): AS: 0 | Bilat: 0 | Mod51: 0 | PC/TC: 0 | Telemed*	NCCI	0.28	$9.77
#	96165	Each additional 15 minutes (List separately in addition to code for primary service) *Indicator(s): AS: 0 | Bilat: 0 | Global: ZZZ | Mod51: 0 | PC/TC: 0 | Telemed*	NCCI	0.13	$4.54

Health and behavior intervention, family (96167-96171)

	Code	Description	NCCI	RVU	SFee
#	96167	(With the patient present), face-to-face; initial 30 minutes *Indicator(s): AS: 0 | Bilat: 0 | Mod51: 0 | PC/TC: 0 | Telemed*	NCCI	2.04	$71.18
#	96168	(With the patient present), face-to-face; each additional 15 minutes (List separately in addition to code for primary service) *Indicator(s): AS: 0 | Bilat: 0 | Global: ZZZ | Mod51: 0 | PC/TC: 0 | Telemed*	NCCI	0.73	$25.47
#	96170	(Without the patient present), face-to-face; initial 30 minute *Indicator(s): Telemed*	NCCI	2.34	$81.65
#	96171	(Without the patient present), face-to-face; each additional 15 minutes (List separately in addition to code for primary service) *Indicator(s): Global: ZZZ | Telemed*	NCCI	0.84	$29.31

Code	Description	NCCI	RVU	$Fee

Administration of health risk assessment instrument (96160-96161)

+ 96160	Administration of patient-focused health risk assessment instrument (eg, health hazard appraisal) with scoring and documentation, per standardized instrument *Indicator(s): Global: ZZZ | PC/TC: 5 | Telemed*	NCCI	0.08	$2.79
+ 96161	Administration of caregiver-focused health risk assessment instrument (eg, depression inventory) for the benefit of the patient, with scoring and documentation, per standardized instrument *Indicator(s): Global: ZZZ | PC/TC: 5 | Telemed*	NCCI	0.08	$2.79

HYDRATION, THERAPEUTIC, PROPHYLACTIC, DIAGNOSTIC INJECTIONS AND INFUSIONS, AND CHEMOTHERAPY AND OTHER HIGHLY COMPLEX DRUG OR HIGHLY COMPLEX BIOLOGIC AGENT ADMINISTRATION (96360-96549)

Therapeutic, Prophylactic, and Diagnostic Injections and Infusions (Excludes Chemotherapy and Other Highly Complex Drug or Highly Complex Biologic Agent Administration) (96365-96379)

Therapeutic, prophylactic, or diagnostic injection (specify substance or drug) (96372-96376)

96372	Subcutaneous or intramuscular *Indicator(s): AS: 0 | Bilat: 0 | Mod51: 0 | PC/TC: 5*	NCCI	0.41	$14.31

PHYSICAL MEDICINE AND REHABILITATION PROCEDURES (97010-97799)

Occupational Therapy Evaluations (97165-97168)

# 97165	Occupational therapy evaluation, low complexity, requiring these components: An occupational profile and medical and therapy history, which includes a brief history including review of medical and/or therapy records relating to the presenting problem; An assessment(s) that identifies 1-3 performance deficits (ie, relating to physical, cognitive, or psychosocial skills) that result in activity limitations and/or participation restrictions; and Clinical decision making of low complexity, which includes an analysis of the occupational profile, analysis of data from problem-focused assessment(s), and consideration of a limited number of treatment options. Patient presents with no comorbidities that affect occupational performance. Modification of tasks or assistance (eg, physical or verbal) with assessment(s) is not necessary to enable completion of evaluation component. Typically, 30 minutes are spent face-to-face with the patient and/or family. *Indicator(s): AS: 0 | Bilat: 0 | Mod51: 5 | PC/TC: 7 | Telemed*	NCCI	2.83	$98.75
# 97166	Occupational therapy evaluation, moderate complexity, requiring these components: An occupational profile and medical and therapy history, which includes an expanded review of medical and/or therapy records and additional review of physical, cognitive, or psychosocial history related to current functional performance; An assessment(s) that identifies 3-5 performance deficits (ie, relating to physical, cognitive, or psychosocial skills) that result in activity limitations and/or participation restrictions; and Clinical decision making of moderate analytic complexity, which includes an analysis of the occupational profile, analysis of data from detailed assessment(s), and consideration of several treatment options. Patient may present with comorbidities that affect occupational performance. Minimal to moderate modification of tasks or assistance (eg, physical or verbal) with assessment(s) is necessary to enable patient to complete evaluation component. Typically, 45 minutes are spent face-to-face with the patient and/or family. *Indicator(s): AS: 0 | Bilat: 0 | Mod51: 5 | PC/TC: 7 | Telemed*	NCCI	2.83	$98.75

Code	Description	NCCI	RVU	$Fee
# 97167	Occupational therapy evaluation, high complexity, requiring these components: An occupational profile and medical and therapy history, which includes review of medical and/or therapy records and extensive additional review of physical, cognitive, or psychosocial history related to current functional performance; An assessment(s) that identifies 5 or more performance deficits (ie, relating to physical, cognitive, or psychosocial skills) that result in activity limitations and/or participation restrictions; and Clinical decision making of high analytic complexity, which includes an analysis of the patient profile, analysis of data from comprehensive assessment(s), and consideration of multiple treatment options. Patient presents with comorbidities that affect occupational performance. Significant modification of tasks or assistance (eg, physical or verbal) with assessment(s) is necessary to enable patient to complete evaluation component. Typically, 60 minutes are spent face-to-face with the patient and/or family. *Indicator(s): AS: 0	Bilat: 0	Mod51: 5	PC/TC: 7	Telemed*	NCCI	2.83	$98.75
# 97168	Re-evaluation of occupational therapy established plan of care, requiring these components: An assessment of changes in patient functional or medical status with revised plan of care; An update to the initial occupational profile to reflect changes in condition or environment that affect future interventions and/or goals; and A revised plan of care. A formal reevaluation is performed when there is a documented change in functional status or a significant change to the plan of care is required. Typically, 30 minutes are spent face-to-face with the patient and/or family. *Indicator(s): AS: 0	Bilat: 0	Mod51: 5	PC/TC: 7	Telemed*	NCCI	1.91	$66.65

Modalities (97010-97039)

Supervised Physical Medicine and Rehabilitation Modalities (97010-97028)

Application of a modality to 1 or more areas

Code	Description	NCCI	RVU	$Fee
97010	Hot or cold packs	NCCI	0.18	$6.28
97014	Electrical stimulation (unattended)	NCCI	0.39	$13.61
97022	Whirlpool *Indicator(s): AS: 0	Bilat: 0	Mod51: 5	PC/TC: 7*	NCCI	0.52	$18.14
97024	Diathermy (eg, microwave) *Indicator(s): AS: 0	Bilat: 0	Mod51: 5	PC/TC: 7*	NCCI	0.21	$7.33
97026	Infrared *Indicator(s): AS: 0	Bilat: 0	Mod51: 5	PC/TC: 7*	NCCI	0.19	$6.63
97028	Ultraviolet *Indicator(s): AS: 0	Bilat: 0	Mod51: 5	PC/TC: 7*	NCCI	0.24	$8.37

Constant Attendance Physical Medicine and Rehabilitation Modalities (97032-97039)

Code	Description	NCCI	RVU	$Fee
97039	Unlisted modality (specify type and time if constant attendance) *Indicator(s): AS: 0	Bilat: 0	Mod51: 0	PC/TC: 7*	NCCI	NE	NE

Application of a modality to 1 or more areas

Code	Description	NCCI	RVU	$Fee
97032	Electrical stimulation (manual), each 15 minutes *Indicator(s): AS: 0	Bilat: 0	Mod51: 5	PC/TC: 7*	NCCI	0.43	$15.00
97033	Iontophoresis, each 15 minutes *Indicator(s): AS: 0	Bilat: 0	Mod51: 5	PC/TC: 7*	NCCI	0.59	$20.59
97034	Contrast baths, each 15 minutes *Indicator(s): AS: 0	Bilat: 0	Mod51: 5	PC/TC: 7*	NCCI	0.43	$15.00
97035	Ultrasound, each 15 minutes *Indicator(s): AS: 0	Bilat: 0	Mod51: 5	PC/TC: 7*	NCCI	0.42	$14.66

Code	Description	NCCI	RVU	$Fee

Therapeutic Procedures (97110-97546)

Code	Description	NCCI	RVU	$Fee
97139	Unlisted therapeutic procedure (specify) Indicator(s): AS: 0 | Bilat: 0 | Mod51: 0 | PC/TC: 7	NCCI	NE	NE
97150	Therapeutic procedure(s), group (2 or more individuals) Indicator(s): AS: 0 | Bilat: 0 | Mod51: 5 | PC/TC: 7 | Telemed	NCCI	0.52	$18.14
97530	Therapeutic activities, direct (one-on-one) patient contact (use of dynamic activities to improve functional performance), each 15 minutes Indicator(s): AS: 0 | Bilat: 0 | Mod51: 5 | PC/TC: 7 | Telemed	NCCI	1.13	$39.43
97533	Sensory integrative techniques to enhance sensory processing and promote adaptive responses to environmental demands, direct (one-on-one) patient contact, each 15 minutes Indicator(s): AS: 0 | Bilat: 0 | Mod51: 5 | PC/TC: 7	NCCI	1.74	$60.71
97535	Self-care/home management training (eg, activities of daily living (ADL) and compensatory training, meal preparation, safety procedures, and instructions in use of assistive technology devices/adaptive equipment) direct one-on-one contact, each 15 minutes Indicator(s): AS: 0 | Bilat: 0 | Mod51: 5 | PC/TC: 7 | Telemed	NCCI	0.97	$33.85
97537	Community/work reintegration training (eg, shopping, transportation, money management, avocational activities and/or work environment/modification analysis, work task analysis, use of assistive technology device/adaptive equipment), direct one-on-one contact, each 15 minutes Indicator(s): AS: 0 | Bilat: 0 | Mod51: 5 | PC/TC: 7	NCCI	0.93	$32.45

Therapeutic procedure, 1 or more areas, each 15 minutes (97110-97124)

Code	Description	NCCI	RVU	$Fee
97110	Therapeutic exercises to develop strength and endurance, range of motion and flexibility Indicator(s): AS: 0 | Bilat: 0 | Mod51: 5 | PC/TC: 7 | Telemed	NCCI	0.87	$30.36
97124	Massage, including effleurage, petrissage and/or tapotement (stroking, compression, percussion) Indicator(s): AS: 0 | Bilat: 0 | Mod51: 5 | PC/TC: 7	NCCI	0.85	$29.66

Therapeutic interventions that focus on cognitive function & compensatory strategies, direct patient contact (97129-97130)

Code	Description	NCCI	RVU	$Fee
97129	Initial 15 minutes Indicator(s): AS: 0 | Bilat: 0 | Mod51: 0 | PC/TC: 0 | Telemed	NCCI	0.67	$23.38
+ 97130	Each additional 15 minutes (List separately in addition to code for primary procedure) Indicator(s): AS: 0 | Bilat: 0 | Global: ZZZ | Mod51: 0 | PC/TC: 0 | Telemed	NCCI	0.65	$22.68

Other Procedures (97799-97799)

Code	Description	NCCI	RVU	$Fee
97799	Unlisted physical medicine/rehabilitation service or procedure Indicator(s): AS: 0 | Bilat: 0 | Mod51: 0 | PC/TC: 7	NCCI	NE	NE

EDUCATION AND TRAINING FOR PATIENT SELF-MANAGEMENT (98960-98962)

Education and training for patient self-management by a qualified, nonphysician health care professional using a standardized curriculum, face-to-face with the patient (could include caregiver/family) each 30 minutes (98960-98962)

Code	Description	NCCI	RVU	$Fee
98960	Individual patient Indicator(s): Telemed	NCCI	0.80	$27.91
98961	2-4 patients Indicator(s): Telemed	NCCI	0.39	$13.61
98962	5-8 patients Indicator(s): Telemed	NCCI	0.29	$10.12

NON-FACE-TO-FACE NONPHYSICIAN SERVICES (98966-98981)

Non-Face-to-Face Nonphysician Telephone Services (98966-98968)

Telephone assessment and management service provided by a qualified nonphysician health care professional to an established patient, parent, or guardian not originating from a related assessment and management service provided within the previous 7 days nor leading to an assessment and management service or procedure within the next 24 hours or soonest available appointment (98966-98968)

Code	Description	NCCI	RVU	$Fee
98966	5-10 minutes of medical discussion Indicator(s): AS: 0 | Bilat: 0 | Mod51: 0 | PC/TC: 0	NCCI	0.40	$13.96
98967	11-20 minutes of medical discussion Indicator(s): AS: 0 | Bilat: 0 | Mod51: 0 | PC/TC: 0	NCCI	0.77	$26.87
98968	21-30 minutes of medical discussion Indicator(s): AS: 0 | Bilat: 0 | Mod51: 0 | PC/TC: 0	NCCI	1.13	$39.43

Qualified Nonphysician Health Care Professional Online Digital Assessment and Management Service (98970-98972)

Code	Description	NCCI	RVU	$Fee
98970	5-10 minutes Indicator(s): AS: 0 | Bilat: 0 | Mod51: 0 | PC/TC: 0	NCCI	0.34	$11.86
98971	11-20 minutes Indicator(s): AS: 0 | Bilat: 0 | Mod51: 0 | PC/TC: 0	NCCI	0.60	$20.94
98972	21 or more minutes Indicator(s): AS: 0 | Bilat: 0 | Mod51: 0 | PC/TC: 0	NCCI	0.94	$32.80

Remote therapeutic monitoring (98975-98981)

Remote therapeutic monitoring treatment management services, physician or other qualified health care professional time in a calendar month requiring at least one interactive communication with the patient or caregiver during the calendar month (98980-98981)

	Code	Description	NCCI	RVU	$Fee
N	98980	First 20 minutes	-	NE	NE
N	98981	Each additional 20 minutes (List separately in addition to code for primary procedure)	-	NE	NE

SPECIAL SERVICES, PROCEDURES AND REPORTS (99000-99082)

Miscellaneous Medicine Services (99000-99082)

Code	Description	NCCI	RVU	$Fee
99000	Handling and/or conveyance of specimen for transfer from the office to a laboratory	NCCI	NE	NE
99050	Services provided in the office at times other than regularly scheduled office hours, or days when the office is normally closed (eg, holidays, Saturday or Sunday), in addition to basic service	NCCI	NE	NE
99051	Service(s) provided in the office during regularly scheduled evening, weekend, or holiday office hours, in addition to basic service	NCCI	NE	NE
99053	Service(s) provided between 10:00 PM and 8:00 AM at 24-hour facility, in addition to basic service	NCCI	NE	NE
99056	Service(s) typically provided in the office, provided out of the office at request of patient, in addition to basic service	NCCI	NE	NE
99058	Service(s) provided on an emergency basis in the office, which disrupts other scheduled office services, in addition to basic service	NCCI	NE	NE
99060	Service(s) provided on an emergency basis, out of the office, which disrupts other scheduled office services, in addition to basic service	NCCI	NE	NE

Code	Description	NCCI	RVU	SFee
® 99070	Supplies and materials (except spectacles), provided by the physician or other qualified health care professional over and above those usually included with the office visit or other services rendered (list drugs, trays, supplies, or materials provided)	NCCI	NE	NE
99071	Educational supplies, such as books, tapes, and pamphlets, for the patient's education at cost to physician or other qualified health care professional	NCCI	NE	NE
® 99072	Additional supplies, materials, and clinical staff time over and above those usually included in an office visit or other nonfacility service(s), when performed during a Public Health Emergency, as defined by law, due to respiratory-transmitted infectious disease	-	NE	NE
99075	Medical testimony	NCCI	NE	NE
99078	Physician or other qualified health care professional qualified by education, training, licensure/regulation (when applicable) educational services rendered to patients in a group setting (eg, prenatal, obesity, or diabetic instructions)	NCCI	NE	NE
99080	Special reports such as insurance forms, more than the information conveyed in the usual medical communications or standard reporting form	NCCI	NE	NE
99082	Unusual travel (eg, transportation and escort of patient) *Indicator(s): AS: 0 | Bilat: 0 | Mod51: 0 | PC/TC: 0*	NCCI	NE	NE

Hospital mandated on call service (99026-99027)

Code	Description	NCCI	RVU	SFee
99026	In-hospital, each hour	NCCI	NE	NE
99027	Out-of-hospital, each hour	NCCI	NE	NE

MODERATE (CONSCIOUS) SEDATION (99151-99157)

Code	Description	NCCI	RVU	SFee
99151	Moderate sedation services provided by the same physician or other qualified health care professional performing the diagnostic or therapeutic service that the sedation supports, requiring the presence of an independent trained observer to assist in the monitoring of the patient's level of consciousness and physiological status; initial 15 minutes of intraservice time, patient younger than 5 years of age	NCCI	2.54	$88.63
99152	Moderate sedation services provided by the same physician or other qualified health care professional performing the diagnostic or therapeutic service that the sedation supports, requiring the presence of an independent trained observer to assist in the monitoring of the patient's level of consciousness and physiological status; initial 15 minutes of intraservice time, patient age 5 years or older	NCCI	1.51	$52.69
+ 99153	Moderate sedation services provided by the same physician or other qualified health care professional performing the diagnostic or therapeutic service that the sedation supports, requiring the presence of an independent trained observer to assist in the monitoring of the patient's level of consciousness and physiological status; each additional 15 minutes intraservice time (List separately in addition to code for primary service) *Indicator(s): Global: ZZZ | PC/TC: 3*	NCCI	0.31	$10.82
99155	Moderate sedation services provided by a physician or other qualified health care professional other than the physician or other qualified health care professional performing the diagnostic or therapeutic service that the sedation supports; initial 15 minutes of intraservice time, patient younger than 5 years of age	NCCI	2.43	$84.79
99156	Moderate sedation services provided by a physician or other qualified health care professional other than the physician or other qualified health care professional performing the diagnostic or therapeutic service that the sedation supports; initial 15 minutes of intraservice time, patient age 5 years or older	NCCI	2.22	$77.46
+ 99157	Moderate sedation services provided by a physician or other qualified health care professional other than the physician or other qualified health care professional performing the diagnostic or therapeutic service that the sedation supports; each additional 15 minutes intraservice time (List separately in addition to code for primary service) *Indicator(s): Global: ZZZ*	NCCI	1.83	$63.85

Code	Description	NCCI	RVU	$Fee

OTHER MEDICINE SERVICES AND PROCEDURES (99170-99199)

Code	Description	NCCI	RVU	$Fee
99199	Unlisted special service, procedure or report *Indicator(s): AS: 0	Bilat: 0	Mod51: 0	PC/TC: 0*	NCCI	NE	NE

HOME HEALTH PROCEDURES AND SERVICES (99500-99602)

Code	Description	NCCI	RVU	$Fee
99509	Home visit for assistance with activities of daily living and personal care	NCCI	NE	NE
99510	Home visit for individual, family, or marriage counseling	NCCI	NE	NE
99600	Unlisted home visit service or procedure	NCCI	NE	NE

Evaluation and Management Services (99091-99499)

COGNITIVE ASSESSMENT AND CARE PLAN SERVICES (99483-99483)

Code	Description	NCCI	RVU	$Fee
® 99483	Assessment of and care planning for a patient with cognitive impairment, requiring an independent historian, in the office or other outpatient, home or domiciliary or rest home, with all of the following required elements: Cognition-focused evaluation including a pertinent history and examination; Medical decision making of moderate or high complexity; Functional assessment (eg, basic and instrumental activities of daily living), including decision-making capacity; Use of standardized instruments for staging of dementia (eg, functional assessment staging test [FAST], clinical dementia rating [CDR]); Medication reconciliation and review for high-risk medications; Evaluation for neuropsychiatric and behavioral symptoms, including depression, including use of standardized screening instrument(s); Evaluation of safety (eg, home), including motor vehicle operation; Identification of caregiver(s), caregiver knowledge, caregiver needs, social supports, and the willingness of caregiver to take on caregiving tasks; Development, updating or revision, or review of an Advance Care Plan; Creation of a written care plan, including initial plans to address any neuropsychiatric symptoms, neuro-cognitive symptoms, functional limitations, and referral to community resources as needed (eg, rehabilitation services, adult day programs, support groups) shared with the patient and/or caregiver with initial education and support. Typically, 50 minutes are spent face-to-face with the patient and/or family or caregiver. *Indicator(s): AS: 0	Bilat: 0	Mod51: 0	PC/TC: 0	Telemed*	NCCI	8.10	$282.63

Category II Codes (0001F-9007F)

DIAGNOSTIC/SCREENING PROCESSES OR RESULTS (3006F-3776F)

Code	Description	NCCI	RVU	$Fee
3720F	Cognitive impairment or dysfunction assessed (Prkns)	-	NE	NE
3755F	Cognitive and behavioral impairment screening performed (ALS)	-	NE	NE

Category III Codes (0042T-0713T)

NEUROLOGY AND NEUROMUSCULAR PROCEDURES/SERVICES (0106T-0590T)

Code	Description	NCCI	RVU	$Fee
0278T	Transcutaneous electrical modulation pain reprocessing (eg, scrambler therapy), each treatment session (includes placement of electrodes) *Indicator(s): AS: 0	Bilat: 0	Mod51: 0	PC/TC: 0*	NCCI	NE	NE

OTHER PROCEDURES/SERVICES (0042T-0703T)

Adaptive Behavior Assessments and Treatment (0362T-0373T)

Code	Description	NCCI	RVU	$Fee
0362T	Behavior identification supporting assessment *Indicator(s): Global: YYY	Telemed*	NCCI	NE	NE
0373T	Adaptive behavior treatment with protocol modification *Indicator(s): Global: YYY	Telemed*	NCCI	NE	NE

Code	Description	NCCI	RVU	SFee
Health and Well-Being Coaching (0591T-0593T)				
Health and well-being coaching face-to-face (0591T-0593T)				
0591T	Individual, initial assessment *Indicator(s): AS: 0	Bilat: 0	Global: YYY	Mod51: 0	PC/TC: 0*	NCCI	NE	NE
0592T	Individual, follow-up session, at least 30 minutes *Indicator(s): AS: 0	Bilat: 0	Global: YYY	Mod51: 0	PC/TC: 0*	NCCI	NE	NE
0593T	Group (2 or more individuals), at least 30 minutes *Indicator(s): AS: 0	Bilat: 0	Global: YYY	Mod51: 0	PC/TC: 0*	NCCI	NE	NE
Remote therapeutic monitoring of a standardized online digital cognitive behavioral therapy program ordered by a physician or other qualified health care professional (0702T-0703T)				
N 0702T	Supply and technical support, per 30 days	-	NE	NE
N 0703T	Management services by physician or other qualified health care professional, per calendar month	-	NE	NE

HCPCS Procedure Codes

Disclaimer: The NCCI flags, RVUs and Fees included here are from October 2021 which were the most current edits at the time of publication. NCCI edits for 2022 will be available by January 1st for FindACode.com subscribers.

Code	Description	NCCI	RVU	$Fee

Transportation Services (A0021-A0999)

Code	Description	NCCI	RVU	$Fee
A0160	Non-emergency transportation: per mile - case worker or social worker	-	NE	NE

Temporary Hospital Outpatient PPS (C1713-C9899)

Code	Description	NCCI	RVU	$Fee
C9756	Intraoperative near-infrared fluorescence lymphatic mapping of lymph node(s) (sentinel or tumor draining) with administration of indocyanine green (ICG) (List separately in addition to code for primary procedure)	-	NE	NE
C9757	Laminotomy (hemilaminectomy), with decompression of nerve root(s), including partial facetectomy, foraminotomy and excision of herniated intervertebral disc, and repair of annular defect with implantation of bone anchored annular closure device, including annular defect measurement, alignment and sizing assessment, and image guidance; 1 interspace, lumbar	NCCI	NE	NE

(G0008-G9987)

QUALITY REPORTING CODES (G0028-G9977)

Code	Description	NCCI	RVU	$Fee
G9012	Other specified case management service not elsewhere classified	-	NE	NE
G9016	Smoking cessation counseling, individual, in the absence of or in addition to any other evaluation and management service, per session (6-10 minutes) [demo project code only]	NCCI	NE	NE

PROCEDURES/PROFESSIONAL SERVICES (G0008-G9949)

Code	Description	NCCI	RVU	$Fee
G0129	Occupational therapy services requiring the skills of a qualified occupational therapist, furnished as a component of a partial hospitalization treatment program, per session (45 minutes or more)	NCCI	NE	NE
G0295	Electromagnetic therapy, to one or more areas, for wound care other than described in g0329 or for other uses	NCCI	NE	NE
G0378	Hospital observation service, per hour	NCCI	NE	NE
G0379	Direct admission of patient for hospital observation care	NCCI	NE	NE
G0451	Development testing, with interpretation and report, per standardized instrument form *Indicator(s): AS: 0 | Bilat: 0 | Mod51: 0 | PC/TC: 5 | PS: 04*	NCCI	0.29	$10.12
G0463	Hospital outpatient clinic visit for assessment and management of a patient	NCCI	NE	NE
G2000	Blinded administration of convulsive therapy procedure, either electroconvulsive therapy (ect, current covered gold standard) or magnetic seizure therapy (mst, non-covered experimental therapy), performed in an approved ide-based clinical trial, per treatment session *Indicator(s): AS: 0 | Bilat: 0 | Global: YYY | Mod51: 0 | PC/TC: 0*	-	NE	NE
G2082	Office or other outpatient visit for the evaluation and management of an established patient that requires the supervision of a physician or other qualified health care professional and provision of up to 56 mg of esketamine nasal self-administration, includes 2 hours post-administration observation *Indicator(s): AS: 0 | Bilat: 0 | Mod51: 0 | PC/TC: 0*	-	24.81	$865.70

Code	Description	NCCI	RVU	$Fee
G2083	Office or other outpatient visit for the evaluation and management of an established patient that requires the supervision of a physician or other qualified health care professional and provision of greater than 56 mg esketamine nasal self-administration, includes 2 hours post-administration observation *Indicator(s): AS: 0 | Bilat: 0 | Mod51: 0 | PC/TC: 0*	-	35.47	$1,237.66
G2211	Visit complexity inherent to evaluation and management associated with medical care services that serve as the continuing focal point for all needed health care services and/or with medical care services that are part of ongoing care related to a patient's single, serious condition or a complex condition. (add-on code, list separately in addition to office/outpatient evaluation and management visit, new or established) *Indicator(s): Global: ZZZ | Telemed*	-	NE	$15.88
+ G2212	Prolonged office or other outpatient evaluation and management service(s) beyond the maximum required time of the primary procedure which has been selected using total time on the date of the primary service; each additional 15 minutes by the physician or qualified healthcare professional, with or without direct patient contact (list separately in addition to cpt codes 99205, 99215 for office or other outpatient evaluation and management services) (do not report g2212 on the same date of service as 99354, 99355, 99358, 99359, 99415, 99416). (do not report g2212 for any time unit less than 15 minutes) *Indicator(s): AS: 0 | Bilat: 0 | Mod51: 0 | PC/TC: 0 | Telemed*	NCCI	0.96	$33.50
G2214	Initial or subsequent psychiatric collaborative care management, first 30 minutes in a month of behavioral health care manager activities, in consultation with a psychiatric consultant, and directed by the treating physician or other qualified health care professional *Indicator(s): AS: 0 | Bilat: 0 | Mod51: 0 | PC/TC: 0*	-	1.85	$64.55

Telehealth Services (G0071-G2025)

Code	Description	NCCI	RVU	$Fee
G0071	Payment for communication technology-based services for 5 minutes or more of a virtual (non-face-to-face) communication between an rural health clinic (rhc) or federally qualified health center (fqhc) practitioner and rhc or fqhc patient, or 5 minutes or more of remote evaluation of recorded video and/or images by an rhc or fqhc practitioner, occurring in lieu of an office visit; rhc or fqhc only *Indicator(s): PC/TC: 0*	NCCI	0.68	$23.73
G0459	Inpatient telehealth pharmacologic management, including prescription, use, and review of medication with no more than minimal medical psychotherapy *Indicator(s): Bilat: 0 | Mod51: 0 | PC/TC: 0 | Telemed*	NCCI	1.22	$42.57
G2010	Remote evaluation of recorded video and/or images submitted by an established patient (e.g., store and forward), including interpretation with follow-up with the patient within 24 business hours, not originating from a related e/m service provided within the previous 7 days nor leading to an e/m service or procedure within the next 24 hours or soonest available appointment *Indicator(s): AS: 0 | Bilat: 0 | Mod51: 0 | PC/TC: 0*	-	0.35	$12.21
G2025	Payment for a telehealth distant site service furnished by a rural health clinic (rhc) or federally qualified health center (fqhc) only *Indicator(s): PC/TC: 0*	-	2.85	$99.45

Telehealth Consultation - cont. (G0425-G0427)

Code	Description	NCCI	RVU	$Fee
G0425	emergency department or initial inpatient, typically 30 minutes communicating with the patient via telehealth *Indicator(s): AS: 0 | Bilat: 0 | Mod51: 0 | PC/TC: 0 | Telemed*	NCCI	2.90	$101.19
G0426	emergency department or initial inpatient, typically 50 minutes communicating with the patient via telehealth *Indicator(s): AS: 0 | Bilat: 0 | Mod51: 0 | PC/TC: 0 | Telemed*	NCCI	3.90	$136.08
G0427	emergency department or initial inpatient, typically 70 minutes or more communicating with the patient via telehealth *Indicator(s): AS: 0 | Bilat: 0 | Mod51: 0 | PC/TC: 0 | Telemed*	NCCI	5.74	$200.29

Code	Description	NCCI	RVU	$Fee

Care Planning/Management Services (G0506-G0512)

+ G0506	Comprehensive assessment of and care planning for patients requiring chronic care management services (list separately in addition to primary monthly care management service) *Indicator(s): AS: 0 | Bilat: 0 | Global: ZZZ | Mod51: 0 | PC/TC: 0 | Telemed*	NCCI	1.77	$61.76
G0511	Rural health clinic or federally qualified health center (rhc or fqhc) only, general care management, 20 minutes or more of clinical staff time for chronic care management services or behavioral health integration services directed by an rhc or fqhc practitioner (physician, np, pa, or cnm), per calendar month *Indicator(s): PC/TC: 0*	NCCI	1.87	$65.25
G0512	Rural health clinic or federally qualified health center (rhc/fqhc) only, psychiatric collaborative care model (psychiatric cocm), 60 minutes or more of clinical staff time for psychiatric cocm services directed by an rhc or fqhc practitioner (physician, np, pa, or cnm) and including services furnished by a behavioral health care manager and consultation with a psychiatric consultant, per calendar month *Indicator(s): PC/TC: 0*	NCCI	4.42	$154.23

Telehealth Services (G0071-G2025)

Telehealth Consultation (G0406-G0509)

G0406	Follow-up inpatient consultation, limited, physicians typically spend 15 minutes communicating with the patient via telehealth *Indicator(s): AS: 0 | Bilat: 0 | Mod51: 0 | PC/TC: 0 | Telemed*	NCCI	1.10	$38.38
G0407	Follow-up inpatient consultation, intermediate, physicians typically spend 25 minutes communicating with the patient via telehealth *Indicator(s): AS: 0 | Bilat: 0 | Mod51: 0 | PC/TC: 0 | Telemed*	NCCI	2.06	$71.88
G0408	Follow-up inpatient consultation, complex, physicians typically spend 35 minutes communicating with the patient via telehealth *Indicator(s): AS: 0 | Bilat: 0 | Mod51: 0 | PC/TC: 0 | Telemed*	NCCI	2.96	$103.28
G0508	critical care, initial, physicians typically spend 60 minutes communicating with the patient and providers via telehealth *Indicator(s): Bilat: 0 | Mod51: 0 | PC/TC: 0 | Telemed*	NCCI	6.03	$210.41
G0509	critical care, subsequent, physicians typically spend 50 minutes communicating with the patient and providers via telehealth *Indicator(s): Bilat: 0 | Mod51: 0 | PC/TC: 0 | Telemed*	NCCI	5.46	$190.52

Prolonged Preventive Service(s) (G0513-G0514)

+ G0513	(beyond the typical service time of the primary procedure), in the office or other outpatient setting requiring direct patient contact beyond the usual service; first 30 minutes (list separately in addition to code for preventive service) *Indicator(s): AS: 0 | Bilat: 0 | Global: ZZZ | Mod51: 0 | PC/TC: 0 | Telemed*	-	1.88	$65.60
+ G0514	(beyond the typical service time of the primary procedure), in the office or other outpatient setting requiring direct patient contact beyond the usual service; each additional 30 minutes (list separately in addition to code g0513 for additional 30 minutes of preventive service) *Indicator(s): AS: 0 | Bilat: 0 | Global: ZZZ | Mod51: 0 | PC/TC: 0 | Telemed*	-	1.88	$65.60

Non-biodegradable Drug Delivery Implants, subdermal (G0516-G0518)

G0516	Insertion of non-biodegradable drug delivery implants, 4 or more (services for subdermal rod implant) *Indicator(s): AS: 0 | Bilat: 0 | Global: 000 | Mod51: 2 | PC/TC: 0*	NCCI	6.38	$222.62
G0517	Removal of non-biodegradable drug delivery implants, 4 or more (services for subdermal implants) *Indicator(s): AS: 0 | Bilat: 0 | Global: 000 | Mod51: 2 | PC/TC: 0*	NCCI	6.35	$221.57
G0518	Removal with reinsertion, non-biodegradable drug delivery implants, 4 or more (services for subdermal implants) *Indicator(s): AS: 0 | Bilat: 0 | Global: 000 | Mod51: 2 | PC/TC: 0*	NCCI	12.02	$419.42

Code	Description	NCCI	RVU	SFee

Drug Tests (G0480-G0659)

Code	Description	NCCI	RVU	SFee
G0480	test(s), definitive, utilizing (1) drug identification methods able to identify individual drugs and distinguish between structural isomers (but not necessarily stereoisomers), including, but not limited to GC/MS (any type, single or tandem) and LC/MS (any type, single or tandem and excluding immunoassays (e.g., IA, EIA, ELISA, EMIT, FPIA) and enzymatic methods (e.g., alcohol dehydrogenase)), (2) stable isotope or other universally recognized internal standards in all samples (e.g., to control for matrix effects, interferences and variations in signal strength), and (3) method or drug-specific calibration and matrix-matched quality control material (e.g., to control for instrument variations and mass spectral drift); qualitative or quantitative, all sources, includes specimen validity testing, per day; 1-7 drug class(es), including metabolite(s) if performed	NCCI	NE	$114.43
G0481	test(s), definitive, utilizing (1) drug identification methods able to identify individual drugs and distinguish between structural isomers (but not necessarily stereoisomers), including, but not limited to GC/MS (any type, single or tandem) and LC/MS (any type, single or tandem and excluding immunoassays (e.g., IA, EIA, ELISA, EMIT, FPIA) and enzymatic methods (e.g., alcohol dehydrogenase)), (2) stable isotope or other universally recognized internal standards in all samples (e.g., to control for matrix effects, interferences and variations in signal strength), and (3) method or drug-specific calibration and matrix-matched quality control material (e.g., to control for instrument variations and mass spectral drift); qualitative or quantitative, all sources, includes specimen validity testing, per day; 8-14 drug class(es), including metabolite(s) if performed	NCCI	NE	$156.59
G0482	test(s), definitive, utilizing (1) drug identification methods able to identify individual drugs and distinguish between structural isomers (but not necessarily stereoisomers), including, but not limited to GC/MS (any type, single or tandem) and LC/MS (any type, single or tandem and excluding immunoassays (e.g., IA, EIA, ELISA, EMIT, FPIA) and enzymatic methods (e.g., alcohol dehydrogenase)), (2) stable isotope or other universally recognized internal standards in all samples (e.g., to control for matrix effects, interferences and variations in signal strength), and (3) method or drug-specific calibration and matrix-matched quality control material (e.g., to control for instrument variations and mass spectral drift); qualitative or quantitative, all sources, includes specimen validity testing, per day; 15-21 drug class(es), including metabolite(s) if performed	NCCI	NE	$198.74
G0483	test(s), definitive, utilizing (1) drug identification methods able to identify individual drugs and distinguish between structural isomers (but not necessarily stereoisomers), including, but not limited to GC/MS (any type, single or tandem) and LC/MS (any type, single or tandem and excluding immunoassays (e.g., IA, EIA, ELISA, EMIT, FPIA) and enzymatic methods (e.g., alcohol dehydrogenase)), (2) stable isotope or other universally recognized internal standards in all samples (e.g., to control for matrix effects, interferences and variations in signal strength), and (3) method or drug-specific calibration and matrix-matched quality control material (e.g., to control for instrument variations and mass spectral drift); qualitative or quantitative, all sources, includes specimen validity testing, per day; 22 or more drug class(es), including metabolite(s) if performed	NCCI	NE	$246.92
G0659	test(s), definitive, utilizing drug identification methods able to identify individual drugs and distinguish between structural isomers (but not necessarily stereoisomers), including but not limited to GC/MS (any type, single or tandem) and LC/MS (any type, single or tandem), excluding immunoassays (e.g., IA, EIA, ELISA, EMIT, FPIA) and enzymatic methods (e.g., alcohol dehydrogenase), performed without method or drug-specific calibration, without matrix-matched quality control material, or without use of stable isotope or other universally recognized internal standard(s) for each drug, drug metabolite or drug class per specimen; qualitative or quantitative, all sources, includes specimen validity testing, per day, any number of drug classes	NCCI	NE	$62.14

Care Management Home Visit or Care Plan Oversight (G0076-G0087)

Home Care Plan Oversight (G0086-G0087)

Code	Description	NCCI	RVU	SFee
G0086	Limited (30 minutes) care management home care plan oversight. for use only in a medicare-approved cmmi model. (services must be furnished within a beneficiary's home, domiciliary, rest home, assisted living and/or nursing facility) *Indicator(s): AS: 0	Bilat: 0	Mod51: 0	PC/TC: 0*	NCCI	2.22	$77.46

Code	Description	NCCI	RVU	$Fee
G0087	Comprehensive (60 minutes) care management home care plan oversight. for use only in a medicare-approved cmmi model. (services must be furnished within a beneficiary's home, domiciliary, rest home, assisted living and/or nursing facility) *Indicator(s): AS: 0 | Bilat: 0 | Mod51: 0 | PC/TC: 0*	NCCI	3.10	$108.17

Existing Patient Home Visit (G0081-G0085)

Code	Description	NCCI	RVU	$Fee
G0081	Brief (20 minutes) care management home visit for an existing patient. for use only in a medicare-approved cmmi model. (services must be furnished within a beneficiary's home, domiciliary, rest home, assisted living and/or nursing facility) *Indicator(s): AS: 0 | Bilat: 0 | Mod51: 0 | PC/TC: 0*	NCCI	1.57	$54.78
G0082	Limited (30 minutes) care management home visit for an existing patient. for use only in a medicare-approved cmmi model. (services must be furnished within a beneficiary's home, domiciliary, rest home, assisted living and/or nursing facility) *Indicator(s): AS: 0 | Bilat: 0 | Mod51: 0 | PC/TC: 0*	NCCI	2.40	$83.74
G0083	Moderate (45 minutes) care management home visit for an existing patient. for use only in a medicare-approved cmmi model. (services must be furnished within a beneficiary's home, domiciliary, rest home, assisted living and/or nursing facility) *Indicator(s): AS: 0 | Bilat: 0 | Mod51: 0 | PC/TC: 0*	NCCI	3.70	$129.10
G0084	Comprehensive (60 minutes) care management home visit for an existing patient. for use only in a medicare-approved cmmi model. (services must be furnished within a beneficiary's home, domiciliary, rest home, assisted living and/or nursing facility) *Indicator(s): AS: 0 | Bilat: 0 | Mod51: 0 | PC/TC: 0*	NCCI	5.12	$178.65
G0085	Extensive (75 minutes) care management home visit for an existing patient. for use only in a medicare-approved cmmi model. (services must be furnished within a beneficiary's home, domiciliary, rest home, assisted living and/or nursing facility) *Indicator(s): AS: 0 | Bilat: 0 | Mod51: 0 | PC/TC: 0*	NCCI	6.32	$220.52

New Patient Home Visit (G0076-G0080)

Code	Description	NCCI	RVU	$Fee
G0076	Brief (20 minutes) care management home visit for a new patient. for use only in a medicare-approved cmmi model. (services must be furnished within a beneficiary's home, domiciliary, rest home, assisted living and/or nursing facility) *Indicator(s): AS: 0 | Bilat: 0 | Mod51: 0 | PC/TC: 0*	NCCI	1.56	$54.43
G0077	Limited (30 minutes) care management home visit for a new patient. for use only in a medicare-approved cmmi model. (services must be furnished within a beneficiary's home, domiciliary, rest home, assisted living and/or nursing facility) *Indicator(s): AS: 0 | Bilat: 0 | Mod51: 0 | PC/TC: 0*	NCCI	2.20	$76.76
G0078	Moderate (45 minutes) care management home visit for a new patient. for use only in a medicare-approved cmmi model. (services must be furnished within a beneficiary's home, domiciliary, rest home, assisted living and/or nursing facility) *Indicator(s): AS: 0 | Bilat: 0 | Mod51: 0 | PC/TC: 0*	NCCI	3.64	$127.01
G0079	Comprehensive (60 minutes) care management home visit for a new patient. for use only in a medicare-approved cmmi model. (services must be furnished within a beneficiary's home, domiciliary, rest home, assisted living and/or nursing facility) *Indicator(s): AS: 0 | Bilat: 0 | Mod51: 0 | PC/TC: 0*	NCCI	5.19	$181.10
G0080	Extensive (75 minutes) care management home visit for a new patient. for use only in a medicare-approved cmmi model. (services must be furnished within a beneficiary's home, domiciliary, rest home, assisted living and/or nursing facility) *Indicator(s): AS: 0 | Bilat: 0 | Mod51: 0 | PC/TC: 0*	NCCI	6.32	$220.52

Home Health/Hospice Services (G0151-G2169)

Code	Description	NCCI	RVU	$Fee
G0155	Services of clinical social worker in home health or hospice settings, each 15 minutes	NCCI	NE	NE
G0337	Hospice evaluation and counseling services, pre-election	NCCI	2.10	$73.28

Behavioral Health Services (G0176-G2011)

Code	Description	NCCI	RVU	$Fee
G0176	Activity therapy, such as music, dance, art or play therapies not for recreation, related to the care and treatment of patient's disabling mental health problems, per session (45 minutes or more)	NCCI	NE	NE

Code	Description	NCCI	RVU	SFee
G0177	Training and educational services related to the care and treatment of patient's disabling mental health problems per session (45 minutes or more)	NCCI	NE	NE
G0396	Alcohol and/or substance (other than tobacco) misuse structured assessment (e.g., audit, dast), and brief intervention 15 to 30 minutes *Indicator(s): AS: 0 | Bilat: 0 | Mod51: 0 | PC/TC: 0 | Telemed*	NCCI	1.04	$36.29
G0397	Alcohol and/or substance (other than tobacco) misuse structured assessment (e.g., audit, dast), and intervention, greater than 30 minutes *Indicator(s): AS: 0 | Bilat: 0 | Mod51: 0 | PC/TC: 0 | Telemed*	NCCI	1.94	$67.69
G0409	Social work and psychological services, directly relating to and/or furthering the patient's rehabilitation goals, each 15 minutes, face-to-face; individual (services provided by a corf-qualified social worker or psychologist in a corf) *Indicator(s): AS: 0 | Bilat: 0 | Mod51: 0*	NCCI	0.41	$14.31
G0410	Group psychotherapy other than of a multiple-family group, in a partial hospitalization setting, approximately 45 to 50 minutes *Indicator(s): Telemed*	NCCI	NE	NE
G0411	Interactive group psychotherapy, in a partial hospitalization setting, approximately 45 to 50 minutes	NCCI	NE	NE
G2011	Alcohol and/or substance (other than tobacco) misuse structured assessment (e.g., audit, dast), and brief intervention, 5-14 minutes *Indicator(s): AS: 0 | Bilat: 0 | Mod51: 0 | PC/TC: 0*	NCCI	0.49	$17.10

Behavioral Screenings/Counseling (G0442-G0473)

Code	Description	NCCI	RVU	SFee
G0442	Annual alcohol misuse screening, 15 minutes *Indicator(s): AS: 0 | Bilat: 0 | Mod51: 0 | PC/TC: 0 | Telemed*	NCCI	0.54	$18.84
G0443	Brief face-to-face behavioral counseling for alcohol misuse, 15 minutes *Indicator(s): AS: 0 | Bilat: 0 | Mod51: 0 | PC/TC: 0 | Telemed*	NCCI	0.77	$26.87
G0444	Annual depression screening, 15 minutes *Indicator(s): AS: 0 | Bilat: 0 | Mod51: 0 | PC/TC: 0 | Telemed*	NCCI	0.54	$18.84
G0445	High intensity behavioral counseling to prevent sexually transmitted infection; face-to-face, individual, includes: education, skills training and guidance on how to change sexual behavior; performed semi-annually, 30 minutes *Indicator(s): AS: 0 | Bilat: 0 | Mod51: 0 | PC/TC: 0 | Telemed*	NCCI	0.81	$28.26
G0446	Annual, face-to-face intensive behavioral therapy for cardiovascular disease, individual, 15 minutes *Indicator(s): AS: 0 | Bilat: 0 | Mod51: 0 | PC/TC: 0 | Telemed*	NCCI	0.77	$26.87
G0447	Face-to-face behavioral counseling for obesity, 15 minutes *Indicator(s): AS: 0 | Bilat: 0 | Mod51: 0 | PC/TC: 0 | Telemed*	NCCI	0.77	$26.87

Brief communication technology-based service, e.g. virtual check-in (G2012-G2252)

Code	Description	NCCI	RVU	SFee
G2012	by a physician or other qualified health care professional who can report evaluation and management services, provided to an established patient, not originating from a related e/m service provided within the previous 7 days nor leading to an e/m service or procedure within the next 24 hours or soonest available appointment; 5-10 minutes of medical discussion *Indicator(s): AS: 0 | Bilat: 0 | Mod51: 0 | PC/TC: 0*	-	0.42	$14.66
G2251	by a qualified health care professional who cannot report evaluation and management services, provided to an established patient, not originating from a related service provided within the previous 7 days nor leading to a service or procedure within the next 24 hours or soonest available appointment; 5-10 minutes of clinical discussion *Indicator(s): AS: 0 | Bilat: 0 | Mod51: 0 | PC/TC: 0*	NCCI	0.42	$14.66
G2252	by a physician or other qualified health care professional who can report evaluation and management services, provided to an established patient, not originating from a related e/m service provided within the previous 7 days nor leading to an e/m service or procedure within the next 24 hours or soonest available appointment; 11-20 minutes of medical discussion *Indicator(s): AS: 0 | Bilat: 0 | Mod51: 0 | PC/TC: 0*	NCCI	0.77	$26.87

Code	Description	NCCI	RVU	SFee

Electrical Stimulation (G0281-G0283)

Code	Description	NCCI	RVU	SFee
G0283	(unattended), to one or more areas for indication(s) other than wound care, as part of a therapy plan of care *Indicator(s): AS: 0	Bilat: 0	Mod51: 5	PC/TC: 7*	NCCI	0.38	$13.26

Opioid Use Disorder Treatment (Office) (G2086-G2088)

Code	Description	NCCI	RVU	SFee
G2086	Office-based treatment for opioid use disorder, including development of the treatment plan, care coordination, individual therapy and group therapy and counseling; at least 70 minutes in the first calendar month *Indicator(s): AS: 0	Bilat: 0	Mod51: 0	PC/TC: 0	Telemed*	-	11.31	$394.64
G2087	Office-based treatment for opioid use disorder, including care coordination, individual therapy and group therapy and counseling; at least 60 minutes in a subsequent calendar month *Indicator(s): AS: 0	Bilat: 0	Mod51: 0	PC/TC: 0	Telemed*	-	10.07	$351.37
G2088	Office-based treatment for opioid use disorder, including care coordination, individual therapy and group therapy and counseling; each additional 30 minutes beyond the first 120 minutes (list separately in addition to code for primary procedure) *Indicator(s): AS: 0	Bilat: 0	Global: ZZZ	Mod51: 0	PC/TC: 0	Telemed*	-	1.91	$66.65

Medication assisted treatment services (Medicare-enrolled opioid treatment program) (G2067-G2080)

Code	Description	NCCI	RVU	SFee
G2067	methadone; weekly bundle including dispensing and/or administration, substance use counseling, individual and group therapy, and toxicology testing, if performed (provision of the services by a medicare-enrolled opioid treatment program)	-	NE	NE
G2068	buprenorphine (oral); weekly bundle including dispensing and/or administration, substance use counseling, individual and group therapy, and toxicology testing if performed (provision of the services by a medicare-enrolled opioid treatment program)	-	NE	NE
G2069	buprenorphine (injectable); weekly bundle including dispensing and/or administration, substance use counseling, individual and group therapy, and toxicology testing if performed (provision of the services by a medicare-enrolled opioid treatment program)	-	NE	NE
G2070	buprenorphine (implant insertion); weekly bundle including dispensing and/or administration, substance use counseling, individual and group therapy, and toxicology testing if performed (provision of the services by a medicare-enrolled opioid treatment program)	-	NE	NE
G2071	buprenorphine (implant removal); weekly bundle including dispensing and/or administration, substance use counseling, individual and group therapy, and toxicology testing if performed (provision of the services by a medicare-enrolled opioid treatment program)	-	NE	NE
G2072	buprenorphine (implant insertion and removal); weekly bundle including dispensing and/or administration, substance use counseling, individual and group therapy, and toxicology testing if performed (provision of the services by a medicare-enrolled opioid treatment program)	-	NE	NE
G2073	naltrexone; weekly bundle including dispensing and/or administration, substance use counseling, individual and group therapy, and toxicology testing if performed (provision of the services by a medicare-enrolled opioid treatment program)	-	NE	NE
G2074	weekly bundle not including the drug, including substance use counseling, individual and group therapy, and toxicology testing if performed (provision of the services by a medicare-enrolled opioid treatment program)	-	NE	NE
G2075	medication not otherwise specified; weekly bundle including dispensing and/or administration, substance use counseling, individual and group therapy, and toxicology testing, if performed (provision of the services by a medicare-enrolled opioid treatment program)	-	NE	NE

Code	Description	NCCI	RVU	SFee
G2076	Intake activities, including initial medical examination that is a complete, fully documented physical evaluation and initial assessment by a program physician or a primary care physician, or an authorized healthcare professional under the supervision of a program physician qualified personnel that includes preparation of a treatment plan that includes the patient's short-term goals and the tasks the patient must perform to complete the short-term goals; the patient's requirements for education, vocational rehabilitation, and employment; and the medical, psycho- social, economic, legal, or other supportive services that a patient needs, conducted by qualified personnel (provision of the services by a medicare-enrolled opioid treatment program); list separately in addition to code for primary procedure	-	NE	NE
G2077	Periodic assessment; assessing periodically by qualified personnel to determine the most appropriate combination of services and treatment (provision of the services by a medicare-enrolled opioid treatment program); list separately in addition to code for primary procedure	-	NE	NE
G2080	Each additional 30 minutes of counseling in a week of medication assisted treatment, (provision of the services by a medicare-enrolled opioid treatment program); list separately in addition to code for primary procedure	-	NE	NE

BUNDLED CARE IMPROVEMENT ADVANCED (BPCI ADVANCED) MODEL VISITS (G9978-G9987)

Code	Description	NCCI	RVU	SFee
G9978	Remote in-home visit for the evaluation and management of a new patient for use only in a medicare-approved bundled payments for care improvement advanced (bpci advanced) model episode of care, which requires these 3 key components: • a problem focused history; • a problem focused examination; and • straightforward medical decision making, furnished in real time using interactive audio and video technology. Counseling and coordination of care with other physicians, other qualified health care professionals or agencies are provided consistent with the nature of the problem(s) and the needs of the patient or the family or both. Usually, the presenting problem(s) are self limited or minor. Typically, 10 minutes are spent with the patient or family or both via real time, audio and video intercommunications technology *Indicator(s): AS: 0 | Bilat: 0 | Mod51: 0 | PC/TC: 0*	-	0.82	$28.61
G9979	Remote in-home visit for the evaluation and management of a new patient for use only in a medicare-approved bundled payments for care improvement advanced (bpci advanced) model episode of care, which requires these 3 key components: • an expanded problem focused history; • an expanded problem focused examination; • straightforward medical decision making, furnished in real time using interactive audio and video technology. Counseling and coordination of care with other physicians, other qualified health care professionals or agencies are provided consistent with the nature of the problem(s) and the needs of the patient or the family or both. Usually, the presenting problem(s) are of low to moderate severity. Typically, 20 minutes are spent with the patient or family or both via real time, audio and video intercommunications technology *Indicator(s): AS: 0 | Bilat: 0 | Mod51: 0 | PC/TC: 0*	-	1.43	$49.90
G9980	Remote in-home visit for the evaluation and management of a new patient for use only in a medicare-approved bundled payments for care improvement advanced (bpci advanced) model episode of care, which requires these 3 key components: • a detailed history; • a detailed examination; • medical decision making of low complexity, furnished in real time using interactive audio and video technology. Counseling and coordination of care with other physicians, other qualified health care professionals or agencies are provided consistent with the nature of the problem(s) and the needs of the patient or the family or both. Usually, the presenting problem(s) are of moderate severity. Typically, 30 minutes are spent with the patient or family or both via real time, audio and video intercommunications technology *Indicator(s): AS: 0 | Bilat: 0 | Mod51: 0 | PC/TC: 0*	-	2.24	$78.16

Code	Description	NCCI	RVU	$Fee
G9981	Remote in-home visit for the evaluation and management of a new patient for use only in a medicare-approved bundled payments for care improvement advanced (bpci advanced) model episode of care, which requires these 3 key components: • a comprehensive history; • a comprehensive examination; • medical decision making of moderate complexity, furnished in real time using interactive audio and video technology. Counseling and coordination of care with other physicians, other qualified health care professionals or agencies are provided consistent with the nature of the problem(s) and the needs of the patient or the family or both. Usually, the presenting problem(s) are of moderate to high severity. Typically, 45 minutes are spent with the patient or family or both via real time, audio and video inter-communications technology *Indicator(s): AS: 0	Bilat: 0	Mod51: 0	PC/TC: 0*	-	3.77	$131.55
G9982	Remote in-home visit for the evaluation and management of a new patient for use only in a medicare-approved bundled payments for care improvement advanced (bpci advanced) model episode of care, which requires these 3 key components: • a comprehensive history; • a comprehensive examination; • medical decision making of high complexity, furnished in real time using interactive audio and video technology. Counseling and coordination of care with other physicians, other qualified health care professionals or agencies are provided consistent with the nature of the problem(s) and the needs of the patient or the family or both. Usually, the presenting problem(s) are of moderate to high severity. Typically, 60 minutes are spent with the patient or family or both via real time, audio and video inter-communications technology *Indicator(s): AS: 0	Bilat: 0	Mod51: 0	PC/TC: 0*	-	5.02	$175.16
G9983	Remote in-home visit for the evaluation and management of an established patient for use only in a medicare-approved bundled payments for care improvement advanced (bpci advanced) model episode of care, which requires at least 2 of the following 3 key components: • a problem focused history; • a problem focused examination; • straightforward medical decision making, furnished in real time using interactive audio and video technology. Counseling and coordination of care with other physicians, other qualified health care professionals or agencies are provided consistent with the nature of the problem(s) and the needs of the patient or the family or both. Usually, the presenting problem(s) are self limited or minor. Typically, 10 minutes are spent with the patient or family or both via real time, audio and video intercommunications technology *Indicator(s): AS: 0	Bilat: 0	Mod51: 0	PC/TC: 0*	-	0.82	$28.61
G9984	Remote in-home visit for the evaluation and management of an established patient for use only in a medicare-approved bundled payments for care improvement advanced (bpci advanced) model episode of care, which requires at least 2 of the following 3 key components: • an expanded problem focused history; • an expanded problem focused examination; • medical decision making of low complexity, furnished in real time using interactive audio and video technology. Counseling and coordination of care with other physicians, other qualified health care professionals or agencies are provided consistent with the nature of the problem(s) and the needs of the patient or the family or both. Usually, the presenting problem(s) are of low to moderate severity. Typically, 15 minutes are spent with the patient or family or both via real time, audio and video intercommunications technology *Indicator(s): AS: 0	Bilat: 0	Mod51: 0	PC/TC: 0*	-	1.62	$56.53

Code	Description	NCCI	RVU	SFee
G9985	Remote in-home visit for the evaluation and management of an established patient for use only in a medicare-approved bundled payments for care improvement advanced (bpci advanced) model episode of care, which requires at least 2 of the following 3 key components: • a detailed history; • a detailed examination; • medical decision making of moderate complexity, furnished in real time using interactive audio and video technology. Counseling and coordination of care with other physicians, other qualified health care professionals or agencies are provided consistent with the nature of the problem(s) and the needs of the patient or the family or both. Usually, the presenting problem(s) are of moderate to high severity. Typically, 25 minutes are spent with the patient or family or both via real time, audio and video intercommunications technology *Indicator(s): AS: 0	Bilat: 0	Mod51: 0	PC/TC: 0*	-	2.46	$85.84
G9986	Remote in-home visit for the evaluation and management of an established patient for use only in a medicare-approved bundled payments for care improvement advanced (bpci advanced) model episode of care, which requires at least 2 of the following 3 key components: • a comprehensive history; • a comprehensive examination; • medical decision making of high complexity, furnished in real time using interactive audio and video technology. Counseling and coordination of care with other physicians, other qualified health care professionals or agencies are provided consistent with the nature of the problem(s) and the needs of the patient or the family or both. Usually, the presenting problem(s) are of moderate to high severity. Typically, 40 minutes are spent with the patient or family or both via real time, audio and video intercommunications technology *Indicator(s): AS: 0	Bilat: 0	Mod51: 0	PC/TC: 0*	-	3.55	$123.87
G9987	Payments for Care Improvement Advanced (BPCI Advanced) model home visit for patient assessment performed by clinical staff for an individual not considered homebound, including, but not necessarily limited to patient assessment of clinical status, safety/fall prevention, functional status/ambulation, medication reconciliation/management, compliance with orders/plan of care, performance of activities of daily living, and ensuring beneficiary connections to community and other services; for use only for a BPCI Advanced model episode of care; may not be billed for a 30-day period covered by a transitional care management code *Indicator(s): Bilat: 0	Mod51: 0	PC/TC: 0*	-	1.29	$45.01

Rehabilitative Services (H0001-H2037)

Code	Description	NCCI	RVU	SFee
H0034	Medication training and support, per 15 minutes	-	NE	NE
H0041	Foster care, child, non-therapeutic, per diem	-	NE	NE
H0042	Foster care, child, non-therapeutic, per month	-	NE	NE
H0043	Supported housing, per diem	-	NE	NE
H0044	Supported housing, per month	-	NE	NE
H0045	Respite care services, not in the home, per diem	-	NE	NE
H1011	Family assessment by licensed behavioral health professional for state defined purposes	-	NE	NE
H2000	Comprehensive multidisciplinary evaluation	-	NE	NE
H2001	Rehabilitation program, per 1/2 day	-	NE	NE
H2010	Comprehensive medication services, per 15 minutes	-	NE	NE

ALCOHOL AND/OR DRUG SERVICES (H0001-H2036)

Code	Description	NCCI	RVU	$Fee
H0001	assessment	-	NE	NE
H0002	Behavioral health screening to determine eligibility for admission to treatment program	-	NE	NE
H0003	screening; laboratory analysis of specimens for presence of alcohol and/or drugs	-	NE	NE
H0004	Behavioral health counseling and therapy, per 15 minutes	-	NE	NE
H0005	group counseling by a clinician	-	NE	NE
H0006	case management	-	NE	NE
H0007	crisis intervention (outpatient)	-	NE	NE
H0008	sub-acute detoxification (hospital inpatient)	-	NE	NE
H0009	acute detoxification (hospital inpatient)	-	NE	NE
H0010	sub-acute detoxification (residential addiction program inpatient)	-	NE	NE
H0011	acute detoxification (residential addiction program inpatient)	-	NE	NE
H0012	sub-acute detoxification (residential addiction program outpatient)	-	NE	NE
H0013	acute detoxification (residential addiction program outpatient)	-	NE	NE
H0014	ambulatory detoxification	-	NE	NE
H0015	intensive outpatient (treatment program that operates at least 3 hours/day and at least 3 days/week and is based on an individualized treatment plan), including assessment, counseling; crisis intervention, and activity therapies or education	-	NE	NE
H0016	medical/somatic (medical intervention in ambulatory setting)	-	NE	NE
H0017	Behavioral health; residential (hospital residential treatment program), without room and board, per diem	-	NE	NE
H0018	Behavioral health; short-term residential (non-hospital residential treatment program), without room and board, per diem	-	NE	NE
H0019	Behavioral health; long-term residential (non-medical, non-acute care in a residential treatment program where stay is typically longer than 30 days), without room and board, per diem	-	NE	NE
H0020	methadone administration and/or service (provision of the drug by a licensed program)	-	NE	NE
H0021	training service (for staff and personnel not employed by providers)	-	NE	NE
H0022	intervention service (planned facilitation)	-	NE	NE
H0023	Behavioral health outreach service (planned approach to reach a targeted population)	-	NE	NE
H0024	Behavioral health prevention information dissemination service (one-way direct or non-direct contact with service audiences to affect knowledge and attitude)	-	NE	NE
H0025	Behavioral health prevention education service (delivery of services with target population to affect knowledge, attitude and/or behavior)	-	NE	NE
H0026	prevention process service, community-based (delivery of services to develop skills of impactors)	-	NE	NE
H0027	prevention environmental service (broad range of external activities geared toward modifying systems in order to mainstream prevention through policy and law)	-	NE	NE
H0028	prevention problem identification and referral service (e.g., student assistance and employee assistance programs), does not include assessment	-	NE	NE
H0029	prevention alternatives service (services for populations that exclude alcohol and other drug use e.g., alcohol free social events)	-	NE	NE
H0030	Behavioral health hotline service	-	NE	NE
H0047	other drug abuse services, not otherwise specified	-	NE	NE
H0048	other drug testing: collection and handling only, specimens other than blood	-	NE	NE
H0049	screening	-	NE	NE
H0050	brief intervention, per 15 minutes	-	NE	NE

Code	Description	NCCI	RVU	$Fee
H2034	abuse halfway house services, per diem	-	NE	NE
H2035	other drug treatment program, per hour	-	NE	NE
H2036	other drug treatment program, per diem	-	NE	NE

BEHAVIORAL HEALTH SERVICES (H0031-H2037)

Code	Description	NCCI	RVU	$Fee
H0031	Mental health assessment, by non-physician	-	NE	NE
H0032	Mental health service plan development by non-physician	-	NE	NE
H0033	Oral medication administration, direct observation	-	NE	NE
H0035	Mental health partial hospitalization, treatment, less than 24 hours	-	NE	NE
H0036	Community psychiatric supportive treatment, face-to-face, per 15 minutes	-	NE	NE
H0037	Community psychiatric supportive treatment program, per diem	-	NE	NE
H0038	Self-help/peer services, per 15 minutes	-	NE	NE
H0039	Assertive community treatment, face-to-face, per 15 minutes	-	NE	NE
H0040	Assertive community treatment program, per diem	-	NE	NE
H0046	Mental health services, not otherwise specified	-	NE	NE
H2011	Crisis intervention service, per 15 minutes	-	NE	NE
H2012	day treatment, per hour	-	NE	NE
H2013	Psychiatric health facility service, per diem	-	NE	NE
H2014	Skills training and development, per 15 minutes	-	NE	NE
H2015	Comprehensive community support services, per 15 minutes	-	NE	NE
H2016	Comprehensive community support services, per diem	-	NE	NE
H2017	Psychosocial rehabilitation services, per 15 minutes	-	NE	NE
H2018	Psychosocial rehabilitation services, per diem	-	NE	NE
H2019	Therapeutic behavioral services, per 15 minutes	-	NE	NE
H2020	Therapeutic behavioral services, per diem	-	NE	NE
H2021	Community-based wrap-around services, per 15 minutes	-	NE	NE
H2022	Community-based wrap-around services, per diem	-	NE	NE
H2027	Psychoeducational service, per 15 minutes	-	NE	NE
H2028	Sexual offender treatment service, per 15 minutes	-	NE	NE
H2029	Sexual offender treatment service, per diem	-	NE	NE
H2030	Mental health clubhouse services, per 15 minutes	-	NE	NE
H2031	Mental health clubhouse services, per diem	-	NE	NE
H2032	Activity therapy, per 15 minutes	-	NE	NE
H2033	Multisystemic therapy for juveniles, per 15 minutes	-	NE	NE
H2037	Developmental delay prevention activities, dependent child of client, per 15 minutes	-	NE	NE

SUPPORTED EMPLOYMENT SERVICES (H2023-H2026)

Code	Description	NCCI	RVU	$Fee
H2023	per 15 minutes	-	NE	NE
H2024	per diem	-	NE	NE
H2025	Ongoing support to maintain employment, per 15 minutes	-	NE	NE
H2026	Ongoing support to maintain employment, per diem	-	NE	NE

Code	Description	NCCI	RVU	$Fee

Temporary Codes (Q0035-Q9992)

Code	Description	NCCI	RVU	$Fee
Q3014	Telehealth originating site facility fee	NCCI	NE	NE

DEPARTMENT OF VETERANS AFFAIRS SERVICES (Q9001-Q9003)

Code	Description	NCCI	RVU	$Fee
Q9001	Assessment by department of veterans affairs chaplain services	-	NE	NE
Q9002	Counseling, individual, by department of veterans affairs chaplain services	-	NE	NE
Q9003	Counseling, group, by department of veterans affairs chaplain services	-	NE	NE
Q9004	whole health partner services	-	NE	NE

HOSPICE CARE (Q5001-Q5010)

Code	Description	NCCI	RVU	$Fee
Q5001	or home health care provided in patient's home/residence	-	NE	NE
Q5002	or home health care provided in assisted living facility	-	NE	NE
Q5003	provided in nursing long term care facility (ltc) or non-skilled nursing facility (nf)	-	NE	NE
Q5004	provided in skilled nursing facility (snf)	-	NE	NE
Q5005	provided in inpatient hospital	-	NE	NE
Q5006	provided in inpatient hospice facility	-	NE	NE
Q5007	provided in long term care facility	-	NE	NE
Q5008	provided in inpatient psychiatric facility	-	NE	NE
Q5009	or home health care provided in place not otherwise specified (nos)	-	NE	NE

Private Payer Codes (S0012-S9999)

S3000 (S3000-S3904)

Code	Description	NCCI	RVU	$Fee
S3005	Performance measurement, evaluation of patient self assessment, depression	-	NE	NE

S5000 (S5000-S5523)

Code	Description	NCCI	RVU	$Fee
S5100	Day care services, adult; per 15 minutes	-	NE	NE
S5101	Day care services, adult; per half day	-	NE	NE
S5102	Day care services, adult; per diem	-	NE	NE
S5105	Day care services, center-based; services not included in program fee, per diem	-	NE	NE
S5110	Home care training, family; per 15 minutes	-	NE	NE
S5111	Home care training, family; per session	-	NE	NE
S5135	Companion care, adult (e.g., iadl/adl); per 15 minutes	-	NE	NE
S5136	Companion care, adult (e.g., iadl/adl); per diem	-	NE	NE
S5140	Foster care, adult; per diem	-	NE	NE
S5141	Foster care, adult; per month	-	NE	NE
S5145	Foster care, therapeutic, child; per diem	-	NE	NE
S5146	Foster care, therapeutic, child; per month	-	NE	NE
S5190	Wellness assessment, performed by non-physician	-	NE	NE
S5199	Personal care item, nos, each	-	NE	NE

Code	Description	NCCI	RVU	$Fee

S8000 (S8030-S8999)

Code	Description	NCCI	RVU	$Fee
S8940	Equestrian/hippotherapy, per session	-	NE	NE

S0000 (S0012-S0813)

Code	Description	NCCI	RVU	$Fee
S0201	Partial hospitalization services, less than 24 hours, per diem	-	NE	NE
S0257	Counseling and discussion regarding advance directives or end of life care planning and decisions, with patient and/or surrogate (list separately in addition to code for appropriate evaluation and management service)	-	NE	NE
S0265	Genetic counseling, under physician supervision, each 15 minutes	-	NE	NE
S0270	Physician management of patient home care, standard monthly case rate (per 30 days)	-	NE	NE
S0271	Physician management of patient home care, hospice monthly case rate (per 30 days)	-	NE	NE
S0272	Physician management of patient home care, episodic care monthly case rate (per 30 days)	-	NE	NE
S0273	Physician visit at member's home, outside of a capitation arrangement	-	NE	NE
S0274	Nurse practitioner visit at member's home, outside of a capitation arrangement	-	NE	NE
S0302	Completed early periodic screening diagnosis and treatment (epsdt) service (list in addition to code for appropriate evaluation and management service)	-	NE	NE
S0311	Comprehensive management and care coordination for advanced illness, per calendar month	-	NE	NE

S9000 (S9001-S9999)

Code	Description	NCCI	RVU	$Fee
S9110	Telemonitoring of patient in their home, including all necessary equipment; computer system, connections, and software; maintenance; patient education and support; per month	-	NE	NE
S9127	Social work visit, in the home, per diem	-	NE	NE
S9433	Medical food nutritionally complete, administered orally, providing 100% of nutritional intake	-	NE	NE
S9444	Parenting classes, non-physician provider, per session	-	NE	NE
S9454	Stress management classes, non-physician provider, per session	-	NE	NE
S9475	Ambulatory setting substance abuse treatment or detoxification services, per diem	-	NE	NE
S9480	Intensive outpatient psychiatric services, per diem	-	NE	NE
S9482	Family stabilization services, per 15 minutes	-	NE	NE
S9484	Crisis intervention mental health services, per hour	-	NE	NE
S9485	Crisis intervention mental health services, per diem	-	NE	NE
S9982	Medical records copying fee, per page	-	NE	NE

DRUGS ADMINISTERED (S0014-S0197)

Code	Description	NCCI	RVU	$Fee
S0109	Methadone, oral, 5 mg	-	NE	NE

State Medicaid Agency Codes (T1000-T5999)

T2000 (T2001-T2101)

Code	Description	NCCI	RVU	$Fee
T2001	Non-emergency transportation; patient attendant/escort	-	NE	NE
T2002	Non-emergency transportation; per diem	-	NE	NE
T2003	Non-emergency transportation; encounter/trip	-	NE	NE
T2010	Preadmission screening and resident review (pasrr) level i identification screening, per screen	-	NE	NE
T2011	Preadmission screening and resident review (pasrr) level ii evaluation, per evaluation	-	NE	NE
T2022	Case management, per month	-	NE	NE
T2023	Targeted case management; per month	-	NE	NE
T2024	Service assessment/plan of care development, waiver	-	NE	NE
T2025	Waiver services; not otherwise specified (nos)	-	NE	NE
T2026	Specialized childcare, waiver; per diem	-	NE	NE
T2027	Specialized childcare, waiver; per 15 minutes	-	NE	NE
T2032	Residential care, not otherwise specified (nos), waiver; per month	-	NE	NE
T2033	Residential care, not otherwise specified (nos), waiver; per diem	-	NE	NE
T2034	Crisis intervention, waiver; per diem	-	NE	NE
T2036	Therapeutic camping, overnight, waiver; each session	-	NE	NE
T2037	Therapeutic camping, day, waiver; each session	-	NE	NE
T2048	Behavioral health; long-term care residential (non-acute care in a residential treatment program where stay is typically longer than 30 days), with room and board, per diem	-	NE	NE

T1000 (T1000-T1999)

Code	Description	NCCI	RVU	$Fee
T1002	Rn services, up to 15 minutes	-	NE	NE
T1006	Alcohol and/or substance abuse services, family/couple counseling	-	NE	NE
T1007	Alcohol and/or substance abuse services, treatment plan development and/or modification	-	NE	NE
T1009	Child sitting services for children of the individual receiving alcohol and/or substance abuse services	-	NE	NE
T1010	Meals for individuals receiving alcohol and/or substance abuse services (when meals not included in the program)	-	NE	NE
T1012	Alcohol and/or substance abuse services, skills development	-	NE	NE
T1013	Sign language or oral interpretive services, per 15 minutes	-	NE	NE
T1014	Telehealth transmission, per minute, professional services bill separately	-	NE	NE
T1016	Case management, each 15 minutes	-	NE	NE
T1017	Targeted case management, each 15 minutes	-	NE	NE
T1018	School-based individualized education program (iep) services, bundled	-	NE	NE
T1023	Screening to determine the appropriateness of consideration of an individual for participation in a specified program, project or treatment protocol, per encounter	-	NE	NE
T1024	Evaluation and treatment by an integrated, specialty team contracted to provide coordinated care to multiple or severely handicapped children, per encounter	-	NE	NE
T1025	Intensive, extended multidisciplinary services provided in a clinic setting to children with complex medical, physical, mental and psychosocial impairments, per diem	-	NE	NE

Code	Description	NCCI	RVU	$Fee
T1026	Intensive, extended multidisciplinary services provided in a clinic setting to children with complex medical, physical, medical and psychosocial impairments, per hour	-	NE	NE
T1027	Family training and counseling for child development, per 15 minutes	-	NE	NE
T1028	Assessment of home, physical and family environment, to determine suitability to meet patient's medical needs	-	NE	NE
T1029	Comprehensive environmental lead investigation, not including laboratory analysis, per dwelling	-	NE	NE
T1040	Medicaid certified community behavioral health clinic services, per diem	-	NE	NE
T1041	Medicaid certified community behavioral health clinic services, per month	-	NE	NE
T1502	Administration of oral, intramuscular and/or subcutaneous medication by health care agency/professional, per visit	-	NE	NE

Hearing Services (V5008-V5364)

SPEECH-LANGUAGE PATHOLOGY SERVICES (V5336-V5364)

Code	Description	NCCI	RVU	$Fee
V5362	Speech screening *Indicator(s): PS: 01*	NCCI	NE	NE
V5363	Language screening *Indicator(s): PS: 01*	NCCI	NE	NE
V5364	Dysphagia screening *Indicator(s): PS: 01*	NCCI	NE	NE

Notes:

5.3 Evaluation & Management Coding

Evaluation and Management (E/M) services are a type of patient encounter between a physician or other qualified healthcare professional (QHP) and a patient seeking medical advice and care for symptoms, conditions, illnesses, or injuries. Commonly, E/M services are face-to-face encounters between the provider and patient, but there are several E/M encounter types that may transpire over the phone, online, or through telehealth/telemedicine (real-time audiovisual) or another form of telecommunication.

Store: See innoviHealth's *Comprehensive Guide to Evaluation & Management* (available in the online store) for more information about properly documenting E/M visits.

Who May Use E/M Codes? Evaluation and Managements codes can only be used by a physician or 'other qualified healthcare professional.' See Resource 402 for more about who is an 'other qualified healthcare professional.'

Tip: In the result of a negative audit finding, seek a second opinion and legal counsel before returning any monies or reporting possible overpayments.

Resource: See Resource 332 for the complete 1995 Documentation Guidelines.
Resource: See Resource 333 for the complete 1997 Documentation Guidelines.

The Basics

E/M Organization and Overview of Components

Organization

According to the American Medical Association's (AMA's) Current Procedural Terminology (CPT) codebook, Evaluation and Management (E/M) codes are organized into broad categories based on their place of service (POS) (e.g., office visits, hospital visits, emergency room visits) which may be further divided into subcategories based on patient status (new or established patient, initial or subsequent encounter, consultation, etc.) Many are further defined by the level of service.

Categories

Patient Status: New vs. Established Patient

Many E/M services are divided into two subcategories of patient types which are defined by the AMA as:

- **New Patient:** One who *has not* received professional services from any physician/qualified healthcare professional in the same group practice, in the exact same specialty and subspecialty, within the last three years (36 months).

- **Established Patient:** One who *has* received professional services from any physician/qualified healthcare professional in the same group practice, in the exact same specialty and subspecialty, within the past three years (36 months).

Tip: In the instance where a physician or other qualified healthcare provider is covering for another provider (e.g., locum tenens), the patient's encounter will be classified as it would have been by the healthcare provider who is not available.

Level of Service

There are more than two dozen types of E/M services in the CPT codebook defined within a category or subcategory. Each subcategory of E/M is further divided into one or more levels of service. The level of service reported is determined by the rules governing the scoring of the specific subcategory of the E/M encounter. It is important to carefully read the applicable category and/or subcategory guidelines and code descriptor before assigning a specific E/M code, as they may change slightly from one subcategory to the next. The requirements of each subcategory may include:

- Location
- Key component details (history, exam, medical decision making) or time, which includes documentation of applicable contributing factors documented in the medical record.

The level of service (except for Office or Other Outpatient Services) is selected based on the following components as outlined in the CPT codebook and shown in *Figure 5.1*. The first three are considered "Key Components" in selecting the level of E/M service, while the next three components are considered "Contributory Factors." The last component, "Time," is discussed on page 318 and page 341.

Figure 5.1

Components for E/M Code Selection	
Key Components	1. History
	2. Examination
	3. Medical Decision Making (MDM)
Contributory Factors	4. Counseling
	5. Coordination of Care
	6. Nature of Presenting Problem (NPP)
Other Component	7. Time

Note: As of 2021, selecting the level of service for Office or Other Outpatient Services only scored based on either Medical Decision Making or Time. However, other payers (e.g., Workers Compensation) might not follow the new scoring guidelines. See the "Office/Other Outpatient E/M Services" segment which begins on page 316.

Nature of Presenting Problem (NPP)

While the majority of this chapter focuses on the three Key Components, the "Nature of the Presenting Problem (NPP)" must be mentioned. In the office setting, physicians and Qualified Healthcare Professionals (QHPs) often use NPP (severity of a patient's condition) to prioritize patient care. When a provider's practice is behind schedule, the NPP can help identify patients with simple or straightforward needs that may streamline patient care and help the provider quickly catch up to the schedule. It allows them to make an educated guess, based on the patient's stated reason for being seen, as to how long or how work intensive a specific patient encounter may be.

Proper use of NPP can facilitate proper and thorough documentation that supports coding at the level of severity identified. A provider who determines a patient with a sore throat and no other chronic conditions is probably a low severity NPP can then identify and document the key components based on a low severity condition, saving time and resources. If during the encounter the provider identifies additional problems that raise the work and decision making level to moderate or high, they can easily add the detail needed to the documentation to match the level of severity.

The CPT codebook identifies five types of NPPs:

Minimal	A problem that may not require the presence of the physician or other qualified healthcare professional, but the service is provided under the physician's or other qualified healthcare professional's supervision.
Self-limited or minor	A problem that runs a definite and prescribed course, is transient in nature, and is not likely to permanently alter health status OR has a good prognosis with management/compliance.
Low severity	A problem where the risk of morbidity without treatment is low; there is little to no risk of mortality without treatment; full recovery without functional impairment is expected.
Moderate severity	A problem where the risk of morbidity without treatment is moderate; there is a moderate risk of mortality without treatment; the prognosis is uncertain.
High severity	A problem where the risk of morbidity without treatment is high to extreme; there is a moderate to high risk of mortality without treatment OR there is a high probability of severe, prolonged functional impairment.

Looking at the above definitions, even to qualify for 99204/99214, the NPP requires at least a moderate level of complexity and risk. Beginning an encounter with an estimated level of NPP in mind helps providers identify documentation requirements which will be needed in order to support the level of service. Adjustments can be made if further evaluation reveals either a lower or higher complexity. For example, a patient who presents with a cold for a day or two may require only over-the-counter remedies and supportive care (low complexity) whereas a patient with multiple, uncontrolled chronic conditions requiring adjustments to prescribed medications and possibly additional testing would be considered moderate complexity. If further evaluation revealed that either of these patients require treatment of a higher level of complexity, the additional documentation requirements showing why their case is more complex is needed to support a higher level. These types of adjustments are easy to make and help providers remember the documentation details required to support the various levels of service more readily.

In the following table, each initial inpatient E/M code has been matched with its corresponding NPP and an example from Appendix C of the current CPT codebook.

Figure 5.2

Code	Nature of Presenting Problem	Example from CPT Appendix C
99221	Low severity	Initial hospital visit for a 14-year-old female with infectious mononucleosis and dehydration.
99222	Moderate severity	Hospital admission for an 18-month-old with 10% dehydration.
99223	High severity	Initial psychiatric visit for an adolescent patient without previous psychiatric history, who was transferred from the medical ICU after an overdose.

Note: Clinical examples for Office or Other Outpatient Services were removed from Appendix C of the CPT codebook beginning in 2021. However, other services are included and reviewing these examples can help understand the levels of care based on the NPP.

By reviewing the information in *Figure 5.2*, it becomes clear that in order to report a moderate to high level E/M code (99204-99205, 99214-99215), the Nature of the Presenting Problem (NPP) must be of at least moderate to high severity, which includes cases with a moderate to high risk of death, and requires the documentation to clearly identify complicating factors that substantiate this level of risk and the associated steps taken to mitigate that risk.

Key Components

CPT guidelines identify rules for scoring the E/M encounter, which includes using either three key components (History, Exam, and Medical Decision Making) or Time (see page 318) to select the level of service as long it is supported by medical necessity (see page 314) as documented in the medical record.

The key components are broken down into additional subcomponents. The number of components required for scoring the encounter also changes depending on the E/M category as shown in the following table:

2022 Key Component Scoring Requirements	
Medical Decision Making or Time (History & Exam are no longer scored)	• **Office or other outpatient** (new/established patient)
Three of the three Key Components are required for the following E/M categories	• Hospital observation services • Initial hospital care • Office consultations (new or established patient) • Initial inpatient consultation • Emergency department services • Initial nursing facility care • Domiciliary care (new patient) • Home (new patient)
Two of the three Key Components are required for the following E/M categories	• Subsequent hospital care • Subsequent nursing facility care • Domiciliary care (established patient) • Home (established patient)

Note: Watch for specific scoring criteria for each subsection of the E/M services, as many changes have taken place and will continue to occur in the future.

Book: See "Office/Other Outpatient E/M Services" on page 316 for more information.

Medical Necessity

Medical necessity is a key factor in determining the overall level of E/M service. CMS states that "Medical necessity of a service is the overarching criterion for payment in addition to the individual requirements of a CPT code."

This means that not only does the E/M level of service reported need to meet the specific code level criteria, that particular level of service must be medically necessary to properly care for the patient's needs according to the normal medical standards of care. One way to look at this is to consider whether or not an equally educated and licensed medical professional of the same specialty/subspecialty would treat the same patient condition in the same way, at the same level of service. This would be an indication of normal medical standard of care and consequently a proper gauge of medical necessity.

Having the best templates and processes in place to ensure a comprehensive history and examination are always documented does not mean the patient actually needed a comprehensive level of service for their current complaint(s). It is recommended to look at medical necessity by assessing how likely the current condition(s) being treated place the patient at risk of severe complications, morbidity, or mortality if left untreated or with implementing the current treatment plan. If the provider consistently documents at the comprehensive level but medical necessity is low, it would be logical to educate the provider on documentation requirements for medical necessity rather than quantity and reduce the documentation burden to free up more time for other patients.

E/M Services with Other Procedures

E/M services are often performed on the same day as a procedure. Sometimes during the performance of an E/M service the decision is made to perform a minor procedure or an urgency is noted in the patient's status requiring a major surgery to be performed immediately. When the decision to perform a procedure (major or minor) is made during the course of an E/M encounter and the documentation clearly indicates so, it may qualify for separate payment along with the procedure performed.

Note: If the decision to perform a surgery was made at a prior encounter, then the E/M service is considered part of the preoperative workup and is not eligible for separate payment so modifiers 25 or 57 should not be reported.

Of importance is the newly revised CPT E/M guidelines that refer to the scoring of data in the MDM portion of an E/M service. The E/M guidelines state (emphasis added) that "[t]he actual performance and/or interpretation of diagnostic tests/studies during a patient encounter are not included in determining the levels of E/M services *when reported separately*." An example would be a healthcare provider evaluating a patient for possible sinus infection who orders a sinus x-ray that is performed in the office and separately billed with a 70000 series CPT code. Any work **related** to the performance or interpretation of the sinus x-ray is *not* counted in the MDM "Data" element used to score the level of E/M service.

Beginning in 2022, CMS has added a new modifier (FT "Unrelated evaluation and management (E/M) visit during a postoperative period, or on the same day as a procedure or another E/M visit") which can help clarify coding in the following circumstances:

- When an E/M service is performed earlier in the day and the provider who performed it (or another provider from the same service, group practice, and specialty) performs a second, unrelated E/M service, the second E/M service is reportable and, based on Medicare policies, may require modifier FT or modifier 25 to indicate they are unrelated and should both be paid.

- When an emergency department provider performs an E/M service which results in a patient admission and later in the day the same provider (or another provider in the same service, group practice, and specialty) performs a critical care service, both providers may bill for both services with modifier 25 appended to the critical care service.

- Critical care services are sometimes required during the global period of a surgery or procedure (whether properatively on the same day, or during the postoperative period). Some CPT code descriptions bundle critical care services into the postoperative global period while others do not. According to CPT and CMS guidelines, as long as the critical care service is unrelated to the procedure performed, it may be separately reimbursed by adding modifier FT. Depending on the specific type of provider and service rendered, consider whether or not modifier 55 (postoperative management only) or modifier 54 (surgical care only) are better suited to the service. In the case where an intensivist accepts the transfer of care postoperatively it may be appropriate to report a combination of all three.

Note: At the time of publication, modifier FT has just been announced so watch for further announcement from payers about its use in conjunction with other modfiers such as 25.

There are many services within the Medicine section of the CPT codebook that are often performed during an E/M service and are reportable together without modifier 25 while others do require it.

Book: See Appendix B — Modifiers for additional information about using modifiers 25 and 57.

Alert: There have been situations where payers automatically deny all E/M services reported with modifier 25. This problem is affecting many specialties and relates to what is considered pre-, intra-, and post-service work for the other procedure billed at the same time as the E/M service. It is recommend that providers work with their professional organization to try resolve problems like this.

Office/Other Outpatient E/M Services

In 2021, Office or Other Outpatient E/M Services (codes 99201-99215) experienced significant changes which almost all payers have adopted. However, many states do not require payers covering Workers Compensation or personal injury to utilize the most current CPT or ICD-10-CM code sets, so when reporting services to these payers, it will be important to identify which CPT guidelines those payers are following, as they may not have begun to follow the changes that started in 2021.

Although these recent changes may eventually lead to the hoped for documentation burden relief many providers are seeking, until Workers Compensation and personal injury payers adopt those changes, providers must ensure that the correct guidelines and their documentation supports those payers' requirements for the E/M code reported. It may be helpful to have customized templates specific to different payers as well as different types of E/M service categories in order to reduce errors on postpayment review.

Alert: Providers should follow the official code set guidelines (CPT), UNLESS their contract with a third-party payer (e.g., Medicare, Blue Cross) specifically states they must follow a specified set of coding guidelines. For example, Medicare requires providers to use their guidelines for reporting prolonged services based on a different set of time criteria.

Store: See innoviHealth's *Comprehensive Guide to Evaluation & Management* (available in the online store) for more comprehensive information about the changes that took place in 2021 which are not included in this publication.

Prolonged E/M Service Codes

CPT Guidelines

The AMA approved a prolonged E/M service add-on code (99417) which may only be used in conjunction with codes 99205 and 99215. This prolonged E/M service code allows the provider to report 1 unit for every 15 minutes of time spent providing patient care (face-to-face and non-face-to-face) beyond the time requirements for these codes. This is a time-based add-on code, so the full time assigned to 99205 (up to 74 minutes) and 99215 (up to 54 minutes) must be exceeded (as noted in the chart below) before 99417 can be reported. For reporting examples based on time, see the following chart:

CPT Office Prolonged Service Reporting

Code	Time in Minutes	Code (s) to Report
99205 (New)	60-74	99205 only
	75-89	99205 + 99417 x 1 unit
	90-104	99205 + 99417 x 2 units
	105 or more	For each additional 15 minutes, report an additional unit of 99417
99215 (Established)	40-54	99215 only
	55-69	99215 + 99417 x 1 units
	70-84	99215 + 99417 x 2 units
	85 or more	For each additional 15 minutes, report an additional unit of 99417

Medicare Guidelines

When CMS identifies a potential issue with a CPT code, description, and/or guideline, they have the option of publishing a HCPCS code (usually a G-code) to replace the CPT code in question ONLY for Medicare beneficiary claims. In the case of prolonged E/M services code 99417, CMS disagrees with the CPT description and guideline that allows providers to report the first unit (1) of 99417 once the *"minimum"* time in the time range has been exceeded by 15 minutes. Instead, CMS requires claims for Medicare beneficiaries to report G2212 instead of 99417 where the code description and guideline indicate that the first unit of G2212 may only be reported once the *"maximum"* time in the time range has been **exceeded** by 15 minutes. As such, providers will need to be very careful when calculating prolonged E/M service units for codes 99205 and 99215 to ensure the guidelines have been adhered to and the proper number of units have been reported.

Medicare Office Prolonged Service Reporting

Code	Time in Minutes	Code (s) to Report
99205 (New)	60-88	99205 only
	89-103	99205 + G2212 x 1 unit
	104-118	99205 + G2212 x 2 units
	119 or more	For each additional 15 minutes, report an additional unit of G2212
99215 (Established)	40-68	99215 only
	69-83	99215 + G2212 x 1 units
	84-98	99215 + G2212 x 2 units
	99 or more	For each additional 15 minutes, report an additional unit of G2212

Tip: Medicare and Medicare Advantage plans are required to adhere to the guidelines for G2212 when reporting prolonged E/M services with code 99205 or 99215. Additionally, watch for published updates by other payers who state they follow Medicare guidelines to determine how they want prolonged E/M services reported.

Note: Do NOT report code 99417 for claims submitted to Medicare. G2212 can only be reported with 99205 or 99215.

Book: See also "Prolonged Service With or Without Direct Patient Contact on the Date of an Office or Other Outpatient Service" on page 360.

Resource: See Resource 52H for more information about code G2212.

> **Alert** — Unlike other timed codes, where an additional unit can be reported once the halfway point of the time interval is reached, reporting a unit of either 99417 or G2212 requires that the full 15 minutes of patient care occurred.

Scoring Based on Time or Medical Decision Making (MDM)

The method used to determine the level of E/M service for codes 99202-99215 allows providers to use either of the following:

- **Time**: Total documented time with or without direct direct patient contact
- **Medical Decision Making (MDM)**: Determined by scoring the elements of diagnosis, data, and risk

Now that the key components of history and examination have been removed from the scoring process, the information documented in these areas is going to be vital for establishing medical necessity (see page 314), properly recording diagnoses, and supporting the reported complexity of care.

The following table identifies the code level selection structure for codes 99202-99215, including the 2022 proposed work relative value units (RVUs): Total RVUs are shown in the code listing that begins on page 348.

Office/Other Outpatient E/M Codes & Scoring Criteria

	Code	History & Exam	MDM	Time	Work RVU	Prolonged Codes
New Patient	99202	Medically appropriate history and exam as determined by the provider	Straightforward	15-29	0.93	n/a
	99203		Low	30-44	1.60	n/a
	99204		Moderate	45-59	2.60	n/a
	99205		High	60-74	3.50	Report 99417 for physician/QHP for each 15 minutes (e.g., one unit for 75-89 minutes)
Established Patient	99211	Ancillary staff service (Document purpose for encounter, what was done, and any patient instructions			0.18	n/a
	99212	Medically appropriate history and exam as determined by the provider	Straightforward	10-19	0.70	n/a
	99213		Low	20-29	1.30	n/a
	99214		Moderate	30-39	1.92	n/a
	99215		High	40-54	2.80	Report 99417 for physician/QHP for each additional 15 minutes (e.g., one unit for 55-69 minutes)

Note: Prolonged clinical staff time supervised by a physician/QHP may be reported (see codes 99415, 99416) but the times and rules are different than what is shown above. See innoviHealth's *Evaluation & Management Coding Cards* (available in the online store) or a CPT codebook for more information.

Time

Time for codes 99202-99215 is scored differently than all other E/M services in that both face-to-face and non-face-to-face services are included in the calculation of time. While it is still recommended that start and stop times are documented, doing so can be difficult when so many activities are considered to be qualifying activities towards the total visit time as shown in the following list:

Physician/other qualified health care professional time includes the following activities when performed:
- preparing to see the patient (eg, review of tests)
- obtaining and/or reviewing separately obtained history
- performing a medically appropriate examination and/or evaluation

- counseling and educating the patient/family/caregiver
- ordering medications, tests, or procedures
- referring and communicating with other healthcare professionals (when not separately reported)
- documenting clinical information in the electronic or other health record
- independently interpreting results (not separately reported) and communicating results to the patient/family/caregiver
- care coordination (not separately reported)

What does "not separately reported" in the above statement mean? The time spent performing care coordination, when that care coordination is separately reportable with an applicable procedure code, should NOT be counted towards the total time of the E/M service, as that time is paid for in the reimbursement of the care coordination service itself. To include that time as part of the E/M service would result in overpayment to the provider.

Example: A provider performs an x-ray during the E/M encounter and reviews the results during the encounter.

The time spent reviewing the results is not counted towards the E/M encounter time as the time spent reviewing the results with the patient is included in the payment for the x-ray service that is billed/reported separately.

The following table compares the times listed in the 2020 CPT codebook code descriptions to the current code descriptions:

New Patient (NP)			Established Patient (EP)		
Code	2020 Time	New Time	Code	2020 Time	New Time
99201	10 min	None - code deleted	99211	5 min	Does not apply
99202	20 min	15-29 min	99212	10 min	10-19 min
99203	30 min	30-44 min	99213	15 min	20-29 min
99204	45 min	45-59 min	99214	25 min	30-39 min
99205	60 min	60-74 min	99215	40 min	40-54 min
		75+ min reported with new Prolonged Services code			55+ min reported with new Prolonged Services code

Pre-, Intra-, Post-Service Time Changes

According to the AMA's *E/M Office Visit Compendium 2021* publication, the E/M codes above consider the total time of the encounter to be inclusive of preservice time (up to 3 days prior), intraservice time (face-to-face), and post-service time (7 days following the E/M service for issues directly related to the reason for the face-to-face intraservice encounter). When the codes were revised, the Relative Value Update Committee (RUC) included a table of time showing the pre-, post-, and intra-service time that made up the recommended times for each code.

Note: Although the RUC stated that these services include all time spent 3 days prior to and 7 days after the service was performed, there is some disagreement about this concept, so it is not a generally accepted guideline except when the specific codes include these instructions in the code description like they do with codes 98966-98968 (telephone assessment and management services), 99441-99443 (telephone E/M services), or G2012 (communication technology-based services).

Generally speaking, if a patient contacts the office to communicate with a provider about a medical condition reportable with a code such as 98966-98968, 99441-99443, or G2012, and the interaction results in an appointment for an E/M service that occurs within seven (7) days of a prior, related E/M encounter or leads to an E/M encounter within the next 24 hours or soonest available appointment, according to the CPT guidelines for these codes, the telephone assessment and management encounter would not be a billable service as it would be bundled into the greater E/M encounter (99202-99215) itself. Although the pre-, intra-, and post-service times were the basis for each E/M service, the CPT guidelines for each individual code should be adhered to and so far, only the telephone assessment and evaluation codes include this specific wording regarding the inclusion of services 3 days prior and 7 days after. This also fits with the guidelines that limit how time is calculated when time is the determining factor for E/M codes 99202-99215. Only time spent by the provider, on the day of the encounter is used to determine the level of service. Time spent on the phone or online communication is simply bundled.

Note: Previous edition(s) of this publication may have included wording indicating that any time spent 3 days prior to and up to 7 days after the E/M service are counted/included in the calculation of time for that E/M encounter. Pay close attention to the revised paragraph above.

Resource: See Resource 540 for more information about what time needs to be included, particularly as it relates to prolonged services.

Medical Decision Making (MDM)

The level of MDM is the second method that may be used to determine an E/M service level. There are some differences in the MDM guidelines for Office or Other Outpatient services which are highlighted, as compared to the previous guidelines, as follows:

> "Medical decision making includes establishing diagnoses, assessing the status of a condition, and/or selecting a management option. Medical decision making in the office and other outpatient services code set is defined by three elements:
>
> 1. The number and complexity of problem(s) that are addressed during the encounter.
>
> 2. The amount and/or complexity of data to be reviewed and analyzed.
>
> 3. The risk of complications, morbidity, and/or mortality of patient management decisions made at the visit, associated with the patient's problem(s), the diagnostic procedure(s), treatment(s)."

Like other E/M services, there are four types of medical decision making: straightforward, low, moderate, and high. However, there are some differences such as the exclusion of the word "complexity" in the official description of the guidelines.

Note: MDM does not apply to code 99211.

1. Number and Complexity of Problems Addressed

This element of MDM is similar to other E/M services but there are some differences which need to be noted. The patient's problem(s) (e.g., condition, illness, injury, symptom, sign, finding, complaint, or other matter addressed at the encounter with or without a final diagnosis being established) should only be reported when it has been either monitored, evaluated, assessed, and/or treated and fully documented in the patient record. Each diagnosis should be documented in a way that it is easy to identify severity, complicating factors, whether it is an acute or chronic condition, an injury, or an illness. The following table describes the type of condition, illness, disease, or injury with a level of severity as explained in the CPT codebook:

Level	Description
Minimal	One self-limited/minor
Low	One of the following: • 2+ self-limited/minor • 1 stable chronic • 1 acute, uncomplicated injury/illness
Moderate	One of the following: • 1+ chronic illness(es), exacerbated, progressing, or side effects of treatment • 2+ stable chronic illnesses • 1 undiagnosed/new problem with uncertain prognosis • 1 acute illness w/systemic symptoms • 1 acute complicated illness/injury
High	One of the following: • 1+ chronic illness(es), w/severe exacerbation, progression, or side effects of treatment • 1 acute or chronic illness/injury posing threat to life or bodily function

Number and Complexity of Problems Addressed

Resource: See Resource 650 for definitions of terms (e.g., self-limited, chronic) in the description column above.

2. Amount and/or Complexity of Data to be Reviewed and Analyzed

Healthcare providers often require additional information from a variety of sources in order to better assess the status of an illness or injury, differentiate between stable and unstable conditions, determine a course of treatment, and/or assess the risk to organ systems or bodily functions, morbidity, and mortality. When scoring the "data" element of MDM, there are three categories of data to be considered which help identify the complexity of the encounter. They are:

1. Quantity of tests ordered or reviewed, number of documents reviewed from external/unique sources, and information obtained from independent historians
2. Independent interpretation of tests performed and interpreted by other providers
3. Discussion of management or test interpretation with an external physician, QHP, or other appropriate source which is defined by CPT as being from a professional who is not a healthcare professional but may be involved in the management of the patient such as a lawyer, case manager, parole officer, or teacher but NOT an informal caregiver or family member.

Where these guidelines differ from other E/M services is in how they are organized for scoring purposes. This element is subdivided into three categories (referred to as Category 1, Category 2, and Category 3 in the tables that follow) with specific tasks associated within each category. When the identified number of tasks are completed within a category, the category requirements have been met. To report higher levels of service, the requirements must be met in more than one category.

The following table summarizes the requirements:

Amount and/or Complexity of Data to be Reviewed and Analyzed	
Code(s)	Criteria
99211 Not applicable (NA)	Not applicable
99202/99212 Minimal	None or minimal
99203/99213 Limited Meet 1 of 2 categories	**Category 1:** Any combination of **2** from the following: ☐☐ Review of prior external note(s) from each unique source* ☐☐ Review result(s) of each unique test* ☐☐ Ordering of each unique test* OR **Category 2** ☐ Assessment requiring an independent historian(s)**
99204/99214 Moderate Meet 1 of 3 categories **99205/99215** High Meet 2 of 3 categories	**Moderate:** Meet 1 of 3 categories **High:** Meet 2 of 3 categories **Category 1:** Any combination of **3** from the following: ☐☐☐ Review of prior external note(s) from each unique source* ☐☐☐ Review of result(s) from each unique test* ☐☐☐ Ordering of each unique test* ☐☐☐ Assessment requiring an independent historian(s)** OR **Category 2:** ☐ Independent interpretation of tests**** (performed by another Physician/QHP [not separately reported]) OR **Category 3:** ☐ Discussion of management or test interpretation (with external MD/QHP, or appropriate source*** [not separately reported])

Notes:

*   A unique test is identified by a CPT or HCPCS code

** An independent historian is a person, other than the patient, who provides a patient history (e.g., spouse, parent, guardian), in addition to the history the patient was (or wasn't) able to provide due to developmental stage, dementia, psychosis, etc.

*** CPT defines an appropriate source as that of a professional who is not a healthcare professional but may be involved in the management of the patient such as a lawyer, case manager, parole officer, or teacher but NOT an informal caregiver or family member

**** An independent interpretation of a test occurs when both the technical and professional components of a test or image have been performed and reported _by an external source_ but the MD/QHP performing the E/M service reviews the image, lab, or study result and documents their own professional opinion. Although they cannot bill for this service, it is counted towards the MDM under Data reviewed.

The AMA states "Each unique test, order, or document contributes to the combination of 2 or combination of 3 in Category 1 below." The following example allows us to see how this would be scored.

Example:

The physician performs a chest x-ray in the office and bills separately for it and then orders an MRI, complete blood count (CBC), and complete metabolic panel (CMP) to be done at an outside lab and imaging center.

Scoring:

Chest X-ray: This is not scored as part of the MDM "Data" element because the provider bills for and is reimbursed for it separately

The following services are represented by a CPT code but they are billed outside the provider's office:

MRI: Counts as ordering of a unique test

CBC: One CPT code represents the individual components of a CBC so it is counted once as ordering of a unique test

CMP: One CPT code represents the individual components of a CMP, so it is counted as ordering of a unique test.

Using the information in the "Amount and/or Complexity of Data to be Reviewed and Analyzed" table, scoring for this patient encounter meets the criteria of Category 1 under "moderate" as 3 unique tests were ordered. This is because the guidelines for "moderate" state that it is necessary to "meet 1 of 3 categories" and Category 1 is met as long as any three boxes are checked in that category.

3. Risk of Complications and/or Morbidity or Mortality of Patient Management

As indicated in the title of this element, scoring is determined by the level of risk associated with treatment. Is there a low or high risk of complications, morbidity, or even death if the patient follows or doesn't follow the recommended treatment plan? For example, an elderly patient with multiple poorly controlled chronic conditions undergoing a major procedure could be considered life-threatening. Conversely, a young, healthy patient with no chronic conditions undergoing the same procedure may have fewer risks.

Traditionally, the Table of Risk, included in the 1995 and 1997 E/M guidelines, was used to determine the third component of risk in the overall MDM score. While much of the information remains the same, some details have been added which clear up some of the previous ambiguity. The risk component for Office or Other Outpatient Services assesses how the diagnostic testing and/or treatment plan for the conditions identified poses a threat of death or loss of bodily function in the individual patient as indicated in the following table:

Risk of Complications and/or Morbidity or Mortality of Patient Management		
Code	Level of Risk	Examples
99211	N/A	No examples are provided in the CPT codebook
99202 99212	Minimal	No examples are provided in the CPT codebook
99203 99213	Low	No examples are provided in the CPT codebook

99204
99214
	Moderate	• Prescription drug management
		• Decision regarding:
		  • Minor surgery with identified patient or procedure risk factors
		  • Elective major surgery without identified patient or procedure risk factors
		• Diagnosis or treatment significantly limited by social determinants of health

99205
99215
	High	• Drug therapy requiring intensive monitoring for toxicity
		• Decision regarding:
		  • Elective major surgery with identified risk factors
		  • Emergency major surgery
		  • Hospitalization
		  • Not to resuscitate or to de-escalate care because of poor prognosis

Tip: ICD-10-CM codes for social determinants of health continue to expand. However, their use in relation to the "moderate" level of risk is dependent on individual payer policies.

Resource: See Resource 651 for a discussion on the new moderate risk level example regarding social determinants of health.

Summary

The following table summarizes the previously discussed levels and components of MDM. To qualify for a level of service, two of the three elements must be met:

Medical Decision Making (MDM) (best 2 of 3)			
Problem(s)	**Data**	**Risk**	**Type of MDM**
Minimal	Minimal/none	Minimal	Straightforward
Low	Limited	Low	Low
Moderate	Moderate	Moderate	Moderate
High	High	High	High

Book: See also "Coding Scenario 2: Current Office E/M Guidelines" on page 343 to see an example using the new MDM guidelines.

Reminder: Although the two key components of history and exam will no longer be used to score the level of an office E/M service, they are still important elements of the patient's medical record and help to support medical necessity. As such, they should be performed and documented regularly. However, the extent of the patient history and examination is left to the discretion of the treating provider.

Coding Scenario 1: 2020 E/M Guidelines

The following example takes a step-by-step approach for each of the key components using the E/M guidelines from 2020. As a reminder, the level selection scoring methodology used may depend on payer policy. According to the CPT codebook and CMS, code level selection is only based on Time (see page 318) or Medical Decision Making (see page 320). At the time of publication, some providers have elected to continue using the old methodology to ensure compliance with all payers.

Use *Figure 5.3* as a helpful reference when navigating the complexity of Evaluation and Management coding throughout this coding scenario.

Figure 5.3

Evaluation & Management								
History (lowest score)				**Exam** (best score)		**MDM** (best 2 of 3)		**Time**
CC	HPI	ROS	PFSH	'95 DGs	'97 DGs	Dx	Data	Risk	>50%

1. **History** identifies the reason the patient is seeking medical attention and provides historical context related to healthcare problems or habits that may have a bearing on diagnosis and treatment. The subcomponents of history include:

- CC: Chief complaint
- HPI: History of Present Illness
- ROS: Review of Systems
- PFSH: Past, Family and Social History

2. **Examination** is established by using either the 1995 or 1997 Documentation Guidelines. In this chapter, both of these approaches will be demonstrated.
   - 95 DGs: The 1995 Documentation Guidelines are more generally defined and base the level of code selected on the number of body areas or systems evaluated. (see *Figure 5.7*)
   - 97 DGs: The 1997 Documentation Guidelines offer eleven system specific Examination requirements as well as a General Multi-System Examination. (see *Figure 5.8*)

3. **Medical Decision Making (MDM)** refers to the complexity of establishing a diagnosis or updating the status of an established diagnosis and determining the correct management option(s), including the risk to the patient if left untreated. Scoring is determined based on:
   - DX: Number of diagnoses and/or management options, as well as the status of the diagnoses (e.g., new, established, stable, worsening, requiring additional testing)
   - DATA: Amount and/or complexity of data to be ordered and/or reviewed
   - RISK: Possibility of complications and/or morbidity or mortality with the current treatment option or if left untreated.

Matrix Selection

Many E/M audit tools are available in the market, but most are overly complex for a typical office encounter. For this reason, innoviHealth developed simplified coding reference tools which should meet the needs of most physicians and QHPs and are used in this coding scenario. *Figure 5.4* shows the "New Patient E/M Matrix," which guides the decision making process for office or outpatient codes. It acts as an audit tool to quickly evaluate whether or not you have selected the appropriate E/M code for the patient encounter.

Store: Helpful two-page color versions of the *E/M Reference Cards* are available with special bundle packages in the online store.

Figure 5.4

ESTABLISHED PATIENT E/M MATRIX (2 OF 3 KEY COMPONENTS)

Office & Outpatient Level of Service		Nature of Presenting Problem (NPP)	History (lowest score)				Exam (best score)		MDM (best 2 of 3)			Time Override
Code	Level	Severity	CC	HPI	ROS	PFSH	'95 DGs	'97 DGs	Dx	Data	Risk	Minutes
99211	n/a	Minimal	Y	Reason for Encounter			Vital Signs/Findings		Instructions			5
99212	Problem Focused (PF)	Self-Limited	Y	1-3	n/a	n/a	1	1-5	1	0-1	min	10
99213	Expanded PF	Low	Y	1-3	1	n/a	2-7	6-11	2	2	low	15
99214	Detailed	Moderate	Y	4+	2-9	1	2x-7x	12 in 2	3	3	mod	25
99215	Comprehensive	High	Y	4+	10+	2+	8+	18 in 9	4	4	high	40

Reminder: Because this particular example is to illustrate the 2020 (and earlier) guidelines, *Figure 5.4* is different than the current office guidelines table as shown in "Coding Scenario 2" which begins on page 343.

This auditing tool facilitates a quick analysis of the E/M service based on the documentation findings. As you can see, code 99211 has the lowest scoring requirements, is used for incident-to encounters with ancillary staff such as medical assistants, registered nurses, etc., and has minimal documentation requirements. The other four are for provider and other qualified healthcare professional (QHP) E/M encounters. For an established patient, scoring within two of the three key components (history, exam, MDM) must reach the required level of service and also meet the medical necessity requirement identified by the level of severity of the NPP.

The NPP column is a reminder that medical necessity must also meet the same level of E/M service. Often we see copy/paste, or pulling forward of information from a prior date of service into the current encounter note, or templates that always include a complete ROS or exam, even when unnecessary. When the NPP matches the key component scoring, the correct E/M level can be reported with confidence.

Clinical Example

The following clinical example is referenced as the New Patient E/M Matrix (*Figure 5.4*) is explained. It is **not** intended to be an example of a perfect clinical record, rather it was formatted this way for teaching purposes to simplify references in this chapter. Note that this matrix was designed to facilitate an audit. Consider modifying your documentation patterns to match these elements so that it is easier to use the matrix, and thus easier for an outside auditor to find what they are looking for as well.

CHIEF COMPLAINT

Facial pain and pressure, nasal congestion, headache.

HISTORY OF PRESENT ILLNESS

Patient is a 45-year old white female, established patient, who presents for evaluation of moderate nasal congestion that began about 10 days ago. She states the congestion is in the bilateral maxillary sinus area. She has tried over the counter Sudafed and nasal spray, which has alleviated congestion enough to help her sleep at night. She states she is constantly congested and the pressure has become intolerable. She thinks she has a sinus infection and would like an antibiotic.

REVIEW OF SYSTEMS

Constitutional: Admits difficulty sleeping due to congestion. Denies fever.

Eyes: Denies eye pain/discharge

ENT: Admits nasal congestion, postnasal drip, and dry mouth from Sudafed and sleeping with mouth open.

Cardiovascular: Denies chest pain, irregular heartbeat, or syncope.

Respiratory: Admits abnormal sputum production. Denies wheezing or cough.

GI: Denies nausea, vomiting, diarrhea.

Skin: Denies rash and itching.

MS: Denies joint pain or swelling.

Endocrine: Denies polyuria, polydipsia, and cold/heat intolerance.

Hem-Lymph: Denies enlarged lymph nodes.

PAST MEDICAL HISTORY

Patient has a history of chronic pain, being treated by pain management with Tramadol and Norco. She had a flu shot two months ago here.

SOCIAL HISTORY

Nonsmoker, nondrinker. She works full-time as a librarian at the local elementary school, where she is often exposed to young children.

PHYSICAL EXAM

Vitals: BP: 138/73 sitting; HR:96-R; RR: 18; temp (F): 97.7; O2 sats: 100% on room air.

Constitutional: Well developed, well nourished female in no acute distress.

Eyes: Conjunctivae normal. No drainage. PERRLA, EOMI.

ENT: External appearance of ears and nose is normal. Otoscopic examination reveals TMs within normal limits bilaterally without perforations. Intranasal exam: Moist with slight clear discharge. Septum is midline. Sinus tenderness on palpation over the maxillary and sphenoid sinuses. Oral mucosa, tongue, palate, and hard palate are all normal appearing. Oropharynx: clear. Tonsils are within normal limits.

Lymphatic: Lymph nodes of the neck are normal appearance. No masses or tenderness.

Neck: Thyroid gland size normal, nontender, no nodules or masses present on palpation, trachea midline.

Respiratory: Unlabored breathing. Normal breath sounds on auscultation.

Cardiovascular: Regular rate and rhythm, no murmurs noted.

ASSESSMENT

Acute maxillary sinusitis.
Acute sphenoidal sinusitis.

PLAN

Zithromax 500 mg oral tablet. Take 1 tablet (500 mg) by oral route once daily for 3 days #3 tablets with 0 refills. Call or return if symptoms worsen or do not improve.

1. History

Chief Complaint (CC)

The first key component to evaluate is the History, which must always include a chief complaint. This is the primary reason for the encounter and is required for every level of E/M code for office visits and should thus always be present in the documentation.

CHIEF COMPLAINT

Facial pain and pressure, nasal congestion, headache.

	History (lowest score)			
	CC	HPI	ROS	PFSH
99211	Y	Reason for Encounter		
99212	Y	1-3	n/a	n/a
99213	Y	1-3	1	n/a
99214	Y	4+	2-9	1
99215	Y	4+	10+	2+

 Tip: The chief complaint (CC) is vital to establishing medical necessity and if missing, it opens the door for claim rejection and/or payer refund demands.

Now that the Chief Complaint has been identified, the remaining three elements of History should be considered together. The criteria for all three must meet or exceed the requirements for any single code, as indicated by the "(lowest score)" in the Matrix.

History of Present Illness (HPI)

Next, use the Matrix (*Figure 5.4*) to determine how many "History of Present Illness" (HPI) elements are present in the clinical example. The elements of HPI, as outlined by the CPT codebook, are listed below.

HISTORY — HPI			
History of Present Illness Elements			
1	Location	5	Duration
2	Quality	6	Context
3	Severity	7	Modifying factors
4	Timing	8	Associated signs & symptoms

History			(lowest score)
	CC	HPI	ROS	PFSH
99211	Y	Reason for Encounter		
99212	Y	1-3	n/a	n/a
99213	Y	1-3	1	n/a
99214	Y	4+	2-9	1
99215	Y	4+	10+	2+

Note that, per the Matrix (*Figure 5.4*), there are only two levels of HPI: brief (1-3 elements) and extended (4 or more elements). The clinical example contains six elements of the HPI. The Matrix in *Figure 5.4* shows that any of the exam codes could be selected because four HPI elements is the minimum required to qualify for the highest level code (99215).

 Tip: Both 99214 & 99215 require 4+ HPI elements. When scoring based on components, always select the highest qualifying code, which in this case would be 99215.

HISTORY OF PRESENT ILLNESS

Patient is a 45-year old white female, established patient, who presents for evaluation of moderate nasal congestion that began about 10 days ago. She states the congestion is in the bilateral maxillary sinus area. She has tried over the counter Sudafed and nasal spray, which has alleviated congestion enough to help her sleep at night. She states she is constantly congested and the pressure has become intolerable. She thinks she has a sinus infection and would like an antibiotic.

HISTORY OF PRESENT ILLNESS

Severity: Moderate **Location:** Nose and sinuses
Duration: 10 days ago **Timing:** Constantly congested
Modifying Factors: Tried OTC sudafed and nasal spray with temporary relief
Associated Signs & Symptoms: Difficulty sleeping, dry mouth

The 1997 DGs state that documentation of the status of three chronic conditions also qualifies for an extended HPI. For many years, this only applied to the 1997 DGs. In 2013, this rule was extended to the 1995 DGs as well. As will be explained in the pages that follow, in order to qualify for the comprehensive History, in addition to documenting the status of three chronic conditions, the provider would also need to document a complete (10+) ROS and at least two areas of the PFSH. It is important to remember that documentation of both the chronic condition and its status are required.

Review of Systems (ROS)

The next element of the History is the Review of Systems (ROS). According to the CPT codebook, there are 14 possible organ systems to review. See *Figure 5.5*

Figure 5.5

HISTORY — ROS			
Review of Systems Elements			
1	Constitutional	8	Musculoskeletal
2	Eyes	9	Integumentary
3	Ears, nose, mouth, throat	10	Neurological
4	Cardiovascular	11	Psychiatric
5	Respiratory	12	Endocrine
6	Gastrointestinal	13	Hematologic / Lymphatic
7	Genitourinary	14	Allergic / Immunologic

Note: A Review of Systems (ROS) is an inventory of the organ systems, obtained through a series of questions to identify signs and/or symptoms which the patient may be experiencing or has experienced. Positive responses and pertinent negatives should be documented.

REVIEW OF SYSTEMS

Constitutional: Admits difficulty sleeping due to congestion. Denies fever.

Eyes: Denies eye pain/discharge

ENT: Admits nasal congestion, postnasal drip, and dry mouth from Sudafed and sleeping with mouth open.

Cardiovascular: Denies chest pain, irregular heartbeat, or syncope.

Respiratory: Admits abnormal sputum production. Denies wheezing or cough.

GI: Denies nausea, vomiting, diarrhea.

Skin: Denies rash and itching.

MS: Denies joint pain or swelling.

Endocrine: Denies polyuria, polydipsia, and cold/heat intolerance.

Hem-Lymph: Denies enlarged lymph nodes.

There were 10 organ systems were reviewed in the clinical example, which, as revealed by a quick glance at the Matrix (*Figure 5.4*), qualifies for 99215. As the Note above states, "Positive responses and pertinent negatives should be documented." This patient's chief complaint is "facial pain and pressure, nasal congestion, and a headache," which means the organ systems we expect to see reviewed should include at least ENT and Neurologic. Additional organ systems that could also have positive findings include Respiratory, Constitutional, Eyes, Hematologic/Lymphatic, and perhaps Gastrointestinal. In other words, for this type of complaint, it would be expected to see these organ systems reviewed instead of Musculoskeletal or Genitourinary, which are not applicable or related to the Chief Complaint. For a new patient, or a patient who has not been seen for six months to a year, a more complete review of systems may be required or desired by the provider to be thorough. Often EHR templates automatically pop up a predetermined list of organ systems to be reviewed, which are not always necessary, and should be carefully reviewed by the provider to ensure they match with the patient responses before signing the record.

Note: A highly common audit finding in E/M encounters is a contradiction between the CC/HPI and the ROS. This is usually caused by the use of templates that are prepopulated with negative findings. When the patient has a positive finding, the provider "theoretically" changes "DENIES" to "ADMITS." However, the majority of providers fail to properly edit and update this information, leading to contradicting information. This is one example of an area in which payers may question documentation inconsistencies.

Past, Family, Social History (PFSH)

The final element of History is made up of the Past Medical, Family, and Social Histories (PFSH). The table below provides examples of what is included in each type of history.

	HISTORY — PFSH	
	Past Medical, Family, and Social History	
1	Past Medical History	A review of the patient's past experiences with illnesses, injuries, and treatments (e.g., operations, hospitalizations, medications, allergies, dietary status).
2	Family History	A review of medical events in the patient's family (e.g., health status of parents, children and siblings, and hereditary diseases). For established patients, a review of the family history should be relevant to the CC/HPI for that encounter.
3	Social History	An age appropriate review of past and current activities (e.g., marital status, employment, drugs, alcohol, tobacco, education, sexual history, and military service).

History (lowest score)

	CC	HPI	ROS	PFSH
99211	Y	Reason for Encounter		
99212	Y	1-3	n/a	n/a
99213	Y	1-3	1	n/a
99214	Y	4+	2-9	1
99215	Y	4+	10+	2+

Just one item needs to be documented in one of the three history areas to qualify for credit. For example, if nothing but the patient's prior surgeries are listed, credit for Past Medical History is given. Likewise, the same credit for Past Medical History would be given if prior surgeries, medications, allergies, and/or dietary status were included. In this case, both Past Medical History and Social History are documented, which is sufficient for a 99215, per the Matrix.

> **PAST MEDICAL HISTORY**
> Patient has a history of chronic pain, being treated by pain management with Tramadol and Norco. She had a flu shot two months ago here.

> **SOCIAL HISTORY**
> Nonsmoker, nondrinker. She works full-time as a librarian at the local elementary school, where she is often exposed to young children.

Tip: As noted in the matrix under history scoring, 99212 and 99213 do not require documentation of any PFSH. Some payers will not accept "unremarkable, noncontributory, or negative" as a valid response for PFSH findings and instead prefer additional information to show the provider asked and had answered a question about family history that is pertinent to the patient's current chief complaint.

Resource: See Resource 604 for more on this subject.

Tip: Another area where risk of recoupment of funds occurs is in a PFSH that has been pulled forward or copied from a prior encounter. When this information is routinely pulled forward or copied and pasted into a note, it can cause upcoding. All PFSH information should be pertinent to the CC/HPI for the current encounter, marked as reviewed and updated, or not included. Many EHR systems now allow providers and staff to verify and update the patient's medical history within a portion of the medical record before pulling it forward into the patient note. When done properly, it removes the negative effects of copy/paste auditing issues. Verifying the information was updated at the time of the service will satisfy the audit process.

Tip: Copying and pasting is being actively addressed in EHR compliance tools, identifying within the body of text where information was pulled or copied from, along with the original author name and date of entry. This allows auditors, coders, and compliance team members to accurately code and educate staff members to support company and payer documentation policies.

History Summary

The overall History must meet or exceed the requirements in all three subcomponents of history. The lowest score within the subcomponents of History determines the overall level of History. In this particular encounter, all of the subcomponents of history qualified for 99215, as seen in *Figure 5.6*. If, for example, the HPI had only scored "Brief" (1-3 in the Matrix) at a 99213, the entire history would be forced to that level.

Figure 5.6

History (lowest score)				
	CC	HPI	ROS	PFSH
99211	Y	Reason for Encounter		
99212	Y	1-3	n/a	n/a
99213	Y	1-3	1	n/a
99214	Y	4+	2-9	1
99215	Y	4+	10+	2+

2. Exam

Exam (best score)	
'95 DGs	'97 DGs
Vital Signs/Findings	
1	1-5
2-7	6-11
2x-7x	12 in 2
8+	18 in 9

The 1995 and 1997 Documentation Guidelines (DGs) define the Exam portion of an E/M encounter differently. The 1995 DGs are calculated based on the quantity of organ systems (OS) and/or body areas (BA) examined, while the 1997 DGs are calculated based on the number of pre-identified examination bullet points documented using either the General Multi-System examination or one of the Single Organ System examinations. Providers may choose between the 1995 or 1997 DGs, to see which one benefits them more. Auditors score the exam using both sets of guidelines and whichever scores higher is used to the benefit of the provider. As the only difference between the 1995 and the 1997 DGs is the exam, it is very important to understand how the documented examination findings fit into each organ system or body area to maximize scoring.

Example: If an encounter scores a 99212 following the 1995 DGs and a 99213 following the 1997 DGs, the provider and the auditor would allow the 99213, as long as the service met the medical necessity requirement.

As we continue in this segment, both the 1995 and 1997 DGs will be used to score our clinical example. Of note when scoring based on the 1997 DGs, you may choose to score using the General Multi-System (GMS) examination or an appropriate Single Organ System (SOS) examination.

The 1995 and 1997 DGs differ in how information is quantified and scored. The 1995 DGs give one point for any amount of information pertaining to an organ system or body area. If six organ systems are documented and only one body area, then the score is either six (detailed) or one (problem focused). Body areas and organ systems are not added together for a score.

In the 1997 DGs, there are pre-identified examination bullet points. These are based on either a General Multi-System examination or one of the Single Organ System examinations. For each bullet point documented within the examination, one point is given. All bullet points are added together for a total score and the number of organ systems examined are also tallied.

In the Single Organ System examinations, the same scoring of documentation using pre-identified bullet points also applies; however, as they are specific to a singular organ system, additional documentation requirements exist to reach the comprehensive service code.

Tip: Any provider, of any specialty or nonspecialty, may score E/M encounters using any of these examination guidelines.

Alert: Although providers may elect to use *either* of the examination guidelines, it is *not* appropriate to combine them on a single case.

The 1995 DGs require an "expanded problem-focused" level examination for 99213 and a detailed level examination for 99214. While both require documentation of 2-7 organ systems or body areas, 99214 requires the affected area to be documented in detail. The guidelines do not quantify the difference, rather they simply state that the exam of this area must be "expanded," as represented by the "x" in the Matrix (*Figure 5.4*).

Resource: See Resource 332 for the complete 1995 Documentation Guidelines.
Resource: See Resource 333 for the complete 1997 Documentation Guidelines.

Figure 5.7

Examination
(1995 Documentation Guidelines)

Body Areas					Organ Systems			
1	Head, face	7	Right upper extremity		1	Constitutional	7	Genitourinary
2	Neck	8	Left upper extremity		2	Eyes	8	Musculoskeletal
3	Chest, breast, axilla	9	Right lower extremity	OR	3	Ears, nose, mouth, throat	9	Skin
4	Abdomen	10	Left lower extremity		4	Cardiovascular	10	Neurological
5	Genitalia, groin, buttocks				5	Respiratory	11	Psychiatric
6	Back				6	Gastrointestinal	12	Hematologic/Lymphatic/Immunologic

The 1995 DGs allow providers to count either organ systems (OS) or body areas (BA), as listed in *Figure 5.7*. Providers may only count from one of the two columns; mixing and matching is not allowed (i.e., it is inappropriate to count abdomen as well as gastrointestinal). Note that each extremity counts as a distinct body area.

Example: Abdomen: Soft, nontender, no hepatosplenomegaly. If counting the abdomen, under the 1995 DGs, one point is counted for BA or one point for OS (not two points). However, if counting this under the 1997 DGs General Multi-System Exam (GMS), two points would be counted for the following bullet points:

- Examination of abdomen with notation of presence of masses or tenderness.
- Examination of liver and spleen

Looking at it this way, the 1997 GMS would be the better way to score this particular examination.

PHYSICAL EXAM

Vitals: BP: 138/73 sitting; HR:96-R; RR: 18; temp (F): 97.7; O2 sats: 100% on room air.

Constitutional: Well developed, well nourished female in no acute distress.

Eyes: Conjunctivae normal. No drainage. PERRLA, EOMI.

ENT: External appearance of ears and nose is normal. Otoscopic examination reveals TMs within normal limits bilaterally without perforations. Intranasal exam: Moist with slight clear discharge. Septum is midline. Sinus tenderness on palpation over the maxillary and sphenoid sinuses. Oral mucosa, tongue, palate, and hard palate are all normal appearing. Oropharynx: clear. Tonsils are within normal limits.

Lymphatic: lymph nodes of the neck are normal appearance. No masses or tenderness.

Neck: Thyroid gland size normal, nontender, no nodules or masses present on palpation, trachea midline.

Respiratory: Unlabored breathing. Normal breath sounds on auscultation.

Cardiovascular: Regular rate and rhythm, no murmurs noted.

Scoring this examination using the 1995 guidelines, the following six (6) organ systems (OS) are identified:

1. Constitutional   2. Eyes   3. ENT
4. Lymphatic   5. Respiratory   6. Cardiovascular

and the following one (1) body area (BA) has been identified:

1. Neck

Note: Some Medicare Administrative Contractors (MACs), Novitas in particular, follow the 4x4 rule for a 99214 "detailed" examination. This rule states that a 99214 is reached when at least four (4) bullet points are documented in four (4) organ systems (OS) or body areas (BA).

Although the overall 1995 score qualifies for 99213 (2-7 body areas or organ systems), it also qualifies for 99214 (2x-7x body areas or organ systems) because six systems were documented and the affected system (ENT) is documented in greater detail than the other systems in this report. To clarify, the detailed examination does not require every examined system to be documented in greater detail. The total number examined must still be 2-7, but only the affected system(s) require the greater detail, even if that is only one system.

In comparison, the 1997 DGs offer a much more detailed list of bulleted items that qualify as part of a General Multi-System Examination. The General Multi-System Examination consists of 14 body areas and organ systems but, for the sake of space, only those that pertain to this example are shown in *Figure 5.8*.

Figure 5.8

Examination
'97 Documentation Guidelines | General Multi-System Examination

System/Body Area	Elements of Examination
Constitutional	Measurement of any three of the following eight vital signs: 1. Sitting or standing blood pressure 2. Supine blood pressure 3. Pulse rate and regularity 4. Respiration 5. Temperature 6. Height 7. Weight (May be measured and recorded by ancillary staff) 8. General appearance of patient (e.g., development, nutrition, body habitus, deformities, attention to grooming)
Eyes	• Inspection of conjunctivae and lids • Examination of pupils and irises (e.g., reaction to light and accommodation, size, and symmetry) • Ophthalmoscopic examination of optic discs (e.g., size, C/D ratio, appearance) and posterior segments (e.g., vessel changes, exudates, hemorrhages)
Ears, Nose, Mouth, Throat	• External inspection of ears and nose (e.g., overall appearance, scars, lesions, masses) • Otoscopic examination of external auditory canals and tympanic membranes • Assessment of hearing (e.g., whispered voice, finger rub, tuning fork) • Inspection of nasal mucosa, septum, and turbinates • Inspection of lips, teeth, and gums • Examination of oropharynx: oral mucosa, salivary glands, hard and soft palates, tongue, tonsils, and posterior pharynx

Examination
'97 Documentation Guidelines | General Multi-System Examination

System/Body Area	Elements of Examination

Lymphatic	• Palpation of lymph nodes in two or more areas:
	  • Neck
	  • Axillae
	  • Groin
	  • Other

Respiratory	• Assessment of respiratory effort (e.g., intercostal retractions, use of accessory muscles, diaphragmatic movement) • Percussion of chest (e.g., dullness, flatness, hyperresonance) • Palpation of chest (e.g., tactile fremitus) • Auscultation of lung (e.g., breath sounds, adventitious sounds, rubs)

Cardiovascular	• Palpation of heart (location, size, thrills)
	• Auscultation of heart with notation of abnormal sounds and murmurs
	• Examination of:
	  • carotid arteries (pulse, amplitude, bruits)
	  • abdominal aorta (size, bruits)
	  • femoral arteries (pulse, amplitude, bruits)
	  • pedal pulses (pulse, amplitude)
	  • extremities for edema and/or varicosities

A comparison of the clinical example to *Figure 5.8* identifies the following body areas and organ system bulleted items:

- **Constitutional:** vital signs
- **Constitutional:** general appearance
- **Eyes:** inspection of conjunctivae
- **Eyes:** examination of pupils
- **ENMT:** external inspection ears/nose
- **ENMT:** otoscopic examination of tympanic membranes
- **ENMT:** inspection nasal mucosa, septum and turbinates
- **ENMT:** examination of oropharynx, oral mucosa, etc.
- **Lymphatic:** palpation of lymph nodes in two or more areas: neck (lacking one area)
- **Neck:** examination of neck (masses, tracheal position)
- **Neck:** examination of thyroid
- **Respiratory:** assessment of effort
- **Respiratory:** auscultation of lungs
- **Cardiovascular:** auscultation of heart

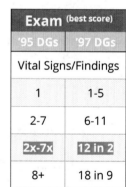

Exam (best score)	
'95 DGs	'97 DGs
Vital Signs/Findings	
1	1-5
2-7	6-11
2x-7x	12 in 2
8+	18 in 9

Therefore, this Exam includes 15 bullets which, according to *Figure 5.4*, qualifies for 99214. This is a "Detailed" exam, which includes at least two elements identified by a bullet from each of six areas/systems OR at least twelve elements identified by a bullet in two or more areas/systems (shown as "12 in 2" in the Matrix.) A comprehensive exam is when the provider performs all elements identified by a bullet in at least nine areas/systems and documents at least two elements identified by a bullet from each of nine areas/systems (shown as "18 in 9" in *Figure 5.4*). The 1995 DGs support the selection of 99214 also, making the PE component the same between 1995 and 1997 scoring. The 1997 DGs are more specific which makes them easier to quantify and audit.

3. MEDICAL DECISION MAKING (MDM)

Medical Decision Making (MDM) is the most complex key component of Evaluation and Management coding. It essentially recognizes the clinical expertise required to appropriately manage patient care. The level of MDM is assessed by answering the following questions:

- How many problems does the patient have and how problematic are they? What is their status (e.g., worse, improved, stable)? (Number of diagnoses or management options)
- How much information needs to be reviewed to properly diagnose and formulate a treatment plan for the case? (Amount and/or complexity of data to be reviewed)
- How risky is the patient's problem? Is this case simple or could the patient lose a limb and/or die if treatment isn't provided? If the patient follows the treatment plan, what is the risk of serious side effects? This should be easily identifiable in the documentation, especially for cases where the provider claims high complexity or severity. (Risk of significant complications, morbidity, and/or mortality)

MDM (best 2 of 3)		
Dx	Data	Risk
Instructions		
1	0-1	min
2	2	low
3	3	mod
4	4	high

The answer to all these questions, scored and brought together, determines the appropriate type of MDM (straightforward, low complexity, moderate complexity, or high complexity). Note that only two of these elements must meet or exceed the level to qualify for the type of MDM selected. This is demonstrated by separately evaluating each of the three elements of MDM. *Figure 5.9* summarizes the three elements of MDM.

Figure 5.9

Medical Decision Making (MDM) (best 2 of 3)			
Diagnoses	Data	Risk	Type of MDM
Minimal (1)	Minimal (0-1)	Minimal	Straightforward
Limited (2)	Limited (2)	Low	Low complexity
Multiple (3)	Moderate (3)	Moderate	Moderate complexity
Extensive (4)	Extensive (4)	High	High complexity

ASSESSMENT
Acute maxillary sinusitis.
Acute sphenoidal sinusitis.

PLAN
Zithromax 500 mg oral tablet. Take 1 tablet (500 mg) by oral route once daily for 3 days #3 tablets with 0 refills. Call or return if symptoms worsen or do not improve.

Number of Diagnoses and/or Management Options

The first element, Number of Diagnoses and/or Management Options, is used to score condition(s) being evaluated, assessed, or managed at the current encounter. It is important to first determine if the problem is self-limited or minor (basically a problem that really didn't need the attention of a healthcare provider but that probably could have been taken care of at home). Next, identify whether a problem (new or established for the patient) is actually new or an established problem for the provider performing the evaluation. If new to the provider, was additional workup (e.g., lab, imaging, testing) needed in order to establish a diagnosis and treatment plan? If the problem isn't new to the provider, is it stable, better, or getting worse? Answers to these questions will help identify the point system applicable to this portion of medical decision making (MDM). Using *Figure 5.10* (Number of Diagnosis or Management Options) helps to score the clinical example and answer these questions.

MDM (best 2 of 3)		
Dx	Data	Risk
Instructions		
1	0-1	min
2	2	low
3	3	mod
4	4	high

There has been controversy over "new problem, with additional workup" in that some believe any workup counts, even when that workup can be done during the same encounter and at the same location with results available during the encounter that effected the workup request. Others have felt additional workup means the patient had to go elsewhere and have a return encounter for results in order to count it as "additional workup." The Medicare Administrative Contractor (MAC) Palmetto GBA responded to this exact issue with the following statement: "'Additional work-up' consists of any diagnostic testing, laboratory testing, etc., and may be performed at the time of visit." It is suggested providers check with the contracted payers to see if they have policies that state otherwise and also with their specific MAC before assuming Palmetto's answer applies to all.

Tip: A "self-limited or minor problem" has a maximum point value of 2, (1 point per with a maximum of 2 allowed) and "new (to examiner) no additional workup required" has a maximum point value of 3, regardless of how many diagnoses may qualify for those levels.

Figure 5.10

Medical Decision Making (MDM) (best 2 of 3)	
Number of Diagnosis or Management Options	
Self-limited or minor problem (max=2)	1 Point
Established (to examiner) stable or improved problem	1 Point
Established (to examiner) worsening problem	2 Points
New (to examiner) problem, no additional work up (max=1)	3 Points
New (to examiner) problem, with additional work up	4 Points

An analysis of this case reveals two diagnoses to manage: acute maxillary sinusitis and acute sphenoid sinusitis. This is an acute condition, which means it is new to the examiner and no additional work up (such as imaging or lab work) is planned. This appears to yield a score of six points, or "extensive" for Number of Diagnosis and/or Management Options. According to the Number of Diagnosis or Management Options Table (*Figure 5.10*), this type of problem (new, no additional work up) has a maximum allowable of just one (1) per encounter. This indicates that instead of a score of six, the score would now only be three, or "multiple," according to *Figure 5.9*.

Tip: Consider using the same wording found in this table when documenting the patient's problems, such as "established" or "new," and "stable" or "worsening." It will make it easier for proper code assignment and auditing, as well as preventing additional provider interruptions or queries.

Amount and/or Complexity of Data to be Reviewed (Data)

The second element of MDM is Amount and/or Complexity of Data to be Reviewed (see *Figure 5.11*). If the healthcare provider needs to review records and lab tests from a dozen different providers, the case has a higher level of decision making. Alternatively, if there is very little data to consider, then the case is fairly straightforward. In this encounter no data was ordered or reviewed, garnering a score of 0, or "Minimal," as depicted in *Figure 5.9*.

But how would scoring be calculated if an x-ray had been ordered during this encounter? Referring to *Figure 5.11* as a guide, the provider would receive 1 point for ordering the imaging. Let's review some scenarios and how they would be scored under "Data."

1. If the provider ordered an x-ray, requiring the patient to return for a follow-up encounter to go over the results of that x-ray, then only one point is garnered for ordering the x-ray at today's encounter.

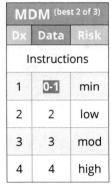

2. When the patient returns for the encounter to review the results of the x-ray (on a different date of service), the provider will garner one point for reviewing the data with the patient at that encounter. If the image is taken at another location and the ordering provider independently visualizes the image and documents an opinion, it is worth 2 points.
3. If the provider owns the imaging equipment, orders an x-ray, has it performed the same day, and bills globally for the x-ray service, only a point for ordering the x-ray would be allowed. The review point and a point for independent visualization are bundled into the global service for the x-ray being billed. Additionally, to bill globally for the x-ray, the provider must create a written report for the imaging being done that includes what was ordered and any findings. To avoid audit issues, this should be easily locatable within the medical record.

Some providers misunderstand how points are garnered in a couple of ways.

- Order/review (same day) of imaging only garners one point
- Order/review (same day) of lab tests only garners one point
- When a provider owns the imaging equipment and bills for the global service (not billing TC or 26 separately), only one point may be garnered for the E/M MDM portion for ordering and/or reviewing during the same encounter. The independent visualization points are not eligible because as part of the global service for the imaging itself, the provider is expected to visualize the image and write up a report with the findings.

Each CPT code has requirements for payment. Imaging performed and billed by the provider carries a requirement to review the images and write a report of any findings. If he gives himself two points credit in the Data section of MDM, "Independent/second visualization of tests with documented summary," for reading the x-rays, he is essentially double dipping or potentially getting paid twice for doing the work once because the increase in his MDM could mean an increase in the final code selection.

Figure 5.11

Medical Decision Making (MDM) (best 2 of 3)	
Amount and/or Complexity of Data to be Reviewed	
Review and/or order of tests in the radiology section (70000)	**1 Point**
Review and/or order of tests in the laboratory section (80000)	**1 Point**
Review and/or order of tests in the medicine section (90000)	**1 Point**
Discussion of test results with performing physician	**1 Point**
Decision to obtain old records or history from someone other than the patient	**1 Point**
Review of old records with documented summary or obtain history from someone other than the patient	**2 Points**
Independent/second visualization of tests with documented summary	**2 Points**

Risk of Significant Complications, Morbidity and/or Mortality

The final element of MDM is Risk of Significant Complications, Morbidity and/or Mortality. The official *Table of Risk* (see *Figure 5.12*) is divided into four levels of complexity: minimal, low, moderate, and high, further identified within three subcategories:

1. Presenting Problem(s): The risk related to the disease processes anticipated between the present encounter and the next one.
2. Diagnostic Procedure(s) Ordered: The risk associated with selecting diagnostic procedures.
3. Management Options: The risk associated with the management option recommended for the patient.

The highest level of risk among all three subcategories determines the overall risk.

Figure 5.12

		Table of Risk	
Level of Risk	Presenting Problem	Diagnostic Procedure(s) Ordered	Management Options
Minimal	• One self-limited or minor problem (cold, insect bite)	• Lab tests req. venipuncture • Chest x-rays • EKG/EEG • Urinalysis • Ultrasound, e.g., Echocardiography • KOH prep	• Rest • Gargles • Elastic bandages • Superficial dressings
Low	• Two or more self-limited or minor problems • One stable chronic illness, e.g., well controlled hypertension, non-insulin dependent diabetes, cataract, BPH • Acute uncomplicated illness or injury, e.g., cystitis, allergic rhinitis, simple sprain	• Physiologic tests not under stress, e.g., pulmonary function tests • Non-cardiovascular imaging studies with contrast, e.g., barium enema • Superficial needle biopsies • Clinical laboratory tests requiring arterial puncture • Skin biopsies	• Over-the-counter drugs • Minor surgery with no identified risk factors • Physical therapy • Occupational therapy • IV fluids without additives
Moderate	• One or more chronic illnesses with mild exacerbation, progression, or side effects of treatment • Two or more stable chronic illnesses • Undiagnosed new problem with uncertain prognosis, e.g., lump in breast • Acute illness with systemic symptoms, e.g., pyelonephritis, pneumonitis, colitis • Acute complicated injury, e.g., head injury with brief loss of consciousness	• Physiologic tests under stress, e.g., cardiac stress test, fetal contraction stress test • Diagnostic endoscopies with no identified risk factors • Deep needle or incisional biopsy • Cardiovascular imaging studies with contrast and no identified risk factors, e.g., arteriogram, cardiac catheterization • Obtain fluid from body cavity, eg lumbar puncture, thoracentesis, culdocentesis	• Minor surgery with identified risk factors • Elective major surgery (open, percutaneous, or endoscopic) with no identified risk factors • Prescription drug management • Therapeutic nuclear medicine • IV fluids with additives • Closed treatment of fracture or dislocation without manipulation
High	• One or more chronic illnesses with severe exacerbation, progression, or side effects of treatment • Acute or chronic illnesses or injuries that pose a threat to life or bodily function, e.g., multiple trauma, acute MI, pulmonary embolus, severe respiratory distress, progressive severe rheumatoid arthritis, psychiatric illness with potential threat to self or others, peritonitis, acute renal failure • An abrupt change in neurologic status, e.g., seizure, TIA, weakness, sensory loss	• Cardiovascular imaging studies with contrast with identified risk factors • Cardiac electrophysiological tests • Diagnostic Endoscopies with identified risk factors • Discography	• Elective major surgery (open, percutaneous, or endoscopic) with identified risk factors • Emergency major surgery (open, percutaneous or endoscopic) • Parenteral controlled substances • Drug therapy requiring intensive monitoring for toxicity • Decision not to resuscitate or to de-escalate care because of poor prognosis

Figure 5.12 indicates that the Level of Risk for the 'Presenting Problem' (the far left column) fits appropriately with "acute uncomplicated illness or injury," which is "low risk." From the middle column (Diagnostic Procedure(s) Ordered), no selection can be made as no diagnostic tests were ordered or reviewed. The determining factor comes from the right column (Management Options), which indicates that a "moderate risk" is associated with "prescription drug management" as our clinical scenario shows the provider wrote a prescription for Zithromax. Only one factor from any one column is necessary to qualify for the overall level of risk.

MDM Summary

When comparing the results (*Figure 5.13*) of the three elements used to determine the overall type of Medical Decision Making (MDM), it is apparent that this case qualifies as 'moderate complexity.' Only two of the three criteria in the MDM table have to meet or exceed the requirements for a given type. In other words, the highest and lowest scores can be dropped and what is left aligns with the level of MDM.

Figure 5.13

Medical Decision Making (MDM) (best 2 of 3)			
Diagnoses	**Data**	**Risk**	**Type of MDM**
Minimal (1)	Minimal (0-1)	Minimal	Straightforward
Limited (2)	Limited (2)	Low	Low Complexity
Multiple (3)	Moderate (3)	Moderate	Moderate Complexity
Extensive (4)	Extensive (4)	High	High Complexity

Note: A rumor was going around for years that the MDM would be considered "moderate complexity" if the provider simply wrote a prescription for the patient. Although "prescription drug management" is a moderate level of risk in the "management options" column, it is only one of the three criteria considered in determining the overall level of MDM.

E/M Decision Summary

Now that all three key components have been examined, they need to be compared to the requirements on the Established Patient E/M Matrix. *Figure 5.14* demonstrates how this is done for an established patient.

Figure 5.14

	ESTABLISHED PATIENT E/M MATRIX (2 OF 3 KEY COMPONENTS)								
	History (lowest score)				**Exam** (best score)		**MDM** (best 2 of 3)		
	CC	HPI	ROS	PFSH	'95 DGs	'97 DGs	Dx	Data	Risk
99211	Y	Reason for Encounter			Vital Signs/Findings		Instructions		
99212	Y	1-3	n/a	n/a	1	1-5	1	0-1	min
99213	Y	1-3	1	n/a	2-7	6-11	2	2	low
99214	Y	4+	2-9	1	2x-7x	12 in 2	3	3	mod
99215	Y	4+	10+	2+	8+	18 in 9	4	4	high

If all the numbers in this table are replaced with the official descriptive terms used in the CPT codebook, the table would look like *Figure 5.15*.

Figure 5.15

	ESTABLISHED PATIENT E/M MATRIX (2 OF 3 KEY COMPONENTS)		
	History (lowest score)	**Exam** (best score)	**MDM** (best 2 of 3)
99211	Reason for Encounter	Vital Signs/Findings	Instructions
99212	Problem focused	Problem focused	Straightforward
99213	Expanded problem focused	Expanded problem focused	Low
99214	Detailed	Detailed	Moderate
99215	Comprehensive	Comprehensive	High

The criteria for code level selection for an established patient encounter is that at least two of the three Key Components must meet or exceed the code requirement. In our clinical example, the History score is comprehensive, the Exam detailed, and the type of Medical Decision Making is of moderate complexity. All three meet or exceed the requirements for 99214.

If this clinical example was for a new patient, all three Key Components would have to meet or exceed the level to qualify. Using our clinical scenario for a new patient would give the following results. See *Figure 5.16*.

Figure 5.16

NEW PATIENT E/M MATRIX (3 OF 3 KEY COMPONENTS)

	History (lowest score)				Exam (best score)		MDM (best 2 of 3)		
	CC	HPI	ROS	PFSH	'95 DGs	'97 DGs	Dx	Data	Risk
99201	Y	1-3	n/a	n/a	1	1-5	1	0-1	min
99202	Y	1-3	1	n/a	2-7	6-11	1	0-1	min
99203	Y	4+	2-9	1-2	2x-7x	12 in 2	2	2	low
99204	Y	4+	10+	3	8+	18 in 9	3	3	mod
99205	Y	4+	10+	3	8+	18 in 9	4	4	high

If the values in this table are replaced with the official descriptive terms used in the CPT codebook, the table would look like *Figure 5.17*. The history can only be scored based on the lowest level in the history section. Only the past medical history and social history were documented, which makes the overall History "detailed," aligning with a 99203. The 1995 DGs support a "detailed" exam, as do the 1997 DGs, so the physical exam would also qualify as 99203. Medical Decision Making would qualify as "moderate" (dropping the highest and lowest scores), making this Key Component qualify for a 99204.

Figure 5.17

NEW PATIENT E/M MATRIX (3 OF 3 KEY COMPONENTS)

	History (lowest score)	Exam (best score)	MDM (best 2 of 3)
99201	Problem focused	Problem focused	Straightforward
99202	Expanded problem focused	Expanded problem focused	Straightforward
99203	Detailed	Detailed	Low
99204	Comprehensive	Comprehensive	Moderate
99205	Comprehensive	Comprehensive	High

Therefore, using the same clinical example, but applying it to a new patient, the figure above demonstrates that the criteria for code 99203 have been met. In this case, the lowest score in any of the three components determines the overall code selection because all three Key Components must either meet or exceed the required criteria for the code. In other words, a "low," or even a "high," complexity type of MDM would not have changed the final code selection.

Code Selection by Counseling Time (2020 Version)

E/M visit code selection is based on either the three Key Component areas OR the Counseling/Time override option, when applicable. Referring back to *Figure 5.1*, the seventh Evaluation and Management component is Time. This component has very specific parameters which must be met in order to be used.

The E/M Guidelines in the CPT codebook divide Time into two categories, as it relates to E/M services in the Outpatient Office setting:

1. Pre- and post- encounter Time: Activities before and after the provider-patient face-to-face time do **not** count in this code selection process.

2. Intra-Service encounter/patient Time: Provider-patient face-to-face time spent performing the key components of an E/M service.

In a typical office visit, the three components of History, Examination and Medical Decision Making are usually the dominant components and counseling Time is nominal. However, on certain occasions, Time could be the overriding component. When counseling and/or coordination of care represents 50% or more of the total E/M encounter (doctor-patient face-to-face time), then Time may become the overriding factor in code selection.

Book: See "Scoring Based on Time or Medical Decision Making (MDM)" on page 318 for information about the current rules for scoring time.

Alert: Do not use time as the basis for an E/M visit to have the patient come back the next day for 'counseling'. There needs to be a reason for a second E/M visit. For example, the patient comes back with imaging from another provider and there needs to be a change in the treatment plan or there is a change in the chief complaint due to another circumstance not discussed in the first encounter.

Tip: It is important to remember that Time (under the 2020 guidelines) can be the over-riding factor **only** when the time spent counseling or coordinating care has taken up 50% (or more) of the face-to-face time spent with the patient, with the remainder spent on performing the three Key Components.

Counseling and Time

The CPT codebook explains that the Time override is frequently used when counseling occurs during the E/M encounter. Counseling is a discussion with the patient and/or family concerning one or more of the following areas:

- Diagnostic results, impressions, and/or recommended diagnostic studies
- Prognosis
- Risks and benefits of management (treatment) options
- Instructions for management (treatment) and/or follow-up
- Importance of compliance with chosen management (treatment) options
- Risk factor reduction
- Patient and family education.

When code selection is determined by Time (and not the three key components), the provider must support this claim with proper documentation. Payers and auditors alike are trained to look for specific documentation elements necessary to support coding based on Time. A summary of what was counseled and/or coordinated with the patient, including terms as listed above, should be well-documented in case the provider needs to support this coding decision at a later date. The appropriate face-to-face time for Office or Other Outpatient E/M codes is as follows:

Figure 5.18

Time Override (2020)	
New Patient	**Established Patient**
99201 - 10 minutes	99211 - 5 minutes
99202 - 20 minutes	99212 - 10 minutes
99203 - 30 minutes	99213 - 15 minutes
99204 - 45 minutes	99214 - 25 minutes
99205 - 60 minutes	99215 - 40 minutes

When Time spent in counseling and coordination of care becomes the deciding factor, because it occupies more than 50% of the total time, simply match the total face-to-face time with the face-to-face time listed above. When documenting Time, the note should include a statement indicating that Time was the overriding factor. An example could be, "I spent 40 minutes face-to-face with the patient and more than 50% of that was spent counseling about the following issues..."

Tip: Some Medicare Advantage Carriers (MACs) require Time spent counseling and/or coordinating care to be documented in the medical record in a specific way. It is smart to know who your MAC is and what their specific Time documentation requirements are.

Suppose the provider entered a patient room at 3:00 PM, gathered a history, performed a physical examination, and as part of the medical decision making process, told the patient he wanted to start her on a new prescription drug that has some associated risks. The provider spent the next 20 minutes (3:10 to 3:30) going over the reasons he wants the patient to take the drug, side effects, restrictions, additional lab testing that will be required to avoid toxicity, and then answered all the patient's questions. The total time was 30 minutes but more than half of that time (20 minutes) was spent in counseling with the patient. The provider could then bill a 99214, based on time alone, even if the key components didn't add up to the level of 99214.

Coding Scenario 2: Current Office E/M Guidelines

This coding scenario uses the Office or Other Outpatient E/M Services guidelines that began in 2021 to score the same new patient encounter in Scenario 1 (not the "Code Selection by Counseling Time (2020 Version)").

Patient SOAP Note Example - Scenario 2

Telehealth Encounter (Audio-Visual): The patient is here for her two-month follow up visit, which is being done live over telemedicine (audio-visual). Consent to perform the encounter via telemedicine was given in writing and is included in the encounter record.

Chief Complaint: Discussion about overall health, comorbid conditions and COVID-19 risk, weight loss, and d upcoming left total knee replacement surgery due to her arthritis.

Subjective: Patient is a 57-year-old Caucasian female, married with 2 children (ages 16 and 18) with history of hypertension, obesity, and is concerned about potential cardiac issues with an upcoming total left knee replacement surgery planned for January (in four months). She is hopeful the surgery will bring relief, as her pain is constant and becomes exacerbated every time she walks. Due to COVID-19, her surgery has been delayed, which will give her some time to lose weight and improve her hypertension. As a CPA, she can work from home and other than trips to the store or to care for her ageing mother who lives alone nearby, her exposure levels are relatively low. She is concerned about her heart health, as she has heard comorbid conditions increase risk of complications from COVID-19 if she were to catch it. She is a nonsmoker, nondrinker, and has been eating more vegetables and protein and reducing carbohydrates. She has lost 13 pounds over the past 3 months. Her main form of exercise is walking on the treadmill but due to her knee pain has been unable to continue. She has a family history of cardiovascular disease and her father died from a heart attack at the age of 72.

Medications: hydrochlorothiazide 12.5 mg a day, Meloxicam 10 mg daily, multivitamin daily, aspirin 81 mg daily, and K2+D3 daily. HEART: Denies chest pain, shortness of breath except when climbing stairs, light-headedness, nausea, vomiting, or diarrhea. Denies current symptoms that could be related to COVID-19 (fever, headache, upper respiratory symptoms, loss of taste). MS (KNEE): Admits to severe osteoarthritis of the left knee, which prevents regular exercise and for which total knee replacement surgery has been put on hold until the pandemic is somewhat controlled. Denies history of diabetes in herself and her family members.

Allergies: No known allergies.

Objective: According to the patient she is 67 inches tall and weighs 187lbs. Other vitals were not checked today due to telehealth encounter. General: No acute distress, alert, and oriented, a little anxious.

Lab/Imaging: EKG last year was normal. The following labs were done last week in preparation for this encounter and reveals a lipid panel including LDL 44, cholesterol 194, triglycerides 118, and A1c 5.1%.

Assessment:
- Hypertension, well controlled on hydrochlorothiazide
- Osteoarthritis, left knee
- Overweight: Patient has recently lost 13 pounds in 3 months
- COVID-19 prevention and discussion

Plan:
- We will send her for a C-reactive protein to check inflammatory processes and determine at that time whether additional intervention needs to take place.
- Continue hydrochlorothiazide; refills provided during today's encounter. Patient will watch stress levels, reduce caffeine intake and try and get 7 hours of sleep.

> - Discussed exercise options, including seated exercises, stretching, and protecting the left knee. Discussed getting adequate protein, reducing all carbohydrates to between 60-90 grams daily, and adding bone broth and collagen to her dietary supplements.
> - COVID-19 Prevention: Keep potentially contaminated objects and body parts out of eyes, nose, and mouth, use of hand cleansers, alcohol wipes and hand sanitizer, public exposure, and other risks discussed to try and prevent exposure while preparing for surgery
> - We will see her back in two weeks with lab results, to review her progress, and discuss her surgery
>
> **Total Time** (with or without direct patient contact): 32 minutes
>
> Provider Signature or attestation statement
> (date and time)

Store: Helpful color *E/M Reference Cards* are available with special bundle packages in the online store.

History: Medically Appropriate

According to the new guidelines for 99202-99215, the physician/QHP has the right to determine what patient history information is considered clinically appropriate based on the patient's complaints and symptoms. As of 2019, ancillary staff (e.g., medical assistant, nurse) may document the patient's history and the physician/QHP may simply review, clarify, or add to it without having to re-document the entire history. For 99202-99215, the amount of history documented from any of the CC, HPI, ROS, and PFSH is entirely left to the clinical judgment of the physician/QHP performing the E/M service.

In this scenario, the provider documented an appropriate history related to the issues the patient wanted to address during this encounter. The physician/QHP has the right to determine the type and quantity of patient history and examination gathered and documented, which helps them eliminate those items that are not pertinent to the immediate evaluation and treatment of the patient and therefore potentially eliminate unnecessary overdocumentation.

Documenting "a medically appropriate history (when performed)" is a vague description, at best. The AMA does not offer any additional advice or interpretation other than specifying that it is up to the physician/QHP to determine what is necessary and appropriate, which begs the question, "What is an inappropriate history?" A physician/QHP should know what information should be documented based on education, training, and medical standards of care related to the presenting condition to provide an accurate diagnosis and safe treatment plan.

Examination: Medically Appropriate

The provider documented an examination that fit within the capabilities of the telemedicine audio-visual encounter and related to those issues being evaluated during this encounter.

The history and examination portions of the E/M Office encounters (99202-99215) are not part of the scoring process for CY 2021 (99202-99215). As such, the physician/QHP can streamline documentation to include only those things necessary for proper treatment and code assignment.

Medical Decision Making OR Total Time

Medical Decision Making

The E/M score for 99202-99215 is determined solely by MDM or all provider time (face to face and other). The guidelines will continue to consider medical necessity as the overarching criteria in combination with the key components when determining the overall level of E/M service reported:

1. **Diagnoses:** The following diagnoses were discussed, evaluated, monitored, or treated during this encounter and therefore may be counted towards the complexity of the E/M service:
   - Hypertension (chronic stable)
   - Osteoarthritis of the left knee (chronic exacerbated)
   - Overweight (BMI 29.3) (chronic, stable)
   - COVID-19 prevention (preventive)
2. **Amount/Complexity of Data:** The provider reviewed three test results (EKG, lipid panel, and A1c) which were not performed during the current encounter and ordered another test (C-reactive protein) which will be reviewed at her follow-up encounter in 2 weeks qualifies this encounter for moderate data.
3. **Risk:** Prescription management (i.e., hydrochlorothiazide) qualifies this encounter for moderate risk.

MDM Score: Moderate = 99214

Diagnoses: Moderate

Data: Moderate

Risk: Moderate

Time

The total time of the encounter was documented at 32 minutes, counting all time the physician/QHP spent in direct patient contact or without direct contact while working on their care. Total time (or Start/Stop) is documented, which qualifies this established E/M service for 99214 (30-39 minutes).

Code Selection

Final E/M Code: 99214 based on MDM and 99214 based on Time

Evaluation and Management Codes

Evaluation and Management codes can only be used by a physician or 'other qualified health care professional.' In this chapter, the acronym QHP is often used for other Qualified Healthcare Professional. Keep in mind that different payers may have different definitions of who is considered a QHP (see Resource 402).

Alert: The RVUs and NCCI edits included here are current as of January 1, 2022. Keep in mind that this information is updated quarterly.

The most current NCCI edits, RVUs, and other code information are available with a FindACode.com subscription.

Coding Conventions

The following coding conventions are used in this procedure section:

Type Styles

CPT code descriptions as listed in the AMA's CPT codebook are in a type style like this.

Explanations added by innoviHealth are in a type style like this.

Code Identifiers

- ●   Identifies a new procedure code
- ▲   Identifies a revised procedure code description
- #   Identifies a re-sequenced code
- +   Identifies CPT add-on codes which describe additional intra-service work associated with the primary procedure.
- ⊘   Identifies codes that are exempt from the use of modifier 51. They are usually performed with another procedure, but may also be performed alone.
- ★   Identifies a code that may be performed via synchronous telemedicine services. For a complete listing, see Appendix C — Telehealth Services.
- ncci   Identifies codes to which NCCI edits apply (see FindACode.com for current NCCI edits.).

Add-on codes mean exactly what the name implies. They indicate that there was an additional service rendered which is related to the primary code. They are always reported after the primary procedure code, are never reported alone, and do not require modifiers (any modifier attached to the primary code automatically applies to the secondary or add-on code). Add-on codes are identified by the plus symbol (+).

For example:

Prolonged service(s) in the outpatient setting requiring direct patient contact beyond the time of the usual service;

★+ 99354   first hour (List separately in addition to code for outpatient Evaluation and Management or psychotherapy service, except with office or other outpatient services [99202, 99203, 99204, 99205, 99212, 99213, 99214, 99215])

★+ 99355   each additional 30 minutes (List separately in addition to the code for prolonged services)

Code 99355 is shown with a "plus" symbol (+), which indicates that in addition to the primary procedure (E/M or psychotherapy), the code listed above it (99354) is considered primary to 99355 and must be reported on a claim before 99355. Be sure to follow the CPT coding instructions for proper usage of these codes (see page 358 for more information on these codes).

RVUs

The RVUs included here are from the 2022 Final Rule, which was the most current information available at the time of publication. Please note that RVUs could be revised prior to January 1st. RVUs differ depending on the location of the service. For the most part, the RVUs listed in this chapter are those for non-facility. If a facility RVU is shown, there is a notation. Complete RVU information is available in FindACode.com (with subscription) and is updated quarterly.

AMA Guidelines

The CPT codebook includes guidelines which explain coding and documentation criteria associated with each individual code. While not presented in this book, Find-A-Code subscribers may view this information online or they may be viewed in the official CPT codebook published by the AMA (available in our online store).

Resource: See Resource 332 for the 1995 E/M documentation guidelines.
Resource: See Resource 333 for the 1997 E/M documentation guidelines.

Patient Status – New or Established

A new patient is one that has not received any face-to-face services from the physician/Qualified Healthcare Professional (QHP) or another provider of the exact same specialty and subspecialty of the same practice, within the last three years. All others are considered an established patient. When a physician/QHP covers for another provider, the patient would be considered the same as if the original provider was available.

For billing purposes, Advanced Practice Registered Nurses (APRNs) and Physician Assistants (PAs) working with providers are considered to be of the same specialty and sub-specialty.

Book: See also "Categories" on page 311 for more information.

Store: See innoviHealth's *Comprehensive Guide to Evaluation & Management* (available in the online store) for more comprehensive information about E/M coding.

Office or Other Outpatient Services

These codes describe the various levels of face-to-face E/M services furnished in the office or other outpatient location, which could include the emergency department (see page 354) or observation services (see page 349) depending on a variety of factors. Services may include counseling and/or coordination of care with other healthcare providers or agencies. See other chapters in this publication for important information on code selection.

Reminder: While History and Examination information is not used to score the level of E/M service for these codes, a medically appropriate history and examination are required to support medical necessity for the service, which is the overarching criteria for the level of E/M service selected.

New Patient

Office or other outpatient visit for the evaluation and management of a new patient, which requires

	CODE	HISTORY	EXAMINATION	COMPLEXITY OF DECISION MAKING	TIME		RVU
★	99202	Medically appropriate	Medically appropriate	Straightforward	15-29	ncci	2.14
★	99203	Medically appropriate	Medically appropriate	Low	30-44	ncci	3.29
★	99204	Medically appropriate	Medically appropriate	Moderate	45-59	ncci	4.90
★	99205	Medically appropriate	Medically appropriate	High	60-74	ncci	6.48

Established Patient

Office or other outpatient visit for the evaluation and management of an established patient, which requires

	CODE	HISTORY	EXAMINATION	COMPLEXITY OF DECISION MAKING	TIME		RVU
▲	99211	no key components are required at this coding level			N/A	ncci	.68
★	99212	Medically appropriate	Medically appropriate	Straightforward	10-19	ncci	1.66
★	99213	Medically appropriate	Medically appropriate	Low	20-29	ncci	2.66
★	99214	Medically appropriate	Medically appropriate	Moderate	30-39	ncci	3.75
★	99215	Medically appropriate	Medically appropriate	High	40-54	ncci	5.29

Prolonged Service: When the provider spends more than the allotted time for a service, prolonged code 99417 or G2212 (depending on payer policy) may be used.

Book: See See "Prolonged E/M Service Codes" on page 316 for more information about these codes.

Note: As of January 1, 2022, the words "Usually, the presenting problem(s) are minimal" were removed from code 99211. This change more closely aligns the description with the key components for that level of service.

Modifier Tips

Modifier 22: Modifier 22 is often incorrectly applied to E/M services and thus denied by payers. Only report modifier 22 with surgical procedure codes.

Modifier 25 for E/M Services: When E/M services are "significant and separately identifiable" they should be billed with modifier 25 appended to the appropriate E/M code. Significant, separately identifiable encounters could include new patients, established patients with a problem unrelated to the diagnosis for the global period they are in, a new problem or injury, exacerbations, counseling, etc.

Book: See Appendix B — Modifiers for a comprehensive listing of modifiers.

Hospital Observation Services

A patient evaluated in the Emergency Department (ED) may be too ill to go home, but not ill enough to require admission as an inpatient and are therefore admitted for observation. Observation allows the patient to continue receiving care and treatment until they are either determined stable enough for release or they need inpatient admission for additional evaluation and treatment. Because the patient in observation hasn't been formally admitted as an inpatient, services rendered to a patient in "observation status" are reported with Observation Care codes. Patients in observation may be located anywhere in the hospital (including the ED).

Do not report Observation Care codes for postoperative recovery services where an outpatient surgical patient is placed under observation during a difficult postoperative recovery. These services are considered part of the global surgical package.

ONLY the _provider or department who admitted the patient for observation_ should report Hospital Observation Services codes. All other providers performing E/M services for a patient in observation should report a code using Office or Other Outpatient E/M service codes.

Note: The RVUs included here for "Hospital Observation Services" are the facility RVUs.

Note: These codes are scheduled for revision in 2023.

Resource: See Resource 819 and search on "midnights rule" for additional information on these services.

OBSERVATION CARE DISCHARGE SERVICES

Code	Description		RVU
99217	Observation care discharge day management (This code is to be utilized to report all services provided to a patient on discharge from outpatient hospital "observation status" if the discharge is on **other than the initial date of "observation status."** To report services to a patient designated as "observation status" or "inpatient status" and discharged on the same date, use the codes for Observation or Inpatient Care Services [including Admission and Discharge Services, 99234-99236 as appropriate.])	ncci	2.07

Report this code for discharge services performed on a day other than the initial date of observation. For same day Observation Admission/Discharge services see codes 99234-99236.

INITIAL OBSERVATION CARE

Initial observation care codes are only reported for a patient placed in observation who remains there overnight. These codes should NOT be reported if a patient is placed in observation and discharged on the same day (see Observation or Inpatient Care Services [including admission and discharge services] codes 99234-99236).

Time includes face-to-face time at the patient's bedside as well as unit/floor time. There are specific rules that apply to these codes, both for E/M services performed by the initiating provider (in their office or elsewhere) and if these patients are, after observation, admitted as an inpatient. See a current CPT codebook or FindACode.com for complete information.

New or Established Patient

Initial observation care, per day, for the evaluation and management of a patient which requires

		Key Component Code Selection - 3 of 3			Average Intra-Service Time		
CODE	SEVERITY OF PROBLEM	HISTORY	EXAMINATION	COMPLEXITY OF DECISION MAKING	COUNSELING OVERRIDE		RVU
99218	Low	Detailed	Detailed	Straightforward or Low	30	ncci	2.83
99219	Moderate	Comprehensive	Comprehensive	Moderate	50	ncci	3.83
99220	High	Comprehensive	Comprehensive	High	70	ncci	5.17

SUBSEQUENT OBSERVATION CARE

These services include reviewing medical records, results of diagnostic tests, and evaluating any changes to the patient status since the last visit by the provider.

Subsequent observation care, per day, for the evaluation and management of a patient, which requires

Key Component Code Selection - 2 of 3

CODE	SEVERITY OF PROBLEM	HISTORY	EXAMINATION	COMPLEXITY OF DECISION MAKING	Average Intra-Service Time COUNSELING OVERRIDE		RVU
# 99224	Stable	Focused	Focused	Straightforward or Low	15	ncci	1.13
# 99225	Minor Complication	Expanded	Expanded	Moderate	25	ncci	2.05
# 99226	Unstable Significant complication Significant new problem	Detailed	Detailed	High	35	ncci	2.92

Hospital Inpatient Services

These services are provided in an inpatient setting which includes partial hospitalizations. Intra-service time includes reviewing medical records, diagnostic tests, and documenting any changes to the patient's status since the previous provider visit. Note that time includes face-to-face time at the patient bedside as well as unit/floor time. Inpatient admissions are reported using initial hospital care service codes. See "Time" on page 318 for more about counting time.

Note: The RVUs included here for these services are the facility RVUs.

Note: These codes are scheduled for revision in 2023.

INITIAL HOSPITAL CARE

New or Established Patient

Initial hospital care, per day, for the evaluation and management of a patient. Counseling and/or coordination of care with other physicians, other qualified health care professionals, or agencies are provided consistent with the nature of the problem(s) and the patient's and/or family's needs.

Key Component Code Selection - 3 of 3

CODE	SEVERITY OF PROBLEM	HISTORY	EXAMINATION	COMPLEXITY OF DECISION MAKING	Average Intra-Service Time COUNSELING OVERRIDE		RVU
99221	Low	Detailed	Detailed	Straightforward or Low	30	ncci	2.91
99222	Moderate	Comprehensive	Comprehensive	Moderate	50	ncci	3.91
99223	High	Comprehensive	Comprehensive	High	70	ncci	5.73

SUBSEQUENT HOSPITAL CARE

According to CPT guidelines (emphasis added), "All levels of subsequent hospital care include reviewing the medical record and reviewing the results of diagnostic studies and changes in the patient's status (ie, changes in history, physical condition and response to management) *since the last assessment*."

This interval history is vital to the determination of the code level.

Subsequent hospital care, per day, for the evaluation and management of a patient. Counseling and/or coordination of care with other physicians, other qualified health care professionals, or agencies are provided consistent with the nature of the problem(s) and the patient's and/or family's needs.

CODE	SEVERITY OF PROBLEM	HISTORY	EXAMINATION	COMPLEXITY OF DECISION MAKING	Average Intra-Service Time / COUNSELING OVERRIDE		RVU
★99231	Stable	Focused	Focused	Straightforward or Low	15	ncci	1.12
★99232	Minor Complication	Expanded	Expanded	Moderate	25	ncci	2.06
★99233	Unstable / Significant complication / Significant new problem	Detailed	Detailed	High	35	ncci	2.96

OBSERVATION OR INPATIENT CARE SERVICES (INCLUDING ADMISSION AND DISCHARGE SERVICES

These codes are used when the patient is admitted and discharged on the same day from either observation or inpatient status.

Special instructions apply. See a current CPT codebook or FindACode.com for the full information.

CODE	SEVERITY OF PROBLEM	HISTORY	EXAMINATION	COMPLEXITY OF DECISION MAKING	Average Intra-Service Time / COUNSELING OVERRIDE		RVU
99234	Low	Detailed	Detailed	Straightforward or Low	40	ncci	3.77
99235	Moderate	Comprehensive	Comprehensive	Moderate	50	ncci	4.78
99236	High	Comprehensive	Comprehensive	High	55	ncci	6.12

HOSPITAL DISCHARGE SERVICES

These codes are used to report inpatient hospital discharge services on a day other than the date of admission. Code selection is determined by the total face-to-face time spent with the patient performing final hospital discharge services.

Intra-service includes final exam, continuing care instructions, prescriptions, etc. If the same provider performs a subsequent inpatient or observation E/M service on the same date as the discharge, only the discharge should be reported. If another provider performs concurrent care on the discharge date, report those services with 99231-99233. When the discharge occurs on the same say as the admission, see codes 99234-99236.

	Hospital discharge day management;		RVU
99238	30 minutes or less	ncci	2.08
99239	more than 30 minutes	ncci	3.04

Consultations

When another physician, or appropriate source (see "Note" below), requests an evaluation and management service to recommend care, or decide who should provide ongoing management for a specific condition or problem, it is known as a consultation. However, the consulting healthcare provider may provide services at the same or a subsequent encounter.

Consultations must be initiated by an appropriate source in order for these codes to apply. See "Note 1" below for some appropriate sources. If the consult is requested by a patient or their family members, consultation service codes would not apply but rather an applicable E/M service code is to be reported from the office (99202-99215), inpatient (99221-99233), domiciliary/rest home (99324-99337), or home care (99341-99350) categories.

Consultations must be supported by a documented request from the appropriate source and a written report created by the consulting healthcare provider which is sent to the requesting source. The consultant's opinion and services provided should also be documented. Be sure that documentation clearly states that this is a consultation by Dr. X with Dr. Y to evaluate a specific condition. Otherwise, it could be inferred that this is a referral which *could* be interpreted by the payer to be a transfer of care.

If the consultation meets the criteria for modifier 32 "Mandated services," append it to the consultation code. Any other service provided on or after the date of the consultation should be reported separately.

If the consultant assumes care for the patient after the consultation is complete (also referred to as a transfer of care), then the typical E/M codes would apply for subsequent encounters (e.g., office or outpatient).

Note 1: Patient/Family requests for a consultation are billed with office/outpatient E/M codes 99202-99215 – not these consultation codes.

Additional instructions apply. See a current CPT codebook or FindACode.com for the full information.

Note 2: These codes are scheduled for revision in 2023.

Alert: Medicare, and some other payers, no longer pay for consultation service codes 99241-99245. Before submitting claims with these codes, check your contracted payer policies to verify coverage.

Note: Consultation codes are different from other primary E/M services in that there must be a written report and there must be a request from an appropriate source documented in the patient file. Appropriate sources other than a physician could include:

physician assistant	occupational therapist	insurance company
nurse practitioner	healthcare agencies	other non-physician health care
employers	lawyers	providers

OFFICE OR OTHER OUTPATIENT CONSULTATIONS

New or Established Patient

These E/M service codes are reported when there is a request for the consulting provider's opinion or advice and that consultation takes place in an outpatient or ambulatory setting (e.g., home, hospital observation. Follow-up visits initiated by either the consulting provider or patient would be billed as an established patient visit (99211-99215, 99334-99337, 99347-99350). This also applies when there is a transfer of care (i.e., where a provider assumes care for the patient either before or after an initial consultation).

Counseling and/or coordination of care with other physicians, other qualified health care professionals, or agencies are provided consistent with the nature of the problem(s) and the patient's and/or family's needs.

Office consultation for a new or established patient, typically face-to-face with the patient and/or family.

		Key Component Code Selection - 3 of 3			Average Intra-Service Time		
CODE	SEVERITY OF PROBLEM	HISTORY	EXAMINATION	COMPLEXITY OF DECISION MAKING	COUNSELING OVERRIDE		RVU
★99241	Minor	Focused	Focused	Straightforward	10	ncci	1.35
★99242	Low	Expanded	Expanded	Straightforward	30	ncci	2.55
★99243	Moderate	Detailed	Detailed	Low	40	ncci	3.51
★99244	Moderate to High	Comprehensive	Comprehensive	Moderate	60	ncci	5.23
★99245	Moderate to High	Comprehensive	Comprehensive	High	80	ncci	6.38

INPATIENT CONSULTATIONS

New or Established Patient

For confirmatory consultation (where one physician confirms the opinion of another physician), see the appropriate E/M service code for the setting and type of service (e.g., consultation).

Counseling and/or coordination of care with other physicians, other qualified health care professionals, or agencies are provided consistent with the nature of the problem(s) and the patient's and/or family's needs.

Inpatient consultation for a new or established patient, at the bedside and on the patient's hospital floor or unit.

		Key Component Code Selection - 3 of 3			Average Intra-Service Time		
CODE	SEVERITY OF PROBLEM	HISTORY	EXAMINATION	COMPLEXITY OF DECISION MAKING	COUNSELING OVERRIDE		RVU
★99251	Self Limited or Minor	Focused	Focused	Straightforward	20	ncci	1.41
★99252	Low	Expanded	Expanded	Straightforward	40	ncci	2.13
★99253	Moderate	Detailed	Detailed	Low	55	ncci	3.31
★99254	Moderate to High	Comprehensive	Comprehensive	Moderate	80	ncci	4.77
★99255	Moderate to High	Comprehensive	Comprehensive	High	110	ncci	5.77

Note: The RVUs included here for codes 99251-99255 are the facility RVUs.

Emergency Department Services

These services are provided in an emergency department providing 24 hour access. For critical care services, see 99291 and 99292. For observation care, see 99217-99220 and 99234-99236.

Note: The RVUs included here for these services are the facility RVUs.

Note: These codes are scheduled for revision in 2023.

New or Established Patient

Counseling and/or coordination of care with other physicians, other qualified health care professionals, or agencies are provided consistent with the nature of the problem(s) and the patient's and/or family's needs.

Emergency department visit for the evaluation and management of a patient.

		Key Component Code Selection - 3 of 3			Average Intra-Service Time		
CODE	SEVERITY OF PROBLEM	HISTORY	EXAMINATION	COMPLEXITY OF DECISION MAKING	COUNSELING OVERRIDE		RVU
99281	Minor	Focused	Focused	Straightforward	NE	ncci	.64
99282	Low to Moderate	Expanded	Expanded	Low	NE	ncci	1.24
99283	Moderate	Expanded	Expanded	Moderate	NE	ncci	2.11
99284	High	Detailed	Detailed	Moderate	NE	ncci	3.56
99285	High, Immed. Threat	Comprehensive	Comprehensive	High	NE	ncci	5.17

Other Emergency Services

Special instructions apply. See a current CPT codebook or FindACode.com for the full information.

			RVU
99288	Physician or other qualified health care professional direction of emergency medical systems (EMS) emergency care, advanced life support	ncci	NE

Critical Care Services

Critical Care services (CCS) are only provided to patients in the inpatient setting (e.g., coronary care unit) who have a "high probability of imminent or life threatening deterioration."

According to CMS, "critical care services encompass both treatment of 'vital organ failure' and 'prevention of further life threatening deterioration of the patient's condition.' Although critical care may be delivered in a moment of crisis or upon being called to the patient's bedside urgently, this is not a requirement for providing critical care service. The treatment and management of the patient's condition, while not necessarily emergent, shall be required based on the threat of imminent deterioration (i.e., the patient shall be critically ill or injured at the time of the physician's visit)."

When rendered by the physician performing critical care services, the following services are considered included (bundled) and not separately billable: 36000, 36410, 36415, 36591, 36600, 43752, 43753, 71045, 71046, 92953, 93561, 93562, 94002-94004, 94660, 94662, 94760-94762.

When counting time, remember that the provider(s) must be *immediately* available to the patient so do **not** count time spent performing activities (e.g., phone calls taken at the office) that occur outside the unit or away from the floor or in activities not contributing to treatment (e.g., meetings). The documentation must attest to the provider giving full attention to the patient during the documented time period.

Special instructions apply. See a current CPT codebook or FindACode.com for the full information.

Alert: Medicare has revised their rules, beginning in 2022, regarding the reporting of these services. See Resource 64A for more information.

Resource: See Resource 352 to review Section 30.6.12 of the *Medicare Claims Processing Manual* for additional guidance by CMS.

Coding Examples

Total Duration of Prolonged Services	Code(s)
less than 30 minutes	appropriate E/M codes
30-74 minutes (30 minutes - 1 hr. 14 min.)	99291 X 1
75-104 minutes (1 hr. 15 min. - 1 hr. 44 min.)	99291 X 1 AND 99292 X 1
105-134 minutes (1 hr. 45 min. - 2 hr. 14 min.)	99291 X 1 AND 99295 X 2
135-164 minutes (2 hr. 15 min. - 2 hr. 44 min.)	99291 X 1 AND 99292 X 3
165-194 minutes (2 hr. 45 min. - 3 hr. 14 min.)	99291 X 1 AND 99292 X 4

Critical care, evaluation and management of the critically ill or critically injured patient; **RVU**

- 99291   first 30-74 minutes   ncci   8.16
- + 99292   each additional 30 minutes (List separately in addition to code for primary service)   ncci   3.56

Note: The RVUs included here for codes 99291 and 99292 are the facility RVUs. For non-facility RVUs and other important fee information, see FindACode.com.

Nursing Facility Services

These services are E/M visits rendered to patients in nursing facilities, whether they be intermediate or long term. They are also used for psychiatric residential treatment centers which provide 24 hour care. When rendered, other services such as psychotherapy may also be reported in addition to these codes.

Providers should oversee the multi-disciplinary care plan. For care plan oversight services only, see 99379-99380.

Medicare requires providers to monitor and evaluate residents at least once every 30 days for the first 90 days after admission and at least once every 60 days thereafter.

Special instructions apply. See a current CPT codebook or FindACode.com for the full information.

Note: These codes are scheduled for revision in 2023.

Tip: Services codes represent a "per day" service and are typically only covered once per day.

INITIAL NURSING FACILITY CARE

New or Established Patient

Counseling and/or coordination of care with other physicians, other qualified health care professionals, or agencies are provided consistent with the nature of the problem(s) and the patient's and/or family's needs.

Initial nursing facility care, per day, at the bedside and on the patient's facility floor or unit.

CODE	SEVERITY OF PROBLEM	HISTORY	EXAMINATION	COMPLEXITY OF DECISION MAKING	COUNSELING OVERRIDE	Average Intra-Service Time		RVU
99304	Low	Detailed	Detailed	Straightfwd or Low	25		ncci	2.57
99305	Moderate	Comprehensive	Comprehensive	Moderate	35		ncci	3.71
99306	High	Comprehensive	Comprehensive	High	45		ncci	4.76

SUBSEQUENT NURSING FACILITY CARE

These per day services include reviewing medical records, results of diagnostic tests, and changes in the patient's status, including psychosocial factors, since the last provider visit.

Counseling and/or coordination of care with other physicians, other qualified health care professionals, or agencies are provided consistent with the nature of the problem(s) and the patient's and/or family's needs.

Subsequent nursing facility care, per day, at the bedside and on the patient's facility floor or unit.

		Key Component Code Selection - 2 of 3			Average Intra-Service Time		
CODE	SEVERITY OF PROBLEM	INTERVAL HISTORY	EXAMINATION	COMPLEXITY OF DECISION MAKING	COUNSELING OVERRIDE		RVU
★99307	Stable	Focused	Focused	Straightforward	10	ncci	1.26
★99308	Minor Complication	Expanded	Expanded	Low	15	ncci	1.99
★99309	Significant complication Significant new problem	Detailed	Detailed	Moderate	25	ncci	2.62
★99310	Unstable Significant complication Significant new problem	Comprehensive	Comprehensive	High	35	ncci	3.86

NURSING FACILITY DISCHARGE SERVICES

These services include the total time (non-continuous) spent discharging the patient from a nursing facility. Providing after care instructions must be face-to-face with the patient. Report the day of the actual provider visit even if the final discharge date differs. Medicare also allows these codes to be used for a patient who expires when the provider is the one who performed the death pronouncement.

	Nursing facility discharge day management;		RVU
99315	30 minutes or less	ncci	2.09
99316	more than 30 minutes	ncci	2.99

OTHER NURSING FACILITY SERVICES

For Medicare, this code may be used in lieu of a subsequent visit to report an annual nursing facility assessment visit on the required schedule of visits on an annual basis. It should not be billed with other nursing facility codes on the same day.

Evaluation and management of a patient involving an annual nursing facility assessment

		Key Component Code Selection - 3 of 3			Average Intra-Service Time		
CODE	SEVERITY OF PROBLEM	INTERVAL HISTORY	EXAMINATION	COMPLEXITY OF DECISION MAKING	COUNSELING OVERRIDE		RVU
99318	Stable	Detailed	Comprehensive	Low to Moderate	30	ncci	2.75

Domiciliary, Rest Home (eg, Boarding Home), or Custodial Care Services

Use these codes to report E/M services provided to patients residing in long-term care facilities which provide room, board, and personal services, but not necessarily medical services (e.g., assisted living facility, group home, custodial care, and intermediate care facilities).

Note: These codes are scheduled for revision in 2023.

Counseling and/or coordination of care with other physicians, other qualified health care professionals, or agencies are provided consistent with the nature of the problem(s) and the patient's and/or family's needs.

New Patient

Domiciliary or rest home visit for the evaluation and management of a new patient, with the patient and/or family or caregiver.

		Key Component Code Selection - 3 of 3			Average Intra-Service Time Counseling Override		RVU
CODE	SEVERITY OF PROBLEM	HISTORY	EXAMINATION	COMPLEXITY OF DECISION MAKING			
99324	Low	Focused	Focused	Straightforward	20	ncci	1.56
99325	Moderate	Expanded	Expanded	Low	30	ncci	2.28
99326	Moderate to High	Detailed	Detailed	Moderate	45	ncci	3.95
99327	High	Comprehensive	Comprehensive	Moderate	60	ncci	5.32
99328	Unstable / Significant complication / Significant new problem	Comprehensive	Comprehensive	High	75	ncci	6.26

Established Patient

Domiciliary or rest home visit for the evaluation and management of an established patient, with the patient and/or family or caregiver.

		Key Component Code Selection - 2 of 3			Average Intra-Service Time Counseling Override		RVU
CODE	SEVERITY OF PROBLEM	HISTORY	EXAMINATION	COMPLEXITY OF DECISION MAKING			
99334	Minor	Focused	Focused	Straightforward	15	ncci	1.75
99335	Low to Moderate	Expanded	Expanded	Low	25	ncci	2.75
99336	Moderate to High	Detailed	Detailed	Moderate	40	ncci	3.89
99337	Moderate to High	Comprehensive	Comprehensive	Moderate to High	60	ncci	5.57

Domiciliary, Rest Home (eg, Assisted Living Facility), or Home Care Plan Oversight Services

Special instructions apply. See a current CPT codebook or FindACode.com for the full information.

Note: These codes are scheduled for revision in 2023.

Individual physician supervision of a patient (patient not present) in home, domiciliary or rest home (eg, assisted living facility) requiring complex and multidisciplinary care modalities involving regular physician development and/or revision of care plans, review of subsequent reports of patient status, review of related laboratory and other studies, communication (including telephone calls) for purposes of assessment or care decisions with health care professional(s), family member(s), surrogate decision maker(s) (eg, legal guardian) and/or key caregiver(s) involved in patient's care, integration of new information into the medical treatment plan and/or adjustment of medical therapy, within a calendar month;

Code	Description		RVU
99339	15-29 minutes	ncci	2.22
99340	30 minutes or more	ncci	3.11

Home Services

The CPT codebook defines home as "a private residence, temporary lodging, or short term accommodation (eg, hotel, campground, hostel, or cruise ship)."

Note: These codes are scheduled for revision in 2023.

Counseling and/or coordination of care with other physicians, other qualified health care professionals, or agencies are provided consistent with the nature of the problem(s) and the patient's and/or family's needs.

New Patient

Home visit for the evaluation and management of a new patient, typically face-to-face with the patient and/or family.

		Key Component Code Selection - 3 of 3			Average Intra-Service Time		
CODE	SEVERITY OF PROBLEM	HISTORY	EXAMINATION	COMPLEXITY OF DECISION MAKING	COUNSELING OVERRIDE		RVU
99341	Low	Focused	Focused	Straightforward	20	ncci	1.56
99342	Moderate	Expanded	Expanded	Low	30	ncci	2.22
99343	Moderate to High	Detailed	Detailed	Moderate	45	ncci	3.61
99344	High	Comprehensive	Comprehensive	Moderate	60	ncci	5.20
99345	Unstable Significant complication Significant new problem	Comprehensive	Comprehensive	High	75	ncci	6.30

Established Patient

Home visit for the evaluation and management of an established patient, typically face-to-face with the patient and/or family.

		Key Component Code Selection - 2 of 3			Average Intra-Service Time		
CODE	SEVERITY OF PROBLEM	INTERVAL HISTORY	EXAMINATION	COMPLEXITY OF DECISION MAKING	COUNSELING OVERRIDE		RVU
99347	Minor	Focused	Focused	Straightforward	15	ncci	1.58
99348	Low to Moderate	Expanded	Expanded	Low	25	ncci	2.40
99349	Moderate to High	Detailed	Detailed	Moderate	40	ncci	3.70
99350	Moderate to High	Comprehensive	Comprehensive	Moderate to High	60	ncci	5.13

Prolonged Services

Alert: There are significant changes to the codes and guidelines for 2021. See See also "Prolonged E/M Service Codes" on page 316 and innoviHealth's *Comprehensive Evaluation & Management* publication (available in the online store) for more information on these services.

Notes:

- Codes 99354 and 99355 were revised in 2021.
- In 2018, CMS added codes G0513 and G0514 for prolonged preventive services in an office or other outpatient setting. Be aware of individual payer requirements.

PROLONGED SERVICE WITH DIRECT PATIENT CONTACT

Prolonged services are those services provided beyond the usual services rendered by a physician or QHP. They are for direct patient contact (both face-to-face and floor/unit of the hospital or nursing facility) and are reported in addition to the primary procedure (i.e., **non-office** E/M service, psychotherapy [90837, 90847]).

Special instructions apply. See a current CPT codebook or FindACode.com for the full information.

Alert: Do NOT use with Office or Other Outpatient Services (99202-99215). See "Prolonged Service With or Without Direct Patient Contact on the Date of an Office or Other Outpatient Service" on page 360.

Resource: See Resource 648 for additional information on properly coding these services.

Example

Total Duration of Prolonged Services	Code(s)
less than 30 minutes	Not reported separately
30-74 minutes (30 minutes - 1 hr. 14 min.)	99356 X 1
75-104 minutes (1 hr. 15 min. - 1 hr. 44 min.)	99356 X 1 AND 99357 X 1
105 or more (1 hr. 45 min. or more)	99356 X 1 AND 99357 X 2 or more for each additional 30 minutes

				RVU
★+	99354	Prolonged service(s) in the outpatient setting requiring direct patient contact beyond the time of the usual service; (List separately in addition to code for outpatient Evaluation and Management or psychotherapy service, except with office or other outpatient services [99202, 99203, 99204, 99205, 99212, 99213, 99214, 99215])	ncci	3.71
★+	99355	each additional 30 minutes (List separately in addition to code for prolonged service)	ncci	2.68

These codes can be used together (or in conjunction with each other). 99354 is an add-on code for 90837, 90847, 99241-99245, 99324-99337, 99341-99350, 99483. Do not use 99354 or 99355 with 99202-99205, 99211-99215, 99415-99417.

+	99356	Prolonged service in the inpatient or observation setting, requiring unit/floor time beyond the usual service; first hour (List separately in addition to code for inpatient or observation Evaluation and Management service)	ncci	2.61
+	99357	each additional 30 minutes (List separately in addition to code for prolonged service)	ncci	2.62

Alert: The RVUs for 99356 and 99357 are the facility RVUs.

PROLONGED SERVICE WITHOUT DIRECT PATIENT CONTACT

Prolonged services are those services provided beyond the usual services provided by a physician or QHP.

Do not use for team conferences, online evaluations, or in place of more specific codes with no time limit. May be used with some non-face-to-face services like medical team conferences. If unsure on usage, check the NCCI edits available by subscription to FindACode.com.

MLN Matters Article MM9905 provides the following guidance: "1) that these codes can only be used to report extended qualifying time of the billing physician or other practitioner (not clinical staff); and 2) Prolonged services cannot be reported in association with a companion E/M code that also qualifies as the initiating visit for CCM services. Practitioners should instead report the add-on code for CCM initiation, if applicable."

Special instructions apply. See a current CPT codebook or FindACode.com for the full information.

Alert: For office or other outpatient services, do NOT use these codes. See "Prolonged Service With or Without Direct Patient Contact on the Date of an Office or Other Outpatient Service" on page 360.

	Prolonged evaluation and management service before and/or after direct patient care;		
99358	first hour	ncci	3.20
+ 99359	each additional 30 minutes (List separately in addition to code for prolonged service)	ncci	1.56

99359 is an add on code for 99358 and may be used in conjunction with other non-face-to-face services which have a time limit (e.g., telephone services.)

Do not report these services in the same month as 99484, 99487-99489, 99490-99494 or with 99495 or 99496.

Do not report these services with any of the following: 99339, 99340, 99374-99380, 99491, 93792, 93793, 99466-99452, 99366-99368, 99421-99423.

Total Duration of Prolonged Services Without Direct Face-to-Face Contact	Code(s)
less than 30 minutes	Not reported separately
30-74 minutes (30 minutes - 1 hr. 14 min.)	99358 X 1
75-104 minutes (1 hr. 15 min. - 1 hr. 44 min.)	99358 X 1 AND 99359 X 1
105 or more (1 hr. 45 min. or more)	99358 X 1 AND 99359 X 2 or more for each additional 30 min

PROLONGED CLINICAL STAFF SERVICES WITH PHYSICIAN OR OTHER QUALIFIED HEALTHCARE PROFESSIONAL SUPERVISION

Prolonged E/M services by clinical staff (e.g., those services beyond the usual face-to-face time E/M service listed) can be coded with 99415 or 99416. They may ONLY be reported with outpatient services (99202-99215).

Special instructions apply. See a current CPT codebook or FindACode.com for the full information.

Prolonged clinical staff service (the service beyond the highest time in the range of total time of the service) during an evaluation and management service in the office or outpatient setting, direct patient contact with physician supervision;   **RVU**

#+ 99415   first hour (List separately in addition to code for outpatient Evaluation and Management service)   ncci   .30

#+ 99416   each additional 30 minutes (List separately in addition to code for prolonged service)   ncci   .17

99416 is an-add on code for 99415.

Do not bill either of these codes with 99354, 99355, 99417, or G2212.

PROLONGED SERVICE WITH OR WITHOUT DIRECT PATIENT CONTACT ON THE DATE OF AN OFFICE OR OTHER OUTPATIENT SERVICE

This new code may only be used in conjunction with 99205 and 99215 when the combined time with and without direct patient on the date of the E/M service exceeds the highest level of service (i.e., 74 minutes for 99205, 54 minutes for 99215). There must be at least 15 minutes to report this code.

Alert: As of January 1, 2021, CMS requires code G2212 instead of 99417 due to potential issues of fraud and abuse. While both codes are valued the same, the Medicare Physician Fee Schedule has reduced the RVU of 99417 to 0.00 indicating that code 99417 will not be paid.

Book: See "Prolonged E/M Service Codes" on page 316 for more important information about properly reporting these services.

Special instructions apply. See a current CPT codebook or FindACode.com for the full information.

Note: In 2018, CMS added codes G0513 and G0514 for prolonged *preventive* services in an office or other outpatient setting. Be aware of individual payer requirements.

★#+ 99417   Prolonged office or other outpatient evaluation and management service(s) beyond the **minimum** required time of the primary procedure which has been selected using total time, requiring total time with or without direct patient contact beyond the usual service, on the date of the primary service, each 15 minutes of total time (List separately in addition to codes 99205, 99215 for office or other outpatient Evaluation and Management services)   .66

			RVU
★+	G2212	Prolonged office or other outpatient evaluation and management service(s) beyond the **maximum** required time of the primary procedure which has been selected using total time on the date of the primary service; each additional 15 minutes by the physician or qualified healthcare professional, with or without direct patient contact (list separately in addition to cpt codes 99205, 99215 for office or other outpatient evaluation and management services) (do not report g2212 on the same date of service as 99354, 99355, 99358, 99359, 99415, 99416). (do not report g2212 for any time unit less than 15 minutes)	.96

STANDBY SERVICES

Do not use these codes to report hospital on-call services (99026, 99027) or with 99464. However, it may be reported with codes 99460 or 99465 where appropriate.

Alert: The RVU included here for code 99360 is the facility RVU.

Special instructions apply. See a current CPT codebook or FindACode.com for the full information.

99360	Standby service, requiring prolonged attendance, each 30 minutes (eg, operative standby, standby for frozen section, for cesarean/high risk delivery, for monitoring EEG)	ncci	1.76

Case Management Services

Management services are provided by the physician or QHP who is responsible for initiating, supervising, and coordinating the direct care of the patient as well as other healthcare services the patient may need.

Special instructions apply to each of the following categories. See a current CPT codebook or FindACode.com for the full information.

Alert: Anticoagulant Management codes 99363 and 99364 are deleted as of 2018. Report with codes 93792, 93793.

MEDICAL TEAM CONFERENCES

These services require at least three participating QHPs. Each are from different specialties and each provide direct patient care. The conference may also include other participants who are actively involved in the patient's care (e.g., patient, family member(s), caregivers, community agencies).

When there is more than one QHP of the same specialty, only one may bill the conference encounter.

Services of less than 30 minutes may not be reported.

Special instructions apply. See a current CPT codebook or FindACode.com for the full information.

Medical Team Conference, Direct (Face-to-Face) Contact With Patient and/or Family

99366	**Medical team conference** with interdisciplinary team of health care professionals, face-to-face with patient and/or family, 30 minutes or more, participation by nonphysician qualified health care professional	ncci	1.25

Medical Team Conference, Without Direct (Face-to-Face) Contact With Patient and/or Family

Medical team conference with interdisciplinary team of health care professionals, patient and/or family not present, 30 minutes or more;

99367	participation by physician	ncci	1.62
99368	participation by nonphysician qualified health care professional	ncci	1.07

Do not report codes 99367-99368 during the same month as 99424-99427, 99437, 99439, 99487, 99489, 99490, or 99491.

Note: The RVUs included here for codes 99367 and 99368 are for facility use only. There are no non-facility RVUs.

Care Plan Oversight Services

Services provided within a 30-day period.

Special instructions apply. See a current CPT codebook or FindACode.com for the full information.

Supervision of a patient under care of **home health agency** (patient not present) in home, domiciliary or equivalent environment (eg, Alzheimer's facility) requiring complex and multidisciplinary care modalities involving regular development and/or revision of care plans by that individual, review of subsequent reports of patient status, review of laboratory and other studies, communication (including telephone calls) for purposes of assessment or care decisions with other health care professional(s), family member(s), surrogate decision maker(s), (eg, legal guardian) and/or key caregiver(s) involved in patient's care, integration of new information into the medical treatment plan and/or adjustment of medical therapy, within a calendar month;

RVU

Code	Description		
99374	15-29 minutes	ncci	2.01
99375	30 minutes or more	ncci	2.99

Supervision of a **hospice** patient (patient not present) requiring complex and multidisciplinary care modalities involving regular development and/or revision of care plans by that individual, review of subsequent reports of patient status, review of related laboratory and other studies, communication (including telephone calls) for purposes of assessment or care decisions with health care professional(s), family member(s), surrogate decision maker(s), (eg, legal guardian) and/or key caregiver(s) involved in patient's care, integration of new information into the medical treatment plan and/or adjustment of medical therapy, within a calendar month;

Code	Description		
99377	15-29 minutes	ncci	2.01
99378	30 minutes or more	ncci	2.99

Supervision of a **nursing facility** patient (patient not present) requiring complex and multidisciplinary care modalities involving regular development and/or revision of care plans by that individual, review of subsequent reports of patient status, review of related laboratory and other studies, communication (including telephone calls) for purposes of assessment or care decisions with health care professional(s), family member(s), surrogate decision maker(s), (eg, legal guardian) and/or key caregiver(s) involved in patient's care, integration of new information into the medical treatment plan and/or adjustment of medical therapy, within a calendar month;

Code	Description		
99379	15-29 minutes	ncci	2.01
99380	30 minutes or more	ncci	2.99

Preventive Medicine Services (Wellness)

This section of the CPT code set is also known as the **health and wellness codes.** These codes are appropriate expressions of annual (initial or periodic) health and wellness encounters for infants, children, adolescents, and adults. The Patient Protection and Affordable Care Act now requires many preventive services to be covered without co-payments, co-insurance, or meeting deductibles.

Resource: See Resource 339 for additional information about preventive services covered by the Affordable Care Act.

Wellness-oriented practices will want to use these codes when appropriate to record the status and growth of these important health promotion services. It will provide valuable management data on the growth of wellness services.

Behavior change interventions should be reported with codes 99406-99409.

For vaccine risk/benefit counseling, see "Immunization Administration for Vaccines/Toxoids" (e.g., 90460, 0001A).

Special instructions apply. See a current CPT codebook or FindACode.com for the full information.

NEW PATIENT

Initial comprehensive preventive medicine evaluation and management of an individual including an age and gender appropriate history, examination, counseling/anticipatory guidance/risk factor reduction interventions, and the ordering of laboratory/diagnostic procedures, new patient; **RVU**

Code	Description		
99381	infant (age under 1 year)	ncci	3.21
99382	early childhood (age 1 through 4 years)	ncci	3.35
99383	late childhood (age 5 through 11 years)	ncci	3.48
99384	adolescent (age 12 through 17 years)	ncci	3.96
99385	18-39 years	ncci	3.84
99386	40-64 years	ncci	4.44
99387	65 years and over	ncci	4.80

ESTABLISHED PATIENT

Periodic comprehensive preventive medicine reevaluation and management of an individual including an age and gender appropriate history, examination, counseling/anticipatory guidance/risk factor reduction interventions, and the ordering of laboratory/diagnostic procedures, established patient;

Code	Description		
99391	infant (age under 1 year)	ncci	2.90
99392	early childhood (age 1 through 4 years)	ncci	3.08
99393	late childhood (age 5 through 11 years)	ncci	3.07
99394	adolescent (age 12 through 17 years)	ncci	3.36
99395	18-39 years	ncci	3.43
99396	40-64 years	ncci	3.69
99397	65 years and over	ncci	3.97

Use of Preventive Medicine Codes

After a patient is discharged or released from active care, these Preventive Service codes could be used. Until then, an established patient E/M code (99211-99215) would be appropriate and reported for the evaluation of outcomes, residuals, and counseling.

The intent of these codes is to report patient services focused on periodic evaluations, reevaluations, counseling risk factor reduction, and change interventions. When the patient encounter is for such services (and not just a treatment modality) then these codes are appropriate.

Wellness Codes and Coverage: The Wellness (Preventive Medicine Services) codes are the least understood and least used codes in most offices that are promoting health and wellness.

PREVENTIVE MEDICINE, INDIVIDUAL COUNSELING

These face-to-face encounters describe encounters with patients with specific conditions who potentially benefit from additional counseling regarding risk factor reductions and interventions (e.g., diet, substance use, injury prevention). E/M services may also be may be provided and reported and must be billed with modifier 25 where appropriate. However, time spent providing these services may NOT be used for E/M code selection.

See also health behavior assessment and intervention services (96156-96171), but do not bill both types of services on the same day.

Special instructions apply. See a current CPT codebook or FindACode.com (with subscription) for the full information.

Preventive medicine counseling and/or risk factor reduction intervention(s) provided to an individual (separate procedure); **RVU**

Code	Description		
99401	approximately 15 minutes	ncci	1.14
99402	approximately 30 minutes	ncci	1.89
99403	approximately 45 minutes	ncci	2.57
99404	approximately 60 minutes	ncci	3.31

These code descriptions are defined as "approximately." Therefore, to select the proper code, follow the general AMA time guidelines which state that unless otherwise noted in code instructions or guidelines, "a unit of time is attained when the midpoint is passed."

Note: Services less than 8 minutes should not be reported because it does not reach the mid-point requirement.

BEHAVIOR CHANGE INTERVENTIONS, INDIVIDUAL

Smoking and tobacco use cessation counseling visit; **RVU**

★ 99406   intermediate, greater than 3 minutes up to 10 minutes   ncci   .45
★ 99407   intensive, greater than 10 minutes   ncci   .83

Alcohol and/or substance (other than tobacco) abuse structured screening (eg, AUDIT, DAST), and brief intervention (SBI) services;

★ G2011   5-14 minutes   ncci   .49
★ 99408   15 to 30 minutes   ncci   1.04
★ 99409   greater than 30 minutes   ncci   2.00

Billing Note: 99408 and 99409 may not be reported together or with 96160, 96161.

SBI services are for the initial screening and brief counseling with the patient/client regarding the results of their AUDIT or DAST and possible interventions needed for treatment. SBI services are not psychotherapy services.

There are also HCPCS rehabilitative codes which could also be used depending on the payer. See also G0396-G0397, H0001-H0003, or H0049.

Note: Code G2011 was created by Medicare; check other payer policies for coverage of this shortened service. Medicare also uses codes G0396 and G0397 to describe these services. As of October 2020, their descriptions changed from "abuse" to "misuse" and we anticipate that the description for 99408 and 99409 will change at some point in the future.

Resource: See Resource 284 for additional information about screening services such as the AUDIT and DAST.

PREVENTIVE MEDICINE, GROUP COUNSELING

Preventive medicine counseling and/or risk factor reduction intervention(s) provided to individuals in a group setting (separate procedure);

99411   approximately 30 minutes   ncci   .61
99412   approximately 60 minutes   ncci   .75

OTHER PREVENTIVE MEDICINE SERVICES

99429   Unlisted preventive medicine service   ncci   NE

Non-Face-to-Face Physician Services

These codes are **only** for physicians or QHPs who may report E/M services. All other providers should use codes 98966-98972. See Resource 402 for more information on who is considered an 'other qualified health care professional.'

Alert: There are very specific guidelines for each of these types of services. It will be critical to carefully review each (e.g., telephone, remote physiological monitoring) to ensure that you are following ALL applicable rules.

Special instructions apply. See a current CPT codebook or FindACode.com (with subscription) for the full information.

TELEPHONE SERVICES

These E/M services for an established patient have specific instructions about when they may be reported. Do not report these services in the following situations because the time would be considered either pre-service or post-service of another service (including telemedicine):

- It results in a visit with the patient within 24 hours or the next available urgent-care appointment
- Is related to a previous visit within the last 7 days for the same or a similar problem
- It occurs during the postoperative period of another procedure

Note: There are many codes that may not be reported with these services for the same patient communication (e.g., 99421, 99442, 99091). See current NCCI edits in FindACode.com (available by subscription) for a comprehensive list.

Book: See Appendix A — NCCI Edits for codes that may not be reported in conjunction with these services.

Telephone evaluation and management service by a physician or other qualified health care professional who may report evaluation and management services provided to an established patient, parent, or guardian not originating from a related E/M service provided within the previous 7 days nor leading to an E/M service or procedure within the next 24 hours or soonest available appointment; **RVU**

Code	Description		
99441	5-10 minutes of medical discussion	ncci	1.64
99442	11-20 minutes of medical discussion	ncci	2.65
99443	21-30 minutes of medical discussion	ncci	3.75

99444 is deleted as of 2020-01-01. See 99421-99423

ONLINE DIGITAL EVALUATION AND MANAGEMENT SERVICES

These codes are only for physicians or QHPs who may report E/M services. All other providers should use codes 98970-98972. Note that codes 98970-98972 also state that they may be used by QHPs, so be aware of state licensing and individual payer requirements regarding which codes should be used.

Do not:

- Include clinical staff time
- Report these services on the same day another physician or QHP reports E/M services 99202-99205, 99212-99215, or 99241-99245

Note: There are many codes that may not be reported with these services (e.g., 99091, 99339).See Appendix A — NCCI Edits or FindACode.com (available by subscription) for a comprehensive list.

In addition to the description of this code, the following important components apply:

- Must be an established patient
- The platform used for correspondence is HIPAA-secure (e.g., EHR portal, secure email)
- May only be reported once every 7 days (may be used again for a different episode)
- The encounter must be documented permanently using electronic or hard copy storage
- A personal timely response by the practitioner is required
- All associated communications, lab orders, phone calls, etc. are included

Alert: The previous instructions for these services were significantly revised as of January 2020. See a current CPT codebook or FindACode.com (with subscription) for the full information.

Coding Example

- An established patient emails the provider through a HIPAA-secure platform about a possible adverse reaction in regards to their treatment plan.
- After secure email correspondence, the provider suggests changes to the treatment plan with instructions to come into the office in 7-10 days.

Resource: See Resource 474 for additional information on these types services.

Tip: Effective January 1, 2021, CMS created a code for the remote assessment of recorded video and/or images by an established patient.

Code	Description
G2250	Remote assessment of recorded video and/or images submitted by an established patient (e.g., store and forward), including interpretation with follow-up with the patient within 24 business hours, not originating from a related service provided within the previous 7 days nor leading to a service or procedure within the next 24 hours or soonest available appointment

Tip: For qualified nonphysician providers, CMS has created the following codes which became effective January 2020:

Qualified nonphysician healthcare professional online assessment and management, for an established patient, for up to seven days, cumulative time during the 7 days;

G2061	5-10 minutes
G2062	11-20 minutes
G2063	21 or more minutes

Online digital evaluation and management service, for an established patient, for up to 7 days, cumulative time during the 7 days;

Code	Description		RVU
# 99421	5-10 minutes	ncci	.44
# 99422	11-20 minutes	ncci	.86
# 99423	21 or more minutes	ncci	1.40

99444 is deleted as of 2020-01-01. See 99421-99423

INTERPROFESSIONAL TELEPHONE/INTERNET/ELECTRONIC HEALTH RECORD CONSULTATIONS

These consultation codes are used in situations where the treating or attending provider (physician or QHP) requests (written or verbal) the opinion of or treatment advice from another healthcare professional, usually a specialist with specific expertise. This provider-to-provider consultation takes place over the telephone, internet, or through the electronic health record (EHR) without a face-to-face patient encounter. For consultations which include the patient and/or family, see 99421-99423, 99441-99443, or 98966-98968.

Typically, these are more complex or urgent situations in which a face-to-face patient-consultant service is not feasible or cannot be attained in a timely manner. There are specific rules governing when these codes can be reported. They are not eligible for reporting if:

- The patient has seen the consulting provider within 14 days of the consultation (before or after)
- A decision to transfer care is made during, or prior to, the consultation (e.g., surgery, hospital visit, scheduled office encounter). However, if the decision is made to transfer care to the consulting provider after the consultation, the service may still qualify, as long as all the other criteria have been met.

Documentation by the treating/attending provider requesting the consultation should support the request and include a summary of the conversation. The consulting provider should document the time spent in the consultation as well as a summary of the information discussed, including any professional opinions or advice rendered to the treating/attending provider.

Review of data including medical records and imaging studies are included in this code and should not be reported separately. Do not report more than once every 7 days and do not report consultations which are less than 5 minutes.

See a current CPT codebook or FindACode.com for full information.

Note: These codes are scheduled for revision in 2023.

Code	Description		RVU
	Interprofessional telephone/Internet/electronic health record assessment and management service provided by a consultative physician including a verbal and written report to the patient's treating/requesting physician or other qualified health care professional;		
99446	5-10 minutes of medical consultative discussion and review	ncci	.54
99447	11-20 minutes of medical consultative discussion and review	ncci	1.06
99448	21-30 minutes of medical consultative discussion and review	ncci	1.59
99449	31 minutes or more of medical consultative discussion and review	ncci	2.13
# 99451	Interprofessional telephone/Internet/electronic health record assessment and management service provided by a consultative physician, including a written report to the patient's treating/requesting physician or other qualified health care professional, 5 minutes or more of medical consultative time	ncci	1.05
# 99452	Interprofessional telephone/Internet/electronic health record referral service(s) provided by a treating/requesting physician or other qualified health care professional, 30 minutes	ncci	1.07

DIGITALLY STORED DATA SERVICES/REMOTE PHYSIOLOGIC MONITORING

These codes may only be reported when the FDA-defined medical device being used has been ordered by a physician or QHP. These services are considered inclusive to E/M services provided on the same day.

Do not report these codes if there are less than 15 days of monitoring.

Note: There are many codes that may not reported with these services (e.g., 99442, 99091). See Appendix A — NCCI Edits for some codes that may not be reported in conjunction with these services. Complete and current NCCI edits can be found in FindACode.com (available by subscription).

Special instructions apply. See a current CPT codebook or FindACode.com for the full information.

	Code	Description		RVU
		Remote monitoring of physiologic parameter(s) (eg, weight, blood pressure, pulse oximetry, respiratory flow rate), initial;		
#	99453	set-up and patient education on use of equipment	ncci	.55
#	99454	device(s) supply with daily recording(s) or programmed alert(s) transmission, each 30 days	ncci	1.61
		Note: Self-measured blood pressure monitoring is reported with codes 99473, 99474.		
#	99091	Collection and interpretation of physiologic data (eg, ECG, blood pressure, glucose monitoring) digitally stored and/or transmitted by the patient and/or caregiver to the physician or other qualified health care professional, qualified by education, training, licensure/regulation (when applicable) requiring a minimum of 30 minutes of time, each 30 day	ncci	1.63
		Do not use code 99091 if a more specific code exists (e.g., 95250 for continuous glucose monitoring.		
		Self-measured blood pressure using a device validated for clinical accuracy;		
#	99473	patient education/training and device calibration		.34
#	99474	separate self-measurements of two readings one minute apart, twice daily over a 30-day period (minimum of 12 readings), collection of data reported by the patient and/or caregiver to the physician or other qualified health care professional, with report of average systolic and diastolic pressures and subsequent communication of a treatment plan to the patient	ncci	.44

Tips:
- Code 99473 can only be used once, regardless of the number of devices.
- Code 99474 may only be reported once per month and not during the same calendar month as ambulatory blood pressure monitoring (e.g., 93784), digitally stored data services/remote physiologic monitoring (e.g., 99091), or chronic care services (e.g., 99490).

REMOTE PHYSIOLOGIC MONITORING TREATMENT MANAGEMENT SERVICES

This code may be used when a healthcare provider (e.g., clinical staff, physician, QHP) utilizes the results of remote physiological monitoring of an FDA-defined medical device to manage a patient under a specific treatment plan ordered by a physician or QHP. Time spent on these services may **not** be included with other services (e.g., E/M).

These codes may be reported with chronic care management services (e.g., 99437, 99487), transitional care management services (e.g., 99495), and behavioral health integration services (e.g., 99484); however, be careful to separate the services and not report time performing these other services twice.

Note: There are many codes that may not reported with these services (e.g., 99442, 99091). See current NCCI edits in FindACode.com (available by subscription) for a comprehensive list.

Special instructions apply. See a current CPT codebook or FindACode.com for the full information.

Remote physiologic monitoring treatment management services, clinical staff/physician/other qualified health care professional time in a calendar month requiring interactive communication with the patient/caregiver during the month **RVU**

#	99457	first 20 minutes	ncci	1.45
#+	99458	each additional 20 minutes (List separately in addition to code for primary procedure)	ncci	1.18

Special Evaluation and Management Services

These services may be provided in an office or other outpatient setting for either new or established patients. They may also be reported with other E/M services where appropriate.

Tip: As of January 1, 2021, CMS added the following two codes for brief technology-based services:

Brief communication technology-based service, e.g. virtual check-in, provided to an established patient, not originating from a related service provided within the previous 7 days nor leading to a service or procedure within the next 24 hours or soonest available appointment;

G2251   by a qualified health care professional who cannot report evaluation and management services; 5-10 minutes of clinical discussion

G2252   by a physician or other qualified health care professional who can report evaluation and management services; 11-20 minutes of medical discussion

Note: In this section, the RVUs with an asterisk (*) have been provided by Find-A-Code and are used for comparative purposes only. Individual payer policies vary on coverage for these services.

BASIC LIFE AND/OR DISABILITY EVALUATION SERVICES

99450   Basic life and/or disability examination that includes: ncci   *1.35
- measurement of height, weight and blood pressure;
- completion of a medical history following a life insurance pro forma;
- collection of blood sample and/or urinalysis complying with "chain of custody" protocols; and
- completion of necessary documentation/certificates.

WORK RELATED OR MEDICAL DISABILITY EVALUATION SERVICES

99455   Work related or medical disability examination by the treating physician that includes: ncci   *2.69
- completion of a medical history commensurate with the patient's condition;
- performance of an examination commensurate with the patient's condition;
- formulation of a diagnosis, assessment of capabilities and stability, & calculation of impairment;
- development of future medical treatment plan; and
- completion of necessary documentation/certificates and report.

			RVU
99456	Work related or medical disability examination by other than the treating physician that includes: • completion of a medical history commensurate with the patient's condition; • performance of an examination commensurate with the patient's condition; • formulation of a diagnosis, assessment of capabilities and stability, and calculation of impairment; • development of future medical treatment plan; and • completion of necessary documentation/certificates and report.	ncci	*6.95

Codes 99455 and 99456 may not be used with 99080 when completing Workers Compensation forms.

Newborn Care Services

Special instructions apply. See a current CPT codebook or FindACode.com for full information.

Note: The RVUs included here for these services (except 99461) are the facility RVUs.

99460	Initial hospital or birthing center care, per day, for evaluation and management of normal newborn infant	ncci	2.75
99461	Initial care, per day, for evaluation and management of normal newborn infant seen in other than hospital or birthing center	ncci	2.70
99462	Subsequent hospital care, per day, for evaluation and management of normal newborn	ncci	1.22
99463	Initial hospital or birthing center care, per day, for evaluation and management of normal newborn infant admitted and discharged on the same date	ncci	3.17

Delivery/Birthing Room Attendance and Resuscitation Services

Special instructions apply. See a current CPT codebook or FindACode.com for full information.

Note: The RVUs included here are the facility RVUs.

99464	Attendance at delivery (when requested by the delivering physician or other qualified health care professional) and initial stabilization of newborn	ncci	2.16

This code may be used with 99460, 99468, and 99477, but not with 99465.

99465	Delivery/birthing room resuscitation, provision of positive pressure ventilation and/or chest compressions in the presence of acute inadequate ventilation and/or cardiac output	ncci	4.21

This code may be used with 99460, 99468, and 99477, but not with 99464. Additional services such as intubation may also be reported as long as they are necessary to the resuscitation.

Inpatient Neonatal Intensive Care Services and Pediatric and Neonatal Critical Care Services

Special instructions apply. See a current CPT codebook or FindACode.com for full information.

Note: The RVUs included here for these services are the facility RVUs.

PEDIATRIC CRITICAL CARE PATIENT TRANSPORT

Critical care face-to-face services, during an interfacility transport of critically ill or critically injured pediatric patient, 24 months of age or younger;

99466	first 30-74 minutes of hands-on care during transport	ncci	6.87
+ 99467	each additional 30 minutes (List separately in addition to code for primary service)	ncci	3.46

				RVU
	Supervision by a control physician of interfacility transport care of the critically ill or critically injured pediatric patient, 24 months of age or younger, includes two-way communication with transport team before transport, at the referring facility and during the transport, including data interpretation and report;			
# 99485	first 30 minutes		ncci	2.19
#+ 99486	each additional 30 minutes (List separately in addition to code for primary procedure)		ncci	1.91

INPATIENT NEONATAL AND PEDIATRIC CRITICAL CARE

99468	Initial inpatient neonatal critical care, per day, for the evaluation and management of a critically ill neonate, 28 days of age or younger	ncci	26.50
99469	Subsequent inpatient neonatal critical care, per day, for the evaluation and management of a critically ill neonate, 28 days of age or younger	ncci	11.48
99471	Initial inpatient pediatric critical care, per day, for the evaluation and management of a critically ill infant or young child, 29 days through 24 months of age	ncci	22.94
99472	Subsequent inpatient pediatric critical care, per day, for the evaluation and management of a critically ill infant or young child, 29 days through 24 months of age	ncci	11.70
99475	Initial inpatient pediatric critical care, per day, for the evaluation and management of a critically ill infant or young child, 2 through 5 years of age	ncci	16.49
99476	Subsequent inpatient pediatric critical care, per day, for the evaluation and management of a critically ill infant or young child, 2 through 5 years of age	ncci	9.89

INITIAL AND CONTINUING INTENSIVE CARE SERVICES

Intensive care services for the neonate or infant (28 days or younger) requires documentation of their present day weight for accurate code assignment.

99477	Initial hospital care, per day, for the evaluation and management of the neonate, 28 days of age or younger, who requires intensive observation, frequent interventions, and other intensive care services	10.03
	Subsequent intensive care, per day, for the evaluation and management of the recovering;	
99478	very low birth weight infant (present body weight less than 1500 grams)	3.96
99479	low birth weight infant (present body weight of 1500-2500 grams)	3.61
99480	infant (present body weight of 2501-5000 grams)	3.46

Cognitive Assessment and Care Plan Services

This code is to be used by a physician or QHP to evaluate a patient (new or existing) showing signs of cognitive impairment. All criteria must be met to bill this code which may only be reported once every 180 days.

Do not report with: 90785, 90791, 90792, 96103, 96120, 96127, 96160-96161, 99605-99607, 99202-99215, 99242-99245, 99324-99337, 99341-99350, 99366-99368, 99497-99498.

Special instructions apply. See a current CPT codebook or FindACode.com for full information.

Note: See the following page for code information.

		RVU
99483	Assessment of and care planning for a patient with cognitive impairment, requiring an independent historian, in the office or other outpatient, home or domiciliary or rest home, with all of the following required elements: • Cognition-focused evaluation including a pertinent history and examination; • Medical decision making of moderate or high complexity; • Functional assessment (eg, basic and instrumental activities of daily living), including decision-making capacity; • Use of standardized instruments for staging of dementia (eg, functional assessment staging test [FAST], clinical dementia rating [CDR]); • Medication reconciliation and review for high-risk medications; • Evaluation for neuropsychiatric and behavioral symptoms, including depression, including use of standardized screening instrument(s); • Evaluation of safety (eg, home), including motor vehicle operation; • Identification of caregiver(s), caregiver knowledge, caregiver needs, social supports, and the willingness of caregiver to take on caregiving tasks; • Development, updating or revision, or review of an Advance Care Plan; • Creation of a written care plan, including initial plans to address any neuropsychiatric symptoms, neuro-cognitive symptoms, functional limitations, and referral to community resources as needed (eg, rehabilitation services, adult day programs, support groups) shared with the patient and/or caregiver with initial education and support. Typically, 50 minutes are spent face-to-face with the patient and/or family or caregiver.	ncci 8.18

Care Management Services

Care Management Services have been significantly revised for 2022. The CPT codebook divides them into "Care Planning," "Chronic Care Management (CCM)," "Complex Chronic Care Management," and "Principle Care Management."

See a current CPT codebook or FindACode.com for full information on each of these types of care management services.

Alert: This subcategory has comprehensive instructional changes for 2022 along with changes to code descriptions and code level guidelines. There is a new guideline for "Care Planning" which details what could be included in a plan of care. Payer policies might also change so watch for notifications.

Notes:

- CMS has different requirements for RHCs and FQHCs reporting these services (e.g., G0511). See Resource 655 for more information. Be aware that there may be updates to this resource as more information becomes available about the changes for 2022.
- There are many codes that may NOT be reported with these services (e.g., 99442, 99091). See Appendix A — NCCI Edits for a specialty-specific selection of codes that may not be reported in conjunction with these services. Complete and current NCCI edits can be found in FindACode.com (available by subscription).

CHRONIC CARE MANAGEMENT SERVICES

Chronic Care Management (CCM) services are for patients with two or more chronic conditions which are expected to last at least 12 months or until the death of the patient. These conditions place them at significant risk of death, acute exacerbation/decompensation, or functional decline. There are comprehensive instructions about the timing and reporting of these services. CMS has created a toolkit to help ensure proper usage of these codes.

Resource: See Resource 627 to review CMS' Chronic Care Management Health Care Professional Toolkit. With the changes to these codes for 2022, changes to this toolkit are likely to be made sometime during the year.

Chronic care management services, per calendar month, with the following required elements:
- multiple (two or more) chronic conditions expected to last at least 12 months, or until the death of the patient;
- chronic conditions place the patient at significant risk of death, acute exacerbation/decompensation, or functional decline;
- comprehensive care plan established, implemented, revised, or monitored

RVU

▲# 99490   first 20 minutes of clinical staff time directed by a physician or other qualified health care professional, per calendar month.   ncci   1.85

▲#+99439   each additional 20 minutes of clinical staff time directed by a physician or other qualified health care professional, per calendar month (List separately in addition to code for primary procedure)   ncci   1.40

> Code 99439 may only be reported with 99490 and cannot be reported more than twice per month.
>
> **Note:** With the addition of code 99439, code G2058 was deleted as of January 1, 2021.

▲# 99491   provided personally by a physician or other qualified health care professional, at least 30 minutes of physician or other qualified health care professional time   ncci   2.49

> Do not report codes 99490 and 99491 together in the same month or with codes 99487 or 99489.

COMPLEX CHRONIC CARE MANAGEMENT SERVICES

Patients requiring *complex* CCM services (CCCM) require moderate or high medical decision making, typically use multiple medications, are unable to perform activities of daily living, require caregiver assistance, and are at a higher risk for acute exacerbation that may quickly lead to a repeat admission or emergency department visit.

The difference between chronic care and *complex* chronic care is the risk of readmission without agressive monitoring and follow-up evaluations. Remember, the entire goal of CCM and CCCM services is to avoid readmission or emergency room visits so it is important to document the severity and risk to the individual patient of this readmission based on the type and severity of the chronic conditions they have. The provider needs to paint a clear picture of the risk, outline the comprehensive (a key word for auditors meaning detailed) care plan and any revisions or alterations made to it. Time must be clearly documented for each encounter, added together for the calendar month (from the 1st to the last day of a specific month), and reported with the following codes.

Complex chronic care management services with the following required elements:
- multiple (two or more) chronic conditions expected to last at least 12 months, or until the death of the patient,
- chronic conditions place the patient at significant risk of death, acute exacerbation/decompensation, or functional decline,
- comprehensive care plan established, implemented, revised, or monitored,
- moderate or high complexity medical decision making;

▲   99487   first 60 minutes of clinical staff time directed by a physician or other qualified health care professional, per calendar month.   ncci   3.88

▲+99489   each additional 30 minutes of clinical staff time directed by a physician or other qualified health care professional, per calendar month (List separately in addition to code for primary procedure)   ncci   2.04

PRINCIPAL CARE MANAGEMENT SERVICES

Principal Care Management Services (PCM) are new for 2022. Unlike CCM services, these may be reported, where applicable, to patients with a *single*, complex chronic condition expected to last a minimum of three (3) months and does not need to last until the death of the patient.

These services include "establishing, implementing, revising, or monitoring a care plan" specific to that single condition.

Unlike CCM and CCCM services, PCM services may be provided for a patient with a _single complex chronic condition_ and requires the service to be provided personally by the physician/QHP.

Documentation must include a description of the chronic condition and what makes it complex in nature, a disease-specific treatment plan, and notes regarding interventions such as frequent adjustments to medications or treatment methods.

As these are time-based codes and the physician/QHP personally provides the services, an accurate portrayal of time is vital to correct code reporting.

Principal care management services, for a single high-risk disease, with the following required elements:
- one complex chronic condition expected to last at least 3 months, and that places the patient at significant risk of hospitalization, acute exacerbation/decompensation, functional decline, or death,
- the condition requires development, monitoring, or revision of disease-specific care plan,
- the condition requires frequent adjustments in the medication regimen and/or the management of the condition is unusually complex due to comorbidities,
- ongoing communication and care coordination between relevant practitioners furnishing care

RVU

●# 99424 first 30 minutes provided personally by a physician or other qualified health care professional, per calendar month — **2.41**

●#+99425 each additional 30 minutes provided personally by a physician or other qualified health care professional, per calendar month (List separately in addition to code for primary procedure) — **1.74**

Code 99425 may only be reported with 99424 and cannot be reported in conjunction with many other services (see Appendix A — NCCI Edits.)

Psychiatric Collaborative Care Management Services

Special instructions apply. See a current CPT codebook or FindACode.com for full information.

Resource: See Resource 647 for more information about these services.

		Psychiatric collaborative care management in a calendar month of behavioral health care manager activities, in consultation with a psychiatric consultant, and directed by the treating physician or other qualified health care professional;		**RVU**
	G2214	initial, first 30 minutes		1.79

> Code G2214 was added in 2021 by CMS and might not be reportable for non-government claims.

	99492	initial, first 70 minutes, first calendar month with the following required elements: • outreach to and engagement in treatment of a patient directed by the treating physician or other qualified health care professional, • initial assessment of the patient, including administration of validated rating scales, with the development of an individualized treatment plan, • review by the psychiatric consultant with modifications of the plan if recommended, • entering patient in a registry and tracking patient follow-up and progress using the registry, with appropriate documentation, and participation in weekly caseload consultation with the psychiatric consultant, and • provision of brief interventions using evidence-based techniques such as behavioral activation, motivational interviewing, and other focused treatment strategies.	ncci	4.44
	99493	subsequent month, first 60 minutes with the following required elements: • tracking patient follow-up and progress using the registry, with appropriate documentation, • participation in weekly caseload consultation with the psychiatric consultant, • ongoing collaboration with and coordination of the patient's mental health care with the treating physician or other qualified health care professional and any other treating mental health providers, • additional review of progress and recommendations for changes in treatment, as indicated, including medications, based on recommendations provided by the psychiatric consultant, • provision of brief interventions using evidence-based techniques such as behavioral activation, motivational interviewing, and other focused treatment strategies, • monitoring of patient outcomes using validated rating scales, and • relapse prevention planning with patients as they achieve remission of symptoms and/or other treatment goals and are prepared for discharge from active treatment	ncci	4.30
	+ 99494	initial or subsequent, each additional 30 minutes (List separately in addition to code for primary procedure)	ncci	1.84

> Code 99494 may only be reported with 99492 or 99493.

Transitional Care Management Services

Special instructions apply. See a current CPT codebook or FindACode.com for full information.

		Transitional Care Management Services with the following required elements: • Communication (direct contact, telephone, electronic) with the patient and/or caregiver within 2 business days of discharge		
★	99495	• Medical decision making of at least **moderate** complexity during the service period • Face-to-face visit, within **14** calendar days of discharge	ncci	6.04
★	99496	• Medical decision making of **high** complexity during the service period • Face-to-face visit, within **7** calendar days of discharge	ncci	8.14

Advance Care Planning

These codes may be used to report face-to-face encounters with patient and/or family members to discuss an advance care plan (e.g., living will, durable power of attorney for health care). Actual forms may or may not be completed at this time.

Use 99497 and 99498 together, when applicable.

These services may be reported on the same day as many E/M services (e.g., 99202-99215). See current NCCI edits, a CPT codebook, or FindACode.com (available with subscription) for a comprehensive listing.

Do not report these services on the same day as: 99291, 99292, 99468, 99469, 99471, 99472, 99475, 99476, 99477, 99478, 99479, 99480, 99483.

Special instructions apply. See a current CPT codebook or FindACode.com for full information.

Advance care planning including the explanation and discussion of advance directives such as standard forms (with completion of such forms, when performed), by the physician or other qualified health care professional;   **RVU**

★ 99497   first 30 minutes, face-to-face with the patient, family member(s), and/or surrogate   ncci   2.47
★+99498   each additional 30 minutes (List separately in addition to code for primary procedure)   ncci   2.14

General Behavioral Health Integration Care Management

Behavioral health integration care management services (99484) are reported by the supervising physician/QHP when services are perfromed by clinical staff for a patient with a behavioral health condition that requires care management services that are both face-to-face and non-face-to-face during a calendar month.

Special instructions apply. See FindACode.com or Resource 647 for more information about these services.

▲# 99484   Care management services for behavioral health conditions, at least 20 minutes of clinical staff time, directed by a physician or other qualified health care professional, per calendar month, with the following required elements: ncci   1.34
- initial assessment or follow-up monitoring, including the use of applicable validated rating scales,
- behavioral health care planning in relation to behavioral/psychiatric health problems, including revision for patients who are not progressing or whose status changes,
- facilitating and coordinating treatment such as psychotherapy, pharmacotherapy, counseling and/or psychiatric consultation, and
- continuity of care with a designated member of the care team.

Other Evaluation and Management Services

99499   Unlisted evaluation and management service   ncci   NE

Notes:

6. Supply Coding

Chapter Contents

6.1 Supply Coding Essentials 379
    About HCPCS Codes 379
    Durable Medical Equipment (DME) 380

6.2 Supply Codes & Tips 383
    Supply Tips 383
    Common Supply Codes 392

6.1 Supply Coding Essentials

About HCPCS Codes

HCPCS (pronounced "hick-picks") is the Healthcare Common Procedure Coding System, maintained by the Centers for Medicare & Medicaid Services (CMS). HCPCS is a 5-character alphanumeric coding system that describes physician and other healthcare provider services and supplies.

It is the Health Insurance Portability and Accountability Act (HIPAA) national standardized coding system used to identify products, supplies, and services that are not included in the CPT code set.

Technically, HCPCS is comprised of three levels or divisions:

1. **Level I - CPT Numeric Codes (00000-99999)**

   This CPT (Current Procedural Terminology) portion is maintained by the American Medical Association (AMA).

2. **Level II - CMS Alpha-numeric Codes (A0000-V9999)**

   This non-CPT portion is maintained by CMS. Codes from the non-CPT portion are easily identifiable. There is a single letter followed by 4 numbers (e.g., A9300 "Exercise equipment"). These codes supplement the CPT codes. They exist because there is a need to more fully identify supplies and services that are not in the CPT codebook.

   These are national codes, and are in the public domain. Decisions regarding additions, revisions, and deletions to codes or descriptors are made annually by a panel comprised of representatives from federal programs such as Medicare and Medicaid, as well as representatives from private insurance agencies.

3. **Level III - Local and State Alpha-numeric Codes (W0000-W9999)**

   Level III codes are not HIPAA approved codes. These codes were formerly reserved for state and local use. With the advent of HIPAA, local codes were no longer permitted. However, Workers Compensation is exempt from HIPAA, and could utilize different modifiers and codes.

Not all HCPCS supply codes are included in this book. The codes included here were selected for this specialized *Reimbursement Guide*.

Website: The most current codes and code information (e.g., NCCI edits and fees), are available to FindACode.com subscribers.

Resource: See Resource 818 for additional information, articles, and webinars about supplies.

Book: See Chapter 5.2 — Procedure Codes & Tips for other non-supply related HCPCS codes.

Tip: New, revised, and deleted codes are implemented quarterly. Depending on the quarter, your specialty may or may not be impacted. FindACode.com always has the most up-to-date codes and also has a list of these updates.

Why You Should Use HCPCS

Mandated Use: The use of HCPCS codes is mandated by CMS on Medicare claims, and many state Medicaid offices also require them.

Improved Communication: A provider can more clearly communicate services and supplies correctly, without the need to use narrative descriptors.

Reduced Claim Resubmissions: Inaccurate codes or incomplete narrative descriptors cause costly time delays. The claims adjudicator must assign a code or return the claim, and the payer's reassignment of the code may be incorrect.

Quick and Efficient: Using up-to-date HCPCS codes on office forms allows office staff to assign fees quickly and easily. This saves time and money.

Faster Processing: Your coding system will be compatible with most insurance companies, speeding up claims processing.

Avoid Audits: Consistent submission of accurate claims will reduce the probability of being targeted for an audit by your carrier.

Accurate Reimbursements: Use HCPCS for accurate and complete reimbursements.
Example: Supplies billed as "over and above those usually included with the office visit" (CPT code 99070) will generally not be reimbursed unless identified with Level II HCPCS codes.

> **Tip 1:** The existence of a code does not imply coverage by third party payers.
> **Tip 2:** Requests for new codes are considered by CMS. See Resource 349 for more about requesting a code change.

Durable Medical Equipment (DME)

Within the Healthcare Common Procedure Coding System (HCPCS) Level II codes set for supplies, there are many items that are classified as Durable Medical Equipment (DME). Generally, such equipment items need to meet all the following requirements:

1. Can be used repeatedly,
2. Primarily used for a medical purpose,
3. Not useful in the absence of an illness/injury and,
4. Appropriate for home use.

DME Application Process

The National Supplier Clearinghouse (NSC) is the national entity contracted by the Centers for Medicare & Medicaid Services (CMS) that issues Medicare DMEPOS supplier authorization numbers. The NSC provides DMEPOS supplier applications, verifies application information, and administers file activity.

> **Resource:** See Resource 354 for information by NSC including webinars.
> **Resource:** See Resource 353 for the official CMS DME website.

Billing Process for DME Items

Once the practitioner or clinic obtains a DMEPOS supplier number, billing commences. However, the billing does not go to the usual Part B MAC. It goes to the Durable Medical Equipment Medicare Administrative Contractors (DME-MAC) in your jurisdiction.

> **Tip:** All DME billing for Medicare is entered on a separate claim form and then transmitted to one of four designated regional DME carriers/contractors.

DME Claim Filing Centers

All DME claims are filed according to jurisdiction into one of four regions (see Resource 355):

- **Jurisdiction A–National Heritage Insurance Company (NHIC)** processes claims for: Connecticut, Delaware, District of Columbia, Maine, Maryland, Massachusetts, New Hampshire, New Jersey, New York, Pennsylvania, Rhode Island, and Vermont.

- **Jurisdiction B–National Government Services** processes claims for: Illinois, Indiana, Kentucky, Michigan, Minnesota, Ohio, and Wisconsin.

- **Jurisdiction C–CGS Administrators, LLC** processes claims for: Alabama, Arkansas, Colorado, Florida, Georgia, Louisiana, Mississippi, New Mexico, North Carolina, Oklahoma, Puerto Rico, South Carolina, Tennessee, Texas, U.S. Virgin Islands, Virginia, and West Virginia.

- **Jurisdiction D–Noridian Administrative Services (NAS)** processes claims for: Alaska, American Samoa, Arizona, California, Guam, Hawaii, Idaho, Iowa, Kansas, Missouri, Montana, Nebraska, Nevada, North Dakota, Northern Mariana Islands, Oregon, South Dakota, Utah, Washington, and Wyoming.

Notes:

6.2 Supply Codes & Tips

The codes included in this chapter are a selection of codes for behavioral health. They are selected from the official Healthcare Common Procedure Coding System (HCPCS) code set. The complete listing of this code set can be found at FindACode.com.

Supply Tips

The following tips for supply codes are taken primarily from Medicare information. Only a few commonly billed supply codes for behavioral health are listed in this "Supply Tips" segment. Additional codes follow these tips.

Book: See Chapter 4.3 — Documentation Tips for information regarding requirements for properly documenting supplies.
Website: Go to FindACode.com for additional information regarding supply codes including fees and third party payer information.

Disclaimer: The information in this chapter contains general information and is the opinion of the authors. It should not be interpreted by providers/payers as official guidance. As such, this information should not be used for claim adjudication. Third party payers should utilize their own payment policies based on clinically sound guidelines.

Conventions

The following conventions are used in this chapter:

Type Styles

Excerpts from official HCPCS descriptions are in a type style like this.

Explanations added by innoviHealth are in a type style like this. Tables are the exception. All text in tables, including codes, notations or explanations by innoviHealth, will be in a type style like this.

Tables like this include official instructions or quotes from payers.

Revision Identifiers

- **N** Signifies a code added this year.
- **R** Signifies a code revised this year. Revised codes may have had a change to their description, inclusion terms, and/or instructional notes.

Code Tip Index

DME Requirements	384
Injections	386
Modifiers	387
Substance Use Medication-Assisted Treatment	388
Supplies — Other	391
Transportation; Non-Emergency (A0080-A0210)	391

DME Requirements

In order to meet medical necessity and other payer requirements, many Durable Medical Equipment (DME) codes must meet very specific requirements, which vary by payer and the actual supply ordered. In most cases, at the minimum, keep a copy of the prescription in the patient's chart.

Reminder: In order to provide DME to Medicare beneficiaries, providers must separately enroll as a DME supplier or payment will be denied.

Book: See Chapter 6.1 — Supply Coding Essentials for more information on becoming a supplier.

Alert: Changes to Medicare rules and regulations regarding DME Orders/Prescriptions became effective on January 1, 2020 and implemented on July 1, 2020. The information presented here includes those changes.

Resource: See Resource 518 to review the complete document.

Face-to-Face Encounter Requirement

Not every DME item requires a face-to-face encounter. However, many payers require a face-to-face encounter before a written order is submitted for certain DME items (e.g., Power Mobility Devices, oxygen, CPAP therapy). Medicare defines this encounter as follows:

> A face-to-face encounter means an in-person or telehealth encounter between the treating practitioner and the beneficiary. The face-to-face encounter must be used for the purpose of gathering subjective and objective information associated with diagnosing, treating, or managing a clinical condition for which the DMEPOS is ordered. Telehealth encounters used to satisfy the face-to-face requirement must meet the requirements of 42 CFR §§ 410.78 and 414.65 for purposes of DMEPOS coverage.
>
> – *Medicare Program Integrity Manual, Chapter 5, Section 5.4*

G0454 Physician documentation of face-to-face visit for durable medical equipment determination performed by nurse practitioner, physician assistant or clinical nurse specialist.

Tip: For Medicare, the face-to-face encounter does not have to be on same date as the creation of the order; however, it must occur within six (6) months prior to the creation of a written order.

Coding Tips

- To streamline the DME ordering process, the 2020 End Stage Renal Disease (ESRD) Prospective Payment System (PPS) Final Rule established the development of a single Master List of DMEPOS items which are potentially subject to a face-to-face encounter, written order prior to delivery, and/or prior authorization requirements as a condition of payment. This list can change annually. See Resource 652 for the Noridian list. Be sure to have appropriate Policies and Procedures in place to ensure that these supplies meet all payer requirements.

- If the prescribing physician is also the supplier, a separate standard written order (SWO) is not required. However, the medical record must still contain all of the required SWO elements.

- Some DME items must have a new SWO regularly issued even if there is no change in the order. Be sure to review the DME medical policy for any specific instructions about when a new SWO is required.

- Rental fees are monthly unless otherwise specified in the description. If the rental period is less than one month, append modifier KR (rental item, partial month).

- Be sure to use appropriate modifiers to indicate the type of purchase (e.g., RR to indicate that this is a rental only or NU for new equipment). See the "Modifiers" segment that follows as well as Appendix B — Modifiers.

Book: See Chapter 4.3 — Documentation Tips for more information regarding DME requirements, including the SWO.
Resource: See Resource 484 for more comprehensive information about DME documentation requirements.
Resource: See Resource 518 for the Medicare Manual instructions for DME claims.

Tip: Rental fees are monthly unless otherwise specified in the description. If the rental period is less than one month, append modifier KR (rental item, partial month).

Note: Be sure to use appropriate modifiers to indicate the type of purchase (e.g., RR to indicate that this is a rental only or NU for new equipment). See also Appendix B — Modifiers.

Modifiers

The following modifiers are commonly associated with DME billing:

- BP The beneficiary has been informed of the purchase and rental options and has elected to purchase the item
- BR The beneficiary has been informed of the purchase and rental options and has elected to rent the item
- BU The beneficiary has been informed of the purchase and after 30 days has not informed the supplier of his/her decision
- GZ Item or service expected to be denied as not reasonable and necessary
- KF Item designated by FDA as class III device
- KR Rental item, billing for partial month
- LL Lease/rental (use the LL modifier when DME equipment rental is to be applied against the purchase price)
- LT Left side (used to identify procedures performed on the left side of the body)
- NR New when rented (use the NR modifier when DME which was new at the time of rental is subsequently purchased)
- NU New equipment
- RA Replacement of a DME, orthotic or prosthetic item
- RB Replacement of a part of DME, orthotic or prosthetic item furnished as part of a repair
- RR Rental (use the RR modifier when DME is to be rented)
- RT Right side (used to identify procedures performed on the right side of the body)
- UE Used durable medical equipment

Injections

When coding drugs, be sure to match the drug accurately by name (brand or generic), strength (ml, mg, gram, units, etc.), and method of administration (IV, IM, inhalant, etc.) Use Item Number 24G (Days or Units) on the *1500 Claim Form* to show multiple units such as in the example below:

Example:
Patient was injected with 3cc of dexamethasone sodium phosphate 1 mg
Code:
J1100 dexamethasone sodium phosphate 1 mg x 3 units.

The following table contains a list of the most commonly reported injectables, listed by brand name for easy reference:

Common Injections Coding Table		
Brand Name(s)	**Generic Name(s)/Code Description**	**Code**
Abilify	Aripiprazole, intramuscular, 0.25 mg	J0400
Abilify Maintena	Aripiprazole, extended release, 1 mg	J0401
Aristada	Aripiprazole lauroxil, 1 mg	J1944
Aristada Initio	Aripiprazole lauroxil, (Aristada Initio), 1 mg	J1943
Ativan	Lorazepam, 2 mg	J2060
Baycadron	Dexamethasone sodium phosphate, 1mg	J1100
Botox	Onabotulinumtoxina, 1 unit	J0585
Decadron	Dexamethasone sodium phosphate, 1mg	J1100
Diazepam	Diazepam, up to 5 mg	J3360
DoubleDex	Dexamethasone sodium phosphate, 1mg	J1100
Duraclon	Clonidine hydrochloride, 1 mg	J0735
Dyloject	Diclofenac sodium, 0.5 mg	J1130
Fluphenazine	Fluphenazine decanoate, up to 25 mg	J2680
Haldol	Haloperidol, up to 5 mg	J1630
Haldol Decanoate	Haloperidol decanoate, per 50 mg	J1631
Haloperidol Lactate	Haloperidol, up to 5 mg	J1630
Invega Sustenna	Paliperidone palmitate extended release, 1 mg	J2426
Lorazepam	Lorazepam, 2 mg	J2060
Mardex	Dexamethasone sodium phosphate, 1mg	J1100
Maxidex	Dexamethasone sodium phosphate, 1mg	J1100
Ozurdex	Dexamethasone sodium phosphate, 1mg	J1100
Probuphine	Buprenorphine implant, 74.2 mg	J0570
Risperdal Consta	Risperidone, (Risperdal Consta), 0.5 mg	J2794
Vitamin B-12	Vitamin b-12 cyanocobalamin, up to 1000 mcg	J3420
Vivitrol	Naltrexone, depot form, 1 mg	J2315
Zulresso	Brexanolone, 1 mg	N J1632
Zyprexa Relprevv	Olanzapine, long-acting, 1 mg	J2358

Modifiers

Most payers require modifiers on many of the supply codes because they describe the type of supply. This is particularly important for supplies that could be either rented or purchased.

Also note that for Medicare, the JW modifier is not used on claims for drugs or biologicals provided under the Competitive Acquisition Program (CAP). Review LCDs for additional requirements.

Book: See Appendix B — Modifiers for a list of modifiers.

Website: Go to FindACode.com to review LCDs and other payer policies (available by subscription) for additional modifier requirements.

Substance Use Medication-Assisted Treatment

Even though the Affordable Care Act requires coverage of substance addiction treatment, there are limits to consider. For example, not every type or dosage of Medication Assisted Treatment (MAT) is covered. Be sure to verify coverage prior to treatment as some payers may require pre-authorizations. This segment only discusses alcohol and opioid substance dependence medications.

Alert: Be aware of payer requirements regarding the separate billing of MAT. If you are billing a bundled service like CMS' bundled opioid use disorder treatment codes G2086-G2088, it is likely that they will not allow you to bill these drugs separately.

Book: See "Alcohol/Substance Use Screening and Counseling" in Chapter 5.2 — Common Procedure Codes & Tips for more about bundled services.

The following medications are FDA-approved for substance dependence treatment:

Alcohol

- Acamprosate (Campral)
- Disulfiram (Antabuse)
- Naltrexone, oral (Revia, Depade)
- Naltrexone extended release injectable (Vivitrol)

Opioid

- Buprenorphine
- Buprenorphine-naloxone
- Methadone
- Naltrexone (oral)
- Naltrexone extended release (injectable)

Tips:

- Buprenorphine is available in several types of formulations: buccal (Belbuca), parenteral (Buprenex), transmucosal film (Bunavail, Suboxone, Zubsolv), sublingual tablet (Subutex), and transdermal patch (Butrans).
- The NDC codes listed in the "Substance Dependence MAT Coding Table" are not all-inclusive. Check the payers preferred drug list to verify coverage.

Website: Search NDC and drug information with a FindACode.com subscription.

Resource: See Resource 615 for information by the Substance Abuse and Mental Health Services Administration (SAMHSA) about MAT.

Book: See "Substance Use Disorders" in Appendix E — Common Diagnosis Code Tips for diagnosis code options.

Coding Tips

- Use Item Number 19 of the *1500 Claim Form* to include important information such as the brand name. Use Item Number 24D (shaded area) for the 11 digit NDC number, Unit of Measurement Qualifier, and Unit Quantity. See Chapter 1.3 — Claims Processing for additional information.
- Suboxone is formulated to be dosed once daily for dependency treatment. Daily doses should be made up of the fewest number of dosage units.
- Dosages may be limited by some payers without prior authorization. For example, according to one payer policy, Suboxone is limited (without prior authorization) to 16 mg per day.
- Disulfiram, Naltrexone (oral), and Buprenorphine-naloxone are covered by most payers without prior authorization.
- Several Medicaid programs require behavioral therapy when billing MATs. Check payer policies to see if it is required by your payer.

- Methadone is a schedule II drug which must be dispensed by a SAMHSA-certified opioid treatment program that is also a DEA-registered narcotics treatment program.
- When opioid agonist treatment is contraindicated, unacceptable, unavailable, or discontinued and the patient has been abstinent for a sufficient period of time, consider using extended-release injectable naltrexone.

Substance Dependence MAT Coding Table

Brand Name(s)	Generic Name(s) Code Description	NDC Code(s)	Unit	Code	Notes*
Antabuse	Disulfiram	51285-0523-02 54868-5034-00	250 mg tablet	J3490	5, 6
Belbuca	Buprenorphine hydrochloride	59385-0021-01	75 ug film	J3490	5
Bunavail	Buprenorphine/naloxone, oral	59385-0014-01 59385-0014-30	4.2-0.7 mg film	J0573-51	7
Bunavail	Injection, baclofen	59385-0016-01 59385-0016-30	6.3-1 mg film	J0475-51	
Campral	Acamprosate	00456-3330-01 00456-3330-63 68151-4760-00	333 mg tablet	J3490	5, 6
Disulfiram	Disulfiram	00093-5035-01 00378-4140-01	250 mg tablet	J3490	5, 6
Dolophine	Methadone hydrochloride tablet	00054-4218-25	5 mg tablet	S0109	
Naltrexone	Naltrexone, depot form	65757-0300-01	380 mg IM	J2315	
Narcan	Naloxonehydrochloride	50090-2422-00 69547-0353-02 55700-0457-01	4 mg spray	J2310	
Revia	Naltrexone, oral	51285-0275-01	50 mg tablet	J2315	4
Subutex	Buprenorphine, oral	00054-0176-13 00093-5378-56 00228-3156-03 00378-0923-93 50383-0924-93	2 mg sublingual tablet	J0571-51	
Subutex	Buprenorphine, oral	00054-0177-13 00093-5379-56 00228-3153-03 00378-0924-93 50383-0930-93	8 mg sublingual tablet	J0571	7
Suboxone	Buprenorphine/naloxone, oral	12496-1202-01 12496-1202-03	2 mg film	J0572	1
Suboxone	Buprenorphine/naloxone, oral	12496-1208-01 12496-1208-03	8 mg film	J0574	
Probuphine	Buprenorphine implant	58284-0100-14	80 mg	J0570	2
Vivitrol	Naltrexone, injection depot form	65757-0300-01	Strength specific	J2315	4
Zubsolv	Buprenorphine/naloxone, oral	54123-0914-30	1.4-0.36 mg sublingual tablet	J0572-51	3
Zubsolv	Buprenorphine/naloxone, oral	54123-0929-30	2.9-0.71 mg sublingual tablet	J0572	3
Zubsolv	Buprenorphine/naloxone, oral	54123-0957-30	5.7-1.4 mg sublingual tablet	J0573	3
See Table Notes Continued on Next Page					

*Notes:
1. Consider using modifier SC to indicate the clinical necessity of this supply
2. Associated procedure codes for drug delivery implants:

Drug Delivery Implant;			
	Insertion	Removal	Removal w/Reinsertion
bioresorbable, biodegradable, non-biodegradable	R 11981	—	—
non-biodegradable 4 or more (services for subdermal rod implant)	— G0516	11982 G0517	11983 G0518
biodegradable or bioresorable	—	—	17999

3. Clinical dose may require multiple strengths per day and may be reimbursed in combinations that reach that clinical dose
4. Maximum of 380 units per dose. Minimum age of use is 18.
5. There are several different NDCs based on the dosage. Verify the dosage and NDC on the packaging.
6. Check with the payer to determine their preferred code to report.
7. If 10 mg of buprenorphine is administered, consider using code J0574 "Buprenorphine/naloxone, oral, greater than 6 mg, but less than or equal to 10 mg buprenorphine"

Supplies — Other

Some supplies, such as dressings, sutures, gauze, betadine preps, drapes, syringes, and needles are required for the performance of certain procedures. As such, these general supplies are usually built into the RVU for the procedure being performed. Occasionally, additional supplies, beyond those considered bundled in the procedure, are required and these supplies may be eligible for separate reimbursement.

The following guidelines from Medicare provide additional guidance:

> A/B MACs (B) make a separate payment for supplies furnished in connection with a procedure only when one of the two following conditions exists:
>
> A. HCPCS code A4300 is billed in conjunction with the appropriate procedure in the Medicare Physician Fee Schedule Data Base (place of service is physician's office). However, A4550, A4300, and A4263 are no longer separately payable as of 2002.
>
> B. . The supply is a pharmaceutical or radiopharmaceutical diagnostic imaging agent (including codes A4641 through A4647); pharmacologic stressing agent (code J1245); or therapeutic radionuclide (CPT code 79900). Other agents may be used which do not have an assigned HCPCS code. The procedures performed are:
>
> - Diagnostic radiologic procedures (including diagnostic nuclear medicine) requiring pharmaceutical or radiopharmaceutical contrast media and/or pharmacologic stressing agent;
> - Other diagnostic tests requiring a pharmacologic stressing agent;
> - Clinical brachytherapy procedures (other than remote after-loading high intensity brachytherapy procedures (CPT codes 77781 through 77784) for which the expendable source is included in the TC RVUs); or
> - Therapeutic nuclear medicine procedures.
>
> – *Medicare Claims Processing Manual, Chapter 12, Section 20.4.4*

Transportation; Non-Emergency (A0080-A0210)

Although non-emergency transportation (codes A0080-A0210) is not covered by Medicare, other payers could cover these types of services as long at it meets the payer's medically necessary guidelines. Be aware of differences in payer policies. For example, one state Medicaid policy says it "covers medically necessary non-emergency ground and air transportation to and from a required medical service for most recipients" and another state policy says that it is covered "only for members with no other means of transportation, to transport members to and from medical appointments for Medicaid covered services."

When billing these services, report the number of miles the patient was transported, round-trip, in Item Number 24G of the *1500 Claim Form*.

Tips:
- If a payer only covers or authorizes a specified number of miles which is less than the number of miles the patient was actually transported, report the authorized miles (units) on a separate line item from the un-authorized miles so that the appropriate total number of miles is reported even if it is noncovered.
- Special types of transportation (e.g., A0425 "Ground mileage" and A0434 "Specialty care transport") may be covered by some Medicare payers. Verify coverage with your local MAC.

Common Supply Codes

Conventions

The following conventions are used in this segment:

Identifiers/Columns

- **N** Signifies a code added this year.
- **R** Signifies a code revised this year. Revised codes may have had a change to their description, inclusion terms, and/or instructional notes.
- **NCCI** Identifies codes to which NCCI edits apply. See Chapter 5.1 — Procedure Coding Essentials for information about NCCI edits. See Appendix A — NCCI Edits for applicable NCCI edits for that code.
- **RVU** This column identifies the total RVU, where applicable, for the code
- **$Fee** This column identifies a Medicare fee for the code. It may be based on the RVU (national, unadjusted amount) or a fee schedule (e.g., laboratory, DME). Where applicable, fees for new equipment (NU) and rentals (RR) are specified separately.

Indicators

Special code edits are included in this code list to assist with accurate code selection and reporting. These edits are identified as "indicators." Appropriately employing them may improve coding accuracy and reduce claim denials. Automatic payer edits can identify and deny claims that fail to meet the basic edits identified here. Become familiar with the edits that affect your organization to avoid unnecessary claim denials.

Note: Not every code will have an associated indicator.

Book: See *Figure F.2* in Appendix F — Coding Reference Tables for a list with explanations of the indicators found in this chapter.

Disclaimer: The NCCI flags, RVUs and Fees included here are from October 2021 which were the most current edits at the time of publication. NCCI edits for 2022 will be available by January 1st for FindACode.com subscribers.

Code	Description	NCCI	RVU	$Fee

Transportation Services (A0021-A0999)

Code	Description	NCCI	RVU	$Fee
A0080	Non-emergency transportation, per mile - vehicle provided by volunteer (individual or organization), with no vested interest	-	NE	NE
A0090	Non-emergency transportation, per mile - vehicle provided by individual (family member, self, neighbor) with vested interest	-	NE	NE
A0100	Non-emergency transportation; taxi	-	NE	NE
A0110	Non-emergency transportation and bus, intra or inter state carrier	-	NE	NE
A0120	Non-emergency transportation: mini-bus, mountain area transports, or other transportation systems	-	NE	NE
A0130	Non-emergency transportation: wheelchair van	-	NE	NE
A0140	Non-emergency transportation and air travel (private or commercial) intra or inter state	-	NE	NE
A0160	Non-emergency transportation: per mile - case worker or social worker	-	NE	NE
A0170	ancillary: parking fees, tolls, other	-	NE	NE
A0180	Non-emergency transportation: ancillary: lodging-recipient	-	NE	NE

Code	Description	NCCI	RVU	SFee
A0190	Non-emergency transportation: ancillary: meals-recipient	-	NE	NE
A0200	Non-emergency transportation: ancillary: lodging escort	-	NE	NE
A0210	Non-emergency transportation: ancillary: meals-escort	-	NE	NE

Medical And Surgical Supplies (A4206-A9598)

REPLACEMENT PARTS (A4630-A4640)

Code	Description	NCCI	RVU	SFee
A4630	batteries, medically necessary, transcutaneous electrical stimulator, owned by patient	-	NE	$6.77 NU

MISCELLANEOUS MEDICAL AND SURGICAL SUPPLIES (A4206-A4290)

Code	Description	NCCI	RVU	SFee
A4206	Syringe with needle, sterile, 1 cc or less, each	-	NE	NE
A4207	Syringe with needle, sterile 2 cc, each	-	NE	NE
A4208	Syringe with needle, sterile 3 cc, each	-	NE	NE
A4209	Syringe with needle, sterile 5 cc or greater, each	-	NE	NE
A4210	Needle-free injection device, each	-	NE	NE
A4211	Supplies for self-administered injections	-	NE	NE
A4455	Adhesive remover or solvent (for tape, cement or other adhesive), per ounce	-	NE	$1.58
A4565	Slings	-	NE	$9.02
A4570	Splint	-	NE	NE
A4595	Electrical stimulator supplies, 2 lead, per month, (e.g., TENS, NMES)	-	NE	$16.52

WOUND DRESSINGS (A2001-A7527)

Code	Description	NCCI	RVU	SFee
A6203	Composite dressing, sterile, pad size 16 sq. in. or less, with any size adhesive border, each dressing	-	NE	$3.95
A6206	Contact layer, sterile, 16 sq. in. or less, each dressing	-	NE	NE
A6216	Gauze, non-impregnated, non-sterile, pad size 16 sq. in. or less, without adhesive border, each dressing	-	NE	$0.05
A6219	Gauze, non-impregnated, sterile, pad size 16 sq. in. or less, with any size adhesive border, each dressing	-	NE	$1.12
A6242	Hydrogel dressing, wound cover, sterile, pad size 16 sq. in. or less, without adhesive border, each dressing	-	NE	$7.09
A6245	Hydrogel dressing, wound cover, sterile, pad size 16 sq. in. or less, with any size adhesive border, each dressing	-	NE	$8.51
A6248	Hydrogel dressing, wound filler, gel, per fluid ounce	-	NE	$19.02
A6251	Specialty absorptive dressing, wound cover, sterile, pad size 16 sq. in. or less, without adhesive border, each dressing	-	NE	$2.32
A6254	Specialty absorptive dressing, wound cover, sterile, pad size 16 sq. in. or less, with any size adhesive border, each dressing	-	NE	$1.40
A6257	Transparent film, sterile, 16 sq. in. or less, each dressing	-	NE	$1.80
A6260	cleansers, any type, any size	-	NE	NE
A6261	filler, gel/paste, per fluid ounce, not otherwise specified	-	NE	NE
A6262	filler, dry form, per gram, not otherwise specified	-	NE	NE
A6413	Adhesive bandage, first-aid type, any size, each	-	NE	NE
A6448	Light compression bandage, elastic, knitted/woven, width less than three inches, per yard	-	NE	$1.35
A6453	Self-adherent bandage, elastic, non-knitted/non-woven, width less than three inches, per yard	-	NE	$0.73

Administrative, Miscellaneous and Experimental (A9150-A9999)

Code	Description	NCCI	RVU	SFee
A9150	Non-prescription drugs	-	NE	NE
A9270	Non-covered item or service	-	NE	NE
A9280	Alert or alarm device, not otherwise classified	-	NE	NE

Durable Medical Equipment (DME) (E0100-E8002)

ULTRAVIOLET CABINET (E0691-E0694)

Code	Description	NCCI	RVU	SFee
E0691	light therapy system, includes bulbs/lamps, timer and eye protection; treatment area 2 square feet or less	-	NE	$1,049.96 NU $104.99 RR
E0692	light therapy system panel, includes bulbs/lamps, timer and eye protection, 4 foot panel	-	NE	$1,318.47 NU $131.74 RR
E0693	light therapy system panel, includes bulbs/lamps, timer and eye protection, 6 foot panel	-	NE	$1,625.29 NU $162.53 RR
E0694	multidirectional light therapy system in 6 foot cabinet, includes bulbs/lamps, timer and eye protection	-	NE	$5,173.17 NU $517.31 RR

TRANSCUTANEOUS AND/OR NEUROMUSCULAR ELECTRICAL NERVE STIMULATORS -- TENS (E0720-E0770)

Code	Description	NCCI	RVU	SFee
E0720	electrical nerve stimulation (tens) device, two lead, localized stimulation	-	NE	$156.39 NU
E0730	electrical nerve stimulation (tens) device, four or more leads, for multiple nerve stimulation	-	NE	$161.75 NU
E0745	Neuromuscular stimulator, electronic shock unit	-	NE	$98.04 RR
E0746	Electromyography (emg), biofeedback device	-	NE	NE

HEAT/COLD APPLICATION (E0200-E0239)

Code	Description	NCCI	RVU	SFee
E0200	Heat lamp, without stand (table model), includes bulb, or infrared element	-	NE	$90.19 NU $12.76 RR
E0202	Phototherapy (bilirubin) light with photometer	-	NE	$72.17 RR
E0203	Therapeutic lightbox, minimum 10,000 lux, table top model	-	NE	NE
E0210	Electric heat pad, standard	-	NE	$37.82 NU $5.47 RR
E0215	Electric heat pad, moist	-	NE	$78.39 NU $10.39 RR

Temporary Procedures & Professional Services (G0008-G9987)

PROCEDURES/PROFESSIONAL SERVICES (G0008-G9949)

Medication assisted treatment services (Medicare-enrolled opioid treatment program) (G2067-G2080)

Code	Description	NCCI	RVU	SFee
G2078	Take-home supply of methadone; up to 7 additional day supply (provision of the services by a medicare-enrolled opioid treatment program); list separately in addition to code for primary procedure	-	NE	NE
G2079	Take-home supply of buprenorphine (oral); up to 7 additional day supply (provision of the services by a medicare-enrolled opioid treatment program); list separately in addition to code for primary procedure	-	NE	NE
® G2215	Take-home supply of nasal naloxone; 2-pack of 4mg per 0.1 ml nasal spray (provision of the services by a medicare-enrolled opioid treatment program); list separately in addition to code for primary procedure	-	NE	NE
G2216	Take-home supply of injectable naloxone (provision of the services by a medicare-enrolled opioid treatment program); list separately in addition to code for primary procedure	-	NE	NE

Drugs Administered (J0120-J9358)

DRUGS ADMINISTERED OTHER THAN ORAL METHOD (J0120-J7402)

Code	Description	NCCI	RVU	SFee
J0400	Injection, aripiprazole, intramuscular, 0.25 mg	-	NE	NE
J0401	Injection, aripiprazole, extended release, 1 mg	-	NE	$6.01
J0475	Injection, baclofen, 10 mg	-	NE	$177.43
J0585	Injection, onabotulinumtoxina, 1 unit	-	NE	$6.09
J0735	Injection, clonidine hydrochloride, 1 mg	-	NE	$23.49
J1130	Injection, diclofenac sodium, 0.5 mg	-	NE	NE
J1630	Injection, haloperidol, up to 5 mg	-	NE	$1.46
J1631	Injection, haloperidol decanoate, per 50 mg	-	NE	$9.57
J1632	Injection, brexanolone, 1 mg	-	NE	NE
J2060	Injection, lorazepam, 2 mg	-	NE	$0.78
J2062	Loxapine for inhalation, 1 mg	-	NE	NE
J2310	Injection, naloxone hydrochloride, per 1 mg	-	NE	$10.93
J2315	Injection, naltrexone, depot form, 1 mg	-	NE	$3.53
J2358	Injection, olanzapine, long-acting, 1 mg	-	NE	$2.91
J2426	Injection, paliperidone palmitate extended release, 1 mg	-	NE	$12.66
J2680	Injection, fluphenazine decanoate, up to 25 mg	-	NE	$10.30
J3360	Injection, diazepam, up to 5 mg	-	NE	$5.79
J3420	Injection, vitamin b-12 cyanocobalamin, up to 1000 mcg	-	NE	$2.12
J3490	Unclassified drugs	-	NE	NE
J3535	Drug administered through a metered dose inhaler	-	NE	NE

Code	Description	NCCI	RVU	$Fee
Buprenorphine (J0570-J0575)				
J0570	implant, 74.2 mg	-	NE	$1,311.75
J0571	oral, 1 mg	-	NE	NE
J0572	Buprenorphine/naloxone, oral, less than or equal to 3 mg buprenorphine	-	NE	NE
J0573	Buprenorphine/naloxone, oral, greater than 3 mg, but less than or equal to 6 mg buprenorphine	-	NE	NE
J0574	Buprenorphine/naloxone, oral, greater than 6 mg, but less than or equal to 10 mg buprenorphine	-	NE	NE
Dexamethasone (J1094-J1100)				
J1100	Injection, dexamethasone sodium phosphate, 1 mg	-	NE	$0.12
Aripiprazole lauroxil (J1943-J1944)				
J1943	Injection, aripiprazole lauroxil, (aristada initio), 1 mg	-	NE	$3.05
J1944	Injection, aripiprazole lauroxil, (aristada), 1 mg	-	NE	$2.99
Inj., Risperidone (J2794-J2798)				
J2794	Injection, risperidone (risperdal consta), 0.5 mg	-	NE	$11.04
J2798	Injection, risperidone, (perseris), 0.5 mg	-	NE	$10.69
INHALATION SOLUTIONS (J7604-J8999)				
J8499	Prescription drug, oral, non chemotherapeutic, nos	-	NE	NE

Private Payer Codes (S0012-S9999)

Code	Description	NCCI	RVU	$Fee
S5000 (S5000-S5523)				
S5199	Personal care item, nos, each	-	NE	NE
S9000 (S9001-S9999)				
S9433	Medical food nutritionally complete, administered orally, providing 100% of nutritional intake	-	NE	NE
DRUGS ADMINISTERED (S0014-S0197)				
S0109	Methadone, oral, 5 mg	-	NE	NE
Nasal spray (S0012-S0013)				
S0013	Esketamine, nasal spray, 1 mg	-	NE	NE

Code	Description	NCCI	RVU	SFee

State Medicaid Agency Codes (T1000-T5999)

Code	Description	NCCI	RVU	SFee
T5999	Supply, not otherwise specified	-	NE	NE

DIAPERS/PADS/WRAPS (T4521-T4545)

Code	Description	NCCI	RVU	SFee
T4543	Adult sized disposable incontinence product, protective brief/diaper, above extra large, each	-	NE	NE
T4544	Adult sized disposable incontinence product, protective underwear/pull-on, above extra large, each	-	NE	NE

Notes:

Appendices

Appendices Content

Appendix A. NCCI Edits 401
    NCCI Edits for CPT 404

Appendix B. Modifiers 419
    Understanding Modifiers 419
    Level I CPT Modifiers 420
    Level II HCPCS Modifiers 434

Appendix C. Provider Documentation Guides 449
    Introduction 449

Appendix D. Telehealth Services 459

Appendix E. Common Diagnosis Code Tips 467
    Coding Conventions & Instructions 468
    Tips 471

Appendix F. Coding Reference Tables 505

Appendix G. Glossary 519

Appendix H. Procedure Code Crosswalks 535

Appendix A. NCCI Edits

The National Correct Coding Initiative (NCCI) was developed by the Centers for Medicare & Medicaid Services (CMS) to promote national correct coding methodologies and to control improper Part B payments resulting from improper coding. Although NCCI edits were not intended for use outside of CMS, some third-party payers have adopted and adapted them for use within their own payment system edits. It is up to the provider to determine whether a third-party payer has published a policy or included wording in the provider's contract that states if they follow the NCCI edits. If they do not, the provider is only required to adhere to the edits published in the CPT codebook.

Book: See "NCCI Coding Edits" in Chapter 5.1 — Procedure Coding Essentials for a more comprehensive information about these edits.

Website: NCCI edits are updated quarterly. The most current NCCI edit information can be found at FindACode.com by clicking on the "NCCI Information" bar on the individual code page.

Resource: To easily verify the codes reported on a claim, use Find-A-Code's *NCCI Edits Validator*™ tool (available by subscription). See Resource 335.

Disclaimer: The NCCI edits included in this appendix are from October 2021 which were the most current edits at the time of publication. As such, new codes for 2022 are not included. NCCI edits for 2022 will be available by January 1st at FindACode.com (with subscription).

Superscript Indicators

The official NCCI data files organize procedure to procedure (P2P) edits by pairing primary and secondary service codes into a table with the primary service code listed in Column 1 and the secondary code(s) in Column 2. When performed at the same time (i.e., same patient, provider, and date of service), the work described by the Column 2 code is considered to be integral to the work described by the Column 1 (primary service) code and therefore bundled into the Column 1 primary service code. This means if billed together, only the primary service (Column 1) code will be paid. However, under certain circumstances, it is appropriate to override the P2P edit, essentially unbundling the secondary service to receive payment for both. Not all secondary procedures (Column 2 codes) are eligible for unbundling. Superscript indicators, located at the end of each Column 2 (secondary service) code, are used to identify which codes pairs may be unbundled under specific circumstances, as explained below:

- A superscript indicator of "0" indicates that the Column 2 code is NOT eligible for unbundling or payment under any circumstance. Do not report it with a modifier to try and override the edit. If the payer requires the provider to follow NCCI edits, then do not include the Column 2 code on the claim, as reporting it may result in a payment error and if not identified until a later audit, may result in fines and penalties or accusations of fraudulent billing practices.

- A superscript indicator of "1" indicates that the service may be eligible for unbundling, but only under certain circumstances identified within the *NCCI Policy Manual* and supported by the medical record.

On the following page is an example of what an NCCI edit might look like **in this appendix**. Where CMS publishes a 2-column table, to identify P2P code pairs, our customized charts list the primary (Column 1) code first followed by the secondary (Column 2) codes and their indicators beneath it. As a reminder, NCCI edits are updated quarterly and this edit is for quarter 3 of 2021.

Example

98968 Nonphysician telephone assessment 21-30 min
36591^0 36592^0 93792^1 93793^1 96523^0 99421^0 99422^0 99446^1 99447^1 $G0250^1$
MUE = 1

Using this example, we will review the meaning of the indicators if 98968 was performed the same day as 36591 and 93792 for payers who follow NCCI edits:

- *Superscript indicator "0" example:* Code 36591 has an indicator of "0" and if performed on the same day, same patient, and by the same provider as 98968, it will be denied. Any effort at an appeal will also result in a denial, even if using a modifier or letter of medical necessity because according to the *NCCI Policy Manual*, 36591 is not reportable with any service other than a laboratory service and 98968 is not a laboratory service.

- *Superscript indicator "1" example:* Code 93792 (patient/caregiver INR training), has a superscript indicator of "1". If performed on the same day, same patient, and by the same provider, it is considered bundled into the 98969 (telephone assessment) assuming the assessment was done to perform the INR training. If, however, the telephone assessment (98968) was performed to address another patient problem and the INR training (93792) just happened to be done at the same time, then according to the *NCCI Policy Manual*, 93792 could be unbundled using modifier 59 or XU (depending on payer preferences) in order to also be eligible for payment. The documentation must support the need for a telephone assessment for a reason other than the INR training to meet all expected criteria to override the edit.

Resource: See Resource 544 for comprehensive information about using NCCI edits including examples.

Alert: Only edits specific to the date of service may be applied. For example, you would not apply edits from 2022 to services performed in 2021.

Note: In this appendix, only the codes included in this publication are listed. To check edits on codes not included in this publication, please visit FindACode.com.

Medically Unlikely Edits

Medically Unlikely Edits (MUE) are the maximum number of units that may be billed on a single session. For example, it is "unlikely" (impossible in some situations) to perform more than one unit in one patient encounter; therefore, the MUE for that service is 1. If you bill 2 units for a single session, the claim is likely to be rejected. Some codes do not have any MUE edits assigned. Those codes with [MUE=N/A] do not have an MUE assigned.

Note: To save space in this appendix, if a code does not show an MUE, the MUE actually is 1. This appendix lists non-facility MUEs; for facility MUE information, go to FindACode.com (with subscription).

NCCI Code Pair (Bundling) Edits

NCCI code pair edits are automated coding edits that prevent improper payment when certain codes are submitted together for Part B covered services. Understanding NCCI edits can help healthcare providers and coders make appropriate coding decisions.

Alert: NCCI edits are only a guide. CMS states that "it is important to understand, however, that the NCCI does not include all possible combinations of correct coding edits or types of unbundling that exist. Providers are obligated to code correctly even if edits do not exist to prevent use of an inappropriate code combination."

There are two types of unbundling: the first is unintentional which results from a misunderstanding of coding, and the second is intentional, when providers deviate from ethical coding to increase payments. Unbundling is essentially the billing of multiple procedures codes for a group of procedures that are covered by a single comprehensive code. Examples of unbundling and improper coding are:

- Fragmenting one service into component parts and coding each component part as if it were a separate service.
- Reporting separate codes for related services when one comprehensive code includes all related services.
- Downcoding a service in order to use an additional code when one higher level and more comprehensive code is appropriate. An example is in laboratory coding with various panels and chemistry test options.

Edit Format

Code pair edits apply to code combinations where one of the codes is either a component of a more comprehensive code or is mutually exclusive. Mutually Exclusive codes are those codes that cannot reasonably be performed in the same session. One example is the reporting of an "initial" service and a "subsequent" service. It is contradictory for a service to be classified as an initial and subsequent service at the same time. CPT codes that are mutually exclusive of one another are based either on the CPT definition or the medical impossibility/improbability that the procedure(s) could be performed at the same session.

Edit Errors Can Happen

While efforts are made to ensure the accuracy of NCCI edits, their official disclaimer states "absolute accuracy cannot be guaranteed." If inaccuracies occur in the future, providers can help resolve the problem by working with associations and payers.

Resource: See Resource 337 for official information on NCCI edits by CMS.

A Simplified Way

FindACode.com includes an NCCI Edits Validator™ tool which is available to subscribers. This tool verifies edits and helps prevent code bundling. Simply enter the codes from your claim, or the codes you plan to report, and click on the "Submit" button. You will get a quick summary of which codes can or cannot be billed together and whether or not they need modifiers.

NCCI Edits for CPT

00104 Anesthesia for electroconvulsive therapy

CCI: 36410^1 64553^1 81000^1 81002^1 81003^1 81005^1 90865^1 95812^0 95813^0 95816^0 95819^0 95822^0 95925^0 95926^0 95927^0 95930^0 95938^0 96372^0 99151^0 99152^0 99153^0 99155^0 99156^0 99157^0 99202^0 99203^0 99204^0 99205^0 99211^0 99212^0 99213^0 99214^0 99215^0 99307^0 99308^0 99309^0 99310^0 99446^0 99447^0 99448^0 99449^0 99451^0 99452^0 99483^0

MUE: N/A

0143U Drug assay, definitive, 120 or more drugs or metabolites, urine, quantitative liquid chromatography with tandem mass spectrometry (LC-MS/MS) using multiple reaction monitoring (MRM), with drug or metabolite description, comments including sample validation, per date of service

CCI: $0144U^0$ $0145U^0$ $0146U^0$ $0147U^0$ $0148U^0$ $0149U^0$ $0150U^0$ 80305^0 80306^0 80307^0 80335^0 80336^0 80337^0 81000^1 81001^1 81002^1 81003^1 81005^1

0144U Drug assay, definitive, 160 or more drugs or metabolites, urine, quantitative liquid chromatography with tandem mass spectrometry (LC-MS/MS) using multiple reaction monitoring (MRM), with drug or metabolite description, comments including sample validation, per date of service

CCI: $0145U^0$ $0146U^0$ $0147U^0$ $0148U^0$ $0149U^0$ $0150U^0$ 80305^0 80306^0 80307^0 80335^0 80336^0 80337^0 81000^1 81001^1 81002^1 81003^1 81005^1

0145U Drug assay, definitive, 65 or more drugs or metabolites, urine, quantitative liquid chromatography with tandem mass spectrometry (LC-MS/MS) using multiple reaction monitoring (MRM), with drug or metabolite description, comments including sample validation, per date of service

CCI: $0146U^0$ $0147U^0$ $0148U^0$ $0149U^0$ $0150U^0$ 80305^0 80306^0 80307^0 80335^0 80336^0 80337^0 81000^1 81001^1 81002^1 81003^1 81005^1

0146U Drug assay, definitive, 80 or more drugs or metabolites, urine, by quantitative liquid chromatography with tandem mass spectrometry (LC-MS/MS) using multiple reaction monitoring (MRM), with drug or metabolite description, comments including sample validation, per date of service

CCI: $0147U^0$ $0148U^0$ $0149U^0$ $0150U^0$ 80305^0 80306^0 80307^0 80335^0 80336^0 80337^0 81000^1 81001^1 81002^1 81003^1 81005^1

0147U Drug assay, definitive, 85 or more drugs or metabolites, urine, quantitative liquid chromatography with tandem mass spectrometry (LC-MS/MS) using multiple reaction monitoring (MRM), with drug or metabolite description, comments including sample validation, per date of service

CCI: $0148U^0$ $0149U^0$ $0150U^0$ 80305^0 80306^0 80307^0 80335^0 80336^0 80337^0 81000^1 81001^1 81002^1 81003^1 81005^1

0148U Drug assay, definitive, 100 or more drugs or metabolites, urine, quantitative liquid chromatography with tandem mass spectrometry (LC-MS/MS) using multiple reaction monitoring (MRM), with drug or metabolite description, comments including sample validation, per date of service

CCI: $0149U^0$ $0150U^0$ 80305^0 80306^0 80307^0 80335^0 80336^0 80337^0 81000^1 81001^1 81002^1 81003^1 81005^1

0149U Drug assay, definitive, 60 or more drugs or metabolites, urine, quantitative liquid chromatography with tandem mass spectrometry (LC-MS/MS) using multiple reaction monitoring (MRM), with drug or metabolite description, comments including sample validation, per date of service

CCI: $0150U^0$ 80305^0 80306^0 80307^0 80335^0 80336^0 80337^0 81000^1 81001^1 81002^1 81003^1 81005^1

0150U Drug assay, definitive, 120 or more drugs or metabolites, urine, quantitative liquid chromatography with tandem mass spectrometry (LC-MS/MS) using multiple reaction monitoring (MRM), with drug or metabolite description, comments including sample validation, per date of service

CCI: 80305^0 80306^0 80307^0 80335^0 80336^0 80337^0 81000^1 81001^1 81002^1 81003^1 81005^1

0173U Psychiatry (ie, depression, anxiety), genomic analysis panel, includes variant analysis of 14 genes

CCI: $0175U^0$

0362T Behavior identification supporting assessment, each 15 minutes of technicians' time face-to-face with a patient, requiring the following components: administration by the physician or other qualified health care professional who is on site; with the assistance of two or more technicians; for a patient who exhibits destructive behavior; completion in an environment that is customized to the patient's behavior.

CCI: 96105^0 96110^0 96125^0 96127^0 96160^1 96161^1 97152^1

MUE: 16

0373T Adaptive behavior treatment with protocol modification, each 15 minutes of technicians' time face-to-face with a patient, requiring the following components: administration by the physician or other qualified health care professional who is on site; with the assistance of two or more technicians; for a patient who exhibits destructive behavior; completion in an environment that is customized to the patient's behavior.

CCI: 96105^0 96110^0 96116^0 96125^0 96127^0

MUE: 24

0591T Health and well-being coaching face-to-face; individual, initial assessment

CCI: $0362T^1$ $0373T^1$ 90839^1 90845^1 96116^1 96127^0 96158^0 96159^0 96164^0 96165^0 96167^0 96168^0 96170^0 96171^0 97151^1 97153^1 97154^1 97155^1 97156^1 97157^1 97158^1 97165^1 97166^1 97167^1 97168^1 99091^0 99202^1 99203^1 99204^1 99205^1 99211^1 99212^1 99213^1 99214^1 99215^1 99307^1 99308^1 99309^1 99310^1 99446^0 99447^0 99448^0 99449^0 99451^0 99452^0

0592T Health and well-being coaching face-to-face; individual, follow-up session, at least 30 minutes

CCI: $0362T^1$ $0373T^1$ $0591T^0$ 90839^1 90845^1 96116^1 96127^0 96164^0 96165^0 96167^0 96168^0 96170^0 96171^0 97151^1 97153^1 97154^1 97155^1 97156^1 97157^1 97158^1 97165^1 97166^1 97167^1 97168^1 99091^0 99202^1 99203^1 99204^1 99205^1 99211^1 99212^1 99213^1 99214^1 99215^1 99307^1 99308^1 99309^1 99310^1 99446^0 99447^0 99448^0 99449^0 99451^0 99452^0

0593T Health and well-being coaching face-to-face; group (2 or more individuals), at least 30 minutes

CCI: $0362T^1$ $0373T^1$ 90839^1 90845^1 96116^1 96127^0 96156^0 96158^0 96159^0 96167^0 96168^0 96170^0 96171^0 97151^1 97153^1 97154^1 97155^1 97156^1 97157^1 97158^1 97165^1 97166^1 97167^1 97168^1 99091^0 99202^1 99203^1 99204^1 99205^1 99211^1 99212^1 99213^1 99214^1 99215^1 99307^1 99308^1 99309^1 99310^1 99446^0 99447^0 99448^0 99449^0 99451^0 99452^0

11981 Insertion, drug-delivery implant (ie, bioresorbable, biodegradable, non-biodegradable)

CCI: 11982^0 36410^1 96372^1

11982 Removal, non-biodegradable drug delivery implant

CCI: 36410^1 96372^1

11983 Removal with reinsertion, non-biodegradable drug delivery implant

CCI: 11981^0 11982^0 36410^1 96372^1

16000 Initial treatment, first degree burn, when no more than local treatment is required

CCI: 36410^1 95812^1 95813^1 95816^1 95819^1 95822^1 96372^1 97022^1 99155^1 99156^1 99157^0 99211^1 99212^1 99213^1 99214^1 99215^1 99307^1 99308^1 99309^1 99310^1 99446^0 99447^0 99448^0 99449^0 99451^0 99452^0

16020 Dressings and/or debridement of partial-thickness burns, initial or subsequent; small (less than 5% total body surface area)

CCI: 16000¹ 36410¹ 95812¹ 95813¹ 95816¹ 95819¹ 95822¹ 96372¹ 97022¹ 99155⁰ 99156⁰ 99157⁰ 99211⁰ 99212¹ 99213¹ 99214¹ 99215¹ 93307¹ 99308¹ 99309¹ 99310¹ 99446⁰ 99447⁰ 99448⁰ 99449⁰ 99451⁰ 99452⁰

29260 Strapping; elbow or wrist

CCI: 36410¹ 95812¹ 95813¹ 95816¹ 95819¹ 95822¹ 96372¹ 99155⁰ 99156⁰ 99157⁰ 99211¹ 99212¹ 99213¹ 99214¹ 99215¹ 99307¹ 99308¹ 99309¹ 99310¹ 99446⁰ 99447⁰ 99448⁰ 99449⁰ 99451⁰ 99452⁰

29280 Strapping; hand or finger

CCI: 36410¹ 95812¹ 95813¹ 95816¹ 95819¹ 95822¹ 96372¹ 99155⁰ 99156⁰ 99157⁰ 99211¹ 99212¹ 99213¹ 99214¹ 99215¹ 99307¹ 99308¹ 99309¹ 99310¹ 99446⁰ 99447⁰ 99448⁰ 99449⁰ 99451⁰ 99452⁰

MUE: 2

29530 Strapping; knee

CCI: 36410¹ 95812¹ 95813¹ 95816¹ 95819¹ 95822¹ 96372¹ 99155⁰ 99156⁰ 99157⁰ 99211¹ 99212¹ 99213¹ 99214¹ 99215¹ 99307¹ 99308¹ 99309¹ 99310¹ 99446⁰ 99447⁰ 99448⁰ 99449⁰ 99451⁰ 99452⁰

29540 Strapping; ankle and/or foot

CCI: 36410¹ 95812¹ 95813¹ 95816¹ 95819¹ 95822¹ 96372¹ 99155⁰ 99156⁰ 99157⁰ 99211¹ 99212¹ 99213¹ 99214¹ 99215¹ 99307¹ 99308¹ 99309¹ 99310¹ 99446⁰ 99447⁰ 99448⁰ 99449⁰ 99451⁰ 99452⁰

30901 Control nasal hemorrhage, anterior, simple (limited cautery and/or packing) any method

CCI: 36410¹ 95812¹ 95813¹ 95816¹ 95819¹ 95822¹ 96372¹ 99155⁰ 99156⁰ 99157⁰ 99211¹ 99212¹ 99213¹ 99214¹ 99215¹ 99307¹ 99308¹ 99309¹ 99310¹ 99446⁰ 99447⁰ 99448⁰ 99449⁰ 99451⁰ 99452⁰

36415 Collection of venous blood by venipuncture

CCI: 99211¹

MUE: 2

64553 Percutaneous implantation of neurostimulator electrode array; cranial nerve

CCI: 36410¹ 95812¹ 95813¹ 95816¹ 95819¹ 95822⁰ 95925⁰ 95926¹ 95927⁰ 95930⁰ 95938⁰ 95970⁰ 96372¹ 99155⁰ 99156⁰ 99157⁰ 99211¹ 99212¹ 99213¹ 99214¹ 99215¹ 99307¹ 99308¹ 99309¹ 99310¹ 99446⁰ 99447⁰ 99448⁰ 99449⁰ 99451⁰ 99452⁰

69200 Removal foreign body from external auditory canal; without general anesthesia

CCI: 36410¹ 95812¹ 95813¹ 95816¹ 95819¹ 95822¹ 96372¹ 99155⁰ 99156⁰ 99157⁰ 99211¹ 99212¹ 99213¹ 99214¹ 99215¹ 99307¹ 99308¹ 99309¹ 99310¹ 99446⁰ 99447⁰ 99448⁰ 99449⁰ 99451⁰ 99452⁰

70371 Complex dynamic pharyngeal and speech evaluation by cine or video recording

CCI: 99446⁰ 99447⁰ 99448⁰ 99449⁰ 99451⁰ 99452⁰

70554 Magnetic resonance imaging, brain, functional MRI; including test selection and administration of repetitive body part movement and/or visual stimulation, not requiring physician or psychologist administration

CCI: 96020¹

70555 Magnetic resonance imaging, brain, functional MRI; requiring physician or psychologist administration of entire neurofunctional testing

CCI: 70554¹ 99446⁰ 99447⁰ 99448⁰ 99449⁰ 99451⁰ 99452⁰

80048 Basic metabolic panel (Calcium, total) This panel must include the following: Calcium, total (82310) Carbon dioxide (bicarbonate) (82374) Chloride (82435) Creatinine (82565) Glucose (82947) Potassium (84132) Sodium (84295) Urea nitrogen (BUN) (84520)

CCI: 82947¹

MUE: 2

80053 Comprehensive metabolic panel This panel must include the following: Albumin (82040) Bilirubin, total (82247) Calcium, total (82310) Carbon dioxide (bicarbonate) (82374) Chloride (82435) Creatinine (82565) Glucose (82947) Phosphatase, alkaline (84075) Potassium (84132) Protein, total (84155) Sodium (84295) Transferase, alanine amino (ALT) (SGPT) (84460) Transferase, aspartate amino (AST) (SGOT) (84450) Urea nitrogen (BUN) (84520)

CCI: 80048⁰ 80076⁰ 82947¹

80061 Lipid panel This panel must include the following: Cholesterol, serum, total (82465) Lipoprotein, direct measurement, high density cholesterol (HDL cholesterol) (83718) Triglycerides (84478)

CCI: 84478⁰

80305 Drug test(s), presumptive, any number of drug classes, any number of devices or procedures; capable of being read by direct optical observation only (eg, utilizing immunoassay [eg, dipsticks, cups, cards, or cartridges]), includes sample validation when performed, per date of service

CCI: 81000¹ 81001¹ 81002¹ 81003¹ 81005¹

80306 Drug test(s), presumptive, any number of drug classes, any number of devices or procedures; read by instrument assisted direct optical observation (eg, utilizing immunoassay [eg, dipsticks, cups, cards, or cartridges]), includes sample validation when performed, per date of service

CCI: 80305⁰ 81000¹ 81001¹ 81002¹ 81003¹ 81005¹

80307 Drug test(s), presumptive, any number of drug classes, any number of devices or procedures; by instrument chemistry analyzers (eg, utilizing immunoassay [eg, EIA, ELISA, EMIT, FPIA, IA, KIMS, RIA]), chromatography (eg, GC, HPLC), and mass spectrometry either with or without chromatography, (eg, DART, DESI, GC-MS, GC-MS/MS, LC-MS, LC-MS/MS, LDTD, MALDI, TOF) includes sample validation when performed, per date of service

CCI: 80305⁰ 80306⁰ 81000¹ 81001¹ 81002¹ 81003¹ 81005¹

81000 Urinalysis, by dip stick or tablet reagent for bilirubin, glucose, hemoglobin, ketones, leukocytes, nitrite, pH, protein, specific gravity, urobilinogen, any number of these constituents; non-automated, with microscopy

CCI: 81002⁰

MUE: 2

81001 Urinalysis, by dip stick or tablet reagent for bilirubin, glucose, hemoglobin, ketones, leukocytes, nitrite, pH, protein, specific gravity, urobilinogen, any number of these constituents; automated, with microscopy

CCI: 81000¹ 81002¹ 81003¹

MUE: 2

81003 Urinalysis, by dip stick or tablet reagent for bilirubin, glucose, hemoglobin, ketones, leukocytes, nitrite, pH, protein, specific gravity, urobilinogen, any number of these constituents; automated, without microscopy

CCI: 81000¹ 81002¹

MUE: 2

81005 Urinalysis; qualitative or semiquantitative, except immunoassays

CCI: 81000⁰ 81002⁰ 81003⁰

MUE: 2

82947 Glucose; quantitative, blood (except reagent strip)

CCI: 82948^1

MUE: 5

85008 Blood count; blood smear, microscopic examination without manual differential WBC count

CCI: 85007^0

85018 Blood count; hemoglobin (Hgb)

CCI: 85008^1

MUE: 2

85025 Blood count; complete (CBC), automated (Hgb, Hct, RBC, WBC and platelet count) and automated differential WBC count

CCI: 85007^0 85008^0 85009^0 85014^1 85018^1 85027^1 85032^0 85048^1

MUE: 2

85027 Blood count; complete (CBC), automated (Hgb, Hct, RBC, WBC and platelet count)

CCI: 85008^0 85014^1 85018^1 85032^0 85048^1

MUE: 2

85032 Blood count; manual cell count (erythrocyte, leukocyte, or platelet) each

CCI: 85008^0

85048 Blood count; leukocyte (WBC), automated

CCI: 85008^0 85032^0

MUE: 2

86580 Skin test; tuberculosis, intradermal

CCI: 96372^1

87081 Culture, presumptive, pathogenic organisms, screening only;

CCI: 87084^1 87088^1

MUE: 2

87084 Culture, presumptive, pathogenic organisms, screening only; with colony estimation from density chart

CCI: 87070^1

87086 Culture, bacterial; quantitative colony count, urine

CCI: 87070^1 87081^1 87084^1

MUE: 3

87088 Culture, bacterial; with isolation and presumptive identification of each isolate, urine

CCI: 87070^1 87084^1

MUE: 3

90632 Hepatitis A vaccine (HepA), adult dosage, for intramuscular use

CCI: 90633^0 90634^0 90636^0

90633 Hepatitis A vaccine (HepA), pediatric/adolescent dosage-2 dose schedule, for intramuscular use

CCI: 90634^0 90636^0

90634 Hepatitis A vaccine (HepA), pediatric/adolescent dosage-3 dose schedule, for intramuscular use

CCI: 90636^0

90785 Interactive complexity (List separately in addition to the code for primary procedure)

CCI: $0362T^0$ $0373T^0$ 96164^0 96165^0 97151^0 97152^0 97153^0 97154^0 97155^0 97156^0 97157^0

MUE: 3

90791 Psychiatric diagnostic evaluation

CCI: $0362T^0$ $0373T^0$ $0591T^0$ $0592T^0$ $0593T^0$ 90832^0 90833^0 90834^0 90836^0 90837^0 90838^0 90839^0 90840^0 90845^0 90846^0 90847^0 90849^0 90853^0 90863^0 90865^0 90867^0 90868^0 90869^0 90870^0 90875^0 90876^0 90880^0 90882^0 90885^0 90887^0 90889^0 96116^0 96127^0 96156^0 96158^0 96159^0 96160^0 96161^0 96164^0 96165^0 96167^0 96168^0 96170^0 96171^0 97151^0 97152^0 97153^0 97154^0 97155^0 97156^0 97157^0 99202^0 99203^0 99204^0 99205^0 99211^0 99212^0 99213^0 99214^0 99215^0 99307^0 99308^0 99309^0 99310^0 99441^0 99442^0 99443^0 99446^0 99447^0 99448^0 99449^0 99451^0 99452^0 99491^0

90792 Psychiatric diagnostic evaluation with medical services

CCI: $0362T^0$ $0373T^0$ $0591T^0$ $0592T^0$ $0593T^0$ 90791^0 90832^0 90833^0 90834^0 90836^0 90837^0 90838^0 90839^0 90840^0 90845^0 90846^0 90847^0 90849^0 90853^0 90863^0 90865^0 90867^0 90868^0 90869^0 90870^0 90875^0 90876^0 90880^0 90882^0 90885^0 90887^0 90889^0 96116^0 96127^0 96156^0 96158^0 96159^0 96160^0 96161^0 96164^0 96165^0 96167^0 96168^0 96170^0 96171^0 97151^0 97152^0 97153^0 97154^0 97155^0 97156^0 97157^0 99202^0 99203^0 99204^0 99205^0 99211^0 99212^0 99213^0 99214^0 99215^0 99307^0 99308^0 99309^0 99310^0 99441^0 99442^0 99443^0 99446^0 99447^0 99448^0 99449^0 99451^0 99452^0 99491^0

90832 Psychotherapy, 30 minutes with patient

CCI: $0362T^0$ $0373T^0$ $0591T^0$ $0592T^0$ $0593T^0$ 90839^0 90840^0 90867^1 90868^1 90869^1 90875^0 90876^0 96116^0 96127^0 96158^0 96159^0 96160^0 96161^0 96164^0 96165^0 96168^0 96171^0 97151^0 97152^0 97153^0 97154^0 97155^0 97156^0 97157^0 99202^0 99203^0 99204^0 99205^0 99211^0 99212^0 99213^0 99214^0 99215^0 99307^0 99308^0 99309^0 99310^0 99441^0 99442^0 99443^0 99446^0 99447^0 99448^0 99449^0 99451^0 99452^0 99483^0 99491^0

MUE: 2

90833 Psychotherapy, 30 minutes with patient when performed with an evaluation and management service (List separately in addition to the code for primary procedure)

CCI: $0362T^0$ $0373T^0$ $0591T^0$ $0592T^0$ $0593T^0$ 90832^0 90839^0 90840^0 90867^1 90868^1 90869^1 90875^0 90876^0 96116^1 96127^0 96158^0 96159^0 96160^0 96161^0 96164^0 96165^0 96168^0 96171^0 97151^0 97152^0 97153^0 97154^0 97155^0 97156^0 97157^0 99446^0 99447^0 99448^0 99449^0 99451^0 99452^0 99491^0

MUE: 2

90834 Psychotherapy, 45 minutes with patient

CCI: $0362T^0$ $0373T^0$ $0591T^0$ $0592T^0$ $0593T^0$ 90832^0 90833^0 90839^0 90840^0 90845^0 90867^1 90868^1 90869^1 90875^0 90876^0 96116^1 96127^0 96158^0 96159^0 96160^0 96161^0 96164^0 96165^0 96167^0 96168^0 96170^0 96171^0 97151^0 97152^0 97153^0 97154^0 97155^0 97156^0 97157^0 99202^0 99203^0 99204^0 99205^0 99211^0 99212^0 99213^0 99214^0 99215^0 99307^0 99308^0 99309^0 99310^0 99441^0 99442^0 99443^0 99446^0 99447^0 99448^0 99449^0 99451^0 99452^0 99483^0 99491^0

MUE: 2

90836 Psychotherapy, 45 minutes with patient when performed with an evaluation and management service (List separately in addition to the code for primary procedure)

CCI: $0362T^0$ $0373T^0$ $0591T^0$ $0592T^0$ $0593T^0$ 90832^0 90833^0 90834^0 90839^0 90840^0 90867^1 90868^1 90869^1 90875^0 90876^0 96116^1 96127^0 96158^0 96159^0 96160^0 96161^0 96164^0 96165^0 96167^0 96168^0 96170^0 96171^0 97151^0 97152^0 97153^0 97154^0 97155^0 97156^0 97157^0 99446^0 99447^0 99448^0 99449^0 99451^0 99452^0 99491^0

MUE: 2

90837 Psychotherapy, 60 minutes with patient

CCI: $0362T^0$ $0373T^0$ $0591T^0$ $0592T^0$ $0593T^0$ 90832^0 90833^0 90834^0 90836^0 90839^0 90840^0 90845^0 90867^1 90868^1 90869^1 90875^0 90876^0 96116^0 96127^0 96156^0 96158^0 96159^0 96160^0 96161^0 96164^0 96165^0 96167^0 96168^0 96170^0 96171^0 97151^0 97152^0 97153^0 97154^0 97155^0 97156^0 97157^0 99202^0 99203^0 99204^0 99205^0 99211^0 99212^0 99213^0 99214^0 99215^0 99307^0 99308^0 99309^0 99310^0 99441^0 99442^0 99443^0 99446^0 99447^0 99448^0 99449^0 99451^0 99452^0 99483^0 99491^0

MUE: 2

90838 Psychotherapy, 60 minutes with patient when performed with an evaluation and management service (List separately in addition to the code for primary procedure)

CCI: $0362T^0$ $0373T^0$ $0591T^0$ $0592T^0$ $0593T^0$ 90832^0 90833^0 90834^0 90836^0 90837^0 90839^0 90840^0 90845^0 90867^1 90868^1 90869^1 90875^0 90876^0 96116^0 96127^0 96156^0 96158^0 96159^0 96160^0 96161^0 96164^0 96165^0 96167^0 96168^0 96170^0 96171^0 97151^0 97152^0 97153^0 97154^0 97155^0 97156^0 97157^0 99446^0 99447^0 99448^0 99449^0 99451^0 99452^0 99491^0

MUE: 2

90839 Psychotherapy for crisis; first 60 minutes

CCI: $0362T^0$ $0373T^0$ 90785^0 90845^0 90846^0 90847^0 90849^0 90853^0 90863^0 90865^0 90867^0 90868^0 90869^0 90870^0 90875^0 90876^0 90880^0 90882^0 90885^0 90887^0 90889^0 96116^0 96127^0 96156^0 96158^0 96159^0 96164^0 96165^0 96167^0 96168^0 96170^0 96171^0 97151^0 97152^0 97153^0 97154^0 97155^0 97156^0 97157^0

90840 Psychotherapy for crisis; each additional 30 minutes (List separately in addition to code for primary service)

CCI: $0362T^0$ $0373T^0$ 90785^0 90845^0 90846^0 90847^0 90849^0 90853^0 90863^0 90865^0 90867^0 90868^0 90869^0 90870^0 90875^0 90876^0 90880^0 90882^0 90885^0 90887^0 90889^0 96116^0 96127^0 96158^0 96159^0 96164^0 96165^0 96168^0 96171^0 97151^0 97152^0 97153^0 97154^0 97155^0 97156^0 97157^0

MUE: 3

90845 Psychoanalysis

CCI: $0362T^0$ $0373T^0$ 90832^0 90833^0 90836^0 90846^1 90847^1 90865^0 96116^0 96127^0 96156^0 96158^0 96159^0 96164^0 96165^0 96167^0 96168^0 96170^0 96171^0 97151^0 97152^0 97153^0 97154^0 97155^0 97156^0 97157^0 99202^0 99203^0 99204^0 99205^0 99211^0 99212^0 99213^0 99214^0 99215^0 99307^0 99308^0 99309^0 99310^0 99483^0

90846 Family psychotherapy (without the patient present), 50 minutes

CCI: $0362T^0$ $0373T^0$ 90832^1 90833^1 90834^1 90836^1 90837^1 90838^1 90847^1 90865^1 90870^1 96116^0 96127^0 96156^0 96158^0 96159^0 96164^0 96165^0 96167^0 96168^0 96170^0 96171^0 97151^0 97152^0 97153^0 97154^0 97155^0 97156^0 97157^0 99202^0 99203^0 99204^0 99205^0 99211^0 99212^1 99213^1 99214^1 99215^1 99307^1 99308^1 99309^1 99310^1 99483^1

90847 Family psychotherapy (conjoint psychotherapy) (with patient present), 50 minutes

CCI: $0362T^0$ $0373T^0$ 90832^1 90833^1 90834^1 90836^1 90837^1 90838^1 90865^1 90870^1 96116^1 96127^0 96156^0 96158^0 96159^0 96164^0 96165^0 96167^0 96168^0 96170^0 96171^0 97151^0 97152^0 97153^0 97154^0 97155^0 97156^0 97157^0 99202^1 99203^1 99204^1 99205^1 99211^1 99212^1 99213^1 99214^1 99215^1 99307^1 99308^1 99309^1 99310^1 99483^1

90849 Multiple-family group psychotherapy

CCI: $0362T^0$ $0373T^0$ 90832^1 90833^1 90834^1 90836^1 90837^1 90838^1 90845^1 90846^1 90847^1 90865^1 90870^1 96116^1 96127^0 96159^0 96164^0 96165^0 96168^0 96171^0 97151^0 97152^0 97153^0 97154^0 97155^0 97156^0 97157^0 99202^1 99203^1 99204^1 99205^1 99211^1 99212^1 99213^1 99214^1 99215^1 99307^1 99308^1 99309^1 99310^1 99483^1

90853 Group psychotherapy (other than of a multiple-family group)

CCI: $0362T^0$ $0373T^0$ 90832^1 90833^1 90834^1 90836^1 90837^1 90838^1 90845^1 90846^1 90847^1 90849^1 90865^1 90870^1 96116^0 96127^0 96159^0 96164^0 96165^0 96168^0 96171^0 97151^0 97152^0 97153^0 97154^0 97155^0 97156^0 97157^0 99202^1 99203^1 99204^1 99205^1 99211^1 99212^1 99213^1 99214^1 99215^1 99307^1 99308^1 99309^1 99310^1 99483^1

90863 Pharmacologic management, including prescription and review of medication, when performed with psychotherapy services (List separately in addition to the code for primary procedure)

CCI: $0362T^0$ $0373T^0$ 96127^0 96164^0 96165^0 96168^0 97151^0 97152^0 97153^0 97154^0 97155^0 97156^0 97157^0

90865 Narcosynthesis for psychiatric diagnostic and therapeutic purposes (eg, sodium amobarbital (Amytal) interview)

CCI: $0362T^0$ $0373T^0$ 90832^0 90833^0 90834^0 90836^0 90837^0 90838^0 96116^0 96127^0 96156^0 96158^0 96159^0 96164^0 96165^0 96167^0 96168^0 96170^0 96171^0 97151^0 97152^0 97153^0 97154^0 97155^0 97156^0 97157^0 99202^0 99203^0 99204^0 99205^0 99211^0 99212^0 99213^0 99214^0 99215^0 99307^0 99308^0 99309^0 99310^0 99483^0

90867 Therapeutic repetitive transcranial magnetic stimulation (TMS) treatment; initial, including cortical mapping, motor threshold determination, delivery and management

CCI: $0362T^0$ $0373T^0$ 90845^1 90846^1 90847^1 90849^1 90853^1 90865^1 90868^1 90869^1 90870^1 90880^1 95925^1 95926^1 95927^1 95930^1 95938^1 96127^0 99202^1 99203^1 99204^1 99205^1 99211^1 99212^1 99213^1 99214^1 99215^1 99307^1 99308^1 99309^1 99310^1 99446^0 99447^0 99448^0 99449^0 99451^0 99452^0 99483^1

90868 Therapeutic repetitive transcranial magnetic stimulation (TMS) treatment; subsequent delivery and management, per session

CCI: $0362T^0$ $0373T^0$ 90845^1 90846^1 90847^1 90849^1 90853^1 90865^1 90870^1 90880^1 95925^1 95926^1 95927^1 95930^1 95938^1 96127^0 99202^1 99203^1 99204^1 99205^1 99211^1 99212^1 99213^1 99214^1 99215^1 99307^1 99308^1 99309^1 99310^1 99446^1 99447^0 99448^0 99449^0 99451^0 99452^0 99483^1

90869 Therapeutic repetitive transcranial magnetic stimulation (TMS) treatment; subsequent motor threshold re-determination with delivery and management

CCI: $0362T^0$ $0373T^0$ 90845^1 90846^1 90847^1 90849^1 90853^1 90865^1 90868^0 90870^1 90880^1 95925^1 95926^1 95927^1 95930^1 95938^1 96127^0 99202^1 99203^1 99204^1 99205^1 99211^1 99212^1 99213^1 99214^1 99215^1 99307^1 99308^1 99309^1 99310^1 99446^0 99447^0 99448^0 99449^0 99451^0 99452^0 99483^1

90870 Electroconvulsive therapy (includes necessary monitoring)

CCI: 00104^0 $0362T^0$ $0373T^0$ 36410^1 90832^0 90833^0 90834^0 90836^0 90837^0 90838^0 90845^0 90865^1 90880^1 95812^1 95813^1 95816^1 95819^1 95822^1 96127^0 96156^0 96158^0 96159^0 96164^0 96165^0 96167^0 96168^0 96170^0 96171^0 96372^1 97151^0 97152^0 97153^0 97154^0 97155^0 97156^0 97157^0 99155^0 99156^0 99157^0 99211^1 99212^1 99213^1 99214^1 99215^1 99307^1 99308^1 99309^1 99310^1 99446^0 99447^0 99448^0 99449^0 99451^0 99452^0

MUE: 2

90875 Individual psychophysiological therapy incorporating biofeedback training by any modality (face-to-face with the patient), with psychotherapy (eg, insight oriented, behavior modifying or supportive psychotherapy); 30 minutes

CCI: $0362T^0$ $0373T^0$ 96159^0 96164^0 96165^0 96168^0 96171^0 97151^0 97152^0 97153^0 97154^0 97155^0 97156^0 97157^0

90876 Individual psychophysiological therapy incorporating biofeedback training by any modality (face-to-face with the patient), with psychotherapy (eg, insight oriented, behavior modifying or supportive psychotherapy); 45 minutes

CCI: $0362T^0$ $0373T^0$ 96158^0 96159^0 96164^0 96165^0 96167^0 96168^0 96170^0 96171^0 97151^0 97152^0 97153^0 97154^0 97155^0 97156^0 97157^0

MUE: N/A

90880 Hypnotherapy

CCI: $0362T^0$ $0373T^0$ 90832^0 90833^0 90834^0 90836^0 90837^0 90838^0 90845^0 90846^0 90847^0 90849^0 90853^0 90865^1 96116^1 96127^0 96156^0 96158^0 96159^0 96164^0 96165^0 96167^0 96168^0 96170^0 96171^0 97151^0 97152^0 97153^0 97154^0 97155^0 97156^0 97157^0 99202^0 99203^0 99204^0 99205^0 99211^0 99212^0 99213^0 99214^0 99215^0 99307^0 99308^0 99309^0 99310^0 99483^0

90882 Environmental intervention for medical management purposes on a psychiatric patient's behalf with agencies, employers, or institutions

CCI: $0362T^0$ $0373T^0$ 97152^0

MUE: N/A

90885 Psychiatric evaluation of hospital records, other psychiatric reports, psychometric and/or projective tests, and other accumulated data for medical diagnostic purposes

CCI: $0362T^0$ $0373T^0$ 96159^0 96164^0 96165^0 96168^0 96171^0 97151^0 97152^0 97153^0 97154^0 97155^0 97156^0 97157^0

MUE: N/A

90887 Interpretation or explanation of results of psychiatric, other medical examinations and procedures, or other accumulated data to family or other responsible persons, or advising them how to assist patient

CCI: $0362T^0$ $0373T^0$ 96159^0 96164^0 96165^0 96168^0 96171^0 97151^0 97152^0 97153^0 97154^0 97155^0 97156^0 97157^0

MUE: N/A

90889 Preparation of report of patient's psychiatric status, history, treatment, or progress (other than for legal or consultative purposes) for other individuals, agencies, or insurance carriers

CCI: $0362T^0$ $0373T^0$

MUE: N/A

90901 Biofeedback training by any modality

CCI: 36410^1 90832^1 90833^1 90834^1 90836^1 90837^1 90838^1 90839^1 90845^1 90846^1 90847^1 90849^1 90853^1 90865^1 90880^1 95812^1 95813^1 95816^1 95819^1 95822^1 96372^1 99155^0 99156^0 99157^0 99211^1 99212^1 99213^1 99214^1 99215^1 99307^1 99308^1 99309^1 99310^1 99446^0 99447^0 99448^1 99449^1 99451^0 99452^0

95800 Sleep study, unattended, simultaneous recording; heart rate, oxygen saturation, respiratory analysis (eg, by airflow or peripheral arterial tone), and sleep time

CCI: 95801^0

95812 Electroencephalogram (EEG) extended monitoring; 41-60 minutes

CCI: 95816^1 95819^1 95822^1

95813 Electroencephalogram (EEG) extended monitoring; 61-119 minutes

CCI: 95812^1 95816^1 95819^1 95822^1

95819 Electroencephalogram (EEG); including recording awake and asleep

CCI: 95816^0 95822^0

95925 Short-latency somatosensory evoked potential study, stimulation of any/all peripheral nerves or skin sites, recording from the central nervous system; in upper limbs

CCI: 95926^0

95938 Short-latency somatosensory evoked potential study, stimulation of any/all peripheral nerves or skin sites, recording from the central nervous system; in upper and lower limbs

CCI: 95925^0 95926^0

95961 Functional cortical and subcortical mapping by stimulation and/or recording of electrodes on brain surface, or of depth electrodes, to provoke seizures or identify vital brain structures; initial hour of attendance by a physician or other qualified health care professional

CCI: 99446^0 99447^0 99448^0 99449^0 99451^0 99452^0

95962 Functional cortical and subcortical mapping by stimulation and/or recording of electrodes on brain surface, or of depth electrodes, to provoke seizures or identify vital brain structures; each additional hour of attendance by a physician or other qualified health care professional (List separately in addition to code for primary procedure)

CCI: 99446^0 99447^0 99448^0 99449^0 99451^0 99452^0

MUE: 5

96020 Neurofunctional testing selection and administration during noninvasive imaging functional brain mapping, with test administered entirely by a physician or other qualified health care professional (ie, psychologist), with review of test results and report

CCI: 95812^1 95813^1 95816^1 95819^1 95925^1 95926^1 95927^1 95930^1 95938^0 96112^0 96113^0 96116^1 96121^0 96125^1 96127^1 96130^1 96131^1 96132^1 96133^1 96136^1 96138^1 96146^1 97165^1 97166^1 97167^1 97168^1 99446^1 99447^1 99448^1 99449^1 99451^1 99452^1

96105 Assessment of aphasia (includes assessment of expressive and receptive speech and language function, language comprehension, speech production ability, reading, spelling, writing, eg, by Boston Diagnostic Aphasia Examination) with interpretation and report, per hour

CCI: 96110^1 96125^1 96127^0 96146^0 96160^0 96161^1 97151^0 97152^0 97153^0 97154^0 97155^0 97156^0 97157^0 97158^0

MUE: 3

96110 Developmental screening (eg, developmental milestone survey, speech and language delay screen), with scoring and documentation, per standardized instrument

CCI: 96125^1 96146^0 97151^0 97152^0 97153^0 97154^0 97155^0 97156^0 97157^0 97158^0

MUE: 3

96112 Developmental test administration (including assessment of fine and/or gross motor, language, cognitive level, social, memory and/or executive functions by standardized developmental instruments when performed), by physician or other qualified health care professional, with interpretation and report; first hour

CCI: $0362T^0$ $0373T^0$ 90791^1 90792^1 90832^1 90833^1 90834^1 90836^1 90837^1 90838^1 90839^1 90845^1 90846^1 90847^1 90849^1 90853^1 90865^1 90870^1 90880^1 96105^1 96110^0 96125^1 96127^1 96130^1 96131^1 96132^1 96133^1 96136^1 96137^0 96138^1 96146^1 96160^1 96161^1 97151^0 97152^0 97153^0 97154^0 97155^0 97156^0 97157^0 97158^0 97165^1 97166^1 97167^1 97168^1 99202^1 99203^1 99204^1 99205^1 99211^1 99212^1 99213^1 99214^1 99215^1 99307^1 99308^1 99309^1 99310^1 99483^1

96113 Developmental test administration (including assessment of fine and/or gross motor, language, cognitive level, social, memory and/or executive functions by standardized developmental instruments when performed), by physician or other qualified health care professional, with interpretation and report; each additional 30 minutes (List separately in addition to code for primary procedure)

CCI: $0362T^0$ $0373T^0$ 90791^1 90792^1 90832^1 90833^1 90834^1 90836^1 90837^1 90838^1 90839^1 90845^1 90846^1 90847^1 90849^1 90853^1 90865^1 90870^1 90880^1 96110^0 96125^1 96127^0 96146^0 96160^1 96161^1 97151^0 97152^0 97153^0 97154^0 97155^0 97156^0 97157^0 97158^0 97165^1 97166^1 97167^1 97168^1 99202^1 99203^1 99204^1 99205^1 99211^1 99212^1 99213^1 99214^1 99215^1 99307^1 99308^1 99309^1 99310^1 99483^1

MUE: 6

96116   Neurobehavioral status exam (clinical assessment of thinking, reasoning and judgment, [eg, acquired knowledge, attention, language, memory, planning and problem solving, and visual spatial abilities]), by physician or other qualified health care professional, both face-to-face time with the patient and time interpreting test results and preparing the report; first hour

CCI: $0362T^1$ 96105^1 96110^1 96112^1 96125^1 96127^0 96146^0 96160^1 96161^1 97151^0 97152^0 97153^0 97154^0 97155^0 97156^0 97157^0 97158^0

96121   Neurobehavioral status exam (clinical assessment of thinking, reasoning and judgment, [eg, acquired knowledge, attention, language, memory, planning and problem solving, and visual spatial abilities]), by physician or other qualified health care professional, both face-to-face time with the patient and time interpreting test results and preparing the report; each additional hour (List separately in addition to code for primary procedure)

CCI: $0362T^0$ $0373T^0$ 96105^1 96110^1 96112^1 96113^0 96125^1 96127^0 96160^1 96161^1 97151^0 97152^0 97153^0 97154^0 97155^0 97156^0 97157^0 97158^0

MUE: 3

96125   Standardized cognitive performance testing (eg, Ross Information Processing Assessment) per hour of a qualified health care professional's time, both face-to-face time administering tests to the patient and time interpreting these test results and preparing the report

CCI: 96127^0 96146^0 96160^1 96161^1 97151^0 97152^0 97153^0 97154^0 97155^0 97156^0 97157^0 97158^0

MUE: 2

96127   Brief emotional/behavioral assessment (eg, depression inventory, attention-deficit/hyperactivity disorder [ADHD] scale), with scoring and documentation, per standardized instrument

CCI: 96146^0 96160^1 96161^1 97151^0 97152^0 97153^0 97154^0 97155^0 97156^0 97157^0 97158^0

MUE: 2

96130   Psychological testing evaluation services by physician or other qualified health care professional, including integration of patient data, interpretation of standardized test results and clinical data, clinical decision making, treatment planning and report, and interactive feedback to the patient, family member(s) or caregiver(s), when performed; first hour

CCI: $0362T^0$ $0373T^0$ 96110^1 96113^0 96125^1 96127^0 96146^1 96160^1 96161^1 97151^0 97152^0 97153^0 97154^0 97155^0 97156^0 97157^0 97158^0

96131   Psychological testing evaluation services by physician or other qualified health care professional, including integration of patient data, interpretation of standardized test results and clinical data, clinical decision making, treatment planning and report, and interactive feedback to the patient, family member(s) or caregiver(s), when performed; each additional hour (List separately in addition to code for primary procedure)

CCI: $0362T^0$ $0373T^0$ 96110^1 96113^1 96125^1 96127^0 96146^1 96160^1 96161^1 97151^0 97152^0 97153^0 97154^0 97155^0 97156^0 97157^0 97158^0

MUE: 7

96132   Neuropsychological testing evaluation services by physician or other qualified health care professional, including integration of patient data, interpretation of standardized test results and clinical data, clinical decision making, treatment planning and report, and interactive feedback to the patient, family member(s) or caregiver(s), when performed; first hour

CCI: $0362T^0$ $0373T^0$ 96110^1 96113^0 96125^1 96127^0 96146^1 96160^1 96161^1 97151^0 97152^0 97153^0 97154^0 97155^0 97156^0 97157^0 97158^0

96133   Neuropsychological testing evaluation services by physician or other qualified health care professional, including integration of patient data, interpretation of standardized test results and clinical data, clinical decision making, treatment planning and report, and interactive feedback to the patient, family member(s) or caregiver(s), when performed; each additional hour (List separately in addition to code for primary procedure)

CCI: $0362T^0$ $0373T^0$ 96110^1 96113^0 96125^1 96127^0 96146^1 96160^1 96161^1 97151^0 97152^0 97153^0 97154^0 97155^0 97156^0 97157^0 97158^0

MUE: 7

96136   Psychological or neuropsychological test administration and scoring by physician or other qualified health care professional, two or more tests, any method; first 30 minutes

CCI: $0362T^0$ $0373T^0$ 96110^1 96113^0 96125^1 96127^0 96138^1 96146^0 96160^1 96161^1 97151^0 97152^0 97153^0 97154^0 97155^0 97156^0 97157^0 97158^0

96137   Psychological or neuropsychological test administration and scoring by physician or other qualified health care professional, two or more tests, any method; each additional 30 minutes (List separately in addition to code for primary procedure)

CCI: $0362T^0$ $0373T^0$ 96110^1 96113^0 96125^1 96127^0 96138^1 96146^0 96160^1 96161^1 97151^0 97152^0 97153^0 97154^0 97155^0 97156^0 97157^0 97158^0

MUE: 11

96138   Psychological or neuropsychological test administration and scoring by technician, two or more tests, any method; first 30 minutes

CCI: $0362T^0$ $0373T^0$ 96110^1 96113^0 96125^1 96127^0 96146^0 96160^1 96161^1 97151^0 97152^0 97153^0 97154^0 97155^0 97156^0 97157^0 97158^0

96139   Psychological or neuropsychological test administration and scoring by technician, two or more tests, any method; each additional 30 minutes (List separately in addition to code for primary procedure)

CCI: $0362T^0$ $0373T^0$ 96110^1 96125^1 96127^0 96146^0 96160^1 96161^1 97151^0 97152^0 97153^0 97154^0 97155^0 97156^0 97157^0 97158^0

MUE: 11

96146   Psychological or neuropsychological test administration, with single automated, standardized instrument via electronic platform, with automated result only

CCI: $0362T^0$ $0373T^0$ 96160^1 96161^1 97151^0 97152^0 97153^0 97154^0 97155^0 97156^0 97157^0 97158^0

96156   Health behavior assessment, or re-assessment (ie, health-focused clinical interview, behavioral observations, clinical decision making)

CCI: $0362T^0$ $0373T^0$ $0591T^0$ $0592T^0$ 90785^0 90832^0 90833^0 90834^0 90836^0 90840^0 90849^0 90853^0 90863^0 90867^0 90868^0 90869^0 90875^0 90876^0 90882^0 90885^0 90887^0 90889^0 96105^0 96110^1 96112^1 96116^1 96125^1 96127^0 96130^1 96132^1 96136^1 96138^1 96146^1 96160^1 96161^0 96164^0 96165^0 96167^1 96168^1 97151^0 97152^0 97153^0 97154^0 97155^0 97156^0 97157^0 97158^0

96158   Health behavior intervention, individual, face-to-face; initial 30 minutes

CCI: $0362T^0$ $0373T^0$ $0592T^0$ 90785^0 90849^0 90853^0 90863^0 90867^0 90868^0 90869^0 90875^0 90882^0 90885^0 90887^0 90889^0 96105^0 96110^1 96112^1 96116^1 96125^1 96127^0 96130^1 96132^1 96136^1 96138^1 96146^1 96160^1 96161^0 96164^0 96165^1 96168^1 97151^0 97152^0 97153^0 97154^0 97155^0 97156^0 97157^0 97158^0

96159 Health behavior intervention, individual, face-to-face; each additional 15 minutes (List separately in addition to code for primary service)

CCI: $0362T^0$ $0373T^0$ $0592T^0$ 90785^0 90863^0 90867^0 90868^0 90869^0 90882^0 90889^0 96105^1 96110^1 96112^1 96116^1 96125^1 96127^0 96130^1 96132^1 96136^1 96138^1 96146^1 96160^0 96161^0 96164^0 96165^0 97151^0 97152^0 97153^0 97154^0 97155^0 97156^0 97157^0 97158^0

MUE: 4

96160 Administration of patient-focused health risk assessment instrument (eg, health hazard appraisal) with scoring and documentation, per standardized instrument

CCI: $0373T^1$ 96110^1 96164^0 96165^0 96167^0 96168^0 96170^0 96171^0 97153^1 97154^1 97155^1 97156^1 97157^1 97158^1 99091^0

MUE: 3

96161 Administration of caregiver-focused health risk assessment instrument (eg, depression inventory) for the benefit of the patient, with scoring and documentation, per standardized instrument

CCI: $0373T^1$ 96110^1 96164^0 96165^0 96167^0 96168^0 96170^0 96171^0 97153^1 97154^1 97155^1 97156^1 97157^1 97158^1 99091^0

96164 Health behavior intervention, group (2 or more patients), face-to-face; initial 30 minutes

CCI: $0362T^0$ $0373T^0$ $0593T^0$ 90867^0 90868^0 90869^0 90882^0 90889^0 96167^0 96168^0 97151^0 97152^0 97153^0 97154^0 97155^0 97156^0 97157^0 97158^0

96165 Health behavior intervention, group (2 or more patients), face-to-face; each additional 15 minutes (List separately in addition to code for primary service)

CCI: $0362T^0$ $0373T^0$ $0593T^0$ 90867^0 90868^0 90869^0 90882^0 90889^0 96167^0 96168^0 97151^0 97152^0 97153^0 97154^0 97155^0 97156^0 97157^0 97158^0

MUE: 6

96167 Health behavior intervention, family (with the patient present), face-to-face; initial 30 minutes

CCI: $0362T^0$ $0373T^0$ 90785^0 90832^0 90833^0 90840^0 90849^0 90853^0 90863^0 90867^0 90868^0 90869^0 90875^0 90882^0 90885^0 90887^0 90889^0 96158^1 96159^1 97151^0 97152^0 97153^0 97154^0 97155^0 97156^0 97157^0 97158^0

96168 Health behavior intervention, family (with the patient present), face-to-face; each additional 15 minutes (List separately in addition to code for primary service)

CCI: $0362T^0$ $0373T^0$ 90785^0 90867^0 90868^0 90869^0 90882^0 90889^0 96159^1 97151^0 97152^0 97153^0 97154^0 97155^0 97156^0 97157^0 97158^0

MUE: 6

96170 Health behavior intervention, family (without the patient present), face-to-face; initial 30 minutes

CCI: $0362T^0$ $0373T^0$ 90785^0 90832^0 90833^0 90840^0 90849^0 90853^0 90863^0 90867^0 90868^0 90869^0 90875^0 90882^0 90885^0 90887^0 90889^0 97151^0 97152^0 97153^0 97154^0 97155^0 97156^0 97157^0 97158^0

96171 Health behavior intervention, family (without the patient present), face-to-face; each additional 15 minutes (List separately in addition to code for primary service)

CCI: $0362T^0$ $0373T^0$ 90785^0 90863^0 90867^0 90868^0 90869^0 90882^0 90889^0 97151^0 97152^0 97153^0 97154^0 97155^0 97156^0 97157^0 97158^0

MUE: 2

96372 Therapeutic, prophylactic, or diagnostic injection (specify substance or drug); subcutaneous or intramuscular

CCI: 99202^1 99203^1 99204^1 99205^1 99211^0 99212^1 99213^1 99214^1 99215^1 99483^1

MUE: 4

97022 Application of a modality to 1 or more areas; whirlpool

CCI: 97168^1

97024 Application of a modality to 1 or more areas; diathermy (eg, microwave)

CCI: 97026^1 97168^1

97026 Application of a modality to 1 or more areas; infrared

CCI: 97022^1 97168^1

97028 Application of a modality to 1 or more areas; ultraviolet

CCI: 97022^1 97026^1 97168^1

97032 Application of a modality to 1 or more areas; electrical stimulation (manual), each 15 minutes

CCI: 97168^1

MUE: 4

97033 Application of a modality to 1 or more areas; iontophoresis, each 15 minutes

CCI: 97168^1

MUE: 4

97034 Application of a modality to 1 or more areas; contrast baths, each 15 minutes

CCI: 97168^1

MUE: 2

97035 Application of a modality to 1 or more areas; ultrasound, each 15 minutes

CCI: 97168^1

MUE: 2

97039 Unlisted modality (specify type and time if constant attendance)

CCI: 97168^1

97124 Therapeutic procedure, 1 or more areas, each 15 minutes; massage, including effleurage, petrissage and/or tapotement (stroking, compression, percussion)

CCI: 97168^1

MUE: 4

97129 Therapeutic interventions that focus on cognitive function (eg, attention, memory, reasoning, executive function, problem solving, and/or pragmatic functioning) and compensatory strategies to manage the performance of an activity (eg, managing time or schedules, initiating, organizing, and sequencing tasks), direct (one-on-one) patient contact; initial 15 minutes

CCI: $0373T^0$ 97153^0 97155^0 97168^1

97130 Therapeutic interventions that focus on cognitive function (eg, attention, memory, reasoning, executive function, problem solving, and/or pragmatic functioning) and compensatory strategies to manage the performance of an activity (eg, managing time or schedules, initiating, organizing, and sequencing tasks), direct (one-on-one) patient contact; each additional 15 minutes (List separately in addition to code for primary procedure)

CCI: $0373T^0$ 97153^0 97155^0 97168^1

MUE: 7

97139 Unlisted therapeutic procedure (specify)

CCI: 97168^1

97150 Therapeutic procedure(s), group (2 or more individuals)

CCI: $0373T^0$ $0593T^0$ 97110^1 97124^1 97153^0 97154^0 97155^0 97156^0 97157^0 97158^0 97530^1 97533^1 97535^1 97537^1

97151 Behavior identification assessment, administered by a physician or other qualified health care professional, each 15 minutes of the physician's or other qualified health care professional's time face-to-face with patient and/or guardian(s)/caregiver(s) administering assessments and discussing findings and recommendations, and non-face-to-face analyzing past data, scoring/interpreting the assessment, and preparing the report/treatment plan

CCI: 90867^0 90868^0 90869^0 90882^0 90889^0 96160^1 96161^1

MUE: 8

97152 Behavior identification-supporting assessment, administered by one technician under the direction of a physician or other qualified health care professional, face-to-face with the patient, each 15 minutes

CCI: 90867^0 90868^0 90869^0 90889^0 96160^1 96161^1

MUE: 16

97153 Adaptive behavior treatment by protocol, administered by technician under the direction of a physician or other qualified health care professional, face-to-face with one patient, each 15 minutes

CCI: 90867^0 90868^0 90869^0 90882^0 90889^0

MUE: 32

97154 Group adaptive behavior treatment by protocol, administered by technician under the direction of a physician or other qualified health care professional, face-to-face with two or more patients, each 15 minutes

CCI: 90867^0 90868^0 90869^0 90882^0 90889^0

MUE: 18

97155 Adaptive behavior treatment with protocol modification, administered by physician or other qualified health care professional, which may include simultaneous direction of technician, face-to-face with one patient, each 15 minutes

CCI: 90867^0 90868^0 90869^0 90882^0 90889^0

MUE: 24

97156 Family adaptive behavior treatment guidance, administered by physician or other qualified health care professional (with or without the patient present), face-to-face with guardian(s)/caregiver(s), each 15 minutes

CCI: 90867^0 90868^0 90869^0 90882^0 90889^0

MUE: 16

97157 Multiple-family group adaptive behavior treatment guidance, administered by physician or other qualified health care professional (without the patient present), face-to-face with multiple sets of guardians/caregivers, each 15 minutes

CCI: 90867^0 90868^0 90869^0 90882^0 90889^0

MUE: 16

97158 Group adaptive behavior treatment with protocol modification, administered by physician or other qualified health care professional, face-to-face with multiple patients, each 15 minutes

CCI: 90785^0 90791^0 90792^0 90832^0 90833^0 90834^0 90836^0 90837^0 90838^0 90839^0 90840^0 90845^0 90846^0 90847^0 90849^0 90853^0 90863^0 90865^0 90867^0 90868^0 90869^0 90870^0 90875^0 90876^0 90880^0 90882^0 90885^0 90887^0 90889^0

MUE: 16

97165 Occupational therapy evaluation, low complexity, requiring these components: An occupational profile and medical and therapy history, which includes a brief history including review of medical and/or therapy records relating to the presenting problem; An assessment(s) that identifies 1-3 performance deficits (ie, relating to physical, cognitive, or psychosocial skills) that result in activity limitations and/or participation restrictions; and Clinical decision making of low complexity, which includes an analysis of the occupational profile, analysis of data from problem-focused assessment(s), and consideration of a limited number of treatment options. Patient presents with no comorbidities that affect occupational performance. Modification of tasks or assistance (eg, physical or verbal) with assessment(s) is not necessary to enable completion of evaluation component. Typically, 30 minutes are spent face-to-face with the patient and/or family.

CCI: $0362T^0$ 96105^1 96125^1 96130^1 96132^1 96136^1 96138^1 96146^1 96156^1 96158^0 96159^0 96164^0 96165^0 96167^0 96168^0 97151^0 97152^0 97168^0 99202^1 99203^1 99204^1 99205^1 99211^1 99212^1 99213^1 99214^1 99215^1 99307^1 99308^1 99309^1 99310^1

97166 Occupational therapy evaluation, moderate complexity, requiring these components: An occupational profile and medical and therapy history, which includes an expanded review of medical and/or therapy records and additional review of physical, cognitive, or psychosocial history related to current functional performance; An assessment(s) that identifies 3-5 performance deficits (ie, relating to physical, cognitive, or psychosocial skills) that result in activity limitations and/or participation restrictions; and Clinical decision making of moderate analytic complexity, which includes an analysis of the occupational profile, analysis of data from detailed assessment(s), and consideration of several treatment options. Patient may present with comorbidities that affect occupational performance. Minimal to moderate modification of tasks or assistance (eg, physical or verbal) with assessment(s) is necessary to enable patient to complete evaluation component. Typically, 45 minutes are spent face-to-face with the patient and/or family.

CCI: $0362T^0$ 96105^1 96125^1 96130^1 96132^1 96136^1 96138^1 96146^1 96156^1 96158^0 96159^0 96164^0 96165^0 96167^0 96168^0 97151^0 97152^0 97165^0 97168^0 99202^1 99203^1 99204^1 99205^1 99211^1 99212^1 99213^1 99214^1 99215^1 99307^1 99308^1 99309^1 99310^1

97167 Occupational therapy evaluation, high complexity, requiring these components: An occupational profile and medical and therapy history, which includes review of medical and/or therapy records and extensive additional review of physical, cognitive, or psychosocial history related to current functional performance; An assessment(s) that identifies 5 or more performance deficits (ie, relating to physical, cognitive, or psychosocial skills) that result in activity limitations and/or participation restrictions; and Clinical decision making of high analytic complexity, which includes an analysis of the patient profile, analysis of data from comprehensive assessment(s), and consideration of multiple treatment options. Patient presents with comorbidities that affect occupational performance. Significant modification of tasks or assistance (eg, physical or verbal) with assessment(s) is necessary to enable patient to complete evaluation component. Typically, 60 minutes are spent face-to-face with the patient and/or family.

CCI: $0362T^0$ 96105^1 96125^1 96130^1 96132^1 96136^1 96138^1 96146^1 96156^1 96158^0 96159^0 96164^0 96165^0 96167^0 96168^0 97151^0 97152^0 97165^0 97166^0 97168^0 99202^1 99203^1 99204^1 99205^1 99211^1 99212^1 99213^1 99214^1 99215^1 99307^1 99308^1 99309^1 99310^1

97168 Re-evaluation of occupational therapy established plan of care, requiring these components: An assessment of changes in patient functional or medical status with revised plan of care; An update to the initial occupational profile to reflect changes in condition or environment that affect future interventions and/or goals; and A revised plan of care. A formal reevaluation is performed when there is a documented change in functional status or a significant change to the plan of care is required. Typically, 30 minutes are spent face-to-face with the patient and/or family.

CCI: $0362T^0$ 96105^1 96125^1 96130^1 96132^1 96136^1 96138^1 96146^1 96156^0 96158^0 96159^0 96164^0 96165^0 96167^0 96168^0 97151^0 97152^0 99202^1 99203^1 99204^1 99205^1 99211^1 99212^1 99213^1 99214^1 99215^1 99307^1 99308^1 99309^1 99310^1

97530 Therapeutic activities, direct (one-on-one) patient contact (use of dynamic activities to improve functional performance), each 15 minutes

CCI: $0373T^0$ 97153^0 97154^0 97155^0 97156^0 97157^0 97158^0 97533^1 97535^1 97537^1

MUE: 6

97533 Sensory integrative techniques to enhance sensory processing and promote adaptive responses to environmental demands, direct (one-on-one) patient contact, each 15 minutes

CCI: $0373T^0$ 97153^0 97154^0 97155^0 97156^0 97157^0 97158^0 97168^1

MUE: 4

97535 Self-care/home management training (eg, activities of daily living (ADL) and compensatory training, meal preparation, safety procedures, and instructions in use of assistive technology devices/adaptive equipment) direct one-on-one contact, each 15 minutes

CCI: 97168^1

MUE: 8

97537 Community/work reintegration training (eg, shopping, transportation, money management, avocational activities and/or work environment/modification analysis, work task analysis, use of assistive technology device/adaptive equipment), direct one-on-one contact, each 15 minutes

CCI: 97168^1

MUE: 6

98960 Education and training for patient self-management by a qualified, nonphysician health care professional using a standardized curriculum, face-to-face with the patient (could include caregiver/family) each 30 minutes; individual patient

CCI: $0592T^0$

MUE: N/A

98961 Education and training for patient self-management by a qualified, nonphysician health care professional using a standardized curriculum, face-to-face with the patient (could include caregiver/family) each 30 minutes; 2-4 patients

CCI: $0593T^0$

MUE: N/A

98962 Education and training for patient self-management by a qualified, nonphysician health care professional using a standardized curriculum, face-to-face with the patient (could include caregiver/family) each 30 minutes; 5-8 patients

CCI: $0593T^0$

MUE: N/A

98968 Telephone assessment and management service provided by a qualified nonphysician health care professional to an established patient, parent, or guardian not originating from a related assessment and management service provided within the previous 7 days nor leading to an assessment and management service or procedure within the next 24 hours or soonest available appointment; 21-30 minutes of medical discussion

CCI: 99446^1 99447^1

99091 Collection and interpretation of physiologic data (eg, ECG, blood pressure, glucose monitoring) digitally stored and/or transmitted by the patient and/or caregiver to the physician or other qualified health care professional, qualified by education, training, licensure/regulation (when applicable) requiring a minimum of 30 minutes of time, each 30 days

CCI: 98970^0 98971^0 98972^0

99151 Moderate sedation services provided by the same physician or other qualified health care professional performing the diagnostic or therapeutic service that the sedation supports, requiring the presence of an independent trained observer to assist in the monitoring of the patient's level of consciousness and physiological status; initial 15 minutes of intraservice time, patient younger than 5 years of age

CCI: 36410^1 96372^1 99152^0 99157^1 99202^1 99203^1 99204^1 99205^1 99211^1 99212^1 99213^1 99214^1 99215^1 99307^1 99308^1 99309^1 99310^1 99483^1

99152 Moderate sedation services provided by the same physician or other qualified health care professional performing the diagnostic or therapeutic service that the sedation supports, requiring the presence of an independent trained observer to assist in the monitoring of the patient's level of consciousness and physiological status; initial 15 minutes of intraservice time, patient age 5 years or older

CCI: 36410^1 96372^1 99157^1 99202^1 99203^1 99204^1 99205^1 99211^1 99212^1 99213^1 99214^1 99215^1 99307^1 99308^1 99309^1 99310^1 99483^1

MUE: 2

99155 Moderate sedation services provided by a physician or other qualified health care professional other than the physician or other qualified health care professional performing the diagnostic or therapeutic service that the sedation supports; initial 15 minutes of intraservice time, patient younger than 5 years of age

CCI: 36410^1 96372^1 99151^0 99153^1 99156^0 99202^0 99203^0 99204^0 99205^0 99211^0 99212^0 99213^0 99214^0 99215^0 99307^0 99308^0 99309^0 99310^0 99483^0

99156 Moderate sedation services provided by a physician or other qualified health care professional other than the physician or other qualified health care professional performing the diagnostic or therapeutic service that the sedation supports; initial 15 minutes of intraservice time, patient age 5 years or older

CCI: 36410^1 96372^0 99152^0 99153^1 99202^0 99203^0 99204^0 99205^0 99211^0 99212^0 99213^0 99214^0 99215^0 99307^0 99308^0 99309^0 99310^0 99483^0

99157 Moderate sedation services provided by a physician or other qualified health care professional other than the physician or other qualified health care professional performing the diagnostic or therapeutic service that the sedation supports; each additional 15 minutes intraservice time (List separately in addition to code for primary service)

CCI: 99153^0

MUE: 6

99202 Office or other outpatient visit for the evaluation and management of a new patient, which requires a medically appropriate history and/or examination and straightforward medical decision making. When using time for code selection, 15-29 minutes of total time is spent on the date of the encounter.

CCI: $0362T^1$ $0373T^1$ 90863^0 96020^1 96105^1 96116^1 96125^1 96130^1 96132^1 96136^1 96138^1 96146^1 96156^0 96158^0 96159^0 96164^1 96165^0 96167^0 96168^0 97151^1 97153^1 97154^1 97155^1 97156^1 97157^1 97158^1 99091^0 99211^1 99212^1 99213^1 99214^1 99215^1 99446^0 99447^0 99448^0 99449^0

99203 Office or other outpatient visit for the evaluation and management of a new patient, which requires a medically appropriate history and/or examination and low level of medical decision making. When using time for code selection, 30-44 minutes of total time is spent on the date of the encounter.

CCI: $0362T^1$ $0373T^1$ 90863^0 96020^1 96105^1 96116^1 96125^1 96130^1 96132^1 96136^1 96138^1 96146^1 96156^0 96158^0 96159^0 96164^1 96165^0 96167^0 96168^0 97151^1 97153^1 97154^1 97155^1 97156^1 97157^1 97158^1 99091^0 99202^0 99211^1 99212^1 99213^1 99214^1 99215^1 99446^0 99447^0 99448^0 99449^0

99204 Office or other outpatient visit for the evaluation and management of a new patient, which requires a medically appropriate history and/or examination and moderate level of medical decision making. When using time for code selection, 45-59 minutes of total time is spent on the date of the encounter.

CCI: $0362T^1$ $0373T^1$ 90863^0 96020^1 96105^1 96116^1 96125^1 96130^1 96132^1 96136^1 96138^1 96146^1 96156^0 96158^0 96159^0 96164^1 96165^0 96167^0 96168^0 97151^1 97153^1 97154^1 97155^1 97156^1 97157^1 97158^1 99091^0 99202^0 99203^0 99211^1 99212^1 99213^1 99214^1 99215^1 99446^0 99447^0 99448^0 99449^0

99205 Office or other outpatient visit for the evaluation and management of a new patient, which requires a medically appropriate history and/or examination and high level of medical decision making. When using time for code selection, 60-74 minutes of total time is spent on the date of the encounter.

CCI: $0362T^1$ $0373T^1$ 90863^0 96020^1 96105^1 96116^1 96125^1 96130^1 96132^1 96136^1 96138^1 96146^1 96156^0 96158^0 96159^0 96164^1 96165^0 96167^0 96168^0 97151^1 97153^1 97154^1 97155^1 97156^1 97157^1 97158^1 99091^0 99202^0 99203^0 99204^0 99211^1 99212^1 99213^1 99214^1 99215^1 99446^0 99447^0 99448^0 99449^0

99211 Office or other outpatient visit for the evaluation and management of an established patient that may not require the presence of a physician or other qualified health care professional

CCI: $0362T^1$ $0373T^1$ 90863^0 96020^1 96105^1 96116^1 96125^1 96130^1 96132^1 96136^1 96138^1 96146^1 96156^0 96158^0 96159^0 96164^1 96165^0 96167^0 96168^0 97151^1 97153^1 97154^1 97155^1 97156^1 97157^1 97158^1 99091^0 99446^0 99447^0 99448^0 99449^0

99212 Office or other outpatient visit for the evaluation and management of an established patient, which requires a medically appropriate history and/or examination and straightforward medical decision making. When using time for code selection, 10-19 minutes of total time is spent on the date of the encounter.

CCI: $0362T^1$ $0373T^1$ 90863^0 96020^1 96105^1 96116^1 96125^1 96130^1 96132^1 96136^1 96138^1 96146^1 96156^0 96158^0 96159^0 96164^1 96165^0 96167^0 96168^0 97151^1 97153^1 97154^1 97155^1 97156^1 97157^1 97158^1 99091^0 99211^1 99446^0 99447^0 99448^0 99449^0

MUE: 2

99213 Office or other outpatient visit for the evaluation and management of an established patient, which requires a medically appropriate history and/or examination and low level of medical decision making. When using time for code selection, 20-29 minutes of total time is spent on the date of the encounter.

CCI: $0362T^1$ $0373T^1$ 90863^0 96020^1 96105^1 96116^1 96125^1 96130^1 96132^1 96136^1 96138^1 96146^1 96156^0 96158^0 96159^0 96164^1 96165^0 96167^0 96168^0 97151^1 97153^1 97154^1 97155^1 97156^1 97157^1 97158^1 99091^0 99211^1 99212^1 99446^0 99447^0 99448^0 99449^0

MUE: 2

99214 Office or other outpatient visit for the evaluation and management of an established patient, which requires a medically appropriate history and/or examination and moderate level of medical decision making. When using time for code selection, 30-39 minutes of total time is spent on the date of the encounter.

CCI: $0362T^1$ $0373T^1$ 90863^0 96020^1 96105^1 96116^1 96125^1 96130^1 96132^1 96136^1 96138^1 96146^1 96156^0 96158^0 96159^0 96164^1 96165^0 96167^0 96168^0 97151^1 97153^1 97154^1 97155^1 97156^1 97157^1 97158^1 99091^0 99211^1 99212^1 99213^1 99446^0 99447^0 99448^0 99449^0

MUE: 2

99215 Office or other outpatient visit for the evaluation and management of an established patient, which requires a medically appropriate history and/or examination and high level of medical decision making. When using time for code selection, 40-54 minutes of total time is spent on the date of the encounter.

CCI: $0362T^1$ $0373T^1$ 90863^0 96020^1 96105^1 96116^1 96125^1 96130^1 96132^1 96136^1 96138^1 96146^1 96156^0 96158^0 96159^0 96164^1 96165^0 96167^0 96168^0 97151^1 97153^1 97154^1 97155^1 97156^1 97157^1 97158^1 99091^0 99211^1 99212^1 99213^1 99214^1 99446^0 99447^0 99448^0 99449^0

99307 Subsequent nursing facility care, per day, for the evaluation and management of a patient, which requires at least 2 of these 3 key components: A problem focused interval history; A problem focused examination; Straightforward medical decision making. Counseling and/or coordination of care with other physicians, other qualified health care professionals, or agencies are provided consistent with the nature of the problem(s) and the patient's and/or family's needs. Usually, the patient is stable, recovering, or improving. Typically, 10 minutes are spent at the bedside and on the patient's facility floor or unit.

CCI: $0362T^1$ $0373T^1$ 90863^0 96020^1 96105^1 96116^1 96125^1 96127^1 96130^1 96132^1 96136^1 96138^1 96146^1 96156^0 96158^0 96159^0 96164^1 96165^0 96167^0 96168^0 96372^0 97151^1 97153^1 97154^1 97155^1 97156^1 97157^1 97158^1 99091^0 99446^0 99447^0 99448^0 99449^0 99451^0 99452^0

99308 Subsequent nursing facility care, per day, for the evaluation and management of a patient, which requires at least 2 of these 3 key components: An expanded problem focused interval history; An expanded problem focused examination; Medical decision making of low complexity. Counseling and/or coordination of care with other physicians, other qualified health care professionals, or agencies are provided consistent with the nature of the problem(s) and the patient's and/or family's needs. Usually, the patient is responding inadequately to therapy or has developed a minor complication. Typically, 15 minutes are spent at the bedside and on the patient's facility floor or unit.

CCI: $0362T^1$ $0373T^1$ 90863^0 96020^1 96105^1 96116^1 96125^1 96127^1 96130^1 96132^1 96136^1 96138^1 96146^1 96156^0 96158^0 96159^0 96164^1 96165^0 96167^0 96168^0 96372^0 97151^1 97153^1 97154^1 97155^1 97156^1 97157^1 97158^1 99091^0 99307^0 99446^0 99447^0 99448^0 99449^0 99451^0 99452^0

99309 Subsequent nursing facility care, per day, for the evaluation and management of a patient, which requires at least 2 of these 3 key components: A detailed interval history; A detailed examination; Medical decision making of moderate complexity. Counseling and/or coordination of care with other physicians, other qualified health care professionals, or agencies are provided consistent with the nature of the problem(s) and the patient's and/or family's needs. Usually, the patient has developed a significant complication or a significant new problem. Typically, 25 minutes are spent at the bedside and on the patient's facility floor or unit.

CCI: $0362T^1$ $0373T^1$ 90863^0 96020^1 96105^1 96116^1 96125^1 96127^0 96130^1 96132^1 96136^1 96138^1 96146^1 96156^0 96158^0 96159^0 96164^0 96165^0 96167^0 96168^0 96372^0 97151^1 97153^1 97154^1 97155^1 97156^1 97157^1 97158^1 99091^0 99307^0 99308^0 99446^0 99447^0 99448^0 99449^0 99451^0 99452^0

99310 Subsequent nursing facility care, per day, for the evaluation and management of a patient, which requires at least 2 of these 3 key components: A comprehensive interval history; A comprehensive examination; Medical decision making of high complexity. Counseling and/or coordination of care with other physicians, other qualified health care professionals, or agencies are provided consistent with the nature of the problem(s) and the patient's and/or family's needs. The patient may be unstable or may have developed a significant new problem requiring immediate physician attention. Typically, 35 minutes are spent at the bedside and on the patient's facility floor or unit.

CCI: $0362T^1$ $0373T^1$ 90863^0 96020^1 96105^1 96116^1 96125^1 96127^0 96130^1 96132^1 96136^1 96138^1 96146^1 96156^0 96158^0 96159^0 96164^0 96165^0 96167^0 96168^0 96372^0 97151^1 97153^1 97154^1 97155^1 97156^1 97157^1 97158^1 99091^0 99307^0 99308^0 99309^0 99446^0 99447^0 99448^0 99449^0 99451^0 99452^0

99439 Chronic care management services with the following required elements: multiple (two or more) chronic conditions expected to last at least 12 months, or until the death of the patient, chronic conditions that place the patient at significant risk of death, acute exacerbation/decompensation, or functional decline, comprehensive care plan established, implemented, revised, or monitored; each additional 20 minutes of clinical staff time directed by a physician or other qualified health care professional, per calendar month (List separately in addition to code for primary procedure)

CCI: 98960^1 98961^1 98962^1 98966^1 98967^1 98968^1 99071^1 99078^1 99080^1 99091^1 99441^0 99442^0 99443^0

MUE: 2

99441 Telephone evaluation and management service by a physician or other qualified health care professional who may report evaluation and management services provided to an established patient, parent, or guardian not originating from a related E/M service provided within the previous 7 days nor leading to an E/M service or procedure within the next 24 hours or soonest available appointment; 5-10 minutes of medical discussion

CCI: $0362T^1$ $0373T^1$ 96127^0 97151^1 97153^1 97154^1 97155^1 97156^1 97157^1 97158^1 98970^1 98971^1 98972^1 99091^0

99442 Telephone evaluation and management service by a physician or other qualified health care professional who may report evaluation and management services provided to an established patient, parent, or guardian not originating from a related E/M service provided within the previous 7 days nor leading to an E/M service or procedure within the next 24 hours or soonest available appointment; 11-20 minutes of medical discussion

CCI: $0362T^1$ $0373T^1$ 96127^0 97151^1 97153^1 97154^1 97155^1 97156^1 97157^1 97158^1 98970^1 98971^1 98972^1 99091^0

99443 Telephone evaluation and management service by a physician or other qualified health care professional who may report evaluation and management services provided to an established patient, parent, or guardian not originating from a related E/M service provided within the previous 7 days nor leading to an E/M service or procedure within the next 24 hours or soonest available appointment; 21-30 minutes of medical discussion

CCI: $0362T^1$ $0373T^1$ 96127^0 97151^1 97153^1 97154^1 97155^1 97156^1 97157^1 97158^1 98970^1 98971^1 98972^1 99091^0 99446^0 99447^0

99446 Interprofessional telephone/Internet/electronic health record assessment and management service provided by a consultative physician, including a verbal and written report to the patient's treating/requesting physician or other qualified health care professional; 5-10 minutes of medical consultative discussion and review

CCI: $0362T^1$ $0373T^1$ 96127^0 97151^1 97152^1 97153^1 97154^1 97155^1 97156^1 97157^1 97158^1 98966^1 98967^1 98970^0 98971^0 98972^0 99091^0 99441^0 99442^0 99451^0 99452^0

99447 Interprofessional telephone/Internet/electronic health record assessment and management service provided by a consultative physician, including a verbal and written report to the patient's treating/requesting physician or other qualified health care professional; 11-20 minutes of medical consultative discussion and review

CCI: $0362T^1$ $0373T^1$ 96127^0 97151^1 97153^1 97154^1 97155^1 97156^1 97157^1 97158^1 98966^1 98967^1 98970^0 98971^0 98972^0 99091^0 99441^0 99442^0 99446^0 99451^0 99452^0

99448 Interprofessional telephone/Internet/electronic health record assessment and management service provided by a consultative physician, including a verbal and written report to the patient's treating/requesting physician or other qualified health care professional; 21-30 minutes of medical consultative discussion and review

CCI: $0362T^1$ $0373T^1$ 96127^0 97151^1 97153^1 97154^1 97155^1 97156^1 97157^1 97158^1 98966^1 98967^1 98968^1 98970^0 98971^0 98972^0 99091^0 99441^0 99442^0 99443^0 99446^0 99447^0 99451^0 99452^0

99449 Interprofessional telephone/Internet/electronic health record assessment and management service provided by a consultative physician, including a verbal and written report to the patient's treating/requesting physician or other qualified health care professional; 31 minutes or more of medical consultative discussion and review

CCI: $0362T^1$ $0373T^1$ 96127^0 97151^1 97153^1 97154^1 97155^1 97156^1 97157^1 97158^1 98966^1 98967^1 98968^1 98970^0 98971^0 98972^0 99091^0 99441^0 99442^0 99443^0 99446^0 99447^0 99448^0 99451^0 99452^0

99451 Interprofessional telephone/Internet/electronic health record assessment and management service provided by a consultative physician, including a written report to the patient's treating/requesting physician or other qualified health care professional, 5 minutes or more of medical consultative time

CCI: $0362T^1$ $0373T^1$ 96127^0 97151^1 97152^1 97153^1 97154^1 97156^1 97157^1 97158^1 99091^0 99452^0

99452 Interprofessional telephone/Internet/electronic health record referral service(s) provided by a treating/requesting physician or other qualified health care professional, 30 minutes

CCI: $0362T^1$ $0373T^1$ 96127^0 99091^0

99453 Remote monitoring of physiologic parameter(s) (eg, weight, blood pressure, pulse oximetry, respiratory flow rate), initial; set-up and patient education on use of equipment

CCI: 99091^0

99454 Remote monitoring of physiologic parameter(s) (eg, weight, blood pressure, pulse oximetry, respiratory flow rate), initial; device(s) supply with daily recording(s) or programmed alert(s) transmission, each 30 days

CCI: 99091^0

99457 Remote physiologic monitoring treatment management services, clinical staff/physician/other qualified health care professional time in a calendar month requiring interactive communication with the patient/caregiver during the month; first 20 minutes

CCI: 99091^0

99483 Assessment of and care planning for a patient with cognitive impairment, requiring an independent historian, in the office or other outpatient, home or domiciliary or rest home, with all of the following required elements: Cognition-focused evaluation including a pertinent history and examination, Medical decision making of moderate or high complexity, Functional assessment (eg, basic and instrumental activities of daily living), including decision-making capacity, Use of standardized instruments for staging of dementia (eg, functional assessment staging test [FAST], clinical dementia rating [CDR]), Medication reconciliation and review for high-risk medications, Evaluation for neuropsychiatric and behavioral symptoms, including depression, including use of standardized screening instrument(s), Evaluation of safety (eg, home), including motor vehicle operation, Identification of caregiver(s), caregiver knowledge, caregiver needs, social supports, and the willingness of caregiver to take on caregiving tasks, Development, updating or revision, or review of an Advance Care Plan, Creation of a written care plan, including initial plans to address any neuropsychiatric symptoms, neuro-cognitive symptoms, functional limitations, and referral to community resources as needed (eg, rehabilitation services, adult day programs, support groups) shared with the patient and/or caregiver with initial education and support. Typically, 50 minutes are spent face-to-face with the patient and/or family or caregiver.

CCI: $0362T^0$ $0373T^1$ $0591T^1$ $0592T^1$ $0593T^1$ 90785^0 90791^0 90792^0 90863^0 96020^1 96105^1 96116^0 96125^0 96127^0 96130^0 96132^0 96136^0 96138^0 96146^0 96156^0 96158^0 96159^0 96160^0 96161^0 96164^0 96165^0 96167^0 96168^0 97151^0 97153^0 97154^1 97155^1 97156^1 97157^1 97158^1 97165^0 97166^0 97167^0 97168^0 99091^0 99202^0 99203^0 99204^0 99205^0 99211^0 99212^0 99213^0 99214^0 99215^0 99446^0 99447^0 99448^0 99449^0 99451^0 99452^0

99491 Chronic care management services with the following required elements: multiple (two or more) chronic conditions expected to last at least 12 months, or until the death of the patient, chronic conditions that place the patient at significant risk of death, acute exacerbation/decompensation, or functional decline, comprehensive care plan established, implemented, revised, or monitored; first 30 minutes provided personally by a physician or other qualified health care professional, per calendar month.

CCI: $0362T^1$ $0373T^1$ 96127^0 97151^1 97152^1 97153^1 97154^1 97156^1 97157^1 97158^1 98960^0 98961^0 98962^0 98966^0 98967^0 98968^0 98970^0 98971^0 98972^0 99071^0 99078^0 99080^0 99091^0 99439^0

99492 Initial psychiatric collaborative care management, first 70 minutes in the first calendar month of behavioral health care manager activities, in consultation with a psychiatric consultant, and directed by the treating physician or other qualified health care professional, with the following required elements: outreach to and engagement in treatment of a patient directed by the treating physician or other qualified health care professional, initial assessment of the patient, including administration of validated rating scales, with the development of an individualized treatment plan, review by the psychiatric consultant with modifications of the plan if recommended, entering patient in a registry and tracking patient follow-up and progress using the registry, with appropriate documentation, and participation in weekly caseload consultation with the psychiatric consultant, and provision of brief interventions using evidence-based techniques such as behavioral activation, motivational interviewing, and other focused treatment strategies.

CCI: $0362T^1$ $0373T^1$ 96127^0 97151^1 97153^1 97154^1 97155^1 97156^1 97157^1 97158^1 98960^0 98961^0 98962^0 98966^0 98967^0 98968^0 98970^0 98971^0 98972^0 99071^0 99078^0 99080^0 99091^0 99441^0 99442^0 99443^0 99493^0

99493 Subsequent psychiatric collaborative care management, first 60 minutes in a subsequent month of behavioral health care manager activities, in consultation with a psychiatric consultant, and directed by the treating physician or other qualified health care professional, with the following required elements: tracking patient follow-up and progress using the registry, with appropriate documentation, participation in weekly caseload consultation with the psychiatric consultant, ongoing collaboration with and coordination of the patient's mental health care with the treating physician or other qualified health care professional and any other treating mental health providers, additional review of progress and recommendations for changes in treatment, as indicated, including medications, based on recommendations provided by the psychiatric consultant, provision of brief interventions using evidence-based techniques such as behavioral activation, motivational interviewing, and other focused treatment strategies, monitoring of patient outcomes using validated rating scales, and relapse prevention planning with patients as they achieve remission of symptoms and/or other treatment goals and are prepared for discharge from active treatment.

CCI: $0362T^1$ $0373T^1$ 96127^0 97151^1 97153^1 97154^1 97155^1 97156^1 97157^1 97158^1 98960^0 98961^0 98962^0 98966^0 98967^0 98968^0 98970^0 98971^0 98972^0 99071^0 99078^0 99080^0 99091^0 99441^0 99442^0 99443^0

99494 Initial or subsequent psychiatric collaborative care management, each additional 30 minutes in a calendar month of behavioral health care manager activities, in consultation with a psychiatric consultant, and directed by the treating physician or other qualified health care professional (List separately in addition to code for primary procedure)

CCI: $0362T^1$ $0373T^1$ 96127^0 97151^1 97153^1 97154^1 97155^1 97156^1 97157^1 97158^1 98960^0 98961^0 98962^0 98966^0 98967^0 98968^0 98970^0 98971^0 98972^0 99071^0 99078^0 99080^0 99091^0 99441^0 99442^0 99443^0

MUE: 2

NCCI Edits for HCPCS Procedures

G0337 Hospice evaluation and counseling services, pre-election
CCI: G0410^1 G0411^1 G0459^0 G0463^0

G0396 Alcohol and/or substance (other than tobacco) misuse structured assessment (e.g., audit, dast), and brief intervention 15 to 30 minutes
CCI: G0442^0 G2011^0

G0397 Alcohol and/or substance (other than tobacco) misuse structured assessment (e.g., audit, dast), and intervention, greater than 30 minutes
CCI: G0396^0 G0442^0 G2011^0

G0406 Follow-up inpatient consultation, limited, physicians typically spend 15 minutes communicating with the patient via telehealth
CCI: G0459^0

G0407 Follow-up inpatient consultation, intermediate, physicians typically spend 25 minutes communicating with the patient via telehealth
CCI: G0406^0 G0459^0

G0408 Follow-up inpatient consultation, complex, physicians typically spend 35 minutes communicating with the patient via telehealth
CCI: G0406^0 G0407^0 G0459^0

G0409 Social work and psychological services, directly relating to and/or furthering the patient's rehabilitation goals, each 15 minutes, face-to-face; individual (services provided by a corf-qualified social worker or psychologist in a corf)
CCI: G0155^1 G0176^1 G0177^1 G0459^1
MUE: N/A

G0410 Group psychotherapy other than of a multiple-family group, in a partial hospitalization setting, approximately 45 to 50 minutes
CCI: G0176^1 G0177^1 G0459^0 G0463^1
MUE: 4

G0411 Interactive group psychotherapy, in a partial hospitalization setting, approximately 45 to 50 minutes
CCI: G0176^1 G0177^1 G0410^1 G0459^0 G0463^1
MUE: 4

G0425 Telehealth consultation, emergency department or initial inpatient, typically 30 minutes communicating with the patient via telehealth
CCI: G0406^0 G0407^0 G0408^0 G0459^0

G0426 Telehealth consultation, emergency department or initial inpatient, typically 50 minutes communicating with the patient via telehealth
CCI: G0406^0 G0407^0 G0408^0 G0425^0 G0459^0 G0508^0 G0509^0

G0427 Telehealth consultation, emergency department or initial inpatient, typically 70 minutes or more communicating with the patient via telehealth
CCI: G0406^0 G0407^0 G0408^0 G0425^0 G0426^0 G0459^0 G0508^0 G0509^0

G0442 Annual alcohol misuse screening, 15 minutes
CCI: G0459^1

G0443 Brief face-to-face behavioral counseling for alcohol misuse, 15 minutes
CCI: G0396^0 G0397^0 G0459^1 G2011^0

G0445 High intensity behavioral counseling to prevent sexually transmitted infection; face-to-face, individual, includes: education, skills training and guidance on how to change sexual behavior; performed semi-annually, 30 minutes
CCI: G0444^0

G0459 Inpatient telehealth pharmacologic management, including prescription, use, and review of medication with no more than minimal medical psychotherapy
CCI: G0444^1 G0445^1 G0446^1 G0447^1

G0463 Hospital outpatient clinic visit for assessment and management of a patient
CCI: G0396^1 G0397^1 G0442^1 G0443^1 G0444^1 G0445^1 G0446^1 G0447^1 G0459^0 G2011^1
MUE: N/A

G0480 Drug test(s), definitive, utilizing (1) drug identification methods able to identify individual drugs and distinguish between structural isomers (but not necessarily stereoisomers), including, but not limited to gc/ms (any type, single or tandem) and lc/ms (any type, single or tandem and excluding immunoassays (e.g., ia, eia, elisa, emit, fpia) and enzymatic methods (e.g., alcohol dehydrogenase)), (2) stable isotope or other universally recognized internal standards in all samples (e.g., to control for matrix effects, interferences and variations in signal strength), and (3) method or drug-specific calibration and matrix-matched quality control material (e.g., to control for instrument variations and mass spectral drift); qualitative or quantitative, all sources, includes specimen validity testing, per day; 1-7 drug class(es), including metabolite(s) if performed
CCI: G0659^0

G0481 Drug test(s), definitive, utilizing (1) drug identification methods able to identify individual drugs and distinguish between structural isomers (but not necessarily stereoisomers), including, but not limited to gc/ms (any type, single or tandem) and lc/ms (any type, single or tandem and excluding immunoassays (e.g., ia, eia, elisa, emit, fpia) and enzymatic methods (e.g., alcohol dehydrogenase)), (2) stable isotope or other universally recognized internal standards in all samples (e.g., to control for matrix effects, interferences and variations in signal strength), and (3) method or drug-specific calibration and matrix-matched quality control material (e.g., to control for instrument variations and mass spectral drift); qualitative or quantitative, all sources, includes specimen validity testing, per day; 8-14 drug class(es), including metabolite(s) if performed
CCI: G0480^0 G0659^0

G0482 Drug test(s), definitive, utilizing (1) drug identification methods able to identify individual drugs and distinguish between structural isomers (but not necessarily stereoisomers), including, but not limited to gc/ms (any type, single or tandem) and lc/ms (any type, single or tandem and excluding immunoassays (e.g., ia, eia, elisa, emit, fpia) and enzymatic methods (e.g., alcohol dehydrogenase)), (2) stable isotope or other universally recognized internal standards in all samples (e.g., to control for matrix effects, interferences and variations in signal strength), and (3) method or drug-specific calibration and matrix-matched quality control material (e.g., to control for instrument variations and mass spectral drift); qualitative or quantitative, all sources, includes specimen validity testing, per day; 15-21 drug class(es), including metabolite(s) if performed
CCI: G0480^0 G0481^0 G0659^0

G0483   Drug test(s), definitive, utilizing (1) drug identification methods able to identify individual drugs and distinguish between structural isomers (but not necessarily stereoisomers), including, but not limited to gc/ms (any type, single or tandem) and lc/ms (any type, single or tandem and excluding immunoassays (e.g., ia, eia, elisa, emit, fpia) and enzymatic methods (e.g., alcohol dehydrogenase)), (2) stable isotope or other universally recognized internal standards in all samples (e.g., to control for matrix effects, interferences and variations in signal strength), and (3) method or drug-specific calibration and matrix-matched quality control material (e.g., to control for instrument variations and mass spectral drift); qualitative or quantitative, all sources, includes specimen validity testing, per day; 22 or more drug class(es), including metabolite(s) if performed

CCI: $G0480^0$ $G0481^0$ $G0482^0$ $G0659^0$

G0508   Telehealth consultation, critical care, initial, physicians typically spend 60 minutes communicating with the patient and providers via telehealth

CCI: $G0406^0$ $G0407^0$ $G0408^0$ $G0459^0$ $G0509^0$

G0509   Telehealth consultation, critical care, subsequent, physicians typically spend 50 minutes communicating with the patient and providers via telehealth

CCI: $G0406^0$ $G0407^0$ $G0408^0$ $G0459^0$

G2011   Alcohol and/or substance (other than tobacco) misuse structured assessment (e.g., audit, dast), and brief intervention, 5-14 minutes

CCI: $G0442^0$

Notes:

Appendix B. Modifiers

Understanding Modifiers

Modifiers provide a way for the practitioner to report or indicate that a procedure or service has been performed, but has been altered by some specific circumstance. The code description for the procedure or service does not change. The appropriate use of modifiers enable practitioners to better communicate with payers and effectively respond to payer policy requirements. For example, there are *some* modifiers which indicate that:

- A procedure or service has both a technical and professional component.
- A procedure or service was performed in more than one location, and/or by more than one practitioner.
- A procedure or service was reduced or increased.
- A bilateral service was performed.
- Unusual events occurred during the procedure or service.

Fee schedules have been developed on the basis of such modifiers. Some payers, such as Medicare and Medicaid, require healthcare providers to use modifiers in some circumstances. Others do not recognize the use of modifiers in coding and billing. Communication with payers ensures accurate coding and expedites payments.

Modifier Applications

The correct use of modifiers is not difficult once a thorough understanding of their application is obtained. Modifiers have two different applications:

- Modifiers may be used to identify circumstances that significantly alter a service or procedure where reimbursement will be altered
- Modifiers may be informational only and have no impact on the normal reimbursement

Modifiers must be in two characters for all insurance claims. The *1500 Claim Form* has space to report up to four modifiers per service line.

Payment Modifiers

As previously mentioned, modifiers may indicate where reimbursement for the service will be different than usual. Some modifiers are referred to as payment modifiers, meaning they are used by payers to help assure accurate and appropriate claims reimbursement. The following statement from Medicare gives some examples of how this works:

> For example, services billed with the assistant at surgery modifier are paid 16 percent of the PFS amount for that service; therefore, the utilization file is modified to only account for 16 percent of any service that contains the assistant at surgery modifier. Similarly, for those services to which volume adjustments are made to account for the payment modifiers, time adjustments are applied as well. For time adjustments to surgical services, the intraoperative portion in the work time file is used; where it is not present, the intraoperative percentage from the payment files used by contractors to process Medicare claims is used instead. Where neither is available, we use the payment adjustment ratio to adjust the time accordingly.
>
> — *Medicare 2022 Physician Fee Schedule Final Rule*

The following table summarizes this statement by Medicare regarding their payment modifiers. Other payers may have different requirements and payment reductions so be aware of any differences.

Modifier	Description	Volume Adjustment	Time Adjustment
80, 81, 82	Assistant at Surgery	16%	Intraoperative portion
AS	Assistant at Surgery — Physician Assistant	14% (85% * 16%)	Intraoperative portion
50 or LT and RT	Bilateral Surgery	150%	150% of work time
51	Multiple Procedure	50%	Intraoperative portion
52	Reduced Services	50%	50%
53	Discontinued Procedure	50%	50%
54	Intraoperative Care only	Preoperative + Intraoperative Pecentages on the payment files used by Medicare contractors to process Medicare claims	Preoperative + Interoperative Portion
55	Postoperative Care only	Postoperative Percentages on the payment files use by Medicare contractors to process Medicare claims	Posoperative portions
62	Co-surgeons	62.5%	50%
66	Team Surgeons	33%	33%
CO, CQ	Physical and Occupational Therapy Assistant Services	88%	88%

Levels of Modifiers

There are three levels of modifiers. Two levels are approved by HIPAA.

- **Level I CPT numeric modifiers:** These two digits codes (ranging from 01-99) are updated by the AMA yearly.
- **Level II HCPCS alphanumeric modifiers:** Ranges AA-ZZ are approved by HIPAA for all payers. They are updated annually by CMS.
- **Level III local modifiers:** Ranges WA-WZ are excluded for HIPAA transactions. However, Workers Compensation is exempt from HIPAA, and could have different modifiers and codes.

Coding Conventions

The following coding conventions are used in this appendix:

Type Styles

Excerpts from the official CPT codebook and HCPCS descriptions are in a type style like this.

> Explanations added by innoviHealth are in a type style like this.

Code Symbols

- ● Identifies a new modifier
- ▲ Identifies a revised modifier

Level I CPT Modifiers

22 Increased Procedural Services

When the work required to provide a service is substantially greater than typically required, it may be identified by adding modifier 22 to the usual procedure code. Documentation must support the substantial additional work and the reason for the additional work (ie, increased intensity, time, technical difficulty of procedure, severity of patient's condition, physical and mental effort required).

Note: This modifier should not be appended to an E/M service.

Reports are required to justify the use of this modifier and as such are closely reviewed by payers. This modifier describes services greater (more complex or time-consuming) than usual for the listed procedure. According to CMS, more "time consuming" means the procedure took at least 50% more time than average to perform and as such could be eligible for modifier 22 as long as there is appropriate supporting documentation. Some experts say it would also be appropriate to add modifier 22 when 25% more work was performed than the procedure usually requires. Because the physician expects greater payment from procedures using modifier 22, third party payers must manually review the documentation to verify it supports additional payment.

The nomenclature of the CPT codes is written to describe the normal, uncomplicated performance of specific procedures. When complications occur, making a procedure more complex or time consuming, modifier 22 should be added to the procedure code to modify the normal description and alert the payer to the unusual circumstances.

It is appropriate to use modifier 22 under the following circumstances:

- The complications cannot be identified by a separate procedure code
- The procedure is lengthy and unusual, or beyond the code's description or RVU
- The services provided by the physician are increased because of unusual circumstances or complications. The work and effort would typically be increased by about 25% or more, and time by 50% or more.

Each procedure carries a risk of complications, estimated level of difficulty, and typical associated time for performance. Sometimes the same procedure performed on different patients can be simple for one and be a bit more difficult for the other, resulting in an average level of difficulty associated with the procedure.

Complications, difficulties, or a longer length of time for performance do not necessarily justify adding modifier 22 for consideration of additional reimbursement. For example, if a procedure has a typical associated time of 1-2 hours and it took the provider a full two hours to complete the surgery, additional payment is not justified any more than the payer paying less because the same procedure only took an hour instead of two. However, if the surgery took three hours (average of 50% more time) or the documentation clearly identifies complications that caused it to be more difficult and time consuming, it would then be reasonable to add modifier 22 and receive additional reimbursement from the payer.

When modifier 22 is submitted, the claim is usually kicked out of the automated processing loop and sent for manual review. That is why an accurate clinical record with appropriate documentation is important.

To facilitate a more efficient manual review, claims with services utilizing modifier 22 should submit (either on paper or electronically) a copy of the procedure note with the claim (depending on payer specific requirements). This enables the manual review process to occur earlier rather than waiting for the payer to request the records.

It is also wise to increase your price to reflect the use of modifier 22, as many payers do not make this increase in payment automatically. Providers should have a process in place to monitor these claims to ensure additional payment was actually made. A payment increase of anywhere from 20-30% could be expected with proper reporting and supporting documentation.

Resource: See Resource 638 for more information.

Alert: This modifier should not be used with an E/M service. It only applies to procedures with a global period of 0, 10, or 90 days.

23 Unusual Anesthesia

Occasionally, a procedure, which usually requires either no anesthesia or local anesthesia, because of unusual circumstances must be done under general anesthesia. This circumstance may be reported by adding modifier 23 to the procedure code of the basic service

Documentation should clearly state what caused the need for general anesthesia.

Example: Although under conscious sedation, the patient could not hold still enough for safe injection of the C4-C5 cervical facet joint. This increased the risk of nicking the spinal cord which could possibly cause paralysis. Therefore, we elected to stop the procedure today and schedule it to be done at XYZ Hospital under general anesthesia

24 Unrelated Evaluation and Management Service by the Same Physician or Other Qualified Health Care Professional During a Postoperative Period

The physician or other qualified health care professional may need to indicate that an evaluation and management service was performed during a postoperative period for a reason(s) unrelated to the original procedure. This circumstance may be reported by adding modifier 24 to the appropriate level of E/M service.

> Do not use modifier 24 in an attempt to obtain payment for the E/M service if the only reason for the service was to provide postoperative care, which is part of the global surgical package.

25 Significant, Separately Identifiable Evaluation and Management Service by the Same Physician on the Same Day of a Procedure or Other Service

It may be necessary to indicate that on the day a procedure or service identified by a CPT code was performed, the patient's condition required a significant, separately identifiable E/M service above and beyond the other service provided or beyond the usual preoperative and postoperative care associated with the procedure that was performed. A significant, separately identifiable E/M service is defined or substantiated by documentation that satisfies the relevant criteria for the respective E/M service to be reported (see **Evaluation and Management Services Guidelines** for instructions on determining level of E/M service). The E/M service may be prompted by the symptom or condition for which the procedure and/or service was provided. As such, different diagnoses are not required for reporting of the E/M services on the same date. This circumstance may be reported by adding modifier 25 to the appropriate level of E/M service.

Note: This modifier is not used to report an E/M service that resulted in a decision to perform surgery. See modifier 57. For significant, separately identifiable non-E/M services, see modifier 59.

> Modifier 25 may ONLY be used in conjunction with E/M services and a handful of HCPCS E/M codes (e.g., G0245). It notifies the payer that the E/M service performed on the same day as a 0 or 10-day global period procedure was done for a significant, separately identifiable reason and should be paid in addition to the procedure and not be bundled into it.
>
> The rules surrounding the proper use of modifier 25 are not complex; however, they tend to cause confusion. The following information should help clarify its use.
>
> As indicated in the official description, pre-service and post-service work pertaining to the global procedure is calculated into the work RVU so an E/M encounter (visit) on the same day as the procedure, to do the pre-service or post-service work, is not payable.
>
> For example, a patient being treated for a head laceration caused by a motor vehicle accident would have typical pre-service/preoperative work that includes a history, pertinent exam (e.g., neurologic exam), and decision making as to the repair of the laceration (which obviously needs repair). This is considered pre-service work to the procedure and is included in the fee for the surgical repair and is not separately payable as an E/M service. Therefore, it would be inappropriate to apply modifier 25 to the E/M service (unbundling it from the procedure) and get paid twice for the E/M service. However, if a more thorough evaluation of the patient was required (of which the pre-service work was just a small part) prior to the repair, modifier 25 may be an appropriate modifier.
>
> If any of the following questions are answered with a yes, then it *might* qualify for usage:
>
> - Could the additional complaint or problem stand alone as a billable service?
> - Is there a different diagnosis for the additional service?
> - If the diagnosis is the same for both conditions, was there extra E/M physician work above and beyond the typical preoperative or postoperative work for the procedure?

Note: Some payers have published policies stating that payments will be reduced (CMS calls a Multiple Procedure Payment Reduction [MPPR]) for E/M services performed during the 0-day and/or 10-day (depending on the payer) global period for another procedure. In light of the upcoming E/M changes, it is likely that more payers will want to implement payment reductions when using this modifier. Check the policies of your contracted payers to see if any payment reduction related to modifier 25 has been implemented.

Alert: Due to a history of inappropriate reporting and over billing, modifier 25 has become the subject of many audit investigations and has repeatedly been included in the Office of Inspector General's (OIG's) Work Plan. It is important for all providers who bill E/M services to understand the appropriate use of modifier 25.

Resource: See Resource 509 for an explanation of the three types of global periods.

Inappropriate Usage

- A new or initial E/M service that results in the decision for major surgery (90-day global period) to be performed the same day or the next day. Use modifier 57 instead of modifier 25.
- An E/M service performed the same day as a 0- or 10-day global procedure, when the decision for surgery has already been made and/or the patient has already been scheduled for the procedure.
- An encounter billed the same day as a surgical procedure (minor or major) when the decision for surgery has already been made.
- Follow-up encounters during the postoperative (global) period of the surgery for issues that are related to recovery from the surgery, including components of the global surgical package (post-surgical pain management by the surgeon; dressing changes; local incision care; removal of sutures, staples, lines, wires, tubes, drains, casts, and splints; insertion, irrigation, and removal of urinary catheters; routine peripheral intravenous lines, nasogastric and rectal tubes; and changes and removal of tracheostomy tubes, etc.)

Appropriate Usage

The following are some examples of when it may be appropriate to use modifier 25 when reporting an E/M service during the global period or on the same day as a procedure:

- Encounters unrelated to the diagnosis for which the surgical procedure is performed, unless the visits occur due to complications of the surgery.
- The patient comes in for a postoperative visit following surgery and the provider performs a history and exam and decision making (as required for postoperative care). Then the provider performs a history, exam, MDM for an issue unrelated to the surgery. As long as the history, exam, or MDM related to the surgery is NOT included in the overall scoring of the other problem, then it may be reported with modifier 25.
- During the process of performing an E/M service the provider identifies a condition, illness, or injury and recommends performance of a 0 or 10-day global procedure for diagnostic or treatment purposes (to be performed during the same encounter), modifier 25 would be appropriate. To assist in identifying the distinct services, the documentation of the E/M service (history, exam, and medical decision making) should be complete and stand on its own merits. This should then be followed by the procedure note, which should also be clearly documented. Sometimes simply separating the two by a few lines and clearly labeling the procedure will aid in any post-procedural audits that may question the validity of the modifier.
- Diagnostic tests and procedures including diagnostic radiological procedures.

Clinical Scenario

Example: During the patient's initial consultation for pain management, the provider ordered a series of four peripheral nerve injections of both feet. The patient had his first injection three days ago and presents today for the second, scheduled injection. The provider takes a brief history, performs a problem focused examination, and determines the patient should continue with the plan to have the second shot in the series today.

Rationale: This is considered normal preoperative and postoperative work which is included in the RVU work units for the procedure being performed, and would be inappropriate to bill separately as an E/M code with modifier 25. The evaluation should still be documented in the medical record, as the RVU for the procedure includes this service and this documentation will help to justify medical necessity for the service being provided.

26 Professional Component

Certain procedures are a combination of a physician or other qualified health care professional component and a technical component. When the physician or other qualified health care professional component is reported separately, the service may be identified by adding modifier 26 to the usual procedure number.

> Radiology is a specialty in which modifier 26 is frequently reported. The work RVUs for any imaging service can be broken down into two components: professional and technical. Professional is represented by modifier 26 and includes interpretation and a report of the image by a radiologist. The technical component (modifier TC) in this case, would be used by the entity that owns the imaging equipment used for the procedure. If the provider both owns the equipment and performs the professional component, no modifier should be used and the provider receives the full payment.

27 Multiple Outpatient Hospital E/M Same Date

For hospital outpatient reporting purposes, utilization of hospital resources related to separate and distinct E/M encounters performed in multiple outpatient hospital settings on the same date may be reported by adding modifier 27 to each appropriate level outpatient and/or emergency department E/M code(s). This modifier provides a means of reporting circumstances involving evaluation and management services provided by physician(s) in more than one (multiple) outpatient hospital setting(s) (eg, hospital emergency department, clinic).

Note: This modifier is not to be used for physician reporting of multiple E/M services performed by the same physician on the same date. For physician reporting of all outpatient evaluation and management services provided by the same physician on the same date and performed in multiple outpatient setting(s) (eg, hospital emergency department, clinic), see Evaluation and Management, Emergency Department, or Preventive Medicine Services codes.

32 Mandated Services

Services related to *mandated* consultation and/or related services (eg, third-party payer, governmental, legislative or regulatory requirement) may be identified by adding the modifier 32 to the basic procedure.

> This modifier flags services required by outside sources other than the patient or the physician. If a court of law, agency, or insurance entity requires that a service be solicited, this modifier indicates such circumstances.
>
> Depending on the payer benefit plans, reimbursement could be made at 100 percent of the allowed amount.
>
> *Example:* The patient's insurance plan requires two opinions. The patient sees another practitioner for a **confirmatory consultation** before the services were scheduled and pre-authorized. Modifier 32 signals to the third party payer that the rules have been followed.

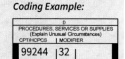

33 Preventive Services

When the primary purpose of the service is the delivery of an evidence based service in accordance with a US Preventive Services Task Force A or B rating in effect and other preventive services identified in preventive services mandates (legislative or regulatory), the service may be identified by adding 33 to the procedure. For separately reported services specifically identified as preventive, the modifier should not be used.

> Do NOT use this modifier on services which are already considered preventative (e.g., immunization, annual wellness visit). It should only be used to clearly identify that the service was performed as a preventive measure (e.g., tobacco cessation counseling).
>
> Reimbursement is typically 100 percent of the allowed amount without co-insurance or deductibles.
>
> **Resource:** See Resource 611 for more information about this modifier.

47 Anesthesia by Surgeon

Regional or general anesthesia provided by the surgeon may be reported by adding modifier 47 to the basic service. (This does not include local anesthesia.)

Note: Modifier 47 would not be used as a modifier for the anesthesia procedures.

> **Tips:**
> - Do not use this modifier with anesthesia procedures (00100-01999)
> - Do not use this modifier if the surgeon is monitoring general anesthesia performed by an anesthesiologist, Certified Registered Nurse Anesthetist (CRNA), resident, or intern
> - Do not use when the surgeon provides moderate sedation

50 Bilateral Procedure

Unless otherwise identified in the listings, bilateral procedures that are performed at the same session, should be identified by adding modifier 50 to the appropriate 5 digit code.

Note: This modifier should not be appended to designated "add-on" codes (see Appendix D in the CPT code book).

> Unless otherwise stated, procedures are considered unilateral in the CPT codebook. In most cases, the addition of modifier 50 is the only way to report that a procedure was done on both sides. For example, when strapping is performed on the ankle of each leg, use 29540-50.
>
> Private insurers may recognize modifier 50 as long as it is used properly. Care must be taken that the code description does not include language that describes "one or both" or "one or more" regions, which, of course, would make modifier 50 unnecessary.
>
> Medicare requires a single line entry for reporting bilateral services such as 29540-50. However, some commercial payers will not accept billing in this manner and either require 29540 and 29540-50 or 29540-RT and 29540-LT as an example. Be aware of individual payer policies. Because of these preferences, it is strongly recommended you carefully review paid claims submitted with bilateral billing to ensure the additional amount for the bilateral side has been added to the payment.
>
> **Note:** For claim submission, depending on the payer policy, either report the procedure on one line using modifier 50 and listing one unit of service, or on two separate lines using modifier RT on one line and LT on the other with one unit of service each.
>
> **Alert:** In 2020, the CPT codebook revised this description to replace the word "surgical" with the word "session." They also added a note that modifier 50 should not be used with add-on codes.
>
> **Note:** Depending on payer reporting policies, bilateral procedures should be reported either on one line using modifier 50 with a single unit of service, or on two separate lines with modifier RT on one line and LT on the other with a single unit of service each.
>
> **Tip:** Carefully review the code description for the service rendered before adding modifier 50. Some procedures are unilateral, unilateral or bilateral, or bilateral. Modifier 50 would only apply to procedures that are unilateral.
>
> **Website:** FindACode.com has an [Additional Code Information] tab which includes the Medicare bilateral code indicator for the code. This can help identify whether or not modifier 50 is applicable.
>
> **Example:** *The patient has bilateral strapping on each side of the upper extremity (e.g., wrist or elbow).*
>
> **Coding Example:**
>
> | D PROCEDURES, SERVICES OR SUPPLIES (Explain Unusual Circumstances) | |
> |---|---|
> | CPT/HCPCS | MODIFIER |
> | 29260 | 50 |
>
> 1 Unit

51 Multiple Procedures

When multiple procedures, other than E/M Services, physical medicine and rehabilitation services, or provision of supplies (eg, vaccines), are performed at the same session by the same provider, the primary procedure or service may be reported as listed. The additional procedure(s) or service(s) may be identified by appending the modifier 51 to the additional procedure or service code(s).

Note: This modifier should not be appended to designated add-on (+) codes.

> **Note:** Add modifier 51 to the surgical procedure code with the lower physician fee schedule amount. Do not use on a procedure code that is described as bilateral or unilateral in its official code description.
>
> **Tip:** Some payer software automatically orders and applies multiple procedure price reductions (MPPR), such as Medicare, making modifier 51 for these payers obsolete. However, it is best to check with all other payers to verify if modifier 51 is required for reporting multiple procedures.

52 Reduced Services

Under certain circumstances a service or procedure is partially reduced or eliminated at the discretion of the physician or other qualified health care provider. Under these circumstances the service provided can be identified by its usual procedure number and the addition of modifier 52, signifying that the service is reduced. This provides a means of reporting reduced services without disturbing the identification of the basic service.

Note: For hospital outpatient reporting of a previously scheduled procedure/service that is partially reduced or cancelled as a result of extenuating circumstances or those that threaten the well-being of the patient prior to or after administration of anesthesia, see modifiers 73 and 74 (see modifiers approved for ASC hospital outpatient use).

> When a procedure is partially reduced, modifier 52 may be used in some situations. This alerts the payer that the service was not completed to its full extent, and as indicated in the description, it enables the provider to report that the services were reduced without changing the official description of the service.
>
> There are very few circumstances where this modifier applies to timed codes since the code description already includes the time limits and a lesser code level would simply be chosen. Some possibilities could be the Acupuncture codes (97810-97814), Medical Nutrition Therapy codes (97802-97804), or special EEG testing (95950-95953; 95956).
>
> **Coding Example:**
>
> | CPT/HCPCS | MODIFIER |
> |---|---|
> | 97810 | 52 |
>
> (PROCEDURES, SERVICES OR SUPPLIES — Explain Unusual Circumstances)
>
> Individual payer policies regarding modifier 52 may vary. A cover letter describing the reduced service along with applicable documentation should accompany the claim.
>
> In addition to the use of modifier 52, it may also be appropriate to use a secondary or tertiary ICD code, along with the primary diagnosis, to document why the procedure was not completed. For example, the codes from the category of Z53 "Persons encountering health services for specific procedures and treatment, not carried out" may be used.
>
> Reimbursement will be reduced, but the amount depends on payer policy. For example, one payer states that it is reduced by 50% of the allowed amount, whereas another payer's policy states that it will be reduced based on the percentage of the full service performed and documented. Therefore, be sure to document the percentage of the service completed.
>
> **Alert:** According to the March 2014 issue of *CPT Assistant*, it is not appropriate to add modifier 52 to Physical Medicine and Rehabilitation time-based codes (97110-97546).

53 Discontinued Procedure

Under certain circumstances, the physician may elect to terminate a surgical or diagnostic procedure. Due to extenuating circumstances or those that threaten the well being of the patient, it may be necessary to indicate that a surgical or diagnostic procedure was started but discontinued. This circumstance may be reported by adding the modifier 53 to the code reported by the physician for the discontinued procedure.

Note: This modifier is not used to report the elective cancellation of a procedure prior to the patient's anesthesia induction and/or surgical preparation in the operating suite. For outpatient hospital/ambulatory surgery center (ASC) reporting of a previously scheduled procedure/service that is partially reduced or cancelled as a result of extenuating circumstances or those that threaten the well being of the patient prior to or after administration of anesthesia, see modifiers 73 and 74 (see modifiers approved for ASC hospital outpatient use).

> Reimbursement is reduced, but the amount depends on payer policy. For example, one Noridian guideline states that the claim amount should be the percentage of the completed procedure. Blue Cross Blue Shield of Massachusetts states that reimbursement is 25% of the allowed amount for all services reported with modifier 53. Be sure to document the percentage of the service completed.

54 Surgical Care Only

When 1 physician or other qualified health care professional performs a surgical procedure and another provides preoperative and/or postoperative management, surgical services may be identified by adding modifier 54 to the usual procedure number.

> This modifier indicates that the surgeon is relinquishing all or part of the post-operative care to another healthcare provider. The healthcare provider rendering post-operative care uses modifier 54. This modifier does not apply to assistant-at-surgery services or Ambulatory Surgical Center (ASC) facility fees.
>
> **Resource:** See Resource 508 for more information on billing surgical services.

55 Postoperative Management Only

When 1 physician or other qualified health care professional performed the postoperative management and another performed the surgical procedure, the postoperative component may be identified by adding modifier 55 to the usual procedure number.

> Use modifier 55 with the procedure code for global periods of 10 or 90 days.
>
> Report the date of surgery as the date of service and indicate the date care was relinquished or assumed in Item Number 19 of the *1500 Claim Form* or the electronic equivalent.
>
> Providers must keep copies of the written transfer agreement in the beneficiary's medical record.
>
> The surgeon does NOT use this code, it is used by a different healthcare provider.
>
> **Resource:** See Resource 508 for more information on billing surgical services.

56 Preoperative Management Only

When 1 physician or other qualified health care professional performed the preoperative care and evaluation and another performed the surgical procedure, the preoperative component may be identified by adding modifier 56 to the usual procedure number.

> This is typically used only for major surgeries which are performed immediately, i.e., on the same day as the decision was made.

57 Decision for Surgery

An evaluation and management service that resulted in the initial decision to perform the surgery may be identified by adding modifier 57 to the appropriate level of E/M service.

> The global period for major surgery is 92 days (the day before and day of the surgery plus the 90 days following the surgery). If the decision to perform the surgery was made the day before or day of the surgery, modifier 57 should be appended to the E/M service to override the edit that would otherwise bundle it into the procedure.

58 Staged or Related Procedure or Service by the Same Physician or Other Qualified Health Care Professional During the Postoperative Period

It may be necessary to indicate that the performance of a procedure or service during the postoperative period was (a) planned or anticipated (staged); (b) more extensive than the original procedure; or (c) for therapy following a surgical procedure. This circumstance may be reported by adding modifier 58 to the staged or related procedure.

Note: For treatment of a problem that requires a return to the operating/procedure room (eg, unanticipated clinical condition), see modifier 78.

59 Distinct Procedural Service

Under certain circumstances, it may be necessary to indicate that a procedure or service was distinct or independent from other non-E/M services performed on the same day. Modifier 59 is used to identify procedures/services, other than E/M services, that are not normally reported together, but are appropriate under the circumstances. Documentation must support a different session, different procedure or surgery, different site or organ system, separate incision/excision, separate lesion, or separate injury (or area of injury in extensive injuries) not ordinarily encountered or performed on the same day by the same individual. However, when another already established modifier is appropriate it should be used rather than modifier 59. Only if no more descriptive modifier is available, and the use of modifier 59 best explains the circumstances, should modifier 59 be used.

Note: Modifier 59 should not be appended to an E/M service. To report a separate and distinct E/M service with a non-E/M service performed on the same date, see modifier 25.

> Do NOT use this modifier with E/M services. It should only be used when there are either NCCI edits (see Appendix A — NCCI Edits) or other payer policies which prohibit the reporting of two services together.
>
> Proper documentation is essential to explain why this service is separate from other non-E/M services performed on the same day. The official description provides examples (e.g., different site, separate lesion).
>
> Medicare created the X{EPSU} modifiers (see also "XU" on page 446) to provide clarity to the appropriateness of overriding the NCCI edit associated with two or more procedures. Although Medicare has not made reporting these instead of modifier 59 mandatory, the definitions and examples provided for them make the circumstances for reporting modifier 59 clearer.
>
> **Note:** Modifiers that identify anatomic positions or laterality (if applicable) should be reported in place of 59 to explain the multiple procedures performed (e.g., RT, LT, E1-E4).
>
> **Alert:** Modifier 59 is often overused and consequently, it has become a target for either pre- or post- payment reviews. Be sure you understand when and where it can be used appropriately. Modifier 59 is reported only to override an NCCI edit. If no NCCI edit exists between the codes, modifier 59 is not reported.
>
> **Resource:** See Resource 401 to read the NCCI instructions regarding modifier 59.
>
> **Warnings:**
> - Documentation in the chart/record should correctly record the parameters of treatment such as location, method of application, intensity, and time. It is fraudulent to alter documentation or billing in order to get paid.
> - Modifier 59 is not reported for surgical procedures performed on contiguous sites. In other words, if the sites of each procedure overlap or connect, modifier 59 should not be reported and the services should not be unbundled.

> **Alert:** In order to address the incorrect usage of modifier 59, four new modifiers (XE, XS, XP, XU) were created in 2015. These modifiers act as a subset of modifier 59 by including additional information to clearly identify the rationale for using a modifier for that service. Not all payers have implemented the use of these modifiers, so verify payer policy to see if they require the use of a modifier other than 59 for the service being billed.
>
> **Resource:** See Resource 392 to read more about the CMS announcement.

62 Two Surgeons

When 2 surgeons work together as primary surgeons performing distinct part(s) of a procedure, each surgeon should report his/her distinct operative work by adding modifier 62 to the procedure code and any associated add-on code(s) for that procedure as long as both surgeons continue to work together as primary surgeons. Each surgeon should report the co-surgery once using the same procedure code. If additional procedure(s) (including add-on procedure(s) are performed during the same surgical session, separate code(s) may also be reported with modifier 62 added.

Note: If a co-surgeon acts as an assistant in the performance of additional procedure(s) other than those reported with the modifier 62, during the same surgical session, those services may be reported using separate procedure code(s) with modifier 80 or modifier 82 added, as appropriate.

> Co-surgeons are two surgeons performing distinct parts of the same procedure during the same surgical session. One surgeon may perform the opening or approach, while the other performs the main procedure and then closes; or any combination of these. A co-surgeon's role may even change mid-procedure, becoming the assistant surgeon for the portion of the surgery performed by the other co-surgeon.
>
> Reimbursement is reduced by a percentage based on payer policy. For example, Noridian pays 62.5% of the Medicare allowed amount for each surgeon.
>
> **Resource:** See Resource 619 for more information.

▲ 63 Procedure Performed on Infants less than 4 kg

Procedures performed on neonates and infants up to a present body weight of 4 kg may involve significantly increased complexity and physician or other qualified health care professional work commonly associated with these patients. This circumstance may be reported by adding modifier 63 to the procedure number.

Note: Unless otherwise designated, this modifier may only be appended to procedures/services listed in the 20100-69990 code series and 92920, 92928, 92953, 92960, 92986, 92987, 92990, 92997, 92998, 93312, 93313, 93314, 93315, 93316, 93317, 93318, 93452, 93505, 93563, 93564, 93568, 93580, 93582, 93590, 93591, 93592, 93593, 93594, 93595, 93596, 93597, 93598, 93615, 93616 from the Medicine/Cardiovascular section. Modifier 63 should not be appended to any CPT codes listed in the **Evaluation and Management** Services, Anesthesia, Radiology, Pathology/Laboratory, or Medicine sections (other than those identified above from the Medicine/Cardiovascular section).

66 Surgical Team

Under some circumstances, highly complex procedures (requiring the concomitant services of several physicians or other qualified health care professionals, often of different specialties, plus other highly skilled, specially trained personnel, various types of complex equipment) are carried out under the "surgical team" concept. Such circumstances may be identified by each participating individual with the addition of modifier 66 to the basic procedure number used for reporting services.

73 Discontinued Out-Patient Hospital/Ambulatory Surgery Center (ASC) Procedure Prior to the Administration of Anesthesia

Due to extenuating circumstances or those that threaten the well being of the patient, the physician may cancel a surgical or diagnostic procedure subsequent to the patient's surgical preparation (including sedation when provided, and being taken to the room where the procedure is to be performed), but prior to the administration of anesthesia (local, regional block(s) or general). Under these circumstances, the intended service that is prepared for but canceled can be reported by its usual procedure number and the addition of modifier 73.

Note: The elective cancellation of a service prior to the administration of anesthesia and/or surgical preparation of the patient should not be reported. For physician reporting of a discontinued procedure, see modifier 53.

74 Discontinued Out-Patient Hospital/Ambulatory Surgery Center (ASC) Procedure After Administration of Anesthesia

Due to extenuating circumstances or those that threaten the well being of the patient, the physician may terminate a surgical or diagnostic procedure after the administration of anesthesia (local, regional block(s), general) or after the procedure was started (incision made, intubation started, scope inserted, etc). Under these circumstances, the procedure started but terminated can be reported by its usual procedure number and the addition of modifier 74.

Note: The elective cancellation of a service prior to the administration of anesthesia and/or surgical preparation of the patient should not be reported. For physician reporting of a discontinued procedure, see modifier 53.

76 Repeat Procedure or Service By Same Physician or Other Qualified Health Care Professional

It may be necessary to indicate that a procedure or service was repeated subsequent to the original procedure or service. This circumstance may be reported by adding the modifier 76 to the repeated procedure or service.

Note: This modifier should not be appended to an E/M service.

> Modifier 76 is used to report a "second" procedure which has been previously reported or performed on the same day. This may occur with interventions which must be aborted due to patient instability, or in cases where a "repeat" of the first minor procedure is necessary because the first minor procedure did not produce the anticipated or optimal results.
>
> This modifier should assist in preventing denials for duplicate submission messages on EOMBs or payment reports. This modifier is usually used for radiology, laboratory, and minor surgical procedures, such as repeat blood sugar tests on the same day.
>
> Commercial payers vary on the use of this modifier. Many do not recognize it at all, stating that they pay based on the procedure alone. Some recognize it during the global surgical period only. Others recognize it at all times when it is appropriate. In all cases the second procedure would be paid for and it would begin a new global surgical package period.
>
> **Note:** Modifiers 76 and 77 are commonly reported with radiology services when multiple chest x-rays or other views are required on the same day by one and/or more providers.
>
> **Reminder:** Informational modifiers (e.g., 76, 77) should NOT be listed before pricing modifiers (e.g., 26).
>
> **Example:** *A 66-year old male presented to the ER at 1 a.m. with symptoms of chest pain, rapid heart rate, and left arm pain. Dr. Jones performed three AP and lateral chest x-rays between 1-7 a.m., then his shift ended and Dr. Smith became his provider from 7 a.m. until 7 p.m., performing two additional AP and lateral chest x-rays.*
>
> This situation would be reported as follows:
>
> Dr. Jones   71045, 71045-76, 71045-76
>
> Dr. Smith   71045-77, 71045-77

77 Repeat Procedure by Another Physician or Other Qualified Healthcare Professional

The physician may need to indicate that a basic procedure or service performed by another physician had to be repeated. This situation may be reported by adding modifier 77 to the repeated procedure/service.

It may be necessary to indicate that a basic procedure or service was repeated by another physician or other qualified health care professional subsequent to the original procedure or service. This circumstance may be reported by adding modifier 77 to the repeated procedure or service.

Note: This modifier should not be appended to an E/M service.

> This modifier is identical to modifier 76 except that it is used when the physician repeating the procedure is not the same as the physician who performed the original service.
>
> Modifiers 76 and 77 are usually not particularly reimbursement oriented, but they are valuable in reporting the circumstances of a procedure correctly and are therefore "informational." They could "save" a claim from pending for an explanation or a denial for duplicate billing. Without this modifier the insurer could view the claim as double billing.
>
> Commercial payers vary on their use of this modifier; many do not recognize it at all and pay only on the first procedure.
>
> **Reminder:** Informational modifiers (e.g., 76, 77) should NOT be listed before pricing modifiers (e.g., 26).
>
> **Coding Example:**
>
> | D PROCEDURES, SERVICES OR SUPPLIES (Explain Unusual Circumstances) | |
> |---|---|
> | CPT/HCPCS | MODIFIER |
> | 72040 | 26 \| 77 |

78 Unplanned Return to the Operating/Procedure Room by the Same Physician or Other Qualified Health Care Professional Following Initial Procedure for a Related Procedure During the Postoperative Period

It may be necessary to indicate that another procedure was performed during the postoperative period of the initial procedure (unplanned procedure following initial procedure). When this procedure is related to the first and requires the use of an operating/procedure room, it may be reported by adding modifier 78 to the related procedure. (For repeat procedures, see modifier 76.)

79 Unrelated Procedure or Service by the Same Physician or Other Qualified Health Care Professional During the Postoperative Period

The individual may need to indicate that the performance of a procedure or service during the postoperative period was unrelated to the original procedure. This circumstance may be reported by using modifier 79. (For repeat procedures on the same day, see modifier 76.)

80 Assistant Surgeon

Surgical assistant services may be identified by adding modifier 80 to the usual procedure number(s).

> Assistant surgeons are not required to dictate a separate or individual operative report. The operative report dictated by the primary surgeon, identifying the assistant surgeon by name, is sufficient.

81 Minimum Assistant Surgeon

Minimum surgical assistant services are identified by adding modifier 81 to the usual procedure number.

> Assistant surgeons are not required to dictate a separate or individual operative report. The operative report dictated by the primary surgeon, identifying the assistant surgeon by name, is sufficient.

82 Assistant Surgeon (when qualified resident surgeon not available)

The unavailability of a qualified resident surgeon is a prerequisite for use of modifier 82 appended to the usual procedure code number(s).

> Documentation should indicate that a qualified resident surgeon was unavailable. Assistant surgeons are not required to dictate a separate or individual operative report. It is sufficient for the operative report dictated by the primary surgeon to simply identify the assistant surgeon by name.

90 Reference (Outside) Laboratory

When laboratory procedures are performed by a party other than the treating or reporting physician, the procedure may be identified by adding the modifier 90 to the usual procedure number.

> This modifier is used to indicate that an outside laboratory rendered the services, rather than the lab of the treating or reporting physician. This notifies the insurer that the lab services were furnished outside the physician's office and the physician is billing for the service.
>
> This modifier could be used differently by non-Medicare payers. Some HMOs require that patients use specific labs with which they contract for services. In this case the physician may draw the blood (code 36415), modify the lab test by adding modifier 90 and send the specimen to the appropriate lab for testing.
>
> Other HMOs will allow the physician to bill them for the testing done in their office if they have CLIA lab certification. If a test still needs to be sent out to a reference lab the HMO may allow the physician to bill the patient for the test and then the physician will reimburse the lab later. Each carrier has their own policy regarding the use of physician labs or outside labs. In all cases payers will request information on who is actually providing the service.
>
> *Example:* The patient went to the reference lab for a fasting glucose test at an integrated multidisciplinary clinic. The laboratory and the physician's office had a billing agreement whereby the office could bill the patient (insurer) and the lab would then bill the physician's office for the service. Lab tests from the office, however, were submitted with modifier 90 (the HMO to which the patient belonged required this billing format).
>
> **Coding Example:**
>
> | D PROCEDURES, SERVICES OR SUPPLIES (Explain Unusual Circumstances) | |
> |---|---|
> | CPT/HCPCS | MODIFIER |
> | 82951 | 90 |
> | 36415 | |
>
> **Note:** Medicare does not allow the above scenario to occur because the physician may only bill for the service that he/she actually provided. The laboratory would bill the Medicare patient and modifier 90 would not be used.

91 Repeat Clinical Diagnostic Laboratory Test

In the course of treatment of the patient, it may be necessary to repeat the same laboratory test on the same day to obtain subsequent (multiple) test results. Under these circumstances, the laboratory test performed can be identified by its usual procedure number and the addition of modifier 91.

Note: This modifier may not be used when tests are rerun to confirm initial results; due to testing problems with specimens or equipment; or for any other reason when a normal, one-time, reportable result is all that is required. This modifier may not be used when other code(s) describe a series of test results (eg, glucose tolerance tests, evocative/suppression testing). This modifier may only be used for laboratory test(s) performed more than once on the same day on the same patient.

92 Alternative Laboratory Platform Testing

When laboratory testing is being performed using a kit or transportable instrument that wholly or in part consists of a single use, disposable analytical chamber, the service may be identified by adding modifier 92 to the usual laboratory procedure code (HIV testing 86701-86703, and 87389). The test does not require permanent dedicated space, hence by its design it may be hand carried or transported to the vicinity of the patient for immediate testing at that site, although location of the testing is not in itself determinative of the use of this modifier.

95 Synchronous Telemedicine Service Rendered Via a Real-Time Interactive Audio and Video Telecommunications System

Synchronous telemedicine service is defined as a real-time interaction between a physician or other qualified health care professional and a patient who is located at a distant site from the physician or other qualified health care professional. The totality of the communication of information exchanged between the physician or other qualified health care professional and the patient during the course of the synchronous telemedicine service must be of an amount and nature that would be sufficient to meet the key components and/or requirements of the same service when rendered via a face-to-face interaction. Modifier 95 may only be ed to the services listed in Appendix P. Appendix P is the list of CPT codes for services that are typically performed face-to-face, but may be rendered via a real-time (synchronous) interactive audio and video telecommunications system.

> This modifier, which was added in 2017, identifies when a service has been provided via telehealth/telemedicine. Be aware of individual payer policies as some may reduce payment. For example, one BC/BS policy states that "Reimbursement is calculated using 50% of the Practice Expense (PE) Relative Value Unit (RVU) for the service."
>
> **Book:** See Appendix D — Telehealth Codes for more information.
>
> **Book:** See also modifier GT on page 438 for more information about telehealth modifiers.

96 Habilitative Services

When a service or procedure that may be either habilitative or rehabilitative in nature is provided for habilitative purposes, the physician or other qualified health care professional may add modifier 96 to the service or procedure code to indicate that the service or procedure provided was a habilitative service. Habilitative services help an individual learn skills and functioning for daily living that the individual has not yet developed, and then keep and/or improve those learned skills. Habilitative services also help an individual keep, learn, or improve skills and functioning for daily living.

> Due to Affordable Care Act requirements, habilitative services are covered differently than other services and thus require the use of an appropriate modifier to notify the payer. This modifier replaces modifier SZ, which was deleted in 2018.
>
> **Resource:** See Resource 128 for more information about this modifier.

97 Rehabilitative Services

When a service or procedure that may be either habilitative or rehabilitative in nature is provided for rehabilitative purposes, the physician or other qualified health care professional may add modifier 97 to the service or procedure code to indicate that the service or procedure provided was a rehabilitative service. Rehabilitative services help an individual keep, get back, or improve skills and functioning for daily living that have been lost or impaired because the individual was sick, hurt, or disabled.

> Due to Affordable Care Act requirements, rehabilitative services are covered differently than other services and thus require the use of an appropriate modifier to notify the payer.
>
> **Resource:** See Resource 128 for more information about this modifier.

99 Multiple Modifiers

Under certain circumstances two or more modifiers may be necessary to completely delineate a service. In such situations modifier 99 should be added to the basic procedure, and other applicable modifiers may be listed as part of the description of the service.

> The paper *1500 Claim Form* has space for up to four modifiers per procedure code. Although not common, if a situation arises where more than four modifiers are needed, check with the payer to determine their preference for reporting this unique situation.
>
> This modifier indicates that multiple modifiers are being attached to a procedure code. Modifier 99 is added immediately after the procedure code itself and signals "more modifiers to come." Modifier 99 would be required if a patient had an unusual circumstance that required a highly specific explanation. Most scenarios which require multiple modifiers also would require a report to clarify the situation. The report would show the legitimacy of using multiple modifiers.
>
> Third party payers recognize the use of modifier 99 and additional modifiers. Reporting such unique circumstances on paper claims is limited to four modifiers. Additional modifiers could be added in the pink supplemental area above the procedure line or by attaching a report. Check with the payer to determine their preference.
>
> The need for more than four modifiers can be explained in Item Number 19 of the *1500 Claim Form*. There is limited space; however, simply listing them in order of importance should suffice. If the payer needs additional information, they will request a copy of the documentation.
>
> **Book:** See Item Number 19 in Chapter 1.3 — Claims Processing for more information.

Level II HCPCS Modifiers

Modifier codes and descriptions are approved by CMS but recommended jointly by the alpha-numeric editorial panel consisting of the American Medical Association (AMA), Health Insurance Association of America (HIAA), and Blue Cross/Blue Shield (BC/BS). Note that these are official descriptions in which capitalization may not necessarily follow grammar rules. These two (2) character codes are added to the basic code. These modifiers are commonly used for reporting Medicare and Medicaid services, however, use of these national modifiers are at the option of private insurance payers.

Note: These modifiers are used with either a procedure or supply code where indicated. Be aware of individual payer requirements.

Reminder: The HCPCS modifiers included here are effective as of January 1, 2022, however, they could change during the year. Any update to these modifiers are available at FindACode.com (with subscription).

A1	Dressing for one wound
A2	Dressing for two wounds
A3	Dressing for three wounds
A4	Dressing for four wounds
A5	Dressing for five wounds
A6	Dressing for six wounds
A7	Dressing for seven wounds
A8	Dressing for eight wounds
A9	Dressing for nine or more wounds
AA	Anesthesia services performed personally by anesthesiologist
AD	Medical supervision by a physician: more than four concurrent anesthesia procedures
AE	Registered dietician
AF	Specialty physician
AG	Primary physician
AH	Clinical psychologist
AI	Principal physician of record
AJ	Clinical social worker
AK	Non participating physician
AM	Physician, team member service
AO	Alternate payment method declined by provider of service
AP	Determination of refractive state was not performed in the course of diagnostic ophthalmological examination
AQ	Physician providing a service in an unlisted health professional shortage area (hpsa)
AR	Physician provider services in a physician scarcity area
AS	Physician assistant, nurse practitioner, or clinical nurse specialist services for assistant at surgery
	Commonly reimbursed at a reduced percentage (e.g., 85%) of assistant surgeon's fee schedule.
AT	Acute treatment (this modifier should be used when reporting service 98940, 98941, 98942)
AU	Item furnished in conjunction with a urological, ostomy, or tracheostomy supply
AV	Item furnished in conjunction with a prosthetic device, prosthetic or orthotic
AW	Item furnished in conjunction with a surgical dressing
AX	Item furnished in conjunction with dialysis services

AY	Item or service furnished to an esrd patient that is not for the treatment of esrd
AZ	Physician providing a service in a dental health professional shortage area for the purpose of an electronic health record incentive payment
BA	Item furnished in conjunction with parenteral enteral nutrition (pen) services
BL	Special acquisition of blood and blood products
BO	Orally administered nutrition, not by feeding tube
BP	The beneficiary has been informed of the purchase and rental options and has elected to purchase the item
BR	The beneficiary has been informed of the purchase and rental options and has elected to rent the item
BU	The beneficiary has been informed of the purchase and rental options and after 30 days has not informed the supplier of his/her decision
CA	Procedure payable only in the inpatient setting when performed emergently on an outpatient who expires prior to admission
CB	Service ordered by a renal dialysis facility (rdf) physician as part of the esrd beneficiary's dialysis benefit, is not part of the composite rate, and is separately reimbursable
CC	Procedure code change (use 'cc' when the procedure code submitted was changed either for administrative reasons or because an incorrect code was filed)
CD	Amcc test has been ordered by an esrd facility or mcp physician that is part of the composite rate and is not separately billable
CE	Amcc test has been ordered by an esrd facility or mcp physician that is a composite rate test but is beyond the normal frequency covered under the rate and is separately reimbursable based on medical necessity
CF	Amcc test has been ordered by an esrd facility or mcp physician that is not part of the composite rate and is separately billable
CG	Policy criteria applied
CH	0 percent impaired, limited or restricted
CI	At least 1 percent but less than 20 percent impaired, limited or restricted
CJ	At least 20 percent but less than 40 percent impaired, limited or restricted
CK	At least 40 percent but less than 60 percent impaired, limited or restricted
CL	At least 60 percent but less than 80 percent impaired, limited or restricted
CM	At least 80 percent but less than 100 percent impaired, limited or restricted
CN	100 percent impaired, limited or restricted

> Prior to January 2019, CMS required the reporting of functional limitation using modifiers CH-CN when billing for outpatient therapy services, including physical therapy (PT), occupational therapy (OT), and speech-language pathology (SLP) services. These severity modifiers were used to reflect the beneficiary's percentage of functional impairment as determined by the clinician furnishing the therapy services.

CO	Outpatient occupational therapy services furnished in whole or in part by an occupational therapy assistant
CP	*Code deleted effective 2018-01-01*
CQ	Outpatient physical therapy services furnished in whole or in part by a physical therapist assistant
CR	Catastrophe/disaster related
CS	Cost-sharing for specified covid-19 testing-related services that result in an order for or administration of a covid-19 test
CT	Computed tomography services furnished using equipment that does not meet each of the attributes of the national electrical manufacturers association (nema) xr-29-2013 standard

> The technical component is commonly reimbursed at a reduced percentage (e.g., 15%).

DA	Oral health assessment by a licensed health professional other than a dentist
E1	Upper left, eyelid

	E2	Lower left, eyelid
	E3	Upper right, eyelid
	E4	Lower right, eyelid
	EA	Erythropoetic stimulating agent (esa) administered to treat anemia due to anti-cancer chemotherapy
	EB	Erythropoetic stimulating agent (esa) administered to treat anemia due to anti-cancer radiotherapy
	EC	Erythropoetic stimulating agent (esa) administered to treat anemia not due to anti-cancer radiotherapy or anti-cancer chemotherapy
	ED	Hematocrit level has exceeded 39% (or hemoglobin level has exceeded 13.0 g/dl) for 3 or more consecutive billing cycles immediately prior to and including the current cycle
	EE	Hematocrit level has not exceeded 39% (or hemoglobin level has not exceeded 13.0 g/dl) for 3 or more consecutive billing cycles immediately prior to and including the current cycle
	EJ	Subsequent claims for a defined course of therapy, e.g., epo, sodium hyaluronate, infliximab
	EM	Emergency reserve supply (for esrd benefit only)
	EP	Service provided as part of medicaid early periodic screening diagnosis and treatment (epsdt) program
	ER	Items and services furnished by a provider-based, off-campus emergency department
	ET	Emergency services
	EX	Expatriate beneficiary
	EY	No physician or other licensed health care provider order for this item or service
	F1	Left hand, second digit
	F2	Left hand, third digit
	F3	Left hand, fourth digit
	F4	Left hand, fifth digit
	F5	Right hand, thumb
	F6	Right hand, second digit
	F7	Right hand, third digit
	F8	Right hand, fourth digit
	F9	Right hand, fifth digit
	FA	Left hand, thumb
	FB	Item provided without cost to provider, supplier or practitioner, or full credit received for replaced device (examples, but not limited to, covered under warranty, replaced due to defect, free samples)
	FC	Partial credit received for replaced device
	FP	Service provided as part of family planning program
●	FQ	The service was furnished using audio-only communication technology
		Resource: See Resource 656 for more information about this new modifier.
●	FR	The supervising practitioner was present through two-way, audio/video communication technology
		Resource: See Resource 657 for more information about this new modifier.
●	FS	Split (or shared) evaluation and management visit
		Resource: See Resource 658 for more information about this new modifier.
●	FT	Unrelated evaluation and management (e/m) visit during a postoperative period, or on the same day as a procedure or another e/m visit. (report when an e/m visit is furnished within the global period but is unrelated, or when one or more additional e/m visits furnished on the same day are unrelated
		Resource: See Resource 659 for more information about this new modifier.
	FX	X-ray taken using film

FY	X-ray taken using computed radiography technology/cassette-based imaging

> Some payers (e.g., Medicare) require modifier FX when reporting conventional film imaging. Medicare also requires modifier FY when the image utilizes computed radiography technology which Medicare defines as "cassette-based imaging which utilizes an imaging plate to create the image involved."
>
> **Resource:** See Resource 630 for more information about using these modifiers, including Medicare's payment reduction amounts.

G0	Telehealth services for diagnosis, evaluation, or treatment, of symptoms of an acute stroke
G1	Most recent urr reading of less than 60
G2	Most recent urr reading of 60 to 64.9
G3	Most recent urr reading of 65 to 69.9
G4	Most recent urr reading of 70 to 74.9
G5	Most recent urr reading of 75 or greater
G6	Esrd patient for whom less than six dialysis sessions have been provided in a month
G7	Pregnancy resulted from rape or incest or pregnancy certified by physician as life threatening
G8	Monitored anesthesia care (mac) for deep complex, complicated, or markedly invasive surgical procedure
G9	Monitored anesthesia care for patient who has history of severe cardio-pulmonary condition
GA	Waiver of liability statement issued as required by payer policy, individual case

> For Medicare, this is a declaration that there is an "ABN on file."
>
> **Book:** See Chapter 2.1 — Medicare Essentials for more information on using this modifier.

GB	Claim being re-submitted for payment because it is no longer covered under a global payment demonstration
GC	This service has been performed in part by a resident under the direction of a teaching physician
GD	Units of service exceeds medically unlikely edit value and represents reasonable and necessary services

> When submitting a claim with this modifier, supporting documentation establishing medical necessity must also be included.
>
> **Book:** See Chapter 6.1 — Procedure Coding Essentials for additional information regarding medically unlikely edits (MUEs).

GE	This service has been performed by a resident without the presence of a teaching physician under the primary care exception
GF	Non-physician (e.g. nurse practitioner (np), certified registered nurse anesthetist (crna), certified registered nurse (crn), clinical nurse specialist (cns), physician assistant (pa)) services in a critical access hospital
GG	Performance and payment of a screening mammogram and diagnostic mammogram on the same patient, same day
GH	Diagnostic mammogram converted from screening mammogram on same day
GJ	"opt out" physician or practitioner emergency or urgent service

> **Book:** See Chapter 2.1 — Medicare Essentials for more about Opting Out of Medicare.

GK	Reasonable and necessary item/service associated with GA or GZ modifier

> According to Medicare, this modifier is used by the provider/supplier to indicate that the service meets reasonable and necessary requirements (e.g., physical therapy, durable medical equipment). It could expand to other providers because it clarifies matters. Non-Medicare payers could possibly use it, as it is an approved HIPAA code set. Accordingly, use by any payer is at their sole discretion.

GL	Medically unnecessary upgrade provided instead of non-upgraded item, no charge, no advance beneficiary notice (abn)
GM	Multiple patients on one ambulance trip

GN	Services delivered under an outpatient speech language pathology plan of care	
GO	Services delivered under an outpatient occupational therapy plan of care	
GP	Services delivered under an outpatient physical therapy plan of care	

> Modifiers GN, GO, and GP are increasingly becoming important and claims will be denied by Medicare and many other payers if not included with physical therapy codes. They are considered secondary modifiers which means that other payment modifiers (e.g., 25, 59) should be reported first.
>
> **Resource:** See Resource 822 for more information.

GQ	Via asynchronous telecommunications system

> Asynchronous "store and forward" technology used in delivering services when the originating site is a federal telemedicine demonstration program in Alaska or Hawaii. Please refer to modifier GT for further qualifications and definitions of the telehealth program.

GR	This service was performed in whole or in part by a resident in a department of veterans affairs medical center or clinic, supervised in accordance with va policy
GS	Dosage of erythropoietin stimulating agent has been reduced and maintained in response to hematocrit or hemoglobin level
GT	Via interactive audio and video telecommunication systems

> Most private payers require modifier 95 instead of modifier GT when reporting telehealth services. Medicare only requires this modifier when telehealth services are provided by Critical Access Hospitals (CAHs). Be aware of individual payer policies regarding reporting these types of services.
>
> **Note:** For asynchronous communication, see modifier GQ.
>
> **Book:** See Appendix D — Telehealth Services for more information.
>
> **Book:** See also modifier 95 on page 432.

GU	Waiver of liability statement issued as required by payer policy, routine notice
GV	Attending physician not employed or paid under arrangement by the patient's hospice provider
GW	Service not related to the hospice patient's terminal condition
GX	Notice of liability issued, voluntary under payer policy

> **Book:** See Chapter 2.1 — Medicare Essentials for more information on using this modifier.

GY	Item or service statutorily excluded or, does not meet the definition of any Medicare benefit or, for non-Medicare insurers, is not a contract benefit

> **Book:** See Chapter 2.1 — Medicare Essentials for more information on using this modifier.

GZ	Item or service expected to be denied as not reasonable and necessary

> No Medicare ABN form was signed by the patient.
>
> **Book:** See Chapter 2.1 — Medicare Essentials for more information on using this modifier.

H9	Court-ordered
HA	Child/adolescent program
HB	Adult program, non geriatric
HC	Adult program, geriatric
HD	Pregnant/parenting women's program
HE	Mental health program
HF	Substance abuse program
HG	Opioid addiction treatment program
HH	Integrated mental health/substance abuse program
HI	Integrated mental health and intellectual disability/developmental disabilities program
HJ	Employee assistance program

HK	Specialized mental health programs for high-risk populations
HL	Intern
HM	Less than bachelor degree level
HN	Bachelors degree level
HO	Masters degree level
HP	Doctoral level
HQ	Group setting
HR	Family/couple with client present
HS	Family/couple without client present
HT	Multi-disciplinary team
HU	Funded by child welfare agency
HV	Funded state addictions agency
HW	Funded by state mental health agency
HX	Funded by county/local agency
HY	Funded by juvenile justice agency
HZ	Funded by criminal justice agency
J1	Competitive acquisition program no-pay submission for a prescription number
J2	Competitive acquisition program, restocking of emergency drugs after emergency administration
J3	Competitive acquisition program (cap), drug not available through cap as written, reimbursed under average sales price methodology
J4	Dmepos item subject to dmepos competitive bidding program that is furnished by a hospital upon discharge
J5	Off-the-shelf orthotic subject to dmepos competitive bidding program that is furnished as part of a physical therapist or occupational therapist professional service

> This modifier became effective on October 1, 2020. Medicare requires physical and occupational therapists to use this modifier when billing OTS back and knee braces (e.g., L0450, L0455, L1812). Watch for further guidance from payers.
>
> **Resource:** See Resource 654 for more information.

JA	Administered intravenously
JB	Administered subcutaneously
JC	Skin substitute used as a graft
JD	Skin substitute not used as a graft
JE	Administered via dialysate
JG	Drug or biological acquired with 340b drug pricing program discount
JW	Drug amount discarded/not administered to any patient
K0	Lower extremity prosthesis functional level 0 - does not have the ability or potential to ambulate or transfer safely with or without assistance and a prosthesis does not enhance their quality of life or mobility.
K1	Lower extremity prosthesis functional level 1 - has the ability or potential to use a prosthesis for transfers or ambulation on level surfaces at fixed cadence. typical of the limited and unlimited household ambulator.
K2	Lower extremity prosthesis functional level 2 - has the ability or potential for ambulation with the ability to traverse low level environmental barriers such as curbs, stairs or uneven surfaces. Typical of the limited community ambulator.
K3	Lower extremity prosthesis functional level 3 - has the ability or potential for ambulation with variable cadence. Typical of the community ambulator who has the ability to transverse most environmental barriers and may have vocational, therapeutic, or exercise activity that demands prosthetic utilization beyond simple locomotion.

	K4	Lower extremity prosthesis functional level 4 - has the ability or potential for prosthetic ambulation that exceeds the basic ambulation skills, exhibiting high impact, stress, or energy levels, typical of the prosthetic demands of the child, active adult, or athlete.
	KA	Add on option/accessory for wheelchair
	KB	Beneficiary requested upgrade for abn, more than 4 modifiers identified on claim
	KC	Replacement of special power wheelchair interface
	KD	Drug or biological infused through dme
	KE	Bid under round one of the dmepos competitive bidding program for use with non-competitive bid base equipment
	KF	Item designated by fda as class iii device
	KG	Dmepos item subject to dmepos competitive bidding program number 1
	KH	Dmepos item, initial claim, purchase or first month rental

> Effective October 1, 2018, the KH modifier is not required for purchased, capped rental durable medical equipment, or parenteral/enteral items and services for Medicare beneficiaries.

	KI	Dmepos item, second or third month rental
	KJ	Dmepos item, parenteral enteral nutrition (pen) pump or capped rental, months four to fifteen
	KK	Dmepos item subject to dmepos competitive bidding program number 2
	KL	Dmepos item delivered via mail
	KM	Replacement of facial prosthesis including new impression/moulage
	KN	Replacement of facial prosthesis using previous master model
	KO	Single drug unit dose formulation
	KP	First drug of a multiple drug unit dose formulation
	KQ	Second or subsequent drug of a multiple drug unit dose formulation
	KR	Rental item, billing for partial month

> See modifier RR for a full month.

	KS	Glucose monitor supply for diabetic beneficiary not treated with insulin
	KT	Beneficiary resides in a competitive bidding area and travels outside that competitive bidding area and receives a competitive bid item
	KU	Dmepos item subject to dmepos competitive bidding program number 3
	KV	Dmepos item subject to dmepos competitive bidding program that is furnished as part of a professional service
	KW	Dmepos item subject to dmepos competitive bidding program number 4
	KX	Requirements specified in the medical policy have been met

> This modifier can be used to specify that although policy caps on the service provided have been met, the provider feels there is evidence that continued care is medically necessary. Medicare requires this modifier (where applicable) when billing therapy services.
>
> No additional information, other than the medical record, is needed to provide support for the KX modifier; however, the medical record should clearly identify the medical necessity for the service. The Medicare Claims Processing Manual states, "Contractors shall not limit medically necessary services that are justified by scientific research applicable to the beneficiary."
>
> Be sure to link the diagnosis code that best supports medical necessity to the therapy service.
>
> **Resource:** See *Section 10.3.1 - Exceptions to Therapy Caps – General* in Resource 618 for more information.
>
> **Alert:** Do not apply KX to all therapy services as this could initiate an audit.

	KY	Dmepos item subject to dmepos competitive bidding program number 5

KZ	New coverage not implemented by managed care
LC	Left circumflex coronary artery
LD	Left anterior descending coronary artery
LL	Lease/rental (use the 'll' modifier when dme equipment rental is to be applied against the purchase price)
LM	Left main coronary artery
LR	Laboratory round trip
LS	Fda-monitored intraocular lens implant
LT	Left side (used to identify procedures performed on the left side of the body)
M2	Medicare secondary payer (msp)
MA	Ordering professional is not required to consult a clinical decision support mechanism due to service being rendered to a patient with a suspected or confirmed emergency medical condition
MB	Ordering professional is not required to consult a clinical decision support mechanism due to the significant hardship exception of insufficient internet access
MC	Ordering professional is not required to consult a clinical decision support mechanism due to the significant hardship exception of electronic health record or clinical decision support mechanism vendor issues
MD	Ordering professional is not required to consult a clinical decision support mechanism due to the significant hardship exception of extreme and uncontrollable circumstances
ME	The order for this service adheres to appropriate use criteria in the clinical decision support mechanism consulted by the ordering professional
MF	The order for this service does not adhere to the appropriate use criteria in the clinical decision support mechanism consulted by the ordering professional
MG	The order for this service does not have applicable appropriate use criteria in the qualified clinical decision support mechanism consulted by the ordering professional
MH	Unknown if ordering professional consulted a clinical decision support mechanism for this service, related information was not provided to the furnishing professional or provider
MS	Six month maintenance and servicing fee for reasonable and necessary parts and labor which are not covered under any manufacturer or supplier warranty
NB	Nebulizer system, any type, fda-cleared for use with specific drug
NR	New when rented (use the 'nr' modifier when dme which was new at the time of rental is subsequently purchased)
NU	New equipment
P1	A normal healthy patient
P2	A patient with mild systemic disease
P3	A patient with severe systemic disease
P4	A patient with severe systemic disease that is a constant threat to life
P5	A moribund patient who is not expected to survive without the operation
P6	A declared brain-dead patient whose organs are being removed for donor purposes
PA	Surgical or other invasive procedure on wrong body part
PB	Surgical or other invasive procedure on wrong patient
PC	Wrong surgery or other invasive procedure on patient
PD	Diagnostic or related non diagnostic item or service provided in a wholly owned or operated entity to a patient who is admitted as an inpatient within 3 days
PI	Positron emission tomography (pet) or pet/computed tomography (ct) to inform the initial treatment strategy of tumors that are biopsy proven or strongly suspected of being cancerous based on other diagnostic testing
PL	Progressive addition lenses
PM	Post mortem

	PN	Non-excepted service provided at an off-campus, outpatient, provider-based department of a hospital
	PO	Excepted service provided at an off-campus, outpatient, provider-based department of a hospital
	PS	Positron emission tomography (pet) or pet/computed tomography (ct) to inform the subsequent treatment strategy of cancerous tumors when the beneficiary's treating physician determines that the pet study is needed to inform subsequent anti-tumor strategy
	PT	Colorectal cancer screening test; converted to diagnostic test or other procedure

> Only use this modifier when a colorectal screening/preventive service turns into a diagnostic/therapeutic service (e.g., colorectal cancer screening becomes diagnostic when a polyp is found and excised for testing).
>
> Typically the deductible is waived, but co-insurance still applies.
>
> **Note:** Do not confuse modifier PT with modifier 33 which is used for other types of preventive services. Also be aware of individual payer policies which may require modifier 33 instead of modifier PT.
>
> **Example:** Patient with a family history of familial adenomatous polyposis, presents for a preventive colonoscopy (G0105). During the course of the screening colonoscopy, a growth is detected and the provider removes the polyp by cold biopsy with forceps.
>
> **Coding Example:**
> | CPT/HCPCS | MODIFIER |
> |---|---|
> | 45385 | PT |

	Q0	Investigational clinical service provided in a clinical research study that is in an approved clinical research study
	Q1	Routine clinical service provided in a clinical research study that is in an approved clinical research study
	Q2	Demonstration procedure/service

> This modifier is to be used when billing services which fall under any of CMS's demonstration projects for Medicare, Medicaid, and the Children's Health Insurance Program (CHIP). Some current projects are Medicaid's Certified Community Behavioral Heath Center (CCBHC) and Medicare's Comprehensive Care for Joint Replacement Model (CJR).

	Q3	Live kidney donor surgery and related services
	Q4	Service for ordering/referring physician qualifies as a service exemption
	Q5	Service furnished under a reciprocal billing arrangement by a substitute physician or by a substitute physical therapist furnishing outpatient physical therapy services in a health professional shortage area, a medically underserved area, or a rural area
	Q6	Service furnished under a fee-for-time compensation arrangement by a substitute physician or by a substitute physical therapist furnishing outpatient physical therapy services in a health professional shortage area, a medically underserved area, or a rural area

> **Resource:** See Resource 609 for more about using modifiers Q5 and Q6 when billing special provider coverage arrangements.

	Q7	One class a finding

> **Resource:** See Resource 507 for more about this modifier for foot care.

	Q8	Two class b findings

> **Resource:** See Resource 507 for more about this modifier for foot care.

	Q9	One class b and two class c findings

> **Resource:** See Resource 507 for more about this modifier for foot care.

	QA	Prescribed amounts of stationary oxygen for daytime use while at rest and nighttime use differ and the average of the two amounts is less than 1 liter per minute (LPM)
	QB	Prescribed amounts of stationary oxygen for daytime use while at rest and nighttime use differ and the average of the two amounts exceeds 4 liters per minute (LPM) and portable oxygen is prescribed

> **Note:** This code was originally deleted in 2005 and reactivated April 2018 with a new description.

	QC	Single channel monitoring

QD	Recording and storage in solid state memory by a digital recorder
QE	Prescribed amount of stationary oxygen while at rest is less than 1 liter per minute (lpm)
QF	Prescribed amount of stationary oxygen while at rest exceeds 4 liters per minute (lpm) and portable oxygen is prescribed
QG	Prescribed amount of stationary oxygen while at rest is greater than 4 liters per minute(lpm)
QH	Oxygen conserving device is being used with an oxygen delivery system
QJ	Services/items provided to a prisoner or patient in state or local custody, however the state or local government, as applicable, meets the requirements in 42 cfr 411.4 (b)
QK	Medical direction of two, three, or four concurrent anesthesia procedures involving qualified individuals
QL	Patient pronounced dead after ambulance called
QM	Ambulance service provided under arrangement by a provider of services
QN	Ambulance service furnished directly by a provider of services
QP	Documentation is on file showing that the laboratory test(s) was ordered individually or ordered as a cpt-recognized panel other than automated profile codes 80002-80019, g0058, g0059, and g0060.
QQ	Ordering professional consulted a qualified clinical decision support mechanism for this service and the related data was provided to the furnishing professional

> **Note:** This code was originally deleted in 2006 and reactivated July 2018 with a new description.

QR	Prescribed amounts of stationary oxygen for daytime use while at rest and nighttime use differ and the average of the two amounts is greater than 4 liters per minute (LPM)

> **Note:** This code was originally deleted in 2007 and reactivated April 2018 with a new description.

QS	Monitored anesthesia care service
QT	Recording and storage on tape by an analog tape recorder
QW	Clia waived test

> The Centers for Medicare and Medicaid Services (CMS) regulates all laboratory testing (except research) performed on humans in the U.S. due to the Clinical Laboratory Improvement Amendments (CLIA). When a simple lab test is exempt from CLIA oversight, add modifier QW.

QX	Crna service: with medical direction by a physician
QY	Medical direction of one certified registered nurse anesthetist (crna) by an anesthesiologist
QZ	Crna service: without medical direction by a physician
RA	Replacement of a dme, orthotic or prosthetic item
RB	Replacement of a part of a dme, orthotic or prosthetic item furnished as part of a repair
RC	Right coronary artery
RD	Drug provided to beneficiary, but not administered "incident-to"
RE	Furnished in full compliance with fda-mandated risk evaluation and mitigation strategy (rems)
RI	Ramus intermedius coronary artery
RR	Rental (use the 'rr' modifier when dme is to be rented)
RT	Right side (used to identify procedures performed on the right side of the body)
SA	Nurse practitioner rendering service in collaboration with a physician

> Be aware of individual payer requirements regarding the use of this modifier. For example, UnitedHealthcare began requiring this modifier, effective September 2017, when billing incident to E/M services rendered by nurse practitioners, physician assistants, and clinical nurse specialists.

SB	Nurse midwife
SC	Medically necessary service or supply
SD	Services provided by registered nurse with specialized, highly technical home infusion training

SE	State and/or federally-funded programs/services	
SF	Second opinion ordered by a professional review organization (pro) per section 9401, p.l. 99-272 (100% reimbursement - no medicare deductible or coinsurance)	
SG	Ambulatory surgical center (asc) facility service	
SH	Second concurrently administered infusion therapy	
SJ	Third or more concurrently administered infusion therapy	
SK	Member of high risk population (use only with codes for immunization)	
SL	State supplied vaccine	
SM	Second surgical opinion	
SN	Third surgical opinion	
SQ	Item ordered by home health	
SS	Home infusion services provided in the infusion suite of the iv therapy provider	
ST	Related to trauma or injury	
SU	Procedure performed in physician's office (to denote use of facility and equipment)	
SV	Pharmaceuticals delivered to patient's home but not utilized	
SW	Services provided by a certified diabetic educator	
SY	Persons who are in close contact with member of high-risk population (use only with codes for immunization)	
T1	Left foot, second digit	
T2	Left foot, third digit	
T3	Left foot, fourth digit	
T4	Left foot, fifth digit	
T5	Right foot, great toe	
T6	Right foot, second digit	
T7	Right foot, third digit	
T8	Right foot, fourth digit	
T9	Right foot, fifth digit	
TA	Left foot, great toe	

> These toe modifiers (T1-TA) are important for reporting podiatry services and orthotics.
>
> **Alert:** Do not use toe modifiers when the code descriptor describes all digits or gives a set number of digits.

TB	Drug or biological acquired with 340b drug pricing program discount, reported for informational purposes
TC	Technical component; under certain circumstances, a charge may be made for the technical component alone; under those circumstances the technical component charge is identified by adding modifier 'tc' to the usual procedure number; technical component charges are institutional charges and not billed separately by physicians; however, portable x-ray suppliers only bill for technical component and should utilize modifier tc; the charge data from portable x-ray suppliers will then be used to build customary and prevailing profiles

> Technical component charges are typically facility or institutional charges. Providers who own the equipment and also perform the professional component (interpret the films and write a report of the findings) do not add any modifier to the procedure code as they will receive full payment for the service provided. Portable x-ray suppliers usually bill for the technical component using this modifier.
>
> When only the technical component is performed, it does not include the interpretation and report (professional component 26). When no modifier is used (TC or 26), it is a declaration that both components of the procedure or service are performed.
>
> **Note:** Do not submit the technical component separately when one physician performs both the professional and technical components on the same day.

TD	Rn
TE	Lpn/lvn
TF	Intermediate level of care
TG	Complex/high tech level of care
TH	Obstetrical treatment/services, prenatal or postpartum
TJ	Program group, child and/or adolescent
TK	Extra patient or passenger, non-ambulance
TL	Early intervention/individualized family service plan (ifsp)
TM	Individualized education program (iep)
TN	Rural/outside providers' customary service area
TP	Medical transport, unloaded vehicle
TQ	Basic life support transport by a volunteer ambulance provider
TR	School-based individualized education program (iep) services provided outside the public school district responsible for the student
TS	Follow-up service
TT	Individualized service provided to more than one patient in same setting
TU	Special payment rate, overtime
TV	Special payment rates, holidays/weekends
TW	Back-up equipment
U1	Medicaid level of care 1, as defined by each state
U2	Medicaid level of care 2, as defined by each state
U3	Medicaid level of care 3, as defined by each state
U4	Medicaid level of care 4, as defined by each state
U5	Medicaid level of care 5, as defined by each state
U6	Medicaid level of care 6, as defined by each state
U7	Medicaid level of care 7, as defined by each state
U8	Medicaid level of care 8, as defined by each state
U9	Medicaid level of care 9, as defined by each state
UA	Medicaid level of care 10, as defined by each state
UB	Medicaid level of care 11, as defined by each state
UC	Medicaid level of care 12, as defined by each state
UD	Medicaid level of care 13, as defined by each state
UE	Used durable medical equipment
UF	Services provided in the morning
UG	Services provided in the afternoon
UH	Services provided in the evening
UJ	Services provided at night
UK	Services provided on behalf of the client to someone other than the client (collateral relationship)
UN	Two patients served
UP	Three patients served
UQ	Four patients served
UR	Five patients served
US	Six or more patients served

V1	Demonstration modifier 1
V2	Demonstration modifier 2
V3	Demonstration modifier 3
V4	Demonstration modifier 4
V5	Vascular catheter (alone or with any other vascular access)
V6	Arteriovenous graft (or other vascular access not including a vascular catheter)
V7	Arteriovenous fistula only (in use with two needles)
VM	Medicare diabetes prevention program (mdpp) virtual make-up session
VP	Aphakic patient
X1	Continuous/broad services: for reporting services by clinicians, who provide the principal care for a patient, with no planned endpoint of the relationship; services in this category represent comprehensive care, dealing with the entire scope of patient problems, either directly or in a care coordination role; reporting clinician service examples include, but are not limited to: primary care, and clinicians providing comprehensive care to patients in addition to specialty care
X2	Continuous/focused services: for reporting services by clinicians whose expertise is needed for the ongoing management of a chronic disease or a condition that needs to be managed and followed with no planned endpoint to the relationship; reporting clinician service examples include but are not limited to: a rheumatologist taking care of the patient's rheumatoid arthritis longitudinally but not providing general primary care services
X3	Episodic/broad services: for reporting services by clinicians who have broad responsibility for the comprehensive needs of the patient that is limited to a defined period and circumstance such as a hospitalization; reporting clinician service examples include but are not limited to the hospitalist's services rendered providing comprehensive and general care to a patient while admitted to the hospital
X4	Episodic/focused services: for reporting services by clinicians who provide focused care on particular types of treatment limited to a defined period and circumstance; the patient has a problem, acute or chronic, that will be treated with surgery, radiation, or some other type of generally time-limited intervention; reporting clinician service examples include but are not limited to, the orthopedic surgeon performing a knee replacement and seeing the patient through the postoperative period
X5	Diagnostic services requested by another clinician: for reporting services by a clinician who furnishes care to the patient only as requested by another clinician or subsequent and related services requested by another clinician; this modifier is reported for patient relationships that may not be adequately captured by the above alternative categories; reporting clinician service examples include but are not limited to, the radiologist's interpretation of an imaging study requested by another clinician

> **Note:** Patient Relationship Code (PRC) modifiers X1-X5 modifiers may be reported as a MIPS quality improvement activity.

XE	Separate encounter, a service that is distinct because it occurred during a separate encounter
XP	Separate practitioner, a service that is distinct because it was performed by a different practitioner
XS	Separate structure, a service that is distinct because it was performed on a separate organ/structure
XU	Unusual non-overlapping service, the use of a service that is distinct because it does not overlap usual components of the main service

> **Alert:** Due to problems with the incorrect usage of modifier 59, CMS added modifiers XE, XP, XS and XU in 2015. These modifiers are considered a subset of modifier 59. Although CMS has stated that they will continue to recognize modifier 59, they also stated that per CPT guidelines, it should not be used when a more descriptive modifier is available.
>
> Individual payer policies vary on the use of these 'X' modifiers.
>
> **Alert:** Claims submitted with an X{EPSU} modifier are commonly subject to either pre- or post-payment reviews.
>
> **Resource:** See Resource 601 for more information on modifier 59.

ZA Code deleted effective 2018-04-01
ZB Code deleted effective 2018-04-01
ZC Code deleted effective 2018-04-01

Notes:

Appendix C. Provider Documentation Guides

Introduction

This section contains a selection of *Provider Documentation Guides (PDGs)*™ which were explained and introduced in Chapter 4.2 – Provider Documentation Training. *PDGs* are simply summaries of all the pertinent information a provider or coder might need to make sure a diagnosis is documented in a manner that allows for correct coding and reporting. ICD-10-CM codes are highly specific, and as such, have more specific criteria. All medical coding is derived from the information healthcare providers document in the medical record. A thorough understanding of the coding rules and options are vital to avoid negative post-payment audits.

1. The condition (i.e., diagnosis), including the ICD-10-CM code or code range

2. Helpful information (e.g., terminology, any applicable HCC categories, what to document list for the provider, and notes for the coder)

3. Applicable instructional notes/guidelines and indicator(s) at the chapter and block levels

4. Information conveyed by each character level with instructional notes, guidelines, and indicators applicable at the category and subcategory levels

If a particular condition is not found in this section, build a *PDG* by hand by looking up the code in The Tabular List and recording the relevant information on a worksheet.

This information is to help facilitate correct documentation to support the diagnoses reported. The *PDG* tool assists the provider by ensuring that all the necessary information is provided and able to be presented in the documentation. It then serves as a guide for the coders/billers by providing the correct codes, guidelines, and even terminology associated with the diagnoses. The *PDGs* in this section have been created for your specialty.

Store: This appendix contains a sample of specialty-specific PDGs. For a larger selection, see innoviHealth's *ICD-10-CM Coding books* or add *Provider Documentation Guides (PDGs)* to your Find-A-Code account for access to thousands of PDGs.

Book: See Appendix F — Coding Reference Tables for lists of the ICD-10-CM Tabular indicators, HAC categories, and HCC codes.

Contents - Provider Documentation Guides

Bipolar Disorder 451

Depressive Episode 453

Major Depressive Disorder, Recurrent 455

Persistent Mood [Affective] Disorders 456

Other Anxiety Disorders 457

Bipolar Disorder

ICD-10-CM: F31.0 - F31.9

What to Document
3rd Character: Mood affective disorder
4th Character: Type of bipolar disorder
5th Character: Severity, other specifications

Chapter Guidelines

5. Mental, Behavioral and Neurodevelopmental disorders (F01-F99)

Includes:
disorders of psychological development
Excludes2:
symptoms, signs and abnormal clinical laboratory findings, not elsewhere classified (R00-R99)
See Guidelines: 1;C.20.a.1

MOOD [AFFECTIVE] DISORDERS (F30-F39)

3rd Character

Document: Mood affective disorder

F30-	Manic episode
F31-	Bipolar disorder
F32-	Major depressive disorder, single episode
F33-	Major depressive disorder, recurrent
F34-	Persistent mood [affective] disorders
F39	Unspecified mood [affective] disorder

4th Character

Document: Type of bipolar disorder

Includes:
bipolar I disorder
bipolar type I disorder
manic-depressive illness
manic-depressive psychosis
manic-depressive reaction
Excludes1:
bipolar disorder, single manic episode (F30.-)
major depressive disorder, single episode (F32.-)
major depressive disorder, recurrent (F33.-)
Excludes2:
cyclothymia (F34.0)
Indicator(s): CMS22: 58 | CMS23: 59 | CMS24: 59 | Rx05: 131 | ESRD21: 58 | HHS04: 88 | HHS05: 88

F31.0 Bipolar disorder, current episode hypomanic
Indicator(s): DSM-5

F31.1- Bipolar disorder, current episode manic without psychotic features

4th Character (continued)

F31.2 Bipolar disorder, current episode manic severe with psychotic features
Including: Current episode with mood-congruent (or mood incongruent) psychotic symptoms; Bipolar 1, current or most recent episode manic with psychotic features
Indicator(s): DSM-5

F31.3- Bipolar disorder, current episode depressed, mild or moderate severity

F31.4 Bipolar disorder, current episode depressed, severe, without psychotic features
Indicator(s): DSM-5

F31.5 Bipolar disorder, current episode depressed, severe, with psychotic features
Including: Current episode depressed with mood-incongruent (or mood congruent) psychotic symptoms; Bipolar 1, current or most recent episode depressed, with psychotic features
Indicator(s): DSM-5

F31.6- Bipolar disorder, current episode mixed

F31.7- Bipolar disorder, currently in remission

F31.8- Other bipolar disorders
Indicator(s): DSM-5

F31.9 Bipolar disorder, unspecified
Including: Manic depression
Indicator(s): DSM-5

5th Character

Document: Severity, other specifications

Indicator(s): DSM-5

Applies to: F31.1-
0 Unspecified
1 Mild
Indicator(s): DSM-5
2 Moderate
Indicator(s): DSM-5
3 Severe
Indicator(s): DSM-5

Applies to: F31.3-
0 Unspecified
1 Mild
Indicator(s): DSM-5
2 Moderate
Indicator(s): DSM-5

Bipolar Disorder (continued)

5th Character (continued)

Applies to: F31.6-

- 0 Unspecified
- 1 Mild
- 2 Moderate
- 3 Severe, without psychotic features
- 4 Severe, with psychotic features
  Including: mixed with mood-congruent (or mood incongruent) psychotic symptoms

Applies to: F31.7-

- 0 Most recent episode unspecified
- 1 In partial remission, most recent episode hypomanic
  Indicator(s): DSM-5
- 2 In full remission, most recent episode hypomanic
  Indicator(s): DSM-5
- 3 In partial remission, most recent episode manic
  Indicator(s): DSM-5
- 4 In full remission, most recent episode manic
  Indicator(s): DSM-5
- 5 In partial remission, most recent episode depressed
  Indicator(s): DSM-5
- 6 In full remission, most recent episode depressed
  Indicator(s): DSM-5
- 7 In partial remission, most recent episode mixed
- 8 In full remission, most recent episode mixed

Applies to: F31.8-

- 1 Bipolar II
  Including: Bipolar disorder, type 2
- 9 Other
  Including: Recurrent manic episodes NOS

6th Character
N/A

7th Character
N/A

Depressive Episode
ICD-10-CM: F32.0 - F32.A

What to Document
3rd Character: Mood affective disorder
4th Character: Severity or remission status, and with or without psychotic features
5th Character: Other depressive episodes

Chapter Guidelines

5. Mental, Behavioral and Neurodevelopmental disorders (F01-F99)

Includes:
 disorders of psychological development
Excludes2:
 symptoms, signs and abnormal clinical laboratory findings, not elsewhere classified (R00-R99)
See Guidelines: 1;C.20.a.1

MOOD [AFFECTIVE] DISORDERS (F30-F39)

3rd Character
Document: Mood affective disorder

- F30- Manic episode
- F31- Bipolar disorder
- **F32-** Depressive episode
- F33- Major depressive disorder, recurrent
- F34- Persistent mood [affective] disorders
- **F39** Unspecified mood [affective] disorder

4th Character
Document: Severity or remission status, and with or without psychotic features

Includes:
 single episode of agitated depression
 single episode of depressive reaction
 single episode of major depression
 single episode of psychogenic depression
 single episode of reactive depression
 single episode of vital depression
Excludes1:
 bipolar disorder (F31.-)
 manic episode (F30.-)
 recurrent depressive disorder (F33.-)
Excludes2:
 adjustment disorder (F43.2)

4th Character (continued)

F32.0 Major depressive disorder, single episode, mild
Indicator(s): CC | DSM-5 | CMS22: 58 | CMS23: 59 | CMS24: 59 | Rx05: 132 | ESRD21: 58

F32.1 Major depressive disorder, single episode, moderate
Indicator(s): CC | DSM-5 | CMS22: 58 | CMS23: 59 | CMS24: 59 | Rx05: 132 | ESRD21: 58

F32.2 Major depressive disorder, single episode, severe without psychotic features
Indicator(s): CC | DSM-5 | CMS22: 58 | CMS23: 59 | CMS24: 59 | Rx05: 132 | ESRD21: 58 | HHS04: 88 | HHS05: 88

F32.3 Major depressive disorder, single episode, severe with psychotic features
Including: Single episode major depression with mood-congruent, mood-incongruent, or psychotic symptoms; Single episode of psychogenic depressive psychosis, psychotic depression, or reactive depressive psychosis
Indicator(s): CC | DSM-5 | CMS22: 58 | CMS23: 59 | CMS24: 59 | Rx05: 132 | ESRD21: 58 | HHS04: 88 | HHS05: 88

F32.4 Major depressive disorder, single episode, in partial remission
Indicator(s): DSM-5 | CMS22: 58 | CMS23: 59 | CMS24: 59 | Rx05: 132 | ESRD21: 58

F32.5 Major depressive disorder, single episode, in full remission
Indicator(s): DSM-5 | CMS22: 58 | CMS23: 59 | CMS24: 59 | Rx05: 132 | ESRD21: 58

F32.8- Other depressive episodes
Including: Atypical depression, Post-schizophrenic depression, Single episode of 'masked' depression NOS
Indicator(s): DSM-5 | DSM-5 | Rx05: 134

F32.9 Major depressive disorder, single episode, unspecified
Including: Major depression NOS
Indicator(s): DSM-5 | Rx05: 134

F32.A Depression, unspecified
Including: Depression NOS, Depressive disorder NOS

Depressive Episode (continued)

5th Character

Document: Other depressive episodes

> Including: Atypical depression, Post-schizophrenic depression, Single episode of 'masked' depression NOS
> *Indicator(s):* DSM-5 | DSM-5 | Rx05: 134

Applies to: F32.8-

1 Premenstrual dysphoric disorder
> *Excludes1:*
> premenstrual tension syndrome (N94.3)
> *Indicator(s):* Female

9 Other specified
> Including: Atypical depression, Post-schizophrenic depression, Single episode of 'masked' depression NOS

6th Character

N/A

7th Character

N/A

Major Depressive Disorder, Recurrent

ICD-10-CM: F33.0 - F33.9

What to Document

3rd Character: Mood affective disorder
4th Character: Severity or remission status, and with or without psychotic features
5th Character: Remission status

Chapter Guidelines

5. Mental, Behavioral and Neurodevelopmental disorders (F01-F99)

Includes:
  disorders of psychological development
Excludes2:
  symptoms, signs and abnormal clinical laboratory findings, not elsewhere classified (R00-R99)
See Guidelines: 1;C.20.a.1

MOOD [AFFECTIVE] DISORDERS (F30-F39)

3rd Character

Document: Mood affective disorder

- F30- Manic episode
- F31- Bipolar disorder
- F32- Major depressive disorder, single episode
- F33- Major depressive disorder, recurrent
- F34- Persistent mood [affective] disorders
- F39   Unspecified mood [affective] disorder

4th Character

Document: Severity or remission status, and with or without psychotic features
Reminder: Final codes are in **BOLD**

Includes:
  recurrent episodes of depressive reaction
  recurrent episodes of endogenous depression
  recurrent episodes of major depression
  recurrent episodes of psychogenic depression
  recurrent episodes of reactive depression
  recurrent episodes of seasonal depressive disorder
  recurrent episodes of vital depression
Excludes1:
  bipolar disorder (F31.-)
  manic episode (F30.-)
Indicator(s): CMS22: 58 | CMS23: 59 | CMS24: 59 | Rx05: 132 | ESRD21: 58

4th Character (continued)

F33.0 Major depressive disorder, recurrent, mild
  Indicator(s): DSM-5

F33.1 Major depressive disorder, recurrent, moderate
  Indicator(s): DSM-5

F33.2 Major depressive disorder, recurrent severe without psychotic features
  Indicator(s): DSM-5

F33.3 Major depressive disorder, recurrent, severe with psychotic symptoms
  Including: Endogenous depression with psychotic symptoms; Recurrent severe episodes of major depression with mood-congruent, mood incongruent, or psychotic symptoms; Recurrent severe episodes of psychogenic depressive psychosis, psychotic depression, or reactive depressive psychosis
  Indicator(s): DSM-5

F33.4- Major depressive disorder, recurrent, in remission

F33.8 Other recurrent depressive disorders
  Including: Recurrent brief depressive episodes

F33.9 Major depressive disorder, recurrent, unspecified
  Including: Monopolar depression NOS
  Indicator(s): DSM-5

5th Character

Document: Remission status

Applies to: F33.4-

0 Unspecified
1 In partial remission
     Indicator(s): DSM-5
2 In full remission
     Indicator(s): DSM-5

6th Character

N/A

7th Character

N/A

Persistent Mood [Affective] Disorders

ICD-10-CM: F34.0 - F34.9

What to Document

4th Character: Type of persistent mood [affective] disorder
5th Character: Other specifications

Terminology:
Dysthymia: A mild but long-term form of depression
Cyclothymic disorder: A rare episodic mood disorder in which your mood shifts up and down from your baseline emotional range, but not as severe as in bipolar I or II disorder

Chapter Guidelines

5. Mental, Behavioral and Neurodevelopmental disorders (F01-F99)

Includes:
disorders of psychological development
Excludes2:
symptoms, signs and abnormal clinical laboratory findings, not elsewhere classified (R00-R99)
See Guidelines: 1;C.20.a.1

MOOD [AFFECTIVE] DISORDERS (F30-F39)

3rd Character

F30-	Manic episode
F31-	Bipolar disorder
F32-	Major depressive disorder, single episode
F33-	Major depressive disorder, recurrent
F34-	**Persistent mood [affective] disorders**
F39	Unspecified mood [affective] disorder

4th Character

Document: Type of persistent mood [affective] disorder
Reminder: All final codes are in **BOLD**

F34.0 Cyclothymic disorder
  Including: Affective personality disorder, Cycloid personality, Cyclothymia, Cyclothymic personality
  Indicator(s): DSM-5 | Rx05: 134

F34.1 Dysthymic disorder
  Including: Depressive neurosis, Depressive personality disorder, Dysthymia, Neurotic depression, Persistent anxiety depression, Persistent depressive disorder
  Excludes2:
  anxiety depression (mild or not persistent) (F41.8)
  Indicator(s): DSM-5 | Rx05: 134

F34.8- Other persistent mood [affective] disorders
  Indicator(s): CMS22: 58 | CMS23: 59 | CMS24: 59 | Rx05: 131 | ESRD21: 58

F34.9 Persistent mood [affective] disorder, unspecified
  Indicator(s): CMS22: 58 | CMS23: 59 | CMS24: 59 | Rx05: 131 | ESRD21: 58

5th Character

Document: Other specifications

  Indicator(s): CMS22: 58 | CMS23: 59 | CMS24: 59 | Rx05: 131 | ESRD21: 58

Applies to: F34.8-

1 Disruptive mood dysregulation disorder
    Indicator(s): DSM-5

9 Other specified

6th Character

N/A

7th Character

N/A

Other Anxiety Disorders

ICD-10-CM: F41.0 - F41.9

What to Document

3rd Character: Type of mental disorder
4th Character: Type of anxiety disorder

Chapter Guidelines

5. Mental, Behavioral and Neurodevelopmental disorders (F01-F99)

Includes:
  disorders of psychological development
Excludes2:
  symptoms, signs and abnormal clinical laboratory findings, not elsewhere classified (R00-R99)
  See Guidelines: 1;C.20.a.1

ANXIETY, DISSOCIATIVE, STRESS-RELATED, SOMATOFORM AND OTHER NONPSYCHOTIC MENTAL DISORDERS (F40-F48)

See Guidelines: 1;C.5.a

3rd Character

Document: Type of mental disorder

F40-	Phobic anxiety disorders
F41-	Other anxiety disorders
F42-	Obsessive-compulsive disorder
F43-	Reaction to severe stress, and adjustment disorders
F44-	Dissociative and conversion disorders
F45-	Somatoform disorders
F48-	Other nonpsychotic mental disorders

4th Character

Document: Type of anxiety disorder

Excludes2:
  anxiety in:
  acute stress reaction (F43.0)
  transient adjustment reaction (F43.2)
  neurasthenia (F48.8)
  psychophysiologic disorders (F45.-)
  separation anxiety (F93.0)

Applies to: F41.-

0   Panic disorder [episodic paroxysmal anxiety]
    Including: Panic attack, Panic state
    Excludes1:
      panic disorder with agoraphobia (F40.01)
    Indicator(s): DSM-5 | Rx05: 135

1   Generalized
    Including: Anxiety neurosis, reaction, or state; Overanxious disorder
    Excludes2:
      neurasthenia (F48.8)
    Indicator(s): DSM-5 | Rx05: 135

3   Mixed

8   Other specified
    Including: Anxiety depression (mild or not persistent), Anxiety hysteria, Mixed anxiety and depressive disorder
    Indicator(s): DSM-5

9   Unspecified
    Including: Anxiety NOS
    Indicator(s): DSM-5

5th Character
N/A

6th Character
N/A

7th Character
N/A

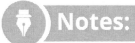

Appendix D. Telehealth Services

Telehealth, also known as telemedicine, has experienced rapid growth over the last few years, particularly in response to the COVID-19 public health emergency (PHE).

Resource: See Resource 641 for additional articles, webinars, and other information regarding telehealth services, including those related to COVID-19.

Explanation

According to the Health Resources and Services Administration (HRSA), telehealth is defined as "the use of electronic information and telecommunications technologies to support and promote long-distance clinical health care, patient and professional health-related education, and public health and health administration. Technologies include videoconferencing, the internet, store-and-forward imaging, streaming media, and landline and wireless communications. Telehealth services may be provided for example, through audio, text messaging, or video communication technology, including videoconferencing software."

It should be noted that different payers may refer to audiovisual communications, store-and-forward, online e-visits, messaging, and telephone communications using different terms (e.g., telehealth, telemedicine, telecommunications, virtual care). Different states may also have differing definitions, although many in the industry differentiate telemedicine as using technology to practice medicine over a distance, while telehealth encompasses all healthcare-related activities.

Note: For the purposes of this appendix, there is no distinction made between the terms telehealth and telemedicine.

Alert: There has been a recent increase in the number of telehealth services being audited. It is recommended the providers conduct their own internal audit on these services to ensure that all necessary requirements have been met and documented.
Resource: See Resource 63A for more information.

There are four basic types of telehealth services:

- **Live (synchronous) videoconferencing:** a two-way audiovisual link between a patient and a healthcare provider.
- **Store-and-forward (asynchronous) videoconferencing:** transmission of a recorded health history to a health practitioner, usually a specialist.
- **Remote patient monitoring (RPM):** the use of connected electronic tools to record personal health and medical data in one location for review by a provider in another location, usually at a different time.
- **Mobile health (mHealth):** healthcare and public health information provided through mobile devices. This can be general educational information, targeted texts, health apps with patient care reminders, or even notifications about disease outbreaks.

Note: Telephone calls may or may not be considered reimbursable telehealth services, depending on the payer. Please note that there are distinct CPT codes for telephone calls by a physician/QHP (99441-99443) or a non physician provider (98966-98968). Be aware that phone calls may be considered inclusive to an E/M service, depending on when the call takes place and if it leads to an E/M encounter.

Before offering telehealth services, healthcare providers need to carefully consider and have documented policies in place regarding all of the following issues:

- **Legal:** licensure, informed consent, malpractice insurance, privacy/confidentiality
- **Ethical:** competencies, documentation, marketing
- **Clinical:** information gathering, handling emergencies, establishing boundaries, provider telepresence
- **Technical:** technologies or platforms employed, cybersecurity, handling repairs
- **Billing:** insurance coverage and requirements, self pay, transmission fees, state and payer-specific requirements

Coding Requirements

There are only a few procedure codes specifically described as telehealth/telemedicine services (See "Other Codes to Consider"). For the most part, modifiers and/or the appropriate Place of Service (POS) code (see next segment) are used in conjunction with certain specified CPT and HCPCS procedure codes to indicate that the service was not provided in the typical location. The list of codes varies by payer so be aware of any differences.

For several years, Medicare has published a list of services which may be rendered via telehealth. The American Medical Association (AMA) also publishes a list of services which they categorize as appropriate to be rendered via telemedicine and used with a specific modifier. This appendix includes both of these lists.

Modifiers and Place of Service

Telehealth is most commonly rendered synchronously and reported with modifier 95. These services are identified in the CPT codebook and in Find-A-Code with a star "★" symbol.

In 2018, Medicare stopped requiring the use of the GT modifier and began to require the use of place of service (POS) 02, except with Critical Access Hospital (CAH) telehealth claims. Some private payers may still prefer the GT modifier over modifier 95, so be aware of individual payer policies. CMS requires asynchronous communication (where simultaneous audiovisual is NOT provided) to be reported with modifier GQ. See "Medicare-specific Requirements" below for additional information.

Note that Place of Service (POS) code 02 has been modified and a new POS code has been added for use when billing telehealth services. Effective January 1, 2022 and implemented April 4, 2022, the following changes are highlighted:

		Telehealth Place of Service Codes	
R	02	Telehealth Provided Other than in Patient's Home	The location where health services and health related services are provided or received, through telecommunication technology. Patient is not located in their home when receiving health services or health related services through telecommunication technology.
N	10	Telehealth Provided in Patient's Home	The location where health services and health related services are provided or received through telecommunication technology. Patient is located in their home (which is a location other than a hospital or other facility where the patient receives care in a private residence) when receiving health services or health related services through telecommunication technology.

Note: Medicare has stated that they will not use the new POS 10. Watch for announcements from other payers to see if they will require the use of this new POS code.

Note: Check individual payer policies for modifier(s) and POS code requirements when reporting telehealth services. During the PHE, payer requirements may be different than their usual policy.

Book: See Appendix B — Modifiers for more information about modifiers 95, FQ, GT, and GQ.

Medicare-Specific Requirements

Medicare requirements may vary from other payers. Under normal circumstances, they do not require the use of either modifier 95 or GT, except for Method II Critical Access Hospitals (CAHs) which need to use modifier GT with certain revenue (i.e., 942, 96X, 97X, 98X) or procedure codes (i.e., Q3014, G0420, G0421). For all other locations, use Place of Service 02 in Item Number 24B on the *1500 Claim Form*. Additionally, modifier GQ should be reported when telehealth services are performed using store-and-forward technology and the provider is certifying that they are at an approved distant site participating in a federal telemedicine demonstration project conducted in Alaska or Hawaii.

Claims for Medicare beneficiaries usually only require the use of Place of Service (POS) code 02 when billing telehealth services. However, during the COVID-19 PHE, at the time of publication, Medicare has instructed providers to use modifier 95 and to report the POS as the location where the services would have taken place under normal circumstances (e.g., office [11]).

Alert: As of January 1, 2022, CMS will require that modifier FQ be appended to the service code to identify that it was furnished via audio-only communication technology for behavioral health services. This change will allow them to more closely monitor utilization and address any potential concerns regarding overutilization.

At the time of publication, information about this new modifier was limited so watch for announcements by payers about it's use.

Resource: See Resource 656 for more information about this modifier.

Provider Types

A provider's board certification(s), taxonomy code(s), and payer-specific credentialing help identify the services which they can perform and be reimbursed for. The CPT's official coding guidelines also provide additional guidance (e.g., E/M services may only be performed by a physician or qualified healthcare professional [QHP]). Be aware of any payer policies which may have additional guidelines regarding performing telehealth services.

During the COVID-19 PHE, Medicare has expanded the types of providers allowed to perform telehealth services to include many additional eligible providers (e.g., physical therapists, speech language pathologists, occupational therapists.)

AMA Telemedicine List

The following is the list of codes that the CPT codebook designates as appropriate to be rendered via telemedicine and reported with modifier 95. They are identified in the CPT codebook and in Find-A-Code with a star "★" symbol.

90785	90791	90792	90832	90833	90834	90836	90837	90838	90839
90840	90845	90846	90847	90863	90951	90952	90954	90955	90957
90958	90960	90961	90963	92227	92228	93228	93229	93268	93270
93271	93272	96040	96116	96160	96161	97110	97112	97116	97161
97162	97165	97166	97530	97535	97750	97755	97760	97761	97802
97803	97804	98960	98961	98962	99202	99203	99204	99205	99212
99213	99214	99215	99231	99232	99233	99241	99242	99243	99244
99245	99251	99252	99253	99254	99255	99307	99308	99309	99310
99354	99355	99356	99357	99406	99407	99408	99409	99417	99495
99496	99497	99498							

Note: Many codes were added to this list for 2022 and the American Medical Association has proposed to add even more codes in 2023.

Digital Medicine Appendix Added

As digital medicine services have increased (e.g., telehealth, remote monitoring, e-visits), there has been some confusion about reporting these services. To address this issue, the 2022 CPT codebook includes a new appendix (i.e., Appendix R) which has a table dividing up the different types of provider services within the context of the CPT codeset. These broad categories are:

- Clinician-to-patient (e.g., visits)
- Clinician-to-clinician (e.g., consultation)
- Patient monitoring and/or therapeutic services
- Digital diagnostic services

It should be noted that information in Appendix R does not supersede government or commercial payer policies and that all guidelines in the codebook still apply and thus services may only be reported if within the scope of practice as allowed by states and individual payers.

Store: See a current CPT codebook or innoviHealth's *Comprehensive Guide to Evaluation & Management* (both are available in the online store) to review Appendix R: Digital Medicine - Services Taxonomy.

CMS Telehealth List

Codes that CMS covers when rendered via telehealth are identified in Find-A-Code with a blue "T" icon. Under normal circumstances, claims for professional telehealth services are reported with POS 02 and do not need a modifier unless the originating site is a federal telemedicine demonstration program in Alaska or Hawaii using asynchronous "store and forward" technology (modifier GQ) or a CAH-specific qualifying facility. See "Medicare-specific Requirements" on the previous page for more information.

Prior to the public health crisis (PHE), CMS limited access to telehealth services based on the location of the patient. CMS identified two locations that qualified beneficiaries to receive telehealth services:

- A county outside a Metropolitan Statistical Area (MSA) designated by the patient's zip code (based on the population of that county as established by the Census Bureau)
- Rural Health Professional Shortage Areas (HPSAs) in a rural census tract (established by the Health Resources and Services Administration [HRSA])

Other than a PHE, there is one notable exception to Medicare's geographic limitations. According to the SUPPORT for Patients and Communities Act, a patient's home may "serve as a telehealth originating site for purposes of treatment of a substance use disorder or a co-occurring mental health disorder, furnished on or after July 1, 2019, to an individual with a substance use disorder diagnosis." The 2022 Medicare Physician Fee Schedule expanded this exception to include the "diagnosis, evaluation, or treatment of a mental health disorder" along with the following requirements:

- An in-person, non-telehealth visit must take place at least once every 12 months
- Exceptions to the in-person visit requirement may be made based on beneficiary circumstances (with the reason documented in the patient's medical record)
- More frequent visits may be allowed as determined by clinical needs on a case-by-case basis

CMS designed a special MSA/HPSA tool that allows a beneficiary to enter their zip code to identify a nearby facility that could act as an originating site. The originating site is the location where a *patient initiates* a telehealth service with the provider.

Originating sites are defined by CMS as: the office of a physician or practitioner, a hospital, a Critical Access Hospital (CAH), a rural health clinic, a Federally Qualified Health Center (FQHC), a hospital or CAH-based renal dialysis center (including satellites), a Skilled Nursing Facility (SNF), or a Community Mental Health Center (CMHC).

The distant site is the location of the healthcare professional providing the service. During the PHE, geographic locations are no longer enforced and the Medicare beneficiary may receive telehealth even in the comfort of their own home. CMS has proposed to continue to expand telehealth coverage as indicated in the table that follows.

The use of a telecommunications system may substitute for a "face-to-face," "hands on" encounter for specified codes which may vary by payer. This simply means a synchronous telehealth encounter is a face-to-face encounter.

CMS currently has three different categories for telehealth services. There are also many Medicare-covered services that are furnished via a telecommunications technology (e.g., G2010, G2012) which are not included on the list that follows. These services are not included on Medicare's list of telehealth services because they are not typically provided in person and are thus telehealth by nature.

In the list that follows, be sure to review the key for additional information about the status of the code for that service. The following codes are on the 2022 CMS-approved telehealth appropriate services available at the time of publication:

77427^P	90785^A	90791^A	90792^A	90832^A	90833^A	90834^A	90836^A	90837^A	90838^A
90839^A	90840^A	90845^A	90846^A	90847^A	90853^A	90875^{N,4}	90951	90952	90953^3
90954	90955	90956^3	90957	90958	90959^3	90960	90961	90962^3	90963
90964	90965	90966	90967	90968	90969	90970	92002^4	92004^4	92012^4
92014^4	92507^{A,3}	92508^{4,A}	92521^{3,A}	92522^{3,A}	92523^{3,A}	92524^{3,A}	92526^7	92550^7	92552^7
92553^7	92555^7	92556^7	92557^7	92563^7	92565^7	92567^7	92568^7	92570^7	92587^7
92588^5	92601^4	92602^4	92603^4	92604^4	92607^7	92608^7	92609^7	92610^7	92625^7
92626^7	92627^7	93750^6	93797^3	93798^3	94002^4	94003^4	94004^4	94005^{4,B}	94664^4
95970^6	95971^6	95972^6	95983^6	95984^6	96105^7	96110^{4,N}	96112^4	96113^4	96116^A
96121^A	96125^7	96127^{4,A}	96130^{3,A}	96131^{3,A}	96132^{3,A}	96133^{3,A}	96136^{3,A}	96137^{3,A}	96138^{3,A}
96139^{3,A}	96156^A	96158^A	96159^A	96160^A	96161^A	96164^A	96165^A	96167^A	96168^A
96170^{4,N}	96171^{4,N}	97110^3	97112^3	97116^3	97129^7	97130^7	97150^4	97151^4	97152^4
97153^4	97154^4	97155^4	97156^4	97157^4	97158^4	97161^3	97162^3	97163^3	97164^3
97165^3	97166^3	97167^3	97168^3	97530^4	97535^{3,A}	97542^4	97750^3	97755^3	97760^3
97761^3	97802^A	97803^A	97804^A	99202	99203	99204	99205	99211	99212
99213	99214	99215	99217^3	99218^P	99219^P	99220^P	99221^P	99222^P	99223^P
99224^3	99225^3	99226^3	99231	99232	99233	99234^P	99235^P	99236^P	99238^3
99239^3	99281^3	99282^3	99283^3	99284^3	99285^3	99291^3	99292^3	99304^P	99305^P
99306^P	99307	99308	99309	99310	99315^3	99316^3	99324^4	99325^4	99326^4
99327^P	99328^P	99334	99335	99336^3	99337^3	99341^P	99342^P	99343^P	99344^P
99345^P	99347	99348	99349^3	99350^3	99354^A	99355^A	99356^A	99357^A	99406^A
99407^A	99441^{4,A}	99442^{4,A}	99443^{4,A}	99468^P	99469^3	99471^P	99472^3	99473^P	99475^P
99476^3	99477^P	99478^3	99479^3	99480^3	99483	99495	99496	99497^A	99498^A
0362T^4	0373T^4	G0108^A	G0109^A	G0270^A	G0296^A	G0396^A	G0397^A	G0406^A	G0407^A
G0408^A	G0410^{4,N}	G0420^A	G0421^A	G0422^3	G0423^3	G0424^3	G0425^A	G0426^A	G0427^A
G0438^A	G0439^A	G0442^A	G0443^A	G0444^A	G0445^A	G0446^A	G0447^A	G0459^A	G0506^A
G0508	G0509	G0513^A	G0514^A	G2086^A	G2087^A	G2088^A	G2211^{A,B}	G2212^A	G9685^4
S9152^{4,N}									

Key:

   3 = Code is a temporary addition available up through December 31, 2023

   4 = Code is a temporary addition only used during the COVID-19 Pandemic PHE as of April 30, 2020

   5 = Code is a temporary addition only used during the COVID-19 Pandemic PHE as of May 10, 2021

   6 = Code is a temporary addition only used during the COVID-19 Pandemic PHE as of October 14, 2020

   7 = Code is a temporary addition only used during the COVID-19 Pandemic PHE as of March 30, 2021

   A = Service may also be provided via audio only

   B = Bundled code

P = Code is a temporary addition only used during the COVID-19 Pandemic PHE

N = Code is not covered by Medicare, but might be billable to secondary or other payers

Notes:
- Although code G2211 shows on this list, it may not be billed to Medicare until 2024.
- CMS reserves the right to add additional services and covered provider types as needed during a PHE so this list could change.

Alert: As of January 1, 2022, two new modifiers have been added by CMS in relation to telehealth:
- FQ "The service was furnished using audio-only communication technology"
- FR "The supervising practitioner was present through two-way, audio/video communication technology"

Resource: See Resources 656 and 657 for more information.

During the PHE, CMS has expanded the list of services that may be provided via telehealth as well as exercising "enforcement discretion" and waiving penalties for HIPAA violations when the provider is acting in good faith when using "everyday communications technologies, such as FaceTime or Skype." Be aware that investigations can, and have occured, so we recommend that organizations take this time to establish appropriate policies and procedures and use ONLY HIPAA-approved technologies. It should be noted that these investigations are likely to become even more prevalent when the PHE is over.

Resource: See Resource 649 to review the information page for Medicare coverage and payment of virtual services.

Other Codes to Consider

The previously listed codes by CMS and the AMA are for services they have approved for being provided via telehealth. Commercial payers may have approved other services to be provided via telehealth. For example, one UnitedHealthcare policy also includes the following codes: G9481-G9489 and G9978-G9986. Be aware of additional payer code listings and requirements.

The following are some HCPCS codes that are described specifically as telehealth services. Payer coverage varies.

Follow-up inpatient consultation; communicating with the patient via telehealth;
- G0406   limited, physicians typically spend 15 minutes
- G0407   intermediate, physicians typically spend 25 minutes
- G0408   complex, physicians typically spend 35 minutes

Telehealth consultation, emergency department or initial inpatient; communicating with the patient via telehealth;
- G0425   typically 30 minutes
- G0426   typically 50 minutes
- G0427   typically 70 minutes or more

Telehealth consultation, critical care, communicating with the patient and providers via telehealth;
- G0508   initial, physicians typically spend 60 minutes
- G0509   subsequent, physicians typically spend 50 minutes

G0459   Inpatient telehealth pharmacologic management, including prescription, use, and review of medication with no more than minimal medical psychotherapy

Coding Tips

- **Face-to-Face Requirements:** For services normally requiring a face-to-face encounter, when the provider meets all the conditions of a payer's telehealth program, the face-to-face requirement is satisfied.

- **Documentation Requirements:** In addition to code-specific documentation requirements, some payers (e.g., Medicaid), require documenting start and stop times as well as the provider and patient site locations. The use of audio and/or video must also be documented. Failure to document these additional items can result in payer payment denials or refund demands.

- **Additional Charges:** Some additional charges that could be billed (where applicable) are codes Q3014 (Telehealth facility fee), G2025 (Distant site fee for RHCs and FQHCs), and T1014 (Telehealth transmission fee). Be aware of individual payer policies regarding the use of these codes.

  - **Facility fees:** Code Q3014 "Telehealth originating site facility fee" is reimbursed by Medicare. The originating site is where the patient is receiving the services – not where the provider is located. Code G2025 was added in July 2020 to be used when the telehealth distant site service is furnished by a Rural Health Clinic (RHC) or a Federally Qualified Health Center (FQHC). Neither of these codes should be reported when the originating site is the patient's home or when the provider and patient are in the same building.

  - **Transmission fees:** Some payers do not separately reimburse code T1014 "Telehealth transmission, per minute, professional services bill separately" because they consider it bundled (included) in the telehealth service.

- **Online medical evaluation (98969, 99444):** Some payers do not cover this because it is an internet response to a patient's online question with no direct, face-to-face patient contact.

- **Interprofessional Telephone/Internet Consultations (99446-99449):** Some payers may not cover these services because they are communications between healthcare providers without any direct, face-to-face patient contact.

- **State-Specific Requirements:** Some states have their own covered services so it is essential to be aware of state-applicable regulations. For example, according to Florida state regulations, codes H0001, H0031, H0046, H0047, H2000, H2010, and H2019 are covered under certain circumstances.

- **Crossing State Lines:** For most states, health care providers are not allowed to provide telehealth services over state lines unless they are licensed in both states. Other than exceptions related to the PHE, there are a few exceptions such as:

  - **Veterans Administration (VA):** VA providers may provide telehealth services across state lines and they are NOT required to be located, licensed, registered, or certified in the state of the patient. See Resource 123 for more information.

  - **Interstate Medical Licensure Compact:** This organization allows for qualifying providers to more easily obtain a medical license for all participating states. See Resource 52D for more information.

  - **Bordering State Laws:** There are some states which have specific laws allowing providers licensed in nearby states to practice in their state. During the COVID-19 PHE, several states waived previous limitations and allowed providers to treat patients over state lines in order to address provider shortages. Medicare also allowed healthcare providers to practice across state lines during that time.

  - **Temporary Exceptions:** Some states allow a short-term, temporary exception to crossing state lines. For example, many states have guest licensure provisions that allow (under certain conditions) an out-of-state-licensed psychologist to provide services for a short period of time — ranging from 10 to 30 days in a calendar year.

Notes:

Appendix E. Common Diagnosis Code Tips

The codes in this appendix are grouped alphabetically by conditions commonly encountered in a behavioral health setting. The correct way to select a code is to look up the main term from the documentation in the Alphabetic Index and then confirm it with the Tabular List. As such, this appendix is just a supplemental reference rather than a replacement to the official code list. Comments and suggestions on this section are welcome. Contact innoviHealth at support@innoviHealth.com.

Disclaimer: The information in this chapter contains general information and is the opinion of the authors. It should not be interpreted by providers/payers as official guidance. As such, this information should not be used for claim adjudication. Third party payers should utilize their own payment policies based on clinically sound guidelines.

Website: Go to FindACode.com to review and search the complete ICD-10-CM code list. You can also download the free Find-A-Code app from the Google Play Store or the Apple Store for your smartphone, iPad, or tablet.

Coding Tips Index

2022 — New Codes	471
Abuse, Neglect, or Maltreatment	473
Adjustment Disorders	476
Anxiety Disorders	477
Attention Deficit Hyperactivity Disorder (ADHD)	478
Autism Spectrum Disorder	479
Bipolar Disorder	480
Borderline Personality Disorder	482
Conduct Disorders	483
Depressive Disorders	484
Developmental Disorders	486
Dissociative Disorders	488
Eating Disorders	489
Factitious Disorder	490
Health Status and Other Contact	491
History "Z" Codes	492
Obsessive-Compulsive Disorder (OCD)	493
Post-COVID-19 Condition	494
Postpartum Depression and Psychosis	495
Post-Traumatic Stress Disorder (PTSD)	496
Rule Out Diagnosis	497
Schizoaffective Disorder	497
Schizophrenia	498
Social Determinants of Health (SDoH)	499
Substance Use Disorders	499

Coding Conventions & Instructions

Conventions

The following conventions are used in this appendix:

Type Styles

Official ICD-10-CM codes and descriptions are in a type style like this.

Explanations added by innoviHealth are in a type style like this. The exception is tables where all text, including codes, notations or explanations by innoviHealth, will be in **a type style like this**.

Tables with official instructions or quotes from payers will be in a table like this.

Revision Identifiers

5 **Signifies a code that is included in the DSM-5 publication by the American Psychiatric Association.** See the "DSM-5" segment that follows for more information. This symbol appears **only** in this chapter. In the Tabular List in the *ICD-10-CM Coding for Behavioral Health* book (available in the online store), they are identified by the DSM-5 indicator.

N Signifies a code added this year.

R Signifies a code revised this year. *

    * Bear in mind that revised codes may have had a change to their description, inclusion terms, and/or instructional notes.

Note — Update Your Codebook Annually: The official ICD-10-CM code set is updated annually with many codes being deleted and revised and new codes added. The guidelines are also often times amended or revised due to the code changes or due to committee and community discussions. As such, it is recommended that your organization keep an ICD-10-CM codebook for the current year.

Code Formatting

Codes found in this appendix that include all the necessary characters are in **bold type**, but those that need additional characters will end with a hyphen (-). To identify the missing characters, search out the codes in the Tabular List. Some of the codes end with an underscore (_). The underscore indicates that a seventh character is required. In most cases, for the codes included in this appendix, the seventh character will be one of the three following options, unless otherwise specified:

    A - initial encounter (use for "active treatment")

    D - subsequent encounter (use for "follow up" care)

    S - sequela (use for "late effects")

Example:

T14.91XA	Suicide attempt, initial encounter
T14.91XD	Suicide attempt, subsequent encounter
T14.91XS	Suicide attempt, sequela

Store: See the *ICD-10-CM Coding for Behavioral Health* book (available in the online store) to learn more about the proper application of these characters.

Alert: Some of these codes include "x" placeholders. Do not delete them if they are included here and do not add them to codes that do not have them listed. The letter "x" is used as a placeholder in certain codes to leave room for future expansion and preserve the format of ICD-10-CM codes (e.g., to ensure that seventh character extensions are indeed the seventh character). There can be more than one placeholder in a code. Officially, it is not case sensitive and thus may be either upper or lowercase; however, be aware of individual payer policies which may differ from this standard.

Instructions

The conditions in this appendix are grouped together by type and may include instructive segments such as, "Codes to Consider," "Coding Tips," etc. As stated in the disclaimer, these segments are general in nature.

Associated Conditions

These coding tips reference conditions which are also commonly associated with the listed condition. Where clinically indicated, be sure to document these conditions in addition to the listed condition.

Diagnostic Criteria

These coding tips reference conditions listed in the DSM manual. As stated previously in the "DSM-5" segment, they are helpful for assessing the patient symptoms to arrive at a diagnostic assessment which is then used to determine the appropriate ICD-10-CM code. Be aware that both code changes and diagnostic changes may not be included in your edition of the DSM-5 book due to updates to the ICD-10-CM code set and criteria updates by the APA.

Tip: Many organizations have recommended using the Clinical Descriptions and Diagnostic Guidelines (sometimes known as the "blue book") which is published by the World Health Organization. See Resource 511 for more information.
FindACode.com subscribers have access to these guidelines at the code level.

DSM-5

The Diagnostic and Statistical Manual (DSM-5) is published by the American Psychiatric Association (APA). Technically, DSM is not an official HIPAA code set, rather, ICD-10-CM is the official HIPAA approved diagnostic code set for billing purposes. The American Psychiatric Association states (emphasis added) that "DSM-5 and the ICD should be thought of as *companion publications.*" Therefore, consider DSM as the criteria which may be utilized for ICD-10-CM code selection. Although a DSM book lists an associated ICD-10-CM code with their criteria, be aware that ICD-10-CM codes change more frequently than DSM book releases. It is up to the provider to ensure that current HIPAA-approved codes are selected for claims submission.

Codes in this chapter, which are also listed in the DSM-5 book and the APA's official DSM-5 update supplement, have been flagged with "⑤" in order to quickly identify them. Remember that payer policies may vary from what is included in DSM-5 so it is important to be aware of these differences. See the segment "ICD-10/DSM Differences" that follows for more information.

Updates to the DSM-5 publication are not made on a regular update schedule. However, any recent updates related to the codes in this chapter are included, where applicable. For example, *Figure E.1* identifies some of the changes listed in the official DSM-5 update dated September 2016 which were not included in this chapter. Please note that there were also changes made to the diagnostic criteria which are not included here for copyright reasons. To review diagnostic criteria changes, see the most recent official update available from the American Psychiatric Association.

Figure E.1

Other Notable DSM Changes		
Disorder	**Change From**	**Change To**
Hypersomnolence disorder	G47.10	F51.11
Insomnia disorder	G47.00	F51.01
Kleptomania	F63.3	F63.2
Language disorder	F80.9	F80.2
Major neurocognitive disorder due to medical condition *Note: code first medical condition (i.e., **G30.9**, **G31.09**, **G31.83**, **G20**)	G31.9	F02.81 F02.80
Trichotillomania (Hair-pulling disorder)	F63.2	F63.3

Book: For easy reference, codes listed in the current DSM-5 publication are noted.

Excludes1

These are the codes which, according to ICD-10-CM, may NOT be coded along with the listed condition. See the *ICD-10-CM Official Guidelines for Coding and Reporting* for additional information.

Note: The *ICD-10-CM Official Guidelines for Coding and Reporting* are not included in this publication. They can be found in the *ICD-10-CM Coding for Behavioral Health* book (available in the online store) or online with a FindACode.com subscription.

ICD-10/DSM Differences

There are many cases where there are coding differences between ICD-10-CM and codes associated with DSM diagnostic criteria. These are noted in the "ICD-10/DSM Differences" segment of the condition. Be aware of individual third-party payer policies regarding these differences and follow the guidelines as outlined by the payer when submitting claims.

Documentation of the patient encounter should include both the diagnostic criteria met as well as the most appropriate ICD-10-CM code along with an explanation of why that code was selected.

> *Example:*
>
> ICD-10/DSM Differences: Catatonia is not classified as a separate disorder under DSM-5. Instead, it is associated with several disorders including schizophrenia, bipolar disorder, autism spectrum disorder, and depression. However, within ICD-10-CM, there are a few codes which include this description. For example: **F06.1** "Catatonic disorder due to known physiologic condition," **F20.2** "Catatonic schizophrenia," and **R40.1** "Catatonic stupor."

Unspecified Codes

There may be situations where an unspecified code is the only appropriate code choice. These codes should be reported when they most accurately reflect what is known about the patient's condition at the time of that specific patient encounter. It would be inappropriate to select a specific code not supported by the medical record or to conduct medically unnecessary diagnostic testing in order to determine a more specific code.

There are three scenarios where reporting an unspecified code is the incorrect approach:

1. The code set is not specific enough. If a diagnosis is confirmed, but ICD-10-CM does not have a specific code that matches the diagnosis, the NEC code should be used, not the unspecified.
2. The provider's documentation does not provide enough detail to select a more specific code. If this is the case, consult the healthcare provider for additional information about the encounter. Ensure that the providers in your organization are familiar with the guidelines and code options needed for complete and accurate documentation. See Appendix C — Provider Documentation Guides.
3. The diagnosis is unconfirmed. If terms such as "rule out," "probable," "suspected," etc. are used, the guidelines pertaining to uncertain diagnoses must be adhered to. It is not as simple as reporting the unspecified code option.

Store: See the *ICD-10-CM Coding for Behavioral Health* book (available in the online store) to learn more about reporting an uncertain diagnosis as well as other important coding guidelines.

Tips

The conditions listed in this segment are those commonly used in a behavioral health setting. They are listed in alphabetical order for easy reference. The codes included in these tips may not be to the highest level of specificity.

Alert: Never code directly from this Tips segment. It is only the first step to finding a probable code. It may be necessary to refer to an official Tabular List for additional required digits and other pertinent coding information such as Notes and Excludes.

Book: See Chapter 5.2 — Common Procedure Codes & Tips for more information about reporting treatment of these conditions.

2022 — New Codes

Effective October 1, 2021, there are some new codes added which could be of interest to a behavioral health practice.

Cannabis

Subcategory T40.7X- was expanded and the placeholder "X" has been removed. Cannabis and synthetic cannabinoids are now reported separately as shown in the following tables:

	Accident*	Assault	Intentional*	Undeterm*
Poisoning by;				
cannabis;	T40.711_	T40.713_	T40.712_	T40.714_
synthetic cannabinoids;	T40.721_	T40.723_	T40.722_	T40.724_

Note: * Accident = accidental (unintentional) / * Intent = intentional self-harm / * Undeterm = undetermined

	Cannabis	Synthetic*
Adverse effect	T40.715_	T40.725_
Underdosing	T40.716_	T40.726_

Note: * Synthetic = synthetic cannabinoids

As with all codes in category T50-, the applicable 7th character should be added to report the type of encounter:

- A - initial encounter
- D - subsequent encounter
- S - sequela

This category includes several instructional notes (i.e., Includes, Code first, Notes, Use additional code(s), Excludes1, Excludes2). Be sure to review and follow this important information when reporting these codes.

Resource: See Resource 543 for more information about codes in this section, including rules and definitions found in the *Official ICD-10-CM Guidelines for Coding and Reporting*.

Website: FindACode.com subscribers can easily view instructional notations at the code level. To see the applicable official guidelines click on the [ICD-10 Official Documentation Guidelines] bar beneath the code.

Depression, Unspecified

Revisions have been made to category F32 and a new code added to describe a situation where the patient is experiencing feelings of depression, but does not meet the criteria for a major depressive disorder. See "Depressive Disorders" on page 484 for more information.

Intellectual Disabilities; Other Genetic Related

Sub-category F78.A- "Other genetic related intellectual disabilities" was added to include the ability to report the linking of an intellectual disability to genetics. See "Developmental Disorders" on page 486 for more information.

Personal History

Several codes were added to report when the patient has a personal history of a condition or action. .See "History "Z" Codes" on page 492 for more information.

Post-COVID-19 Condition

While many practices won't need to use the confirmed COVID-19 code (**U07.1**), there were new rules for COVID-19 which became effective in April 2020. See Resource 52G for more comprehensive information on those rule changes. The rules have changed again due to a new code for reporting conditions related to COVID-19. See also "Post-COVID-19 Condition" on page 494.

Self-Harm

Some interesting changes took place in relation to the reporting of self-harm to address the "intent" of the action by separating suicidal behavior from other actions which are included in sub-category R45.85- "Homicidal and suicidal ideations." Two new personal history codes were also added (see "History "Z" Codes" on page 492 for more information) and the following code was added to sub-category R45.8- "Other symptoms and signs involving emotional state":

 R45.88 Nonsuicidal self-harm

  Nonsuicidal self-injury

  Nonsuicidal self-mutilation

  Self-inflicted injury without suicidal intent

  Code also injury, if known

Social Determinants of Health

Social Determinants of Health are beginning to play a more important role in health care. See page 499 for more information about the new codes that were added.

Abuse, Neglect, or Maltreatment

Explanation

Properly coding abuse, neglect, or maltreatment requires differentiating between confirmed and suspected cases. Alleged and suspected are terms used to describe conditions that have not yet been substantiated or proven, while confirmed is a term that indicates there is evidence that proves (confirms) the allegation to be true. For abuse, it is also necessary to document the type (i.e., physical, sexual, psychological). Some healthcare providers have expressed concern about the legal implications of reporting these codes even when required by either state or federal law. There are statutes for reporting domestic violence, which vary from state to state. Typically it is required for documentation to include the type of violence, the source (e.g., police report, legal entity) and the relationship of the abuser to the patient. Misreporting a "suspected" versus a "confirmed" case can have severe ramifications such as the victim and family losing coverage or being denied coverage for certain types of insurance. Therefore, it is important that your healthcare organization's active compliance program has a clear process in place for reporting abuse, neglect, or maltreatment.

It is likely that your organization already has policies outlining documentation criteria for these types of cases. Policies should include guidelines on confirmed versus suspected as well as what constitutes maltreatment since that is defined at the state level within civil and criminal statutes.

Federal law provides the following definition of child abuse and neglect:

- Any recent act or failure to act on the part of a parent or caretaker which results in death, serious physical or emotional harm, sexual abuse or exploitation; or
- An act or failure to act which presents an imminent risk of serious harm.

- The Federal Child Abuse Prevention and Treatment Act (CAPTA) (42 U.S.C.A. § 5106g)

Codes to Consider

Abuse, Neglect, Maltreatment Coding Table

	confirmed	suspected	Personal history of (in childhood)
Maltreatment	adult T74.91x_ child T74.92x_	adult T76.01x_ child T76.02x_	
Neglect or abandonment	adult T74.01x_ child T74.02x_	adult T74.01x_ child T74.02x_	Z62.812
Physical abuse	adult T74.11x_ child T74.12x_	adult T74.11x_ child T74.12x_	Z62.810
Psychological abuse	adult T74.31x_ child T74.32x_	adult T74.31x_ child T74.32x_	Z62.811
Sexual abuse	adult T74.21x_ child T74.22x_	adult T74.21x_ child T74.22x_	Z62.810
Encounter for mental health services for;		victim	perpetrator
child abuse (parental)		Z69.010	Z69.011
child abuse (non-parental)		Z69.020	Z69.021
spousal or partner abuse		Z69.11	Z69.12
other (e.g., rape victim)		Z69.81	Z69.82

Book: See Resource 528 for more information about domestic violence, including state-specific requirements.

Book: See the segment "Health Status and Other Contact" on page 491 for other external cause codes not related to abuse, neglect, or maltreatment.

Alert: Official ICD-10-CM Guidelines direct the coder to report a confirmed code when the record simply states "abuse" or "neglect." Therefore, it is important that providers are educated on this guideline so they are aware of this rule and its potential ramifications.

Note: Although not included on the table above, there are codes for confirmed and suspected exploitation: sexual (T74.5-, T76.5-) and labor (T74.6-, T76.6-).

Coding Tips

<u>Diagnostic Criteria</u>: Codes with the ⑤ flag are listed in DSM-5. See DSM-5 diagnostic criteria for additional information on coding these conditions.

<u>ICD-10/DSM Differences</u>: The DSM-5 book does not separate maltreatment into its own category with associated codes so be aware of individual payer and/or state-specific requirements.

<u>Sequencing</u>: There is a sequencing rule, specific to External Cause codes, which states that abuse codes should be reported before *all other external cause* codes (see the official explanation that follows for more information). Use the following sequence for abuse, neglect, or maltreatment:

1. An appropriate code from category T74- (confirmed) or T76- (suspected)
2. Any accompanying mental health or injury code(s) related to the abuse
3. An external cause code, where applicable, (X92-Y09) to identify the cause of any physical injuries
4. A perpetrator code (Y07-) for confirmed cases, if the perpetrator is known

> Sequence first the appropriate code from categories T74, Adult and child abuse, neglect and other maltreatment, confirmed) or T76, Adult and child abuse, neglect and other maltreatment, suspected) for abuse, neglect and other maltreatment, followed by any accompanying mental health or injury code(s).
>
> If the documentation in the medical record states abuse or neglect it is coded as confirmed (T74-). It is coded as suspected if it is documented as suspected (T76-).
>
> For cases of confirmed abuse or neglect an external cause code from the assault section (X92-Y09) should be added to identify the cause of any physical injuries. A perpetrator code (Y07) should be added when the perpetrator of the abuse is known. For suspected cases of abuse or neglect, do not report external cause or perpetrator code.
>
> If a suspected case of abuse, neglect or mistreatment is ruled out during an encounter code Z04.71, Encounter for examination and observation following alleged physical adult abuse, ruled out, or code Z04.72, Encounter for examination and observation following alleged child physical abuse, ruled out, should be used, not a code from T76.
>
> If a suspected case of alleged rape or sexual abuse is ruled out during an encounter code Z04.41, Encounter for examination and observation following alleged adult rape or code Z04.42, Encounter for examination and observation following alleged child rape, should be used, not a code from T76.
>
> If a suspected case of forced sexual exploitation or forced labor exploitation is ruled out during an encounter, code Z04.81, Encounter for examination and observation of victim following forced sexual exploitation, or code Z04.82, Encounter for examination and observation of victim following forced labor exploitation, should be used, not a code from T76.
>
> – *ICD-10-CM Official Guidelines for Coding and Reporting Section I.C.19.f*

Updates: Several changes have been made to these codes over the last few years. Be aware of the following:

- Effective October 1, 2018:
  - A new code was added for Factitious disorder to differentiate between self-imposed and imposed by someone else (e.g., caregiver). See Factitious Disorder on page 490 for more information.
  - New guidelines were added to the *ICD-10-CM Official Guidelines for Coding and Reporting* regarding forced sexual exploitation. See the last paragraph of the official guidelines listed previously.
  - Screening encounters are becoming more common and new codes were added to describe these services. Be sure to use the appropriate Z13- code for screenings.
  - Although not included in the Codes to Consider table, there were new codes for confirmed and suspected exploitation: sexual (T74.5-, T76.5-) and labor (T74.6-, T76.6-).
- Effective October 1, 2017, a substantial number of inclusion terms (e.g., neglect, psychological abuse, physical abuse, sexual abuse) were added to codes in category Z69-. See the *ICD-10-CM Coding for Behavioral Health* publication or FindACode.com to review these codes.

Adjustment Disorders

Explanation

Adjustment disorders are maladaptive reactions to identifiable psychosocial stressor(s) (e.g., loss of job or loved one) occurring within a short time (up to 3 months) after onset of the stressor(s). They are manifested by either impairment in social or occupational functioning or by symptoms (depression, anxiety, etc.) that are above and beyond a normal and/or expected reaction to the stressor(s) or triggering event(s). Specify the type of symptom(s) manifested (e.g., anxiety, conduct disturbance).

Codes to Consider	
Adjustment disorder with;	
anxiety	⑤ F43.20
conduct disturbance	⑤ F43.24
depressed mood	⑤ F43.21
mixed anxiety and depressed mood	⑤ F43.23
mixed disturbance of emotions and conduct	⑤ F43.25
other symptoms	F43.29
Adjustment disorder, unspecified	⑤ F43.20

Coding Tips

Diagnostic Criteria: Codes with the ⑤ flag are listed in DSM-5. See DSM-5 diagnostic criteria for additional information on coding these conditions. The September 2016 DSM-5 update noted that the condition should be specified as either acute or chronic (persistent).

ICD-10/DSM Differences: nothing significant to note

Associated Conditions: Adjustment disorders can accompany most other mental disorders and/or medical conditions. When DSM-5 diagnostic criteria for more than one mental disorder are met, it is appropriate to code both conditions.

Excludes1: None

Other:

- As indicated by the Excludes2 note, **F93.0** "Separation anxiety disorder of childhood" may also be reported, where applicable.

- According to DSM-5 diagnostic criteria, Adjustment disorders are noted immediately following a stressful event, whereas posttraumatic stress disorder (PTSD) is not diagnosed until at least one month has passed since the stressor(s) occured. Be aware of timelines and other diagnositic criteria before reporting diagnosis code(s).

- When depression symptoms meet the diagnostic criteria of major depressive disorder (MDD), do not code this condition. See "Depressive Disorders" on page 484.

- If symptoms persist longer than 6 months after the stressor is no longer present, another diagnosis should be considered.

- For sleep disturbances related to this condition, ICD-10-CM includes code **F51.02** "Adjustment insomnia" and **Z72.820** "Lack of adequate sleep" which could be reported, as applicable. Neither of these codes are included in the DSM publication.

Anxiety Disorders

Explanation

Anxiety includes feelings of uncontrollable nervousness, fear, apprehension, and worry ranging from mildly unsettling to severe debilitation. Those suffering from anxiety disorders tend to avoid situations that trigger or worsen their symptoms. This in turn impacts job performance, school work, and personal relationships.

In general, for a person to be diagnosed with an anxiety disorder, the fear or anxiety must:

- Be out of proportion to the situation or age inappropriate
- Last six months or longer
- Negatively impact normal functioning.

Codes to Consider	
Acute stress disorder	F43.0
Anxiety disorder due to:	
another medical condition	F06.4
known physiological condition	F06.4
Generalized anxiety disorder (GAD)	F41.1
Obsessive-compulsive disorder (OCD) (See "Obsessive-Compulsive Disorder" segment)	
Other specified anxiety disorders	F41.8
Panic disorder	F41.0
Phobias	F40-
Post-traumatic stress disorder (PTSD)	F43.10
Social anxiety disorder (SAD)	F40.10
Separation anxiety disorder	F93.0

Coding Tips

Diagnostic Criteria: Codes with the ⑤ flag are listed in DSM-5. See DSM-5 diagnostic criteria for additional information on coding these conditions.

ICD-10/DSM Differences: ICD-10-CM includes additional designations to consider such as:

- Agoraphobia: Agoraphobia has only one DSM code option (**F40.00**), but ICD-10-CM also includes Agoraphobia with panic disorder (**F40.01**) or without panic disorder (**F40.02**).
- Other phobias such as Claustrophobia (**F40.240**) and Arachnophobia (**F40.210**). See F40- in the Tabular List in the *ICD-10-CM Coding for Behavioral Health* book (available in the online store) for additional options.

Associated Conditions:

- Anxiety disorders often manifest with substance use and abuse. See the segment on "Substance Use Disorders" for more information on coding these conditions.
- For the F41- codes: acute stress reaction (**F43.0**), transient adjustment reaction (F43.2-), neurasthenia (**F48.8**), psychophysiologic/somatoform disorders (F45-), separation anxiety (**F93.0**)

Excludes1: For code **F41.0**: Panic disorder with agoraphobia (**F40.01**)

Other: Specific phobias all need to have 6 characters to be billable. In other words, 6 characters are needed to meet highest level of specificity requirements.

Attention Deficit Hyperactivity Disorder (ADHD)

Explanation

Attention deficit hyperactivity disorder (ADHD) is a behavioral disorder which typically begins in early childhood (typically 2-5 years of age) and tends to diminish during late adolescence although it can continue into adulthood. It is characterized by distractibility, impulsivity, hyperactivity, inattention and often trouble organizing tasks and projects, difficulty going to sleep, and social problems caused by being aggressive, loud, or impatient. ADHD lasts more than 6 months and causes problems in school, at home and in social situations. The National Institute of Mental Health (NIMH) describes this disorder the following way:

> Attention-deficit/hyperactivity disorder (ADHD) is a brain disorder marked by an ongoing pattern of inattention and/or hyperactivity-impulsivity that interferes with functioning or development.
>
> Inattention means a person wanders off task, lacks persistence, has difficulty sustaining focus, and is disorganized; and these problems are not due to defiance or lack of comprehension.
>
> Hyperactivity means a person seems to move about constantly, including situations when it is not appropriate, excessively fidgets, taps, or talks. In adults, it may be extreme restlessness or wearing others out with their activity.
>
> Impulsivity means a person makes hasty actions that occur in the moment without first thinking about them and that may have high potential for harm; or a desire for immediate rewards or inability to delay gratification. An impulsive person may be socially intrusive and excessively interrupt others or make important decisions without considering the long-term consequences.

Codes to Consider

ADHD;	
combined type	F90.2
hyperactive type	F90.1
inattentive type	F90.0
other type	F90.8
unspecified type	F90.9

Coding Tips

Diagnostic Criteria: Codes **F90.0-F90.9** are all listed in DSM-5. See DSM-5 diagnostic criteria for additional information on coding these conditions.

ICD-10/DSM Differences: nothing significant to note

Associated Conditions: anxiety disorders (F40-, F41-), mood [affective] disorders (F30-F39), pervasive developmental disorders (F84-), schizophrenia (F20-), learning disabilities, oppositional defiant disorder (**F91.3**), depression (see "Depressive Disorders"), social anxiety (**F40.10**), substance abuse (see "Substance Use Disorders"), bipolar disorder (F31-)

Excludes1: None

Other: According to the APA, "ADHD symptoms must not occur exclusively during the course of schizophrenia or another psychotic disorder and must not be better explained by another mental disorder, such as a depressive or bipolar disorder, anxiety disorder, dissociative disorder, personality disorder, or substance intoxication or withdrawal."

Coverage: Payers typically cover the following services:

- Behavior modification services
- Pharmacological treatment

Autism Spectrum Disorder

Explanation

Autism spectrum disorder (ASD) is a neurological and developmental disorder that begins early in childhood and lasts throughout a person's life. It affects how a person acts and interacts with others, communicates, and learns. According to DSM-5, it includes what used to be known as Asperger syndrome and pervasive developmental disorders.

It is called a "spectrum" disorder because people with ASD can have a range of symptoms. People with ASD might have problems talking with you, or they might not look you in the eye when you talk to them. They may also have restricted interests and repetitive behaviors. They may spend a lot of time putting things in order, or they may say the same sentence again and again. They may often seem to be in their "own world."

Diagnosis is made through various tests and evaluations. The causes of ASD are currently not known. Research suggests that both genes and environment play important roles.

Treatment typically includes behavior and communication therapies, skills training, and/or medication.

Note: Be sure to review the "Coding Tips" segment since there are coding differences to consider.

Codes to Consider	
Asperger's syndrome	F84.5
Autistic disorder	⑤ F84.0
Other childhood disintegrative disorder	F84.3
Other pervasive developmental disorders	F84.8
Rett's syndrome	F84.2
Unspecified pervasive developmental disorder	F84.9

Coding Tips

Diagnostic Criteria: Only **F84.0** is listed in DSM-5. See DSM-5 diagnostic criteria for additional information on coding this condition.

ICD-10/DSM Differences: The DSM-5 publication states that Autism Spectrum Disorder includes autistic disorder, Asperger's syndrome, or Pervasive developmental disorder not otherwise specified. However, ICD-10-CM guidelines exclude Asperger's syndrome (**F84.5**) from Autistic disorder (**F84.0**) and from some other codes as listed above. Due to these differences, be aware of individual payer policies and coding guidelines. Also of note, in 2017, ICD-10-CM added the description "Autism Spectrum Disorder" to code **F84.0**.

Associated Conditions: As of October 1, 2021, the "Use additional code to identify any associated medical condition and intellectual disabilities" was changed to "Code also any associated medical condition and intellectual disabilities."

Other: Consider evaluation for social (pragmatic) communication disorder (**F80.82**) for patients with marked deficits in social communication, but do not otherwise meet criteria for autism spectrum disorder.

Bipolar Disorder

Explanation

Bipolar Disorder is characterized by severe and unusual mood changes consisting of alternating manic (very happy and active) and depressive episodes separated by periods of normal mood. It is necessary to evaluate the changes in activity and energy, not just mood. The depressive mood may be accompanied by loss of energy and libido. The manic mood and grandiosity may be accompanied by overactivity, decreased attention span, irritability, or pressured speech (speaking rapidly and in a disorganized manner which is difficult to understand or follow). The patient may alternate rapidly between depressive symptoms and symptoms of mania, from day to day or from hour to hour.

Notes:
- Manic episodes begin abruptly and last 2 weeks to 4 or 5 months (4 months is typical)
- Depressions last, on average, 6 months.
- Use the mixed state code when manic episodes include depressive symptoms and for depression that includes mania or hypomania.
- Hypomania involves mild-to-moderate mood elevation, often with optimism rather than grandiosity, slight pressure of speech, increased activity level, and decreased need for sleep.
- ICD-10-CM added "Manic depression" as an inclusion term to code **F31.9** effective October 1, 2017.

Book: For other types of depressive disorders, see the "Depressive Disorders" segment on page 484.

Bipolar Disorders Coding Table

Current or most recent episode	Depressed	Hypomanic	Manic	Manic w/o psychotic features	Mixed	Unspec
Mild	F31.31			F31.11	F31.61	
Moderate	F31.32			F31.12	F31.62	
Severe				F31.13		
Severe w/o psychotic features	F31.4				F31.63	
Severe w/ psychotic features	F31.5		F31.2		F31.64	
Partial remission	F31.75	F31.71	F31.73		F31.77	
Full remission	F31.76	F31.72	F31.74		F31.78	F31.70
Unspecified	F31.30			F31.10	F31.60	F31.9
N/A		F31.0				

Other codes:
- F31.81 Bipolar II
- F31.89 Other bipolar disorder

Coding Tips

Diagnostic Criteria: Codes with the 5 flag in the "Bipolar Disorders Coding Table" are listed in DSM-5. See DSM-5 diagnostic criteria for additional information on coding these conditions.

ICD-10/DSM Differences:
- Effective August 2015, there were a few code reference changes in the DSM-5 update:
  - Bipolar I, hypomanic, in partial remission was changed from **F31.73** to **F31.71**
  - Bipolar I, hypomanic, in full remission was changed from **F31.74** to **F31.72**
- Effective October 1, 2017, ICD-10-CM added the following inclusion terms to category F31-: Bipolar I disorder and Bipolar type I disorder.

Associated Conditions: cyclothymia (**F34.0**)

Excludes1: bipolar disorder, single manic episode (F30-), major depressive disorder, single episode (F32-), major depressive disorder, recurrent (F33-)

Other:
- When there are only repeated episodes of mania without depression, it is still appropriate to code this condition as bipolar.
- A diagnosis of mixed bipolar affective disorder should be made only if the two sets of symptoms are both prominent for the greater part of the current episode of illness, and if that episode has lasted for at least two weeks.
- Single manic episodes (**F30.0-F30.9**) are not included in this segment.
- Major Depressive Disorders are not included here (see "Depressive Disorders" on page 484).

Borderline Personality Disorder

Explanation

A personality disorder characterized by difficulty regulating emotions which is evidenced by mood instability, poor self-image or sense of self, and flawed interpersonal relationships. Symptoms include:

- impulsive and self-damaging acts
- uncontrolled anger
- fears of abandonment
- chronic feelings of emptiness
- recurrent self-mutilating behavior and/or suicide threats
- short-term stress-induced periods of paranoia and/or dissociation.

Treatment typically includes therapy and/or medication. However, hospitalization may be necessary where safety is a concern during periods of extreme stress, impulsive behaviors, or suicidal behaviors.

Codes to Consider		
Borderline personality disorder	5	F60.3

Coding Tips

Diagnostic Criteria: **F60.3** is listed in DSM-5. See DSM-5 diagnostic criteria for additional information on coding this condition.

ICD-10/DSM Differences: nothing significant to note

Associated Conditions:

- Antisocial personality disorder (**F60.2**), Homicidal ideations (**R45.850**), Suicidal ideations (**R45.851**)
- Addictive behaviors: e.g., overeating (see "Eating Disorders"), gambling (**F63.0**, **Z72.6**), spending sprees, shoplifting, promiscuous sexual behavior
- See also the following segments: "Anxiety Disorder," "Bipolar Disorder," "Depressive Disorders," "Eating Disorders," "Post-Traumatic Stress Disorder (PTSD)," "Substance Use Disorders"

Excludes1: None

Conduct Disorders

Explanation

According to DSM, these conditions are unique in that the manifested behaviors violate the rights of others (e.g., aggression, destruction of property) and/or bring the individual into significant conflict with societal norms or authority figures. At least 3 symptoms must be present in the past 12 months with one symptom having been present in the past 6 months. To be diagnosed with conduct disorder, the symptoms must cause significant impairment in social, academic, or occupational functioning.

Codes to Consider	
Conduct disorder;	
confined to family context	F91.0
childhood-onset type	F91.1
adolescent-onset type	F91.2
other	F91.8
unspecified	F91.9
Oppositional defiant disorder	F91.3

Coding Tips

Diagnostic Criteria: All codes except **F91.0** are listed in DSM-5. See DSM-5 diagnostic criteria for additional information on coding these conditions.

ICD-10/DSM Differences: In 2017, ICD-10-CM added the following inclusion terms to **F91.8**:

- Other specified conduct disorder, and
- Other specified disruptive disorder.

Associated Conditions: conduct problems associated with attention-deficit hyperactivity disorder (F90-), mood [affective] disorders (F30-F39), pervasive developmental disorders (F84-), schizophrenia (F20-)

Excludes1: antisocial behavior (Z72.81-), antisocial personality disorder (**F60.2**)

Depressive Disorders

Explanation

According to the APA:

> Depressive disorders include disruptive mood dysregulation disorder, major depressive disorder (including major depressive episode), persistent depressive disorder (dysthymia), premenstrual dysphoric disorder, substance/medication-induced depressive disorder, depressive disorder due to another medical condition, other specified depressive disorder, and unspecified depressive disorder. The common feature of all of these disorders is the presence of sad, empty, or irritable mood, accompanied by somatic and cognitive changes that significantly affect the individual's capacity to function. What differs among them are issues of duration, timing, or presumed etiology.

Patients with a depressive disorder often benefit from seeing a psychiatrist, psychologist, or other mental health counselor. If medication is needed, the person must see a psychiatrist or other healthcare professional with prescribing privileges.

Store: Not all depressive and mood disorders are included in this common codes chapter. See the *ICD-10-CM Coding for Behavioral Health* book for the Alphabetic Index and Tabular List (generally F30 through F39). For a complete listing of the entire code set, see the *ICD-10-CM Comprehensive CodeBook*. Both are available in the online store.

Alert: As of October 1, 2021, use new code **F32.A** to report "Depression, unspecified." This new code makes a specific distinction between major depressive disorder (MDD) and a patient who is experiencing feelings of depression, but does not meet the criteria for another, more specific type of depression (e.g., postpartum, MDD).

Codes to Consider	
Depression, unspecified	N F32.A
Depressive disorder	
due to another medical condition	(multiple coding options)
due to substance or medication	(multiple coding options)
Disruptive mood dysregulation disorder	5 F34.81
Major depressive disorder (see the "Major Depressive Disorder (MDD) Coding Table")	F32.0 - F33.9
Persistent depressive disorder (dysthymia)	5 F34.1
Postpartum depression	F53.0
Premenstrual dysphoric disorder	5 F32.81

Major Depressive Disorder (MDD) Coding Table		
	Single Episode	Recurrent*
Mild	F32.0	F33.0
Moderate	F32.1	F33.1
Severe w/o psychotic features	F32.2	F33.2
Severe w/psychotic features	F32.3	F33.3
Partial remission	F32.4	F33.41
Full remission	F32.5	F33.42
Remission, unspecified	No Code	F33.40
Unspecified	F32.9	F33.9
*To be considered recurrent, there must be at least 2 consecutive months between episodes.		

Coding Tips

<u>Diagnostic Criteria</u>: Codes with the ⑤ flag are listed in DSM-5. See DSM-5 diagnostic criteria for additional information on coding these conditions.

<u>ICD-10/DSM Differences</u>:

- Effective October 1, 2021, code **F32.A** was added to ICD-10-CM. At the time of publication, an official update has not been released by the APA about whether or not this code will be part of the DSM-5 publication. As such, code **F32.A** does not have the DSM-5 icon in the "Codes to Consider" table. However, since the APA expressed support for this new code, it is likely that this code may eventually be added to their publication.

- Effective October 1, 2018, a new code (**F53.0**) was added for postpartum depression. The DSM-5 book only includes a specifier for postpartum (peripartum) depression and no distinct code. At the time of publication, no updates had been released by the APA regarding this new code, so be aware of payer requirements regarding its use. See also "Postpartum Depression and Psychosis" on page 495 for more information.

<u>Associated Conditions</u>: adjustment disorder (F43.2-), separation anxiety disorder of childhood (**F93.0**)

- **Disruptive Mood Regulation Disorder**: Symptoms of disruptive mood dysregulation disorder are common to other disorders such as bipolar disorder, oppositional defiant disorder, and conduct disorder. The disorder often co-occurs with depression, anxiety, or attention deficit hyperactivity disorder.

- **Depressive Disorder Due to Another Medical Condition**: When coding conditions due to a medical condition, two codes are required: one to identify the underlying condition and another to identify the depressive condition. Sequencing of codes is determined by the reason for admission/encounter.

- **Dysthymia**: Persistent depression (mild or moderate, lasting two years or longer in adults) (**F34.1**). Note that there are four additional symptoms included for a diagnosis of MDD. If all of the symptoms of Major Depression Disorder (MDD) are present during the current period of the depression, a diagnosis of MDD should be made instead of dysthymia.

<u>Excludes1</u>:

- For category F32-: bipolar disorder (F31-), manic episode (F30-), recurrent depressive disorder (F33-)

- For category F33-: bipolar disorder (F31-), manic episode (F30-)

<u>Other</u>:

- **Major Depressive Disorder (MDD)** has very specific diagnostic requirements that must be met in order to report these codes. According to the Diagnostic and Statistical Manual (DSM-5) which is published by the APA, there must be at least five symptoms (one of which is depressed mood or loss of interest or pleasure) which occur during the same two-week period and are documented by the provider (including severity as indicated in the "Major Depressive Disorder (MDD) Coding Table."

Resource: See Resource 51B for more information about the diagnostic criteria for MDD.

- **Disruptive mood dysregulation disorder (F34.81)** was listed in DSM-5 as F34.8. However, the American Psychiatric Association's (APA) September 2016 update included code **F34.81** which is no longer an unspecific code and should thus potentially reduce payer problems.
- **Premenstrual dysphoric disorder (F32.81)** was listed in DSM-5 as **N94.3**. However, the American Psychiatric Association's (APA) September 2016 update included code **F32.81**.
- At some point during the treatment visits, the patient will no longer need active care. For example, when treating cases of major depression, the APA defines three separate phases:
    - Acute Phase – Remission is induced (minimum 6 - 8 weeks in duration).
    - Continuation Phase – Remission is preserved and relapse prevented (usually 16 - 20 weeks in duration).
    - Maintenance Phase – Susceptible patients are protected against recurrence or relapse of subsequent major depressive episodes (duration varies with frequency and severity of previous episodes).

Book: See Chapter 4.1 — Documentation Essentials for more information about documenting the type of care.

Developmental Disorders

Explanation

This section is for some other developmental disorders not included elsewhere in this chapter. According to DSM-5, Neurodevelopmental Disorders "typically manifest early in development, often before the child enters grade school, and are characterized by developmental deficits that produce impairments of personal, social, academic, or occupational functioning."

Codes to Consider	
Dyslexia, developmental	F81.0
Intellectual disabilities	F70, F71, F72, F73, F78-, F79
Mathematics disorder	F81.2
Other development disorders of scholastic skills	F81.89
Social pragmatic communication disorder	F80.82
Specific reading disorder	F81.0
Speech sound disorder	F80.0
Written expression disorder	F81.81

Store: Not all developmental disorders are listed here. See the *ICD-10-CM Coding for Behavioral Health* book for the Alphabetic Index and Tabular List for other code options. For a complete listing of the entire code set, see the *ICD-10-CM Comprehensive CodeBook*. Both are available in the online store.

Coding Tips

<u>Diagnostic Criteria</u>: Codes with the ⑤ flag are listed in DSM-5. See DSM-5 diagnostic criteria for additional information on coding these conditions.

<u>ICD-10/DSM Differences</u>: nothing notable (n/a)

<u>Associated Conditions</u>: attention deficit hyperactivity disorder (see page 478), autism spectrum disorder (see page 479), developmental coordination disorder (**F82**), social pragmatic communication disorder (**F80.82**), and a family history of developmental disorders (no applicable ICD-10-CM codes)

<u>Excludes1</u>:

- For codes **F70-F79**: borderline intellectual functioning, IQ above 70 to 84 (**R41.83**)
- For code **F81.0**: alexia NOS (**R48.0**), dyslexia NOS (**R48.0**)
- For code **F81.2**: acalculia NOS (**R48.8**)

<u>Other</u>:

- As of October 1, 2021 F78 was expanded to include a new sub-category F78.A- "Other genetic related intellectual disabilities" which includes a new code to differentiate "SYNGAP1-related intellectual disability" from other types of genetic intellectual disabilities. Other associated conditions (e.g., Autism spectrum disorder [**F84.0**]) may also be reported with these codes. See Resource 54A for more information.
- Social pragmatic communication disorder (**F80.82**) was added in 2017.
- Codes **F70-F79** may not be listed as the primary diagnosis if there are any associated physical or developmental disorders.

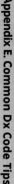

Dissociative Disorders

Explanation

Dissociative Disorders (also known as conversion disorders) are characterized by alterations in normal functions (e.g., memory, awareness, identity, or perception) which typically manifest after some form of trauma as an involuntary coping or defense mechanism. They are categorized by the manifested symptoms (e.g., amnesia, conversion disorder, fugue, stupor).

Codes to Consider	
Amnesia	F44.0
Conversion disorder	F44.4-F44.7
Fugue	F44.1
Other	F44.81-F44.89
Stupor	F44.2
Unspecified	F44.9

Coding Tips

Diagnostic Criteria: All but **F44.2** are listed in DSM-5. See DSM-5 diagnostic criteria for additional information on coding these conditions. The World Health Organization describes diagnostic criteria for dissociative stupor (**F44.2**) as meeting the general criteria for dissociative disorder with "profound diminution or absence of voluntary movements and speech, and of normal responsiveness to light, noise and touch," and "maintenance of normal muscle tone, static posture, and breathing (and often limited coordinated eye movements)."

ICD-10/DSM Differences: In 2017, ICD-10-CM revised codes **F44.0** and **F44.1**. Dissociative amnesia with dissociative fugue was added to **F44.1** and excluded from **F44.0** (see Excludes1 below). None of these changes are noted in DSM-5 updates documents; however, that is the way they are listed in the official DSM-5 manual.

Associated Conditions: malingering [conscious simulation] (**Z76.5**)

- For code **F44.0**, also consider: alcohol or other psychoactive, substance-induced amnestic disorder (F10, F13, F19 with .26, .96), amnestic disorder due to known physiological condition (**F04**), postictal amnesia in epilepsy (G40-)

- For code **F44.2**, also consider: catatonic disorder due to known physiological condition (**F06.1**), depressive stupor (F32-, F33-), manic stupor (F30-), bipolar disorder (F31-)

Excludes1:

- For code **F44.0**: amnesia NOS (**R41.3**), anterograde amnesia (**R41.1**), dissociative amnesia with dissociative fugue (**F44.1**), retrograde amnesia (**R41.2**)

- For code **F44.2**: catatonic stupor (**R40.1**), stupor NOS (**R40.1**)

Eating Disorders

Explanation

Eating Disorders go beyond restricting caloric intake. Rather, they are potentially life-threatening illnesses which are simultaneously psychological and physical and are often based on feelings of self-control and emotions. All conditions are characterized by a range of abnormal and harmful eating behaviors which are typically accompanied and motivated by unhealthy beliefs, perceptions, and expectations concerning eating, weight, and body shape.

Codes to Consider	
Anorexia NOS	R63.0
Anorexia nervosa;	
unspecified	F50.00
restricting type	⑤ F50.01
binge eating/purging type	⑤ F50.02
Avoidant/restrictive food intake disorder	⑤ F50.82
Binge eating disorder	⑤ F50.81
Bulimia nervosa	⑤ F50.2
Pica;	
child	⑤ F98.3
adult	⑤ F50.89
Unspecified eating disorder	⑤ F50.9

Coding Tips

<u>Diagnostic Criteria</u>: Codes with the ⑤ flag are listed in DSM-5. See DSM-5 diagnostic criteria for additional information on coding these conditions.

<u>ICD-10/DSM Differences</u>:

- Prior to the American Psychiatric Association's (APA) September 2016 update, the DSM manual only listed F50.8- as the ICD-10-CM crosswalk for binge eating and pica. However, the update shows the new codes as listed in the "Codes to Consider" table.

- The DSM September 2016 update listed Avoidant/Restrictive Food Intake Disorder as code **F50.89**. However, effective October 1, 2017, code **F50.82** "Avoidant/restrictive food intake disorder" was added and was listed in the DSM October 2017 update as the code to use instead of **F50.89**.

<u>Associated Conditions</u>: Anxiety disorders, obsessive-compulsive disorder, and neurodevelopmental disorders including autism spectrum disorder, attention-deficit/hyperactivity disorder, and intellectual disability.

- For F50- codes: feeding disorder in infancy or childhood (F98.2-), pica of infancy and childhood (**F98.3**)

- For F98- codes: breath-holding spells (**R06.89**), gender identity disorder of childhood (**F64.2**), Kleine-Levin syndrome (**G47.13**), obsessive-compulsive disorder (F42-), sleep disorders not due to a substance or known physiological condition (F51-)

Excludes1:

- For category F50-: anorexia NOS (**R63.0**), feeding difficulties (**R63.3**), feeding problems of newborn (**P92-**), polyphagia (**R63.2**)

 Note: As of October 1, 2021, feeding difficulties (R63.3) was changed from an Excludes1 to and Excludes2 for category F50-. As such, a patient may have both conditions at the same time even if it isn't part of the condition described by codes in category F50-.

- For subcategory F50.0-: loss of appetite (**R63.0**), psychogenic loss of appetite (**F50.89**)
- For code **F50.2**: anorexia nervosa, binge eating/purging type (**F50.02**)

Other:

- Childhood eating disorders are in a different chapter of ICD-10-CM than adult eating disorders. They are found in category F98-.
- Be aware of payer policies regarding treatment programs. Differing levels of impairment determine whether treatment needs to take place in an inpatient, partial hospital, or even intensive outpatient program setting.

Factitious Disorder

Explanation

Factitious Disorder, previously known as Munchausen's syndrome, is characterized by an individual's intentional falsification (e.g., feigning, purposely created or inflicted) of physical or psychological signs and/or symptoms. These falsified signs or symptoms are imposed on either themselves or another individual (previously called factitious disorder by proxy). This deception occurs even when there is no obvious external benefit (e.g., economic gain). They are willing to subject themselves or others (e.g., their child) to painful or risky tests and operations in order to obtain sympathy and/or attention. This behavior cannot be otherwise explained by another disorder such as a delusional disorder or another psychotic disorder.

Codes to Consider	Self	Proxy
Unspecified	⑤ F68.10	⑤ F68.A
w/ psychological signs and symptoms	F68.11	--
w/ physical signs and symptoms	F68.12	--
Combined psychological and physical symptoms	F68.13	--

Coding Tips

Diagnostic Criteria: Codes with the ⑤ flag are listed in DSM-5. See DSM-5 diagnostic criteria for additional information on coding these conditions.

ICD-10/DSM Differences:

- Only code **F68.10** has diagnostic criteria listed in the DSM-5 publication. The October 2018 update by the American Psychiatric Association (APA) states to use code **F68.A** to report "Factitious disorder imposed on another."

Associated Conditions:

- Personality or identity disorders

Other:

- Documentation should specify whether this is a single or recurring episode.
- According to the *ICD-10-CM Official Guidelines for Coding and Reporting*, "Munchausen's syndrome by proxy (MSBP) is a disorder in which a caregiver (perpetrator) falsely reports or causes an illness or injury in another person (victim) under his or her care, such as a child, an elderly adult, or a person who has a disability." In this situation, the perpetrator is reported with code **F68.A** and the victim should be assigned an abuse diagnosis (e.g., T74.1-). See the "Abuse, Neglect, or Maltreatment" segment on page 473 for abuse coding options.
- When there is an obvious motivation, consider using code **Z76.5** "Malingerer [conscious simulation]."

Health Status and Other Contact

Explanation

Codes found in Chapter 21 "Factors influencing health status and contact with health services (Z00-Z99)" describe both the health status of a patient as well as other reasons for patient encounters. They should be used when circumstances other than a disease, injury, or external cause needs to be recorded in the patient record, particularly if there is a circumstance or problem that affects their health status.

Book: See the "Abuse, Neglect, or Maltreatment" segment on page 473 for more information.

Note: Effective October 1, 2018, new codes were added for certain types of screening encounters. Be aware of payer requirements and use the appropriate Z13- code where applicable.

Codes to Consider	
Examination and observation for other specified reasons	Z04.89
Observation for other suspected diseases and conditions ruled out	Z03.89
Other specified counseling	Z71.89
Parent child conflict;	
adopted child	Z62.821
biological child	Z62.820
foster child	Z62.822
Screening;	
alcoholism	Z13.39
autism	Z13.41
depression	Z13.31
depression, maternal	Z13.32
developmental delays;	
global (milestones)	Z13.42
other	Z13.49
unspecified	Z13.40
intellectual disabilities	Z13.39
mental health and behavioral disorders, other	Z13.39
mental health and behavioral disorders, unspecified	Z13.30

Coding Tips

<u>Diagnostic Criteria</u>: Codes with the flag are listed in DSM-5. See DSM-5 diagnostic criteria for additional information on coding these conditions.

<u>ICD-10/DSM Differences</u>:

- DSM-5 only includes a small number of coding options for external causes whereas ICD-10-CM has significantly more. Those included here are only a small sampling of the more common codes. Be aware of individual payer requirements which may require other code options. See the Tabular List in the *ICD-10-CM Coding for Behavioral Health* book (available in the online store) or visit FindACode.com.
- Several new screening codes were added in 2019 to category Z13-. The DSM-5 book doesn't discuss codes for screenings.

History "Z" Codes

There are two types of history "Z" codes: personal and family. Personal history codes explain a patient's past medical condition that <u>no longer exists</u> and for which the patient is <u>not receiving any treatment</u>. The potential for recurrence may be there and require monitoring, but monitoring encounters are reported using the personal history code and not the condition that no longer exists. Be careful not to assign conditions the patient is currently being treated for long-term as "history" just because the current encounter did not address the condition. Prostate cancer is commonly miscoded as "history" when long-term treatment is being given but only addressed infrequently.

Family history codes are for use when a patient has a family member(s) who has had a particular disease that causes the patient to be at higher risk of also contracting the disease. Common family history conditions may include mental health disorders, degenerative disorders, cancer, etc. As screening tests are usually performed to rule out a possible problem, many times they are performed to rule out a condition that runs in the patient's family such as heart disease or breast cancer, so a combination of screening services and family history ICD-10-CM codes will be commonly seen.

History codes are also acceptable on any medical record regardless of the reason for visit. A history of an illness, even if no longer present, is important information that may alter the type of treatment ordered.

Book: See Chapter 4 — Tabular List for personal history code options. They are also available on FindACode.com.

Effective October 1, 2021, the following personal history codes were added:

Personal history of;

N	**Z91.51**	suicidal behavior
N	**Z91.52**	nonsuicidal self-harm

Reference: *ICD-10-CM Official Guidelines for Coding and Reporting 1.C.21.c.4*

Obsessive-Compulsive Disorder (OCD)

Explanation

According to the APA: "DSM-5 has created a new chapter for a cluster of disorders that involve obsessional thoughts and/or compulsive behaviors. These include obsessive-compulsive disorder (OCD), body dysmorphic disorder (BDD), hoarding disorder, trichotillomania (hair-pulling disorder), and excoriation (skin-picking) disorder. There are also categories for patients whose symptoms are secondary to medications or substances, are due to another medical condition, or do not quite meet criteria for one of the named disorders."

Codes to Consider		
Mixed obsessional thoughts and acts	⑤	F42.2
Hoarding disorder	⑤	F42.3
Excoriation (skin-picking) disorder	⑤	F42.4
Other obsessive-compulsive disorder	⑤	F42.8
Obsessive-compulsive disorder, unspecified	⑤	F42.9

Store: The remainder of this segment only discusses OCD and not the other disorders in this category. See the Alphabetic Index in the *ICD-10-CM Coding for Behavioral Health* book or FindACode.com to find the other conditions.

Coding Tips

Diagnostic Criteria: There are unique diagnostic requirements for each disorder as listed in the "Explanation." See DSM-5 diagnostic criteria for additional information on coding these conditions.

ICD-10/DSM Differences: The original DSM-5 book lists F42 as the only ICD-10-CM code for all these disorders. However, the September 2016 update by the APA revised these codes as listed in the "Codes to Consider" table.

Associated Conditions: obsessive-compulsive personality (disorder) (**F60.5**), obsessive-compulsive symptoms occurring in depression (F32-F33), obsessive-compulsive symptoms occurring in schizophrenia (F20-)

Excludes1: For category F42-: obsessive-compulsive symptoms occurring in depression (F32-F33) or schizophrenia (F20-)

Post-COVID-19 Condition

Due to a need to track conditions related to a previous COVID-19 infection, code **U09.9** "Post COVID-19 condition, unspecified" was created in Chapter 22 "Provisional assignment of new diseases of uncertain etiology or emergency use (U00-U85)."

The creation of this new code facilitates tracking and linking of problems/conditions associated with a previous infection from COVID-19. The following important instructional notes apply to this new code:

Note: This code enables establishment of a link with COVID-19.

This code is not to be used in cases that are still presenting with active COVID-19. However, an exception is made in cases of re-infection with COVID-19, occurring with a condition related to prior COVID-19.

Post-acute sequela of COVID-19

Code first the specific condition related to COVID-19 if known, such as:

chronic respiratory failure (J96.1-)

loss of smell (**R43.8**)

loss of taste (**R43.8**)

multisystem inflammatory syndrome (**M35.81**)

pulmonary embolism (I26.-)

pulmonary fibrosis (**J84.10**)

The *Official ICD-10-CM Guidelines for Coding and Reporting* include the following instructions about this code (emphasis added):

> For sequela of COVID-19, or associated symptoms or conditions that develop following a ***previous*** COVID-19 infection, assign a code(s) for the specific symptom(s) or condition(s) related to the previous COVID-19 infection, if known, and code U09.9, Post COVID-19 condition, unspecified.
>
> Code U09.9 should not be assigned for manifestations of an active (current) COVID-19 infection.
>
> If a patient has a condition(s) associated with a ***previous*** COVID-19 infection **and** develops a new active (current) COVID-19 infection, code U09.9 may be assigned in conjunction with code U07.1, COVID-19, to identify that the patient also has a condition(s) associated with a previous COVID-19 infection. Code(s) for the specific condition(s) associated with the previous COVID-19 infection and code(s) for manifestation(s) of the new active (current) COVID-19 infection should also be assigned.
>
> — *Section I;C.1.g.1.m*

Postpartum Depression and Psychosis

Explanation

Postpartum depression (PPD) typically emerges over the first two to three postpartum months but may occur anytime after delivery. Some women may even note the onset of milder depressive symptoms during pregnancy. Symptoms include several of the following: depressed or sad mood; tearfulness; loss of interest in usual activities; significant anxiety; sleep disturbances; feelings of guilt, worthlessness, incompetence; fatigue; change in appetite; panic attacks; suicidal thoughts.

It may be difficult to detect postpartum depression because many of the symptoms used to diagnose depression (e.g., sleep disturbance, appetite disturbance, fatigue) also occur in postpartum women in the absence of depression. Using an appropriate screening tool (e.g., Edinburgh Postnatal Depression Scale) can help to identify this condition.

Puerperal psychosis is rare, and is the most severe form of postpartum psychiatric illness. It is characterized by a typically dramatic onset of symptoms as early as the first 48 to 72 hours after delivery. The majority of women with puerperal psychosis develop symptoms within the first two postpartum weeks. Women with this disorder exhibit the following: 1) a rapidly shifting depressed or elated mood; 2) disorientation or confusion; and 3) erratic or disorganized behavior. For a diagnosis of psychosis, there must be delusions, hallucinations, or both. Delusional beliefs are common and often center on the infant. Auditory hallucinations that instruct the mother to harm herself or her infant may also occur.

Codes to Consider	
Postpartum;	
depression	F53.0
psychosis	F53.1

Coding Tips

<u>Diagnostic Criteria</u>: There are unique diagnostic requirements as listed in the "Explanation."

<u>ICD-10/DSM Differences</u>: The original DSM-5 book only includes a specifier for postpartum (peripartum) depression and no specific code. At the time of publication, no guidelines or updates had been released by the APA regarding the use of these codes.

<u>Excludes1</u>:

- Mood disorders with psychotic features (**F30.2, F31.2, F31.5, F31.64, F32.3, F33.3**)
- Postpartum dysphoria (**O90.6**)
- Psychosis in schizophrenia, schizotypal, delusional, and other psychotic disorders (F20-F29)

Book: See "Depressive Disorders" on page 484 for reporting other types of depression.

Post-Traumatic Stress Disorder (PTSD)

Explanation

PTSD was listed in DSM-IV as an Anxiety Disorder. In DSM-5, it is included in the Trauma- and Stressor-Related Disorders category. The criteria for PTSD includes identification of the traumatic events, four sets of symptom clusters, and two subtypes. There are also requirements regarding the duration of symptoms, how it impacts one's functioning, and ruling out substance use and medical illnesses.

Codes to Consider	
PTSD;	
acute	F43.11
chronic	F43.12
unspecified	F43.10

Coding Tips

Diagnostic Criteria: Only **F43.10** is listed in DSM-5. See DSM-5 diagnostic criteria for additional information on coding this condition.

ICD-10/DSM Differences:

- PTSD has only one code in DSM-5 (**F43.10**) but there are three options in ICD-10-CM. Since the DSM code association is an 'unspecified' code, be aware of payer requirements.

- According to the APA, "DSM-5 will include the addition of two subtypes: PTSD in children younger than 6 years and PTSD with prominent dissociative symptoms (either experiences of feeling detached from one's own mind or body, or experiences in which the world seems unreal, dreamlike or distorted)." These sub-types are not identified within ICD-10-CM code options.

Associated Conditions: Always document the triggering or external event(s) and where applicable, include an appropriate ICD-10-CM code (e.g., **T76.12XD** "Child physical abuse, suspected, subsequent encounter"). Not all triggering events will have an associated ICD-10-CM code. Use the Alphabetic Index in the *ICD-10-CM Coding for Behavioral Health* book or visit FindACode.com to find applicable codes.

Excludes1: none

Other:

- Functional Impairment: Assess and document the PTSD-related functional impairment according to standardized clinical practice guidelines.

- Acute stress disorder has the same criteria as PTSD but is of a shorter duration. Symptoms of intrusion, avoidance, negative cognitive and mood alteration, and persistent arousal appear within 4 weeks of the trauma and last for 2 days to 4 weeks.

Rule Out Diagnosis

When the clinical documentation indicates uncertainty of a diagnosis with words such as: "probable," "suspected," "likely," "questionable," "possible," "still to be ruled out," "compatible with," or "consistent with," do not report it as definitive or confirmed **unless** you are coding for inpatient admissions to short-term, acute, long-term care, or a psychiatric hospital.

According to the *ICD-10-CM Official Guidelines for Coding and Reporting*, correct coding would be to code the signs, symptoms, and/or abnormal clinical and lab findings using codes R00-R99. These are the only acceptable outpatient codes when a diagnosis has not been firmly established.

Choose the most appropriate code(s) from Chapter 18 "Symptoms, Signs and Abnormal Clinical and Laboratory Findings, Not Elsewhere Classified (R00-R99)." Be aware that not all symptoms have a code.

Store: See the *ICD-10-CM Coding for Behavioral Health* book (available in the online store) for more information on this and other important coding guidelines.

Schizoaffective Disorder

Explanation

Schizoaffective disorder is indicated when the patient has symptoms of both schizophrenia and a mood disorder – but does not strictly meet diagnostic criteria for either alone. Typically, symptoms occur during the same episode (or at least within a few days of each other) and cannot be attributed to a substance (drug) or another medical condition. Specify the type of mood disorder (i.e., bipolar, depressive, other, unspecified) for final code selection.

Codes to Consider	
Bipolar type	F25.0
Depressive type	F25.1
Other	F25.8
Unspecified	F25.9

Coding Tips

Diagnostic Criteria: Only **F25.0** and **F25.1** are listed in DSM-5. See DSM-5 diagnostic criteria for additional information on coding these conditions.

ICD-10/DSM Differences: DSM-5 only includes two types (bipolar and depressive) even though other options are available within ICD-10-CM. Be aware of payer policies.

Note: Schizophreniform psychosis was removed as an ICD-10-CM inclusion term for codes **F25.0** and **F25.1** effective October 1, 2017.

Associated Conditions: Anxiety disorders, Posttraumatic stress disorder (PTSD), Attention-deficit hyperactivity disorder (ADHD), Substance abuse

Excludes1: mood [affective] disorders with psychotic symptoms (**F30.2**, **F31.2**, **F31.5**, **F31.64**, **F32.3**, **F33.3**), schizophrenia (F20-)

Schizophrenia

Explanation

Schizophrenia is a disorder characterized by delusions and hallucinations (hearing voices or sounds, or sensations like smell or taste) which begins between the ages 16 and 30 and continues throughout adulthood. Symptoms cause significant social or occupational dysfunction/impairment and must have been present for a minimum of six months, and include at least one month of active symptoms. Symptoms may include disorganized speech and behavior (disorganized or catatonic), and delusions (typically of control, influence, or persecutory beliefs of various kinds).

Schizophreniform is a type of schizophrenia in which symptoms last **less than** six months AND also include a mood episode (e.g., depression, mania).

Codes to Consider	
Schizophrenia;	
catatonic	**F20.2**
disorganized	**F20.1**
paranoid	**F20.0**
residual	**F20.5**
other	**F20.89**
undifferentiated	**F20.3**
unspecified	**F20.9**
Schizophreniform disorder	**F20.81**

Coding Tips

Diagnostic Criteria: Only **F20.9** and **F20.81** are listed in DSM-5. See DSM-5 diagnostic criteria for additional information on coding these conditions.

ICD-10/DSM Differences:

- **Schizophrenia**: According to DSM-5, **F20.9** is the only ICD-10-CM code for all types of schizophrenia. DSM-5 discontinued the subtypes of paranoid, disorganized, catatonic, undifferentiated, and residual. However, the ICD-10-CM Tabular List continues to use these descriptions in the available coding options. Since **F20.9** is an 'unspecified' code, payers may likely require more specificity unless they adhere closely to DSM-5 criteria.

- **Catatonic Disorders**: DSM-5 includes a 'specifier' for catatonia which also applies to depressive, bipolar, and psychotic disorders.

Associated Conditions: schizophrenic reaction in: alcoholism (F10.15-, F10,25-, F10.95-), brain disease (**F06.2**), epilepsy (**F06.2**), psychoactive drug use (F11-F19 with .15, .25, .95), schizotypal disorder (**F21**)

Excludes1: brief psychotic disorder (**F23**), cyclic schizophrenia (**F25.0**), mood [affective] disorders with psychotic, symptoms (**F30.2, F31.2, F31.5, F31.64, F32.3, F33.3**), schizoaffective disorder (F25-), schizophrenic reaction NOS (**F23**)

Other:

- Do not use this diagnosis if symptoms can be attributed to another condition or substance (drug)

- Document the status of the condition as one of the following: episodic, with partial or complete remissions, or chronic

- Treatment includes medication as well as therapy, family education, rehabilitation, and/or skills training

Social Determinants of Health (SDoH)

According to coding and reporting rules, any member of a person's care team can collect SDoH data during an encounter. This includes providers, social workers, community health workers, case managers, patient navigators, and clinical staff. Common data collection tools may be used to collect this information such as health risk assessments, screening tools, self-reporting, and even in-person interactions. Note that SDoH should not be limited to just what ICD-10-CM codes currently exist for reporting as there are ongoing efforts to continue expanding these codes for SDoH data collection and reporting. To report SDoH codes, the information must be documented in the medical record. Efforts should continue within every organization to not only identify and document SDoH, but to also identify ways in which coordination of care, additional services, or referrals may be incorporated into the patient's treatment plan to improve SDoH outcomes. Codes for reporting SDoH are located in categories Z55-Z65. Effective October 1, 2021, the following are available for reporting:

- [N] **Z55.5** — Less than a high school diploma
- [N] **Z58.6** — Inadequate drinking-water supply
- [N] **Z59.-** — Situations related to homelessness
- [N] **Z59.48** — Other specified lack of adequate food
- [N] **Z59.8-** — Housing instability

Note: SDoH was added to the Risk portion of "Medical Decision Making" scoring for Office or Other Outpatient Services (99202-99215) in 2021.

Book: See Chapter 5.3 — Evaluation & Management Coding for more information about properly documenting E/M visits including the scoring of the Risk component.

Substance Use Disorders

Explanation

A Substance Use Disorder (SUD) occurs when an individual's use of a substance (e.g., alcohol, drug) causes problems at work, school, and/or home and often leads to health problems or disability. It is characterized by impaired control, social impairment, risky substance use behaviors, and other pharmacological criteria. Within DSM-5 (but not ICD-10-CM), SUDs are categorized by their level of severity (e.g., mild, moderate, severe) which is determined by the number of diagnostic criteria that are met. In ICD-10-CM, the characters are descriptive with a unique presentation which facilitates accurate reporting of all SUD disorders even when only three-character categories are used:

- the third character indicates the substance
- the fourth and fifth characters describe the psychopathological syndrome (e.g., intoxication, residual states)
- the sixth character describes the associated symptom(s) (e.g., delusion, hallucination, anxiety)

Defining Remission

For appropriate clinical treatment and statistical reporting it is necessary to properly distinguish between a current SUD and one that is in remission (i.e., full criteria have been met in the past but currently the patient is no longer experiencing symptoms). To meet this need, in 2018, new diagnosis codes were added (all ending in .11) along with inclusion terms which match DSM-5 terminology for SUD severity as well as to indicate whether the remission is "early" or "sustained." The October 2017 DSM-5 update included those new codes.

There are two types of remission described by DSM-5 (i.e., early, sustained), but they are not coded separately for ICD-10-CM. *Section I.C.5.b* of the *ICD-10-CM Official Guidelines for Coding and Reporting* provides the following guidance:

"Mild substance use disorders in early or sustained remission are classified to the appropriate codes for substance abuse in remission, and moderate or severe substance use disorders in early or sustained remission are classified to the appropriate codes for substance dependence in remission." Both types of remission recognize that cravings or strong desires to use the substance do not count toward determining remission status.

Abuse vs. Dependence vs. Use

Code selection is based on the level of impairment in social, occupational, or recreational functioning. Abuse is the most severe, followed by dependence and then use. Only choose a "Use" code when the impairment level does not meet the complete criteria for either abuse or dependence.

Dependence is characterized by a compulsive or obsessive pattern of substance use (i.e., inability to stop) whereas abuse is characterized by using it too much or too often.

Note: None of the criteria for SUD have been met for the following period of time:
- early: 3-12 months
- sustained: 12+ months

Alert: Effective October 1, 2018, "Cannabis dependence with withdrawal" was removed as an inclusion term for **F12.288** and assigned code **F12.23**. There was also another new cannabis code: **F12.93** "Cannabis use, unspecified with withdrawal."

Substance Use Disorders Coding Table

3rd character					
Alcohol	(F10)	Inhalants	(F18)	Other psychoactive substances drug use and multiple	(F19)
Cannabis	(F12)	Nicotine	(F17)	Sedatives, hypnotics, anxiolytics	
Cocaine	(F14)	Opioids	(F11)	Stimulants, other, including caffeine	(F13)
Hallucinogens	(F16)				(F15)

*Note: Not all the 3 character code blocks have 6th character options. Because the 5th and 6th characters may NOT apply to all 3rd and 4th character categories, always check Chapter 4 — Tabular List or FindACode.com before deciding which code to use.

4th character		5th character		6th character	
Abuse	(.1)	with induced:			
		mood disorder	(.14)	n/a	
		psychotic disorder	(.15)	with delusions	(.150)
				with hallucinations	(.151)
				unspecified	(.159)
		with intoxication	(.12)	uncomplicated	(.120)
				delirium	(.121)
				w/ perceptual disturbance	(.122)
				unspecified	(.129)
		with substance-induced dementia	(.17)	n/a	
		with other induced disorder	(.18)	anxiety disorder	(.180)
				sexual disorder	(.181)
				sleep disorder	(.182)
				other induced disorder	(.188)
		in remission	(.11)	n/a	
		uncomplicated	(.10)	n/a	
		with unspecified induced disorder	(.19)	n/a	

4th character		5th character		6th character	
Dependence	(.2)	in remission	(.21)	n/a	
		with induced mood disorder	(.24)	n/a	
		with induced persisting amnestic disorder	(.26)	n/a	
		with induced persisting dementia	(.27)	n/a	
		with induced psychotic disorder	(.25)	with delusions	(.250)
				with hallucinations	(.251)
				unspecified	(.259)
		with intoxication	(.22)	uncomplicated	(.220)
				delirium	(.221)
				w/ perceptual disturbance	(.222)
				unspecified	(.229)
		with withdrawal	(.23)	uncomplicated	(.230)
				delirium	(.231)
				w/ perceptual disturbance	(.232)
				unspecified	(.239)
		with substance-induced dementia	(.27)	n/a	
		with other induced disorders	(.28)	anxiety disorder	(.280)
				sexual dysfunction	(.281)
				sleep disorder	(.282)
				other induced disorder	(.288)
		uncomplicated	(.20)	n/a	
		with unspecified induced disorder	(.29)	n/a	
Use, unspecified	(.9)	with induced mood disorder	(.94)	n/a	
		with induced psychotic disorder	(.95)	with delusions	(.950)
				with hallucinations	(.951)
				sleep disorder	(.959)
		with induced persisting amnestic disorder	(.96)	n/a	
		with induced persisting dementia	(.97)	n/a	
		with other induced disorders	(.98)	anxiety disorder	(.980)
				sexual dysfunction	(.981)
				sleep disorder	(.982)
				other induced disorder	(.988)
		with intoxication	(.92)	uncomplicated	(.920)
				delirium	(.921)
				w/ perceptual disturbance	(.922)
				unspecified	(.929)
		with substance-induced dementia	(.97)	n/a	
		with unspecified induced disorder	(.99)	n/a	
		with withdrawal	(.93)	uncomplicated	(.930)
				delirium	(.931)
				w/ perceptual disturbance	(.932)
				unspecified	(.939)

Coding Tips

<u>Diagnostic Criteria</u>: See DSM-5 diagnostic criteria for additional information on coding these conditions. Note that unlike other tables in this chapter, the "Substance Use Disorders Coding Table" does not include the DSM-5 flag next to applicable code(s). All **EXCEPT** the following are listed in DSM-5:

F10.120	F10.150	F10.151	F10.188	F10.19	F10.21	F10.220	F10.230	F10.250	F10.251
F10.29	F10.920	F10.950	F10.951						
F11.120	F11.150	F11.151	F11.159	F11.19	F11.21	F11.220	F11.250	F11.251	F11.259
F11.29	F11.90	F11.920	F11.93	F11.950	F11.951	F11.959			
F12.120	F12.150	F12.151	F12.19	F12.21	F12.220	F12.250	F12.251	F12.29	F12.90
F12.920	F12.950	F12.951							
F13.120	F13.150	F13.151	F13.188	F13.19	F13.21	F13.220	F13.230	F13.250	F13.251
F13.26	F13.29	F13.90	F13.920	F13.93-	F13.950	F13.951	F13.96		
F14.120	F14.150	F14.151	F14.19	F14.21	F14.220	F14.250	F14.251	F14.29	F14.90
F14.920	F14.950	F14.951							
F15.120	F15.150	F15.151	F15.19	F15.21	F15.220	F15.250	F15.251	F15.29	F15.90
F15.920	F15.950	F15.951							
F16.120	F16.122	F16.150	F16.151	F16.183	F16.188	F16.19	F16.21	F16.250	F16.251
F16.283	F16.288	F16.29	F16.90	F16.920	F16.950	F16.951	F16.988		
F17.201	F17.210	F17.21-	F17.22-	F17.29-					
F18.120	F18.150	F18.151	F18.19	F18.21	F18.220	F18.250	F18.251	F18.29	F18.90
F18.920	F18.950	F18.951							
F19.120	F19.122	F19.150	F19.151	F19.16	F19.19	F19.21	F19.220	F19.222	F19.230
F19.232	F19.250	F19.251	F19.26	F19.29	F19.90	F19.920	F19.922	F19.93-	F19.950
F19.951	F19.96								

<u>ICD-10/DSM Differences</u>: There are far fewer disorders listed in DSM-5 than ICD-10-CM. Please follow payer guidelines for code usage.

- Caffeine use is included with category F15- "Other stimulant related disorders."

- Effective October 1, 2018 some new codes for cannabis withdrawal (**F12.23** and **F12.93**) were created so it is likely that one or both of these codes may be included in future official DSM-5 updates.

- Several substance use code descriptions were updated, effective October 1, 2016. These inclusion term additions more closely align with DSM-5 diagnostic criteria descriptions. For example, **F10.10** added the inclusion term: "Alcohol use disorder, mild."

<u>Associated Conditions</u>: attention deficit disorder (see "Attention Deficit Hyperactivity Disorder (ADHD)"), depression (see "Depressive Disorders"), post-traumatic stress disorder (see "Post-Traumatic Stress Disorder (PTSD)"), other behavioral disorder (e.g., psychotic disorder)

<u>Other</u>:

- When the symptoms are related to an SUD, do NOT report it separately unless it was a condition existing prior to the substance use. For example, typically **F16.180** "Hallucinogen abuse with hallucinogen-induced anxiety disorder" should not also report **F41.1** "Generalized anxiety disorder."

- For subcategory F10-: use an additional code for blood alcohol level, if applicable (Y90-)

Note: There are many pertinent includes and excludes at various levels throughout this section. Be sure to review the selected code in a Tabular listing to ensure proper code selection.

Store: See innoviHealth's *ICD-10-CM Coding for Behavioral Health* (available in the online store) for a Tabular List. They are also available with a FindACode.com subscription.

- Counseling codes: There is a separate category in ICD-10-CM (Z71-) for reporting when a patient seeks medical advice. Some of these are associated with the treatment for substance use disorders. Also consider including the following codes (as indicated) to ensure accurate reimbursement:
  - Alcohol abuse counseling and surveillance (Z71.4-)
  - Drug abuse counseling and surveillance (Z71.5-)
  - Tobacco abuse counseling (**Z71.6**)

Notes:

Appendix F. Coding Reference Tables

Figure F.1

__ICD-10-CM Tabular Indicators__			
Abbreviation	**Title**	**Source**	**Description**
Adult	Adult	CMS	Age range 15-24 years inclusive
CC	Complication or Comorbidity	MS-DRG v38.1	Presence of a complication or condition that increases the severity of a patient's condition, affects DRG assignment, and increases the resources needed to care for the patient appropriately.
DSM-5	DSM-5	APA	Codes mentioned in the American Psychiatric Association's DSM-5 publication. This indicator is useful for those working in the field of behavioral health or in an integrated care practice.
Female	Female only	CMS	Female-related diagnoses only
HAC: #	Hospital Acquired Condition	MS-DRG v38.1	A condition that arises during a hospital stay that affects the patient negatively and may affect DRG assignment.
CMS22: # **CMS23: #** **CMS24: #**	CMS Hierarchical Condition Categories; v22, v23, v24	CMS	Payment model for Medicare Advantage plans used to identify and calculate enrollee health status; versions 22, 23, and 24
ESRD21: #	CMS-ESRD Hierarchical Condition Categories	CMS	Payment model for Medicare ESRD plans used to identify and calculate enrollee health status
HHS04: # **HHS05: #**	HHS Hierarchical Condition Categories; v04, v05	HHS	Payment model for Affordable Care Act plans used to identify and calculate enrollee health status; versions 04, 05
Male	Male only	CMS	Male-related diagnoses only
Manifestation	Manifestation	CMS	Describes the manifestation of an underlying disease, not the disease itself. Code first the underlying disease followed by the manifestation code.
Maternity	Maternity	CMS	Age-range 12-55 years only
MCC	Major Complication or Comorbidity	MS-DRG v38.1	Presence of a major complication or condition that increases the severity of the patient's condition, affects DRG assignment, and significantly increases the resources needed to care for the patient appropriately.
Newborn	Newborn	CMS	Only reported for newborns 0-28 days old
NoPDx/M	Unacceptable principal diagnosis (for Medicare)	CMS	There are selected codes that describe a circumstance which influences an individual's health status, but not a current illness or injury, or codes that are not specific manifestation but they may be due to an underlying cause. These codes are considered unacceptable as a principal diagnosis. The following unacceptable principal diagnosis code is considered "acceptable" when a secondary diagnosis is also coded on the record. Example: **Z51.89** "Encounter for other specified aftercare"
PDx/CC	Primary diagnosis is its own CC	MS-DRG v38.1	Diagnosis is a combination code in ICD-10-CM, which also represents the CC. In ICD-9-CM, it was represented by two or more codes, one of which was the CC.
PDx/MCC	Primary diagnosis is its own MCC	MS-DRG v38.1	Diagnosis is a combination code in ICD-10-CM, which also represents the MCC. In ICD-9-CM, it was represented by two or more codes, one of which was the MCC.
Pediatric	Pediatric	CMS	Age range 0-17 inclusive
POAEx	Present on Admission Exempt	CDC/CMS	Diagnosis codes that cannot be listed as Present on Admission. They are exempt from POA use.
QAdmit	Questionable Admission	CMS	Some diagnoses are not usually sufficient justification for admission to an acute care hospital. For example, if a patient is given code **R03.0** for elevated blood pressure reading, without diagnosis of hypertension, then the patient would have a questionable admission, since an elevated blood pressure reading is not normally sufficient justification for admission to a hospital.
RxHCC: #	Prescription Drug Hierarchical Condition Categories	MS-DRG v38.1	A risk adjustment payment model utilized by prescription drug plans for Medicare Part D beneficiaries.
Z-PDx	Only as Principal/First-Listed Diagnosis	ICD-10-CM Guidelines	Codes located in Chapter 21 that begin with the letter "Z" and can only be reported as first-listed or principal diagnosis.

Figure F.2

Procedure/Supply Code Indicators			
Abbreviation	Title	Source	Description
Add On	CPT Add on code	AMA	Codes which may only be billed in conjunction with a primary procedure which was also performed by the same provider rendering the primary procedure. They must never be reported alone. CPT Guidelines will indicate which codes it should be used with.
AS: #	Assistant Surgeon (80, 82)	CMS	The key below explains the number that follows "AS:" 0 This indicator will be initially denied if billed with modifier 80 or 82, but if there is a valid reason for the assistant, clearly documented in the operative report, the claim may be appealed with written documentation and considered for payment 1/9 Either indicator identifies codes that may NOT be reported with modifier 80 or 82 and will be denied if submitted with those modifiers. 2 This indicator identifies codes that are 80/82 assistant surgeon eligible. Medicare pays 16% of the global surgery fee when billed with modifier 80 or 82. If a PA, NP, or CNS perform the assistant at surgery service, payment is 85% of the 16% for the assistant at surgery portion. Only teaching hospitals may report modifier 82. Some commercial payers may pay a little more (20%).
Bilat	Bilateral Surgery (50)	CMS	The key below explains the number that follows "Bilat:" 0 Physiology or anatomy doesn't permit a bilateral service or the service is specifically unilateral and a bilateral service code exists that should be used instead. 1 150% Bilateral payment adjustment. 150% payment adjustment for bilateral procedures applies. 2 Bilateral procedure. 150% payment adjustment does not apply. RVUs are already based on the procedure being performed as a bilateral procedure. 3 No bilateral payment adjustment. Services in this category are generally radiology and diagnostic services which are not subject to laterality. 9 Concept does not apply.
DxImage	Diagnostic Imaging	CMS	Subject to the Multiple Procedure Payment Reduction (MPPR) of 50% on the TC of the imaging procedure.
FDA	Product pending FDA approval	AMA	Codes are assigned to products/vaccines that are awaiting approval from the Food and Drug Administration (FDA). Once the approval is granted by the FDA, this flag is removed. FindACode.com always has the current approval status in the "Code History."
Female	Female Only	CMS	Gender-specific supply/procedure (female): The performance of certain procedures may require significantly different approaches when performed in a male as opposed to a female. Also, some HCPCS code descriptions designate if the supply/service is to be reported for a male or a female or by anatomical description.
Global: #	Global Days	CMS	A global period is a period of time which begins with a surgical procedure and ends at a specified time after the procedure. Many procedures have a follow-up period in which normal post-operative care is considered bundled into the global surgery fee. This indicator identifies codes for which the global concept applies and if so, for how many days. See Resource 508 for more information. The key below explains what follows the word Global: 010 Minor procedure: Total global period is 11 days (the day of the surgery + 10 days postoperative). 090 Major surgery: Total global period is 92 days (the day prior to the surgery + the day of the surgery + 90 days postoperative). YYY Carrier determined: The local Medicare carrier determines whether the global concept applies and establishes the postoperative period, if appropriate, at time of pricing. MMM Maternity: This is a maternity code; the usual global period does not apply.
IP	Inpatient Only	CMS	Codes that are only covered when performed in an inpatient setting.

Procedure/Supply Code Indicators

Abbreviation	Title	Source	Description
Male	Male Only	CMS	Gender-specific supply/procedure (male): The performance of certain procedures may require significantly different approaches when performed in a male as opposed to a female. Also, some HCPCS code descriptions designate if the supply/service is to be reported for a male or a female or by anatomical description.
M-Status	Medicare Status Codes	CMS	This important indicator is for identifying Medicare's payment status for the code. The key below explains the value that follows the abbreviation "M-Status." **A** — Active code. These codes are separately paid under the physician fee schedule if covered. There will be RVUs and payment amounts for codes with this status. The presence of an "A" indicator does not mean that Medicare has made a national coverage determination regarding the service; carriers remain responsible for coverage decisions in the absence of a national Medicare policy. **B** — Payment for covered services are always bundled into payment for other services not specified. There will be no RVUs or payment amounts for these codes and no separate payment is ever made. When these services are covered, payment for them is subsumed by the payment for the services to which they are incident (an example is a telephone call from a hospital nurse regarding care of a patient. **C** — Carriers price the code. Carriers will establish RVUs and payment amounts for these services, generally on an individual case basis following review of documentation such as an operative report. Carriers may also gap-fill payment based on a comparable code(s) or value of multiple codes. When this occurs, RVUs are not maintained for these codes; instead, the carrier fee is indexed each year using the MPFSDB update factor. The update factor is located on the display screen and on the MPFSDB Indicator Download file. **D** — Deleted/discontinued codes. Codes with this indicator had a 90 day grace period before January 1, 2005. **E** — Excluded from physician fee schedule by regulation. These codes are for items and/or services that CMS chose to exclude from the fee schedule payment by regulation. No RVUs or payment amounts are shown and no payment may be made under the fee schedule for these codes. Payment for them, when covered, continues under reasonable charge procedures. **I** — Not valid for Medicare purposes. Medicare uses another code for reporting of, and payment for, these services. (Code NOT subject to a 90 day grace period.) **J** — Anesthesia services (no relative value units or payment amounts for anesthesia codes on the database, only used to facilitate the identification of anesthesia services.) **M** — Measurement codes, used for reporting purposes only. **N** — Non-covered service. These codes are carried on the HCPCS tape as noncovered services. **P** — Bundled/excluded codes. There are no RVUs and no payment amounts for these services. No separate payment is made for them under the fee schedule. If the item or service is covered as incident to a physician service and is provided on the same day as a physician service, payment for it is bundled into the payment for the physician service to which it is incident (an example is an elastic bandage furnished by a physician incident to a physician service). If the item or service is covered as other than incident to a physician service, it is excluded from the fee schedule (for example, colostomy supplies) and is paid under the other payment provision of the Act.

More on next page

Procedure/Supply Code Indicators

Abbreviation	Title	Source	Description
M-Status (continued)	Medicare Status Codes	CMS	Q — Therapy functional information code (used for required reporting purposes only.) R — Restricted coverage. Special coverage instructions apply. T — There are RVUs and payment amounts for these services, but they are only paid if there are no other services payable under the physician fee schedule billed on the same date by the same provider. If any other services payable under the physician fee schedule are billed on the same date by the same provider, these services are bundled into the physician services for which payment is made. X — Statutory exclusion. These codes represent an item or service that is not in the statutory definition of "physician services" for fee schedule payment purposes. No RVUs or payment amounts are shown for these codes and no payment may be made under the physician fee schedule. (Examples are ambulances services and clinical diagnostic laboratory services.)
Mod51: #	Multiple Procedures	CMS	Multiple procedures performed at the same encounter often overlap in pre-, intra-, and post-procedure work and as such, reimbursement is slightly reduced because this work is not repeated. The indicators below identify the method used to determine payment reduction. The key below explains the number that follows "Mod51:" 0 — No payment adjustment rules for multiple procedures apply. 1 — Standard payment adjustment rules in effect for multiple procedures apply. Reduction is 100%, 50%, 25%, 25%, 25%, and by report. 2 — Standard payment adjustment rules for multiple procedures apply. Standard reduction is 100%, 50%, 50%, 50%, 50%, and then by report. 3 — Special payment adjustment rules for multiple endoscopic procedures apply. 4 — Special payment adjustment rules on the TC of multiple diagnostic imaging. 5 — Subject to 50% of the practice expense component for certain therapy services. 6 — Special payment adjustment rules on the TC of multiple cardiovascular Dx services. 7 — Special payment adjustment rules on the TC of multiple ophthalmology Dx services apply.
PC/TC: #	Professional/Technical Indicator	CMS	Some codes are divided into their professional and/or technical component for reimbursement. When submitting claims, be sure to apply the appropriate modifier(s) as needed to clarify the service rendered. See *Appendix B — Modifiers* for additional information on modifiers 26, PC, and TC. The key below explains the number that follows "PC/TC:" 0 — Physician Service Code 1 — Diagnostic Tests for Radiology Services 2 — Professional Component Only Code 3 — Technical Component Only Code 4 — Global Test Only Code 5 — Incident To Code 6 — Laboratory Physician Interpretation Code 7 — Physical Therapy Service, for which Payment may not be Made 8 — Physician Interpretation Code

Procedure/Supply Code Indicators			
Abbreviation	Title	Source	Description
PS: #	Physician Supervision Status	CMS	This indicator identifies the level of supervision required for services that may be performed by midlevels/QHPs. The key below explains the number that follows the letters "PS:" 01 Procedure must be performed under the general supervision of a physician. 02 Procedure must be performed under the direct supervision of a physician. 03 Procedure must be performed under the personal supervision of a physician. 04 Does not apply when procedure is performed by an independent psychologist or a clinical psychologist. 05 Physician supervision policy does not apply when procedure is furnished by a qualified audiologist. 06 Physician/Physical Therapist (PT) must be certified by the American Board of Physical Therapy Specialties (ABPTS) as electrophysiological specialist & permitted by state law. 21 May be performed by technician with certification under general supervision of a physician. 22 May be performed by a technician with online real-time contact with physician. 66 May be performed by a physician/PT with ABPTS certification and certification in this specific procedure. 6A Level 66 plus PT with ABPTS certification may supervise another PT; only the certified PT may bill. 77 Performed by a PT with ABPTS certification, PT without certification under physician, or by technologist with certification under physician. 7A Level 77 plus the PT with ABPTS certification may supervise another PT, but only the PT with ABPTS certification may bill.
Reseq	Resequenced CPT Code	AMA	Resequenced codes are out of numerical order in the CPT code book. This is done because there are not enough code options available to continue the same numerical sequence.
Telemed	Telemedicine covered service	AMA/CMS	This service may be performed via synchronous telehealth/telemedicine services. CPT and CMS designate different codes, but in this listing, both are identified with the same indicator. See Appendix D — Telehealth Codes for the separate lists.

Figure F.3

HCC Codes and Descriptions (CMS-HCC v22)

1	HIV/AIDS	82	Respirator Dependence/Tracheostomy Status
2	Septicemia, Sepsis, Systemic Inflammatory Response Syndrome/Shock	83	Respiratory Arrest
6	Opportunistic Infections	84	Cardio-Respiratory Failure and Shock
8	Metastatic Cancer and Acute Leukemia	85	Congestive Heart Failure
9	Lung and Other Severe Cancers	86	Acute Myocardial Infarction
10	Lymphoma and Other Cancers	87	Unstable Angina and Other Acute Ischemic Heart Disease
11	Colorectal, Bladder, and Other Cancers	88	Angina Pectoris
12	Breast, Prostate, and Other Cancers and Tumors	96	Specified Heart Arrhythmias
17	Diabetes with Acute Complications	99	Cerebral Hemorrhage
18	Diabetes with Chronic Complications	100	Ischemic or Unspecified Stroke
19	Diabetes without Complication	103	Hemiplegia/Hemiparesis
21	Protein-Calorie Malnutrition	104	Monoplegia, Other Paralytic Syndromes
22	Morbid Obesity	106	Atherosclerosis of the Extremities with Ulceration or Gangrene
23	Other Significant Endocrine and Metabolic Disorders	107	Vascular Disease with Complications
27	End-Stage Liver Disease	108	Vascular Disease
28	Cirrhosis of Liver	110	Cystic Fibrosis
29	Chronic Hepatitis	111	Chronic Obstructive Pulmonary Disease
33	Intestinal Obstruction/Perforation	112	Fibrosis of Lung and Other Chronic Lung Disorders
34	Chronic Pancreatitis	114	Aspiration and Specified Bacterial Pneumonias
35	Inflammatory Bowel Disease	115	Pneumococcal Pneumonia, Empyema, Lung Abscess
39	Bone/Joint/Muscle Infections/Necrosis	122	Proliferative Diabetic Retinopathy and Vitreous Hemorrhage
40	Rheumatoid Arthritis and Inflammatory Connective Tissue Disease	124	Exudative Macular Degeneration
46	Severe Hematological Disorders	134	Dialysis Status
47	Disorders of Immunity	135	Acute Renal Failure
48	Coagulation Defects and Other Specified Hematological Disorders	136	Chronic Kidney Disease, Stage 5
54	Drug/Alcohol Psychosis	137	Chronic Kidney Disease, Severe (Stage 4)
55	Drug/Alcohol Dependence	157	Pressure Ulcer of Skin with Necrosis Through to Muscle, Tendon, or Bone
57	Schizophrenia	158	Pressure Ulcer of Skin with Full Thickness Skin Loss
58	Major Depressive, Bipolar, and Paranoid Disorders	161	Chronic Ulcer of Skin, Except Pressure
70	Quadriplegia	162	Severe Skin Burn or Condition
71	Paraplegia	166	Severe Head Injury
72	Spinal Cord Disorders/Injuries	167	Major Head Injury
73	Amyotrophic Lateral Sclerosis and Other Motor Neuron Disease	169	Vertebral Fractures without Spinal Cord Injury
74	Cerebral Palsy	170	Hip Fracture/Dislocation
75	Myasthenia Gravis/Myoneural Disorders, Inflammatory and Toxic Neuropathy	173	Traumatic Amputations and Complications
76	Muscular Dystrophy	176	Complications of Specified Implanted Device or Graft
77	Multiple Sclerosis	186	Major Organ Transplant or Replacement Status
78	Parkinson's and Huntington's Diseases	188	Artificial Openings for Feeding or Elimination
79	Seizure Disorders and Convulsions	189	Amputation Status, Lower Limb/Amputation Complications
80	Coma, Brain Compression/Anoxic Damage		

HCC Codes and Descriptions (CMS-HCC v24)

1	HIV/AIDS	79	Seizure Disorders and Convulsions
2	Septicemia, Sepsis, Systemic Inflammatory Response Syndrome/Shock	80	Coma, Brain Compression/Anoxic Damage
6	Opportunistic Infections	82	Respirator Dependence/Tracheostomy Status
8	Metastatic Cancer and Acute Leukemia	83	Respiratory Arrest
9	Lung and Other Severe Cancers	84	Cardio-Respiratory Failure and Shock
10	Lymphoma and Other Cancers	85	Congestive Heart Failure
11	Colorectal, Bladder, and Other Cancers	86	Acute Myocardial Infarction
12	Breast, Prostate, and Other Cancers and Tumors	87	Unstable Angina and Other Acute Ischemic Heart Disease
17	Diabetes with Acute Complications	88	Angina Pectoris
18	Diabetes with Chronic Complications	96	Specified Heart Arrhythmias
19	Diabetes without Complication	99	Intracranial Hemorrhage
21	Protein-Calorie Malnutrition	100	Ischemic or Unspecified Stroke
22	Morbid Obesity	103	Hemiplegia/Hemiparesis
23	Other Significant Endocrine and Metabolic Disorders	104	Monoplegia, Other Paralytic Syndromes
27	End-Stage Liver Disease	106	Atherosclerosis of the Extremities with Ulceration or Gangrene
28	Cirrhosis of Liver	107	Vascular Disease with Complications
29	Chronic Hepatitis	108	Vascular Disease
33	Intestinal Obstruction/Perforation	110	Cystic Fibrosis
34	Chronic Pancreatitis	111	Chronic Obstructive Pulmonary Disease
35	Inflammatory Bowel Disease	112	Fibrosis of Lung and Other Chronic Lung Disorders
39	Bone/Joint/Muscle Infections/Necrosis	114	Aspiration and Specified Bacterial Pneumonias
40	Rheumatoid Arthritis and Inflammatory Connective Tissue Disease	115	Pneumococcal Pneumonia, Empyema, Lung Abscess
46	Severe Hematological Disorders	122	Proliferative Diabetic Retinopathy and Vitreous Hemorrhage
47	Disorders of Immunity	124	Exudative Macular Degeneration
48	Coagulation Defects and Other Specified Hematological Disorders	134	Dialysis Status
51	Dementia With Complications	135	Acute Renal Failure
52	Dementia Without Complication	136	Chronic Kidney Disease, Stage 5
54	Substance Use with Psychotic Complications	137	Chronic Kidney Disease, Severe (Stage 4)
55	Substance Use Disorder, Moderate/Severe, or Substance Use with Complications	138	Chronic Kidney Disease, Moderate (Stage 3)
56	Substance Use Disorder, Mild, Except Alcohol and Cannabis	157	Pressure Ulcer of Skin with Necrosis Through to Muscle, Tendon, or Bone
57	Schizophrenia	158	Pressure Ulcer of Skin with Full Thickness Skin Loss
58	Reactive and Unspecified Psychosis	159	Pressure Ulcer of Skin with Partial Thickness Skin Loss
59	Major Depressive, Bipolar, and Paranoid Disorders	161	Chronic Ulcer of Skin, Except Pressure
60	Personality Disorders	162	Severe Skin Burn or Condition
70	Quadriplegia	166	Severe Head Injury
71	Paraplegia	167	Major Head Injury
72	Spinal Cord Disorders/Injuries	169	Vertebral Fractures without Spinal Cord Injury
73	Amyotrophic Lateral Sclerosis and Other Motor Neuron Disease	170	Hip Fracture/Dislocation
74	Cerebral Palsy	173	Traumatic Amputations and Complications
75	Myasthenia Gravis/Myoneural Disorders and Guillain-Barre Syndrome/Inflammatory and Toxic Neuropathy	176	Complications of Specified Implanted Device or Graft
76	Muscular Dystrophy	186	Major Organ Transplant or Replacement Status
77	Multiple Sclerosis	188	Artificial Openings for Feeding or Elimination
78	Parkinson's and Huntington's Diseases	189	Amputation Status, Lower Limb/Amputation Complications

HCC Codes and Descriptions (HHS-HCC v07)

#	Description	#	Description
1	HIV/AIDS	62	Congenital/Developmental Skeletal and Connective Tissue Disorders
2	Septicemia, Sepsis, Systemic Inflammatory Response Syndrome/Shock	63	Cleft Lip/Cleft Palate
3	Central Nervous System Infections, Except Viral Meningitis	64	Major Congenital Anomalies of Diaphragm, Abdominal Wall, and Esophagus, Age < 2
4	Viral or Unspecified Meningitis	66	Hemophilia
6	Opportunistic Infections	67	Myelodysplastic Syndromes and Myelofibrosis
8	Metastatic Cancer	68	Aplastic Anemia
9	Lung, Brain, and Other Severe Cancers, Including Pediatric Acute Lymphoid Leukemia	69	Acquired Hemolytic Anemia, Including Hemolytic Disease of Newborn
10	Non-Hodgkin's Lymphomas and Other Cancers and Tumors	70	Sickle Cell Anemia (Hb-SS)
11	Colorectal, Breast (Age < 50), Kidney, and Other Cancers	71	Beta Thalassemia Major
12	Breast (Age 50+) and Prostate Cancer, Benign/Uncertain Brain Tumors, and Other Cancers and Tumors	73	Combined and Other Severe Immunodeficiencies
13	Thyroid Cancer, Melanoma, Neurofibromatosis, and Other Cancers and Tumors	74	Disorders of the Immune Mechanism
18	Pancreas Transplant Status/Complications	75	Coagulation Defects and Other Specified Hematological Disorders
19	Diabetes with Acute Complications	81	Drug Use with Psychotic Complications
20	Diabetes with Chronic Complications	82	Drug Use Disorder, Moderate/Severe, or Drug Use with Non-Psychotic Complications
21	Diabetes without Complication	83	Alcohol Use with Psychotic Complications
23	Protein-Calorie Malnutrition	84	Alcohol Use Disorder, Moderate/Severe, or Alcohol Use with Specified Non-Psychotic Complications
26	Mucopolysaccharidosis	87_1	Schizophrenia
27	Lipidoses and Glycogenosis	87_2	Delusional and Other Specified Psychotic Disorders, Unspecified Psychosis
28	Congenital Metabolic Disorders, Not Elsewhere Classified	88	Major Depressive and Bipolar Disorders
29	Amyloidosis, Porphyria, and Other Metabolic Disorders	90	Personality Disorders
30	Adrenal, Pituitary, and Other Significant Endocrine Disorders	94	Anorexia/Bulimia Nervosa
34	Liver Transplant Status/Complications	96	Prader-Willi, Patau, Edwards, and Autosomal Deletion Syndromes
35_1	Acute Liver Failure/Disease, Including Neonatal Hepatitis	97	Down Syndrome, Fragile X, Other Chromosomal Anomalies, and Congenital Malformation Syndromes
35_2	Chronic Liver Failure/End-Stage Liver Disorders	102	Autistic Disorder
36	Cirrhosis of Liver	103	Pervasive Developmental Disorders, Except Autistic Disorder
37_1	Chronic Viral Hepatitis C	106	Traumatic Complete Lesion Cervical Spinal Cord
37_2	Chronic Hepatitis, Except Chronic Viral Hepatitis C	107	Quadriplegia
41	Intestine Transplant Status/Complications	108	Traumatic Complete Lesion Dorsal Spinal Cord
42	Peritonitis/Gastrointestinal Perforation/Necrotizing Enterocolitis	109	Paraplegia
45	Intestinal Obstruction	110	Spinal Cord Disorders/Injuries
46	Chronic Pancreatitis	111	Amyotrophic Lateral Sclerosis and Other Anterior Horn Cell Disease
47	Acute Pancreatitis	112	Quadriplegic Cerebral Palsy
48	Inflammatory Bowel Disease	113	Cerebral Palsy, Except Quadriplegic
54	Necrotizing Fasciitis	114	Spina Bifida and Other Brain/Spinal/Nervous System Congenital Anomalies
55	Bone/Joint/Muscle Infections/Necrosis	115	Myasthenia Gravis/Myoneural Disorders and Guillain-Barre Syndrome/Inflammatory and Toxic Neuropathy
56	Rheumatoid Arthritis and Specified Autoimmune Disorders	117	Muscular Dystrophy
57	Systemic Lupus Erythematosus and Other Autoimmune Disorders	118	Multiple Sclerosis
61	Osteogenesis Imperfecta and Other Osteodystrophies	119	Parkinson's, Huntington's, and Spinocerebellar Disease, and Other Neurodegenerative Disorders

HCC Codes and Descriptions (HHS-HCC v07)

Code	Description	Code	Description
120	Seizure Disorders and Convulsions	204	Miscarriage with Complications
121	Hydrocephalus	205	Miscarriage with No or Minor Complications
122	Non-Traumatic Coma, Brain Compression/Anoxic Damage	207	Pregnancy with Delivery with Major Complications
123	Narcolepsy and Cataplexy	208	Pregnancy with Delivery with Complications
125	Respirator Dependence/Tracheostomy Status	209	Pregnancy with Delivery with No or Minor Complications
126	Respiratory Arrest	210	(Ongoing) Pregnancy without Delivery with Major Complications
127	Cardio-Respiratory Failure and Shock, Including Respiratory Distress Syndromes	211	(Ongoing) Pregnancy without Delivery with Complications
128	Heart Assistive Device/Artificial Heart	212	(Ongoing) Pregnancy without Delivery with No or Minor Complications
129	Heart Transplant Status/Complications	217	Chronic Ulcer of Skin, Except Pressure
130	Congestive Heart Failure	218	Extensive Third Degree Burns
131	Acute Myocardial Infarction	219	Major Skin Burn or Condition
132	Unstable Angina and Other Acute Ischemic Heart Disease	223	Severe Head Injury
135	Heart Infection/Inflammation, Except Rheumatic	226	Hip and Pelvic Fractures
137	Hypoplastic Left Heart Syndrome and Other Severe Congenital Heart Disorders	228	Vertebral Fractures without Spinal Cord Injury
138	Major Congenital Heart/Circulatory Disorders	234	Traumatic Amputations and Amputation Complications
139	Atrial and Ventricular Septal Defects, Patent Ductus Arteriosus, and Other Congenital Heart/Circulatory Disorders	242	Extremely Immature Newborns, Birthweight < 500 Grams
142	Specified Heart Arrhythmias	243	Extremely Immature Newborns, Including Birthweight 500-749 Grams
145	Intracranial Hemorrhage	244	Extremely Immature Newborns, Including Birthweight 750-999 Grams
146	Ischemic or Unspecified Stroke	245	Premature Newborns, Including Birthweight 1000-1499 Grams
149	Cerebral Aneurysm and Arteriovenous Malformation	246	Premature Newborns, Including Birthweight 1500-1999 Grams
150	Hemiplegia/Hemiparesis	247	Premature Newborns, Including Birthweight 2000-2499 Grams
151	Monoplegia, Other Paralytic Syndromes	248	Other Premature, Low Birthweight, Malnourished, or Multiple Birth Newborns
153	Atherosclerosis of the Extremities with Ulceration or Gangrene	249	Term or Post-Term Singleton Newborn, Normal or High Birthweight
154	Vascular Disease with Complications	251	Stem Cell, Including Bone Marrow, Transplant Status/Complications
156	Pulmonary Embolism and Deep Vein Thrombosis	253	Artificial Openings for Feeding or Elimination
158	Lung Transplant Status/Complications	254	Amputation Status, Lower Limb/Amputation Complications
159	Cystic Fibrosis		
160	Chronic Obstructive Pulmonary Disease, Including Bronchiectasis		
161_1	Severe Asthma		
161_2	Asthma, Except Severe		
162	Fibrosis of Lung and Other Lung Disorders		
163	Aspiration and Specified Bacterial Pneumonias and Other Severe Lung Infections		
174	Exudative Macular Degeneration		
183	Kidney Transplant Status/Complications		
184	End Stage Renal Disease		
187	Chronic Kidney Disease, Stage 5		
188	Chronic Kidney Disease, Severe (Stage 4)		
203	Ectopic and Molar Pregnancy		

HCC Codes and Descriptions (ESRD-HCC v21)

#	Description	#	Description
1	HIV/AIDS	86	Acute Myocardial Infarction
2	Septicemia, Sepsis, Systemic Inflammatory Response Syndrome/Shock	87	Unstable Angina and Other Acute Ischemic Heart Disease
6	Opportunistic Infections	88	Angina Pectoris
8	Metastatic Cancer and Acute Leukemia	96	Specified Heart Arrhythmias
9	Lung, Brain, and Other Severe Cancers	99	Cerebral Hemorrhage
10	Lymphoma and Other Cancers	100	Ischemic or Unspecified Stroke
11	Colorectal, Bladder, and Other Cancers	103	Hemiplegia/Hemiparesis
12	Breast, Prostate, and Other Cancers and Tumors	104	Monoplegia, Other Paralytic Syndromes
17	Diabetes with Acute Complications	106	Atherosclerosis of the Extremities with Ulceration or Gangrene
18	Diabetes with Chronic Complications	107	Vascular Disease with Complications
19	Diabetes without Complication	108	Vascular Disease
21	Protein-Calorie Malnutrition	110	Cystic Fibrosis
22	Morbid Obesity	111	Chronic Obstructive Pulmonary Disease
23	Other Significant Endocrine and Metabolic Disorders	112	Fibrosis of Lung and Other Chronic Lung Disorders
27	End-Stage Liver Disease	114	Aspiration and Specified Bacterial Pneumonias
28	Cirrhosis of Liver	115	Pneumococcal Pneumonia, Empyema, Lung Abscess
29	Chronic Hepatitis	122	Proliferative Diabetic Retinopathy and Vitreous Hemorrhage
33	Intestinal Obstruction/Perforation	124	Exudative Macular Degeneration
34	Chronic Pancreatitis	134	Dialysis Status
35	Inflammatory Bowel Disease	135	Acute Renal Failure
39	Bone/Joint/Muscle Infections/Necrosis	136	Chronic Kidney Disease, Stage 5
40	Rheumatoid Arthritis and Inflammatory Connective Tissue Disease	137	Chronic Kidney Disease, Severe (Stage 4)
46	Severe Hematological Disorders	138	Chronic Kidney Disease, Moderate (Stage 3)
47	Disorders of Immunity	139	Chronic Kidney Disease, Mild or Unspecified (Stages 1-2 or Unspecified)
48	Coagulation Defects and Other Specified Hematological Disorders	140	Unspecified Renal Failure
51	Dementia With Complications	141	Nephritis
52	Dementia Without Complication	157	Pressure Ulcer of Skin with Necrosis Through to Muscle, Tendon, or Bone
54	Drug/Alcohol Psychosis	158	Pressure Ulcer of Skin with Full Thickness Skin Loss
55	Drug/Alcohol Dependence	159	Pressure Ulcer of Skin with Partial Thickness Skin Loss
57	Schizophrenia	160	Pressure Pre-Ulcer Skin Changes or Unspecified Stage
58	Major Depressive, Bipolar, and Paranoid Disorders	161	Chronic Ulcer of Skin, Except Pressure
70	Quadriplegia	162	Severe Skin Burn or Condition
71	Paraplegia	166	Severe Head Injury
72	Spinal Cord Disorders/Injuries	167	Vertebral Fractures without Spinal Cord Injury
73	Amyotrophic Lateral Sclerosis and Other Motor Neuron Disease	169	Pathological Fractures, Except of Vertebrae, Hip, or Humerus
74	Cerebral Palsy	170	Hip Fracture/Dislocation
75	Polyneuropathy	173	Traumatic Amputations and Complications
76	Muscular Dystrophy	176	Complications of Specified Implanted Device or Graft
77	Multiple Sclerosis	186	Major Organ Transplant or Replacement Status
78	Parkinson's and Huntington's Diseases	188	Artificial Openings for Feeding or Elimination
79	Seizure Disorders and Convulsions	189	Amputation Status, Lower Limb/Amputation Complications
80	Coma, Brain Compression/Anoxic Damage		
82	Respirator Dependence/Tracheostomy Status		
83	Respiratory Arrest		
84	Cardio-Respiratory Failure and Shock		
85	Congestive Heart Failure		

HCC Codes and Descriptions (Rx-HCC v05)

1	HIV/AIDS	148	Mild or Unspecified Intellectual Disability/Developmental Disorder
5	Opportunistic Infections	156	Myasthenia Gravis, Amyotrophic Lateral Sclerosis and Other Motor Neuron Disease
15	Chronic Myeloid Leukemia	157	Spinal Cord Disorders
16	Multiple Myeloma and Other Neoplastic Disorders	159	Inflammatory and Toxic Neuropathy
17	Secondary Cancers of Bone, Lung, Brain, and Other Specified Sites; Liver Cancer	160	Multiple Sclerosis
18	Lung, Kidney, and Other Cancers	161	Parkinson's and Huntington's Diseases
19	Breast and Other Cancers and Tumors	163	Intractable Epilepsy
30	Diabetes with Complications	164	Epilepsy and Other Seizure Disorders, Except Intractable Epilepsy
31	Diabetes without Complication	165	Convulsions
40	Specified Hereditary Metabolic/Immune Disorders	166	Migraine Headaches
41	Pituitary, Adrenal Gland, and Other Endocrine and Metabolic Disorders	168	Trigeminal and Postherpetic Neuralgia
42	Thyroid Disorders	185	Primary Pulmonary Hypertension
43	Morbid Obesity	186	Congestive Heart Failure
45	Disorders of Lipoid Metabolism	187	Hypertension
54	Chronic Viral Hepatitis C	188	Coronary Artery Disease
55	Chronic Viral Hepatitis, Except Hepatitis C	193	Atrial Arrhythmias
65	Chronic Pancreatitis	206	Cerebrovascular Disease, Except Hemorrhage or Aneurysm
66	Pancreatic Disorders and Intestinal Malabsorption, Except Pancreatitis	207	Spastic Hemiplegia
67	Inflammatory Bowel Disease	215	Venous Thromboembolism
68	Esophageal Reflux and Other Disorders of Esophagus	216	Peripheral Vascular Disease
80	Aseptic Necrosis of Bone	225	Cystic Fibrosis
82	Psoriatic Arthropathy and Systemic Sclerosis	226	Chronic Obstructive Pulmonary Disease and Asthma
83	Rheumatoid Arthritis and Other Inflammatory Polyarthropathy	227	Pulmonary Fibrosis and Other Chronic Lung Disorders
84	Systemic Lupus Erythematosus, Other Connective Tissue Disorders, and Inflammatory Spondylopathies	241	Diabetic Retinopathy
87	Osteoporosis, Vertebral and Pathological Fractures	243	Open-Angle Glaucoma
95	Sickle Cell Anemia	260	Kidney Transplant Status
96	Myelodysplastic Syndromes and Myelofibrosis	261	Dialysis Status
97	Immune Disorders	262	Chronic Kidney Disease Stage 5
98	Aplastic Anemia and Other Significant Blood Disorders	263	Chronic Kidney Disease Stage 4
111	Alzheimer's Disease	311	Chronic Ulcer of Skin, Except Pressure
112	Dementia, Except Alzheimer's Disease	314	Pemphigus
130	Schizophrenia	316	Psoriasis, Except with Arthropathy
131	Bipolar Disorders	355	Narcolepsy and Cataplexy
132	Major Depression	395	Lung Transplant Status
133	Specified Anxiety, Personality, and Behavior Disorders	396	Major Organ Transplant Status, Except Lung, Kidney, and Pancreas
134	Depression	397	Pancreas Transplant Status
135	Anxiety Disorders	395	Lung Transplant Status
145	Autism	396	Major Organ Transplant Status, Except Lung, Kidney, and Pancreas
146	Profound or Severe Intellectual Disability/Developmental Disorder	397	Pancreas Transplant Status
147	Moderate Intellectual Disability/Developmental Disorder		

515

Figure F.4

	Hospital-acquired Condition (HAC)
01	Foreign Object Retained After Surgery
02	Air Embolism
03	Blood Incompatibility
04	Stage III and IV Pressure Ulcers
05	Falls and Trauma
06	Catheter-Associated Urinary Tract Infection (UTI)
07	Vascular Catheter-Associated Infection
08	Surgical Site Infection, Mediastinitis following Coronary Artery Bypass Graft (CABG)
09	Manifestations of Poor Glycemic Control
10	Deep Vein Thrombosis (DVT) / Pulmonary Embolism (PE) with Total Knee or Hip Replacement
11	Surgical Site Infection Following Bariatric Surgery
12	Surgical Site Infection Following Certain Orthopedic Procedures of Spine, Shoulder and Elbow
13	Surgical Site Infection (SSI) Following Cardiac Implantable Electronic Device (CIED)
14	Iatrogenic Pneumothorax with Venous Catheterization

Notes:

Notes:

Appendix G. Glossary

#

1500 Health Insurance Claim Form The industry standard used by healthcare professionals and suppliers to submit claims for reimbursement.

A

Abdomen The front part of the body that lies between the chest and pelvis (stomach).

ABN Advanced Beneficiary Notice of Noncoverage.

Abulia A lack of will or initiative. The patient is unable to act or make decisions independently. It may range from subtle to overwhelming in severity.

Abuse Billing third-party payers such as Medicare for services that are not covered or are not correctly coded.

Accept assignment A provider agrees to have the insurance payment come directly to the office instead of the patient. Generally, preferred (contracted) providers are required to accept assignment.

Accreditation Process by which an organization recognizes a program of study or an institution as meeting predetermined standards.

Acquired Produced by influences outside an organism, not genetic.

Active Care Modes of treatment requiring "active" involvement, participation, and responsibility on the part of the patient.

Activities of Daily Living (ADLs) Daily habits such as bathing, dressing and eating. ADLs are often used as an assessment tool to determine an individual's ability to function at home or in a less restricted environment of care.

Actual Charge A provider's usual fee for a service as indicated on a *1500 Claim Form*. This is not the charge billed to the patient, which may be limited by contract with that payer.

Acupuncture A practice in which needles are inserted into specific acupoints and manipulated for induction of anesthesia, relief of pain and other various conditions.

Acute Refers to the condition that is the primary reason for the current encounter. Of short duration and relatively severe.

Acute Condition Conditions are considered "acute" within the first 4-8 weeks post-injury/illness.

Acute Headache or Migraine abrupt, severe

Adaptive Behavior A collection of conceptual, social, and practical skills that people learn in order to function in their daily lives.

Add-on Code Describes additional intra-service work associated with the primary procedure.

Addenda Official updates to HIPAA approved code sets.

Adverse Any response to a drug that is noxious, unintended, and occurs with proper dosage.

Afferent Carrying impulses towards a center; when sensory nerve impulses are sent toward the brain.

Aftercare An encounter for something planned in advance, for example, cast removal.

Aggravation Worsening of a preexisting impairment in such a way that the degree of permanent impairment is increased.

-algia A suffix meaning "pain," as in neuralgia.

Alignment Establishing a straight line between structures.

Allowed (approved) amount The amount a third-party payer determines is their fee for a procedure or service. It may be less than the provider's actual charge.

Anesthesia Loss of sensation caused by administration of a drug or other medical intervention.

Ankylosis Stiffness of a joint due to abnormal adhesion and rigidity of the bones of the joint, which may be the result of injury or disease

APM An Alternative Payment Model (APM) is a Medicare payment model which includes incentive payments for providing high-quality and cost-efficient care. APMs can apply to a specific clinical condition, a care episode, or a population. Advanced APMs are part of the Quality Payment Program.

Appeals process Legal means by which a provider may dispute reimbursements or determinations made by a third-party payer.

Apportionment Distribution or allocation of causation among multiple factors that caused or significantly contributed to the injury or disease and existing impairment.

Assisted Living Care A living arrangement for individuals who are unable to live independently. Provides mid-level custodial care, medication management and transportation.

Aquatic Therapy with Therapeutic Exercises "any type of exercise performed in a water environment. DO NOT code the water modality (eg, hubbard tank, whirlpool) and the type of therapeutic exercise (eg, neuromuscular reeducation) separately. Code only the aquatic therapy with therapeutic exercise, 97113." - *AMA CPT Assistant; Summer 1995*

ARRA American Recovery and Reinvestment Act of 2009 is the legislation which created HITECH and added funding for many other programs, including incentives for adopting health information technology.

Assessment An evaluation or appraisal.

Atrophy The wasting away or gradual decline of effectiveness, usually due to degeneration of cells.

Automobile Medical Expense Insurance (Med-Pay) Component of automobile insurance that provides compensation for healthcare services rendered for injuries to the driver and passengers of the subscriber's automobile, or to the subscriber if injured in another party's automobile.

Autonomic Nervous System The part of the nervous system that regulates involuntary action, e.g., the intestines, heart, and glands; comprised of the sympathetic and parasympathetic nervous systems.

B

Balance Billing Procedure of billing a patient for the remaining amount, after the payer has completed payment and any required/appropriate write-offs have been taken.

Bilateral Pertaining to both sides of the body or structure.

Biofeedback A training technique that enables an individual to gain some element of voluntary control over autonomic body functions.

Biomechanics The application of mechanical laws to living structures.

Brace An orthopedic device used to align or hold parts of the body in place.

Brain Stem The "primitive" (oldest) area of the brain that extends down into the cervical area of the spinal cord.

Bundling (CPT Codes) process in which the submitted CPT Code is incorporated by the payer into another submitted CPT code.

C

Capitation Reimbursement system where a payer reimburses a provider a predetermined list of services to an insured for a specified number of days.

Carrier Insurer that underwrites or administers life, health, or other insurance programs.

Case Management Method designed to monitor and coordinate specific health services of an insured to achieve the desired health outcome in a cost-effective manner.

Cast An artificial reproduction of a body part; a rigid dressing.

Category Refers to ICD-10-CM diagnosis codes listed within a specific three-character category, for example, category E10 Type 1 diabetes mellitus.

Cause That which brings about any condition or produces any effect.

Central Nervous System The brain and spinal cord.

Cerebellum The "hind" brain.

Centers for Medicare and Medicaid Services (CMS) The federal agency which administers Medicare, Medicaid, and the Children's Health Insurance Program.

CERT Comprehensive Error Rate Testing. Helps determine the national error rate for Medicare Fee-For-Service programs.

Certified Community Behavioral Health Clinic (CCBHC) A new type of payment model created by section 223 of the Protecting Access to Medicare Act (PAMA). Currently undergoing a two-year demonstration program.

CHAMPUS and CHAMPVA The Civilian Health and Medical Program of the Uniformed Services, and the Medical Program of the Veteran Services.

Charge Price of a service provided by a practitioner.

Chief Complaint A concise statement describing the symptom, problem, condition, diagnosis or other factor that is reason for the encounter.

Chronic Continuing over a long period of time or recurring frequently.

Chronic Care Management Primary care services that contribute to better health and care for individuals with chronic conditions, as well as reduced spending. CMS does not recognize these services for patients who reside in a facility.

Chronic Headache or Migraine Occurring 15 or more days per month for at least six months.

Cloud Computing Using a network of remote servers hosted on the Internet to store, manage, and process data, rather than a local server or a personal computer.

Cluster Headache Occurs in cyclical patterns or clusters, usually over a period of several weeks. Pain is usually limited to one side of the head and around the eye.

Combination Code In ICD-10-CM, a single code which classifies two or more diagnoses or a diagnosis with an associated complication or manifestation.

Community Mental Health Center (CMHC) A healthcare facility or network of agencies organized to provide a coordinated program of providing mental health care services.

Comorbidity Is the simultaneous presence of two chronic diseases or conditions in a patient. Example: "the comorbidity of anxiety and depression in Parkinson's disease."

Conscious Sedation *See Moderate (conscious sedation)*

Constant Attendance Requires direct (one-on-one) patient contact by physician or other qualified healthcare professional. Involves visual, verbal, and/or manual contact with patient during service.

Contracture Stiffness or constriction in muscles, joints, tendons, ligaments, or skin, that restricts normal movement.

Contrast Bath "Alternate immersion of a body part in hot water (98-112 degrees fahrenheit) and cold water (60-75 degrees fahrenheit)." - *AMA CPT Assistant; Summer 1995*

Co-Payment The portion that an insurance policy designates as the amount for which the patient is responsible. New legislation waives co-pays for some preventive services.

Corporate Integrity Agreement (CIA) A document that outlines the obligations an individual practitioner or small group practice agrees to as part of a civil settlement in order to be able to continue to participate in federal healthcare programs.

CPT Current Procedural Terminology (CPT) is the HIPAA-approved coding system developed by the American Medical Association.

Credentialing Payer review procedure where an applying, or participating provider must meet payer network participation standards in order to begin, or continue participation, in the payer network.

Cryo- A prefix meaning "low temperature," as in cryotherapy.

CT Scan Computed Tomography, formerly known as CAT Scan or Computer Aided Tomography, which uses pencil-thin X-ray beams and a computer to create a type of three-dimensional X-ray.

D

Date of Service (DOS) Date a healthcare service was rendered by the provider to an insured.

Deductible The amount that the beneficiary is responsible for during each calendar year before health insurance benefits begin. This applies only to services and supplies covered by the health insurance policy approved amounts–not actual charges.

Department of Defense (DOD) The federal agency which administers the healthcare programs for the military and their families. This includes DOD, TriCare and the Department of Veterans Affairs Hospitals and programs.

Department of Veterans Affairs (VA) The federal agency that provides patient care and federal benefits to veterans and their dependents.

derma- A prefix meaning "skin," as in dermatome.

Dermatomes Areas of skin sensitivity that reflect the function of specific nerves distributed from the spinal cord.

Detailed An extended history or examination of the affected body area(s) and other symptomatic or related organ system(s).

Diagnosis An expert opinion identifying the nature and cause of a patient's concern or complaint, and/or abnormal finding(s).

Diagnostic Statement The problem statement or clinical impression of the assessment worded in a manner that correlates with ICD-10-CM terminology.

Diathermy The therapeutic use of high frequency electrical current to create a heat response within an area of the body. diathermy (eg, microwave) (1 or more areas) "Creates heat in the soft tissues, due to the resistance offered by the tissues, by the passage of high frequency electrical currents. The objective of this treatment is to cause vasodilatation and/or muscle relaxation, with subsequent pain relief. Diathermy energy can cause a greater rise in deep tissue temperature than any form of infrared energy." - *AMA CPT Assistant; Summer 1995*

Differential Diagnosis The determination of which of two or more disorders with similar symptoms is the one from which the patient is suffering, by a systematic comparison and contrasting of the clinical findings.

Disability Alternation of an individual's capacity to meet personal, social, or occupational demands or statutory or regulatory requirements because of an impairment.

Disease Any deviation from or interruption of the normal structure or function of any part, organ, or system of the body that is manifested by a characteristic set of symptoms whose prognosis may be known or unknown.

Documentation The recording of pertinent facts and observations about a patient's health history and physical examination of the system(s) applicable to the current encounter.

DOD *See Department of Defense.*

Domiciliary Care A supervised living arrangement in a home-like environment for individuals who are unable to live alone due to age-related impairments or physical, mental or visual disabilities.

Downcoding The process whereby insurance carriers reduce the value of a procedure and the resulting reimbursement, due to either 1) a mismatch of CPT code and description or 2) ICD-10-CM code does not justify the procedure or level of service.

Drug Induced Headache Also known as medication-overuse headache. Occurs more than 15 days per month for at least three months and develops or is markedly worse during medication overuse.

DSM-5 Diagnostic and Statistical Manual of Mental Disorders (DSM) is a standard classification of mental disorders utilizing a set of diagnostic criteria to arrive at a diagnosis. It is not a HIPAA-approved code set for diagnostic reporting, but DSM codes refer to ICD-10-CM codes.

Dys- A prefix meaning "abnormal," as in dysfunction.

E

-ectomy A suffix meaning "cutting out," as in hysterectomy.

Edema A condition in which fluid fills a damaged joint area with excessive fluid, causing swelling, similar to that of a sprained ankle.

Efferent Carrying away from a central organ; nerve impulses leaving the brain to peripheral tissues.

Electronic Data Interchange (EDI) Automated exchange of data and documents in a standardized format. In health care, some common uses of this technology include claims submission and payment, eligibility, and referral authorization.

Electronic Health Record (EHR) An electronic record of health-related information for an individual that conforms to national standards for interoperability, which can be created, managed, and consulted by authorized clinicians and staff across more than one healthcare organization.

Electronic Medical Record (EMR) An electronic record of health-related information for an individual, which can be created, gathered, managed, and consulted by authorized clinicians and staff within one healthcare organization. The data does not need to conform to any standards.

ePHI Electronic Protected Health Information ePHI is any electronic version of protected health information as defined by HIPAA/HITECH regulations. *See also PHI.*

EMG Electromyograph a device used to measure muscle contraction resulting from electrical stimulation.

Employer Liability Employers can be held liable for their own actions or any actions committed by their employees that are within the scope of employment.

EMS Electro-Muscle Stimulation; a form of electrical stimulation designed to help reduce swelling and inflammation.

Episode of Care For ICD-10-CM, this refers to the 7th characters indicating the type of the encounter (e.g., initial, subsequent). From a procedural perspective, it is the set of all clinically-related services provided to treat a clinical condition or procedure from the onset of symptoms until maximum therapeutic benefit is reached.

Episodic Headache Occurring greater than one but less than 15 days per month for at least three months. Lasting a minimum of 30 minutes per headache. Does not include nausea or vomiting.

Eponyms Medical procedures or conditions named after a person or place.

ERISA The Employee Retirement Income Security Act is a federal law that sets standards of protection for individuals in most voluntarily established, private-sector retirement plans. This includes requirements for employer sponsored benefits such as pension and health plans.

ERISA appeals The process for appealing incorrectly adjudicated claims for employee sponsored health plans.

Established patient One who has received professional services from the physician or another physician of the same specialty who belongs to the same group practice, within the past three years.

Ethical behavior boundaries Fulfilling responsibilities with integrity and honesty.

Etiology The cause(s) or origin of a disease.

Evaluation and Management (E/M) A category of service in the CPT to express various patient encounters.

Exacerbation An exacerbation is a temporary, marked deterioration of the patient's condition because of an acute flare-up of the condition being treated.

Examination The process of inspecting and testing the body and its systems to determine the presence or absence of disease or injury.

Exertional Headache A headache that is brought on by any form of exercise. May last from five minutes to 48 hours and may be accompanied by the following: sensitivity to light, sensitivity to sound, nausea, vomiting.

Explanation of Benefits (EOB) also referred to as Explanation of Medical Benefits (EOMB). Statement from the payer sent to a provider and an insured explaining services provided, services denied, amount billed, amount owed by the insured, amount not paid, amount paid by the insurer, denial reasons, etc.

External Appeal An appeal made to request the right of an independent review of a patient's case.

F

False Claims Act (FCA) Helps prevent persons and companies from defrauding government programs.

Federal Bureau of Investigation (FBI) The FBI investigates violations of federal criminal law and provides law enforcement assistance to federal, state, local, and international agencies. The FBI has investigated practitioners for fraud and abuse.

Federal Trade Commission (FTC) This commission deals with both consumer protection and competition jurisdiction in broad sectors of the economy. The FTC pursues vigorous and effective law enforcement, and shares its expertise with other federal and state agencies, such as HHS.

Fee for Service (FFS) Specific payment amounts for specified services rendered/received.

Fee Schedule List of established fees, or maximum amounts allowed, for specified healthcare services.

Fraud The intentional deception or misrepresentation that the individual knows to be false or does not believe to be true, perpetrated to gain some unauthorized benefit.

Frontal Pertaining to the front.

Functional Brain Mapping Testing of language, memory, motor skills, memory, sensation and other functions. Performed during the imaging procedure.

Functional limitation Inability to completely perform a task due to an impairment.

G

Gait Training "training of the manner or style of walking, including rhythm and speed. Three phases of gait include the stance phase, the swing phase, and the double support phase." - *AMA CPT Assistant; Summer 1995*

Gatekeeper Entity responsible for overseeing and coordinating all aspects of an insured's healthcare including preauthorizing a referral to a specialist.

Global Fee Comprehensive reimbursement, for one or more related services, rendered on a date of service.

-graph A suffix meaning "record," as in radiograph.

Grievance Procedure Formal appeal process by which an insured or provider can voice a complaint and seek a remedy.

H

Habilitation Refers to health care services that help a person acquire, keep or improve, partially or fully, and at different points in life, skills related to communication and activities of daily living. These services address the competencies and abilities needed for optimal functioning in interaction with their environments. Habilitative services include physical therapy, occupational therapy, speech-language pathology, audiology and other services for people with disabilities in a variety of inpatient and/or outpatient settings.

HCPCS Healthcare Common Procedure Coding System is the HIPAA-approved code set for specified supplies and services.

Health A state of optimal physical, mental, and social well-being and not merely the absence of disease and infirmity.

Health Information Exchange (HIE) The electronic movement of health-related information among organizations according to nationally recognized standards.

Health Information Organization (HIO) An organization that oversees and governs health information exchange among organizations, according to nationally recognized standards.

Health Insurance Portability and Accountability Act of 1996 This law is comprised of two sections. The first title protects workers' health insurance coverage when they change or lose their job. The second title establishes national standards for electronic health transactions.

HHS Department of Health and Human Services

Hierarchy A system that ranks items one above another.

HIPAA *See Health Insurance Portability and Accountability Act of 1996.*

History of Present Illness A chronological description of the development of the patient's present illness from the first sign and/or symptom to the present.

HITECH Enforcement Rule A section of the American Recovery and Reinvestment Act of 2009 that contains breach notification provisions and increases fines and penalties for all HIPAA violations.

Homeostasis A state of physiological equilibrium produced by a balance of functions and chemical composition within an organism.

Hubbard Tank "A tank designed for full immersion of the body for hydrotherapy. A narrow section at the middle of the tank allows the provider to reach the patient, and a wider section at each end permits full abduction of the patient's legs and arms. The tank is fitted with an aerator that agitates the water and provides gentle massage and debridement of wounds. Useful in the treatment of burns and chronic multiple joint disorders." - AMA CPT Assistant; Summer 1995

Hyper- A prefix meaning "over," as in hypertension.

Hypermobility Excess movement of an area.

Hypnic Headache Type of headache that most commonly occurs at night during dreaming. Onset is usually after the age of 50. May occur 15 or more times per month with no known trigger. Headaches may last from 15 minutes to 3 hours and are most often felt on both sides of the head. Other symptoms may include nausea and sensitivity to light or sound.

Hypo- A prefix meaning "under," as in hypoglycemic.

Hypomobility Restricted movement of an area.

I

ICD-10-CM International Classification of Diseases, 10th Revision, Clinical Modification. Use of ICD-10-CM codes began on October 1, 2015.

ICD-9-CM International Classification of Diseases, 9th Revision, Clinical Modification (ICD-9-CM) is the current HIPAA approved code set for diagnoses up to September 30, 2015.

Idiopathic Of uncertain or unknown origin

Imaging Radiological production of a clinical image using X-rays, ultrasound, computed tomography, magnetic resonance, radionuclide scanning, thermography, etc.

Immobilization The process of holding a joint or bone in place with a device such as splint, cast, or brace in order to prevent an injured area from moving while it heals.

Impairment An impairment is considered permanent when it has reached maximum medical improvement. Loss, loss of use, or derangement of any body part, organ system, or organ function.

Indemnity Insurance Healthcare insurance that relies on fee-for-service reimbursement and defines the maximum amounts reimbursed for covered services.

Independent Medical Examination (IME) Evaluation performed by an independent examiner, who evaluates but does not provide care for the individual.

Independent Practice Association (IPA) or Organization (IPO) Delivery model in which an insurer contracts with a physician organization, which in turn contracts with individual physicians. The IPA physicians practice in their own offices and continue to also see their fee-for-service patients. The insurer reimburses the IPA on a capitated basis; however, the IPA may reimburse the physicians on an FFS or capitated basis.

Infrared "Modality which uses light and heat to raise the tissue temperature 5 to 10 degrees centigrade in the area of application." - AMA CPT Assistant; Summer 1995

Inferior Lower in position.

Inflammation A reaction of soft tissue due to injury that may include malfunction, discomfort, rise in temperature, swelling, and increased blood supply.

Indian Health Service (IHS) The federal agency which administers the healthcare programs for American Indians and Alaska Natives. It is a division of the Department of Health and Human Services (HHS).

Inpatient Care Care given a registered bed patient in a hospital, nursing home, or other medical institution.

Insurance Reform A term broadly used to encompass legislative discussions and laws intended to improve the healthcare system in the U.S.

Insurance Reimbursement The process by which providers request compensation from insurance companies.

Insurance Verification Process by which you determine if the patient has insurance coverage before providing any services.

Insurer Underwrites or administers life, health or other insurance programs.

Inter- A prefix meaning "between," as in intersegmental.

Interactive Complexity Specific communication factors such as high anxiety and the use of interpreters which complicate the delivery of psychiatric procedures. *See Chapter 5.3 for additional information.*

Interference Damage or deficit to the nervous system.

Intractable Not easily managed (such as with medications).

Iontophoresis The process of using a small electric charge to deliver medicine through the skin. "The introduction of ions of soluble salts into the body by an electric current." - *AMA CPT Assistant; Summer 1995*

-itis A suffix meaning "inflammation," as in arthritis.

L

Late Effect A residual effect (condition produced) after the acute phase of an illness or injury has ended.

Lateral The side view of the body.

Liens and Assignment Legal process by which providers receive reimbursement for treatment provided to a patient.

Letters of Appeal Letter which contains a compelling case for medical necessity, and thus payment of a claim.

Limiting Charge A cap on how much Non-Participating physicians may bill Medicare patients.

Listing A system used to describe the motion or position of vertebral segments in relation to adjacent vertebral segments.

-lysis The breaking down of a membrane by cell, often by viral, enzymic, or osmotic mechanisms.

M

MACRA The Medicare Access and CHIP Reauthorization Act of 2015 repealed the SGR physician payment formula and combined parts of the Physician Quality Reporting System (PQRS), Value-based Payment Modifier (VBM), and the Medicare Electronic Health Record (EHR) incentive program into one single program called the Merit-based Incentive Payment System (MIPS).

Maintenance Care This therapy includes services that seek to prevent disease, promote health and prolong and enhance the quality of life, or maintain or prevent deterioration of a chronic condition.

Managed Care Techniques intended to reduce unnecessary health costs.

Manifestation Characteristic signs or symptoms of an illness.

Manual Therapy Procedure by which the hands directly contact the body to treat articulations and/or soft tissues.

Massage Methodical pressure, friction and kneading of the body upon bare skin.

Maximum Medical Improvement (MMI) Condition or state that is well stabilized and unlikely to change substantially in the next year, with or without treatment.

Maximum Therapeutic Benefit (MTB) Return to pre-injury/illness status or failure to improve beyond a certain level of symptomatology or disability, whatever the treatment/care approach.

Medicaid Health insurance program that provides financial medical assistance to those who can't afford to pay for coverage according to state specified levels of poverty.

Medical Decision Making (MDM) A term by the American Medical Association for Clinical Decision Making to describe the process of establishing a diagnosis and/or selecting one of four different management option levels of service.

Medical Ethics Moral principles that apply to practicing medicine.

Medical Necessity Related to activities which may be justified as reasonable treatment for a given condition.

Medical Payments Coverage (Med-Pay) Component of automobile insurance that provides compensation for healthcare services rendered for injuries as defined by policy.

Medical Record Also known as health record. The documentation of a patient's medical history, care and treatment by a provider.

Medicare The federal health insurance program for people over the age of 65 and other individuals with disabilities due to specific diseases.

Medicare Administrative Contractor (MAC) Formerly known as "carriers," they produce Local Coverage Determinations (LCDs) for the jurisdictions they serve.

Medicare Non-Par fee allowance Medicare non-participating provider allowance. This is 95% of the Par Fee Allowance.

Medicare Par Fee allowance Medicare participating provider allowance.

Medicare Supplemental Insurance (MediGap)/Supplement Health insurance sold by private insurance companies to fill the "gaps" in Original Medicare Plan coverage. Medigap policies help pay some of the healthcare costs that the Original Medicare Plan doesn't cover – normally, this would be the deductible and coinsurance for covered services. Medigap policies must follow Federal and state laws and the front of a Medigap policy must clearly identify it as "Medicare Supplement Insurance".

Medigap A supplemental private insurance policy for extra benefits not covered or not fully covered by Medicare.

Menstrual Migraine Migraines that affect women around the time of their menstrual cycle.

MIPS The Merit-Based Incentive Payment System is a program legislated by MACRA that replaced the three current incentive programs (EHR, PQRS, and Value Based Payment Modifier (VBM)).

Modifiers Codes that modify a procedure code without changing the actual code.

Moderate (Conscious) Sedation Uses drugs to depress patient consciousness to the level that the patient can still respond purposefully to verbal commands. Can be given alone or accompanied with light tactile stimulation. Different than minimal or deep sedation or monitored anesthesia care.

MRI Magnetic Resonance Imaging The use of strong magnets and radio waves to create an image of the internal structures of the body.

Multiple Codes Refers to the need to use more than one ICD-10-CM code to fully identify and code a condition. Use a combination code if one exists.

Mutually Exclusive Edits Identifies code pairs that are unlikely to be performed on a patient on the same day, according to the NCCI.

Myalgia Pain in a muscle or group of muscles

Myo- A prefix meaning "muscle," as in myofascitis.

N

NA Not applicable.

National Committee for Quality Assurance (NCQA) Non-profit managed care organization accreditation agency created to improve patient care quality and health plan performance in partnership with managed care plans, purchasers, consumers, and the public sector.

National Correct Coding Initiative (NCCI) Rules provided by CMS to control improper coding that leads to incorrect payment on Part B insurance claims.

National Practitioner Data Bank (NPDB) Computerized data bank maintained by the Federal Government that compiles information on providers against whom malpractice claims have been paid or certain disciplinary actions have been taken.

NE Not Established.

NEC Not Elsewhere Classified.

Neural Canal The opening in the spine through which the spinal cord passes.

Neuritis The inflammation of a nerve.

Neuro- A prefix meaning "nerve," as in neurocanal.

Neuralgia Pain along the course of a nerve

Neurological Pertaining to the nervous system.

Neuropathy Pain, weakness, numbness or difficulty controlling specific muscles due to nerve damage

New Daily Persistent Headache (NDPH) Daily headache that does not relax or lessen from onset or from less than three days from onset. Includes the following criteria: sensitivity to light, sound and mild nausea. Will include at least two of the following pain characteristics: bilateral location, pressing/tightening (non-pulsating) quality, mild or moderate intensity, not aggravated by routine physical activity.

New Patient One who has not received any professional services from the physician or another physician of the same specialty who belongs to the same group practice, within the past three years (this does not apply in all situations, such as an emergency department revisit).

No-Fault Insurance Automobile insurance that provides coverage under the subscriber's policy regardless of who was at fault in an automobile accident.

Non-Participating Provider A provider who chooses not to sign the Medicare Participation agreement. These providers can choose to accept assignment on a case-by-case basis; however, services that are unassigned are subject to the "limiting charge" restriction.

NOS Not Otherwise Specified.

Not Intractable Responds well to some treatment - manageable

NPI National Provider Identifier A 10-digit number that is required for all electronic HIPAA transactions.

NUCC National Uniform Claim Committee

Nursing Facility A licensed health-care facility providing long term medical/nursing care, or short term rehabilitation services for injured, disabled or sick individuals.

O

Objective Findings What the healthcare provider finds by examination and evaluation.

Oblique Slanting; diagonal.

Occipital Pertaining to the lower, posterior (back) portion of the head or skull.

Office of Audit Services (OAS) The federal agency responsible for overseeing auditing services designed to examine the performance of HHS programs in order to reduce waste, abuse, mismanagement, and to promote HHS economy and efficiency.

Office of Civil Rights (OCR) The federal agency responsible for enforcing the HIPAA Privacy and Security Rules.

Office of Counsel to the Inspector General (OCIG) The federal agency responsible for providing general legal services (including fraud and abuse cases) to the OIG. Office of Evaluation and Inspections (OEI) Conducts national evaluations to provide information and recommendations to prevent fraud, waste, or abuse, and to promote the economy, efficiency, and effectiveness of federal programs.

Office of Investigations (OI) Conducts criminal, civil, and administrative investigations of fraud and misconduct related to HHS programs. OI investigative efforts often lead to criminal convictions, administrative sanctions, and/or civil monetary penalties.

Office of Inspector General (OIG) The federal agency responsible for protecting the integrity of HHS programs by eliminating waste and fraud in these programs.

Offset The recovery by Medicare of a non-Medicare debt by reducing present or future Medicare payments and applying the amount withheld to the debt incurred.

-ology A suffix meaning "study of," as in biology.

Open Panel Designation indicating a payer is currently accepting new providers to participate in a payer network.

Opt Out An official designation for a provider who agrees to operate outside the Medicare system. When a provider opts out of Medicare, he or she opts out of all Medicare programs and plans for a two year period. This option is only available to certain types of healthcare providers.

-osis A suffix meaning functional disease or condition. Abnormal increase.

-opathy A suffix meaning a disease or disorder.

Osteo- A prefix meaning "bone," as in osteoarthritis.

Other Qualified Healthcare Provider An individual who by education, training, licensure/regulation, and facility privileging (when applicable) who performs a professional service within his/her scope of practice and in accordance with third-party payer requirements. *See Resource 475 for information.*

Out-of-Area Benefits Healthcare benefits available to an insured patient while the insured is outside the payer network geographic service area.

Out-of-Network Benefits Healthcare benefits available to an insured while the insured is in the payer's geographic service area and receives service from a non-participating provider.

Out-of-Network Provider Healthcare provider who is not participating in a payer network.

Outcomes Assessment Process by which quality of health care is researched and measured.

Overpayment Assessment A decision that an incorrect amount of money has been paid for Medicare services and a determination of what that amount is.

P

Palliative Treatment Treatment that relieves symptoms but not the cause of the symptom.

Palpation Physical examination with your fingers; the art of feeling with the hand.

Part A Medicare insurance that covers institutional services for inpatients that are then billed by the hospital to the Medicare contractor. Individual providers do not submit claims for Part A services.

Part B Medicare insurance which helps to pay for all physician services that are medically necessary, outpatient hospital care and some other medical services that Part A does not cover. Also known as fee-for-service.

Part C Also known as Medicare Advantage, this program allows Medicare-approved private insurance companies to provide Part A, B, and D benefits but with different rules, costs, and coverage restrictions. With this program, there could be lower costs and extra benefits. Does not always include the same benefits as traditional Medicare.

Participating Provider A provider who agrees to "accept assignment" for all services provided to all Medicare patients for the following year. The provider signs a Participation agreement and accepts the Participating provider fee schedule.

Passive care Application of treatment procedures by the caregiver to the patient who "passively" submits to and receives care.

Patho- A prefix meaning "disease," as in pathology.

Pathology Structural and functional manifestations of disease.

Patient Liability Amount an insured is legally obligated to pay for services rendered.

Payer (or payor) Insurer that underwrites or administers life, health, or other insurance programs.

PECOS (Provider Enrollment Chain and Ownership System) Medicare's electronic provider and supplier enrollment system.

Pediatrics The care of infants and children and the treatment or prevention of their common health disorders.

Peer Review Evaluation of healthcare services, by healthcare personnel of similar training, to evaluate quality and appropriateness (e.g., necessity, frequency, efficacy) of care provided.

Peer Review Organization (PRO) Organizations that review medical records and claims to evaluate quality and appropriateness (e.g., necessity, frequency, efficacy) of care provided.

Periodic Headache Recurring headache at regular or intermittent intervals. May or may not be accompanied by symptoms. Intensity and duration may vary as well.

Peripheral Nervous System The nervous system that connects the central nervous system with every cell, tissue, and organ of the body.

Personal Health Record (PHR) An electronic record of health-related information for an individual that conforms to national standards for interoperability, which can be managed, shared, and controlled by the individual.

Personal Injury (PI) Case involving medical conditions arising from an automobile crash or an accident occurring in a home or at a business site.

Personal Injury Protection (PIP) component of automobile insurance that provides compensation for healthcare services rendered for injuries as defined by policy.

PHI *See Protected Health Information.*

Physical Therapy Modalities and treatments within the Physical Medicine Rehabilitation section of the CPT codebook.

Physiology The biological science of essential and characteristic life processes, activities, and functions; the vital processes of an organism.

Physiotherapy Treatment with physical and/or mechanical means, such as massage, electricity, etc.

-plegia A suffix meaning "paralysis," as in paraplegia.

Point-of-Service (POS) Health insurance benefits program in which subscribers can select between different delivery systems (e.g., HMO, PPO, and fee-for-service) at the time of accessing services rather than making the selection at time of open enrollment.

Policy Limits Maximum coverage allowed by a benefits policy. It usually refers to a "dollar limit" or a "visit limit" for a specific service or category of care.

POMR (Problem Oriented Medical Record) A record-keeping methodology for reporting the health status of a patient. SOAP is one component of the POMR.

Post-Examination An examination used to monitor the healing process and the patient's progress towards recovery.

Post-Traumatic Headache Commonly follows a mild to severe head injury.

Posterior Toward the back of the body.

Post-Payment Audit An audit that is conducted after claims have been paid. Typically performed by the payer to discover and recover overpayments.

PPACA The Patient Protection and Affordable Care Act (PPACA) of 2010. Also known as the Affordable Care Act (ACA) or "Obamacare."

Pre-Existing Condition Condition developed prior to issuance of a health insurance policy that may result in the limitation of coverage or benefits.

Preventative Care Any management plan that seeks to prevent disease, prolong life, promote health and enhance the quality of life. *See also Maintenance Care.*

Primary Care Physician (PCP) Clinician who is accountable for addressing a large majority of personal healthcare needs, developing a sustained partnership with patients, and practicing in the context of family and community.

Primary Diagnosis Code The ICD-10-CM code that defines the main reason for the current patient encounter.

Primary Coverage Policy that reimburses costs before any other insurance policy under coordination of benefits rules.

Prior Authorization Formal process requiring providers to obtain approval to provide particular services or procedures before they are provided.

Private Contract A contract between a Medicare beneficiary and a provider who has opted out of Medicare. The beneficiary agrees to give up all Medicare payments for services furnished by the provider and to pay the provider directly without regard to any limits that would otherwise apply to what the provider could charge. The contract must by in writing and must be signed before any service is provided.

Private Insurance Companies Insurance companies which are funded and administered in the private sector.

Problem Focused A limited history or examination of the affected area or organ system.

Prognosis A prediction of the probable course and outcome of a disease or the likelihood of recovery from a disease.

Prolonged Service when E/M service is prolonged or greater than the highest level of E/M service.

Prone Lying horizontal with the face downward.

Proximal Closer to reference point.

Protected Health Information (PHI) Information held by a covered entity which concerns health status, provision of healthcare, or payment for healthcare that can be linked to an individual. PHI is protected by HIPAA/HITECH and may not be disclosed or used, except in specific situations.

Q

Quality Measure A reported code(s) used by payers to measure or quantify healthcare processes, outcomes, patient perceptions, and organizational structure and/or systems that are associated with the ability to provide high-quality health care and/or that relate to one or more quality goals for health care.

Quality Payment Program (QPP) The new CMS payment program which includes the Merit-based Incentive Payment System (MIPS) and Advanced Alternative Payment Models (APMs).

Qui Tam Law that allows for an individual to bring suit for fraud committed against the federal government.

R

RAC Recovery Audit Contractors Program that was created to detect and correct improper payments under the Medicare program.

Radiograph A specially sensitized film that records the internal structures of the body by the passage of X-rays. An X-ray film.

Radiology The scientific discipline of medical imaging using ionization radiation, radionuclides, nuclear magnetic resonance, and ultrasound waves.

Reconsideration *See Redetermination.*

Recoupment The recovery by Medicare of Medicare debt by reducing present or future Medicare payments and applying the amount withheld to the debt incurred.

Recurrence A return of symptoms from a previously treated condition that has been quiescent for 30 or more days.

Redetermination Medicare review process that is performed after the initial determination and denial.

Referral Process of sending a patient from one practitioner to another for healthcare services. Health plans may require designated primary care providers authorize a referral for coverage of specialty services.

Reflex An involuntary action resulting from stimulus.

Refractory Headache Resistant to treatments, which usually refers to "standard" preventative medications.

Regional Health Information Organization (RHIO) An organization that brings together healthcare providers and organizations that govern health information exchange among them for the purpose of improving health care in a geographic region.

Rehabilitative Care Services that help a person keep, restore or improve skills and functioning for daily living and skills related to communication that have been lost or impaired because a person was sick, injured or disabled. These services include physical therapy, occupational therapy, speech-language pathology and psychiatric rehabilitation services in a variety of inpatient and/or outpatient settings.

Reimbursement Financial compensation by a third-party payer such as an insurance company for a service or treatment.

Relief care *See Initial Intensive Care.*

Residual The long-term condition(s) resulting from a previous acute illness or injury.

Resource-Based Relative Value Scale (RBRVS) System whereby payments for services are determined by the resource costs needed to provide that service. The value of code is divided into three components: physician work, practice expense and professional liability insurance expense.

Retrospective Review Procedure that verifies and analyzes the medical necessity and appropriateness of healthcare services previously rendered to the insured.

Risk Management Prioritization of risks, used to minimize liability.

Rule Out Refers to a method used to indicate that a condition is probable, suspected, or questionable, but unconfirmed.

RVU (Relative Value Unit) Numeric expression of the probable intrinsic worth of one procedure/ service to another. The RVU is converted into a fee by a dollar conversion factor.

S

-scope A suffix meaning "to see," as in microscope.

Secondary Diagnosis Code(s) listed after the primary code that indicates additional condition(s) or cause(s) for the current encounter which further define and clarify the patient status.

Secondary Payer When coordinating benefits, the health plan that pays benefits only after the primary payer has paid its full benefits. It will pay the lesser of a) its benefits in full, or b) an amount that when added to the benefits payable by the primary payer equals 100% of covered charges.

Sections Refers to portions of the ICD-10-CM Tabular List that are organized in groups of three-character codes. For example, Endocrine, nutritional and metabolic diseases (E00-E89).

Self-insurance A situation where the consumer pays for healthcare expenses on their own.

Sequencing The process of listing ICD-10-CM codes in the proper order.

Significant, Separately Identifiable Service A service that is above and beyond the other service provided or beyond the usual service associated with the procedure that was performed. It is expressed with the modifier 25 for E/M services and other modifiers for other services.

Signed Consent Form Primary purpose is to maintain legality for doctor and patient.

SOAP (Subjective, Objective, Assessment, Plan) Note A record-keeping methodology for documenting patient encounters.

Solo Practice Healthcare provider who practices alone or with others but does not pool income or expenses.

Spasm An abnormal or prolonged contraction of muscle tissue.

Specialty Care Provider (SCP) Providers other than a Primary Care Physician.

Specificity Refers to the requirement to code to the highest number of characters possible: from 3 to up to 7 characters, when choosing an ICD-10-CM code.

Stabbing Headache Also known as "Ice Pick Headaches". Identified as intense, sharp, stabbing pain. Headaches last for up to a few seconds and recur irregularly, ranging from one to many per day. There are no other accompanying symptoms.

State Departments of Labor and Industries State agencies responsible for regulating workers' compensation, workplace safety, labor and consumer protection, and licensing within their state.

Status Migrainosus Debilitating migraine headache lasting for more than 72 hours

Stem Portion of word which gives the basic meaning.

Stereoradiography Preparing a radiograph such that the depth, width and height can be viewed.

Structural Quality Measure A measure that reflects the organizational, technological, and human resources infrastructure of a system necessary for the delivery of quality health care (such as the use of health information technology for the submission of measures).

Sub- A prefix meaning "less than," as in subluxation.

Subcategories Refers to groupings of ICD-10-CM codes listed under three-character categories.

Subdural Hemorrhage A bleeding underneath the dural and arachnoidal membranes, usually due to trauma which can produce abnormal function, aberra. Acute and chronic forms occur; chronic hematomas may become encapsulated by neomembranes.

Subjective Complaint Problem identified by the patient, such as lethargy, anxiety, etc.

Subrogation Process where an insurer recovers funds from a third party when the action (e.g., auto accident) resulting in medical treatment was the fault of another person.

Suffix Portion of word which modifies the root word.

Superior Upper, or higher in position.

Supportive Care Treatment for patients who have reached maximum therapeutic benefit from care.

Symptom Magnification Conscious and willful feigning or exaggeration of a disease or effect of an injury in order to obtain external gain.

T

Tabular List The portion of ICD-10-CM which list codes and definitions in alphanumeric order.

Technical Component Portion of a healthcare service that associates extra provisions other than the professional service. Reported with modifier TC.

Technique The manner of performance or the details of any procedure, method, or maneuver.

Telehealth/Telemedicine Performing a healthcare service via synchronous communication. Some states use both terms interchangeably. Conversely, in some cases, "telehealth" is used to reflect a broader definition, while "telemedicine" is used mainly to define the delivery of medical services. Services considered appropriate to be rendered via telehealth are shown in Appendix D – Telehealth Codes.

Tension Headache Most common type of headache. Can last from minutes to days, average is 4-6 hours in length. Pain can radiate from the lower back of head, neck, eyes and other muscle groups.

Therapy Methods used to assist in the relief of pain, rehabilitation, and restoration of normal body functions.

Third Party Administrator (TPA) Independent organization that provides administrative services including claims processing and underwriting for other entities such as insurance companies or employers.

Third Party Claim Situation where insurance coverage applies to a party not listed in the policy, but may receive reimbursement due to negligence or fault of another.

Timely Filing Designated number of calendar days in which services must be billed to be eligible for reimbursement.

Trans- A prefix meaning "across," as in transverse.

Transitional Care Management Services services for an established patient from an inpatient hospital setting to the patient's community setting. Requires moderate or high complexity medical decision making during the transition.

Treatment Plan A written document which outlines the plan for helping the patient return to optimal health. It includes the progression of therapy and milestones of progress. It is a key element in establishing medical necessity.

Trigger Point An involuntarily tight band of muscle that is painful when pressed and can cause referred pain in other parts of the body.

U

UB-04 The industry claim submission standard used by facilities/institutions for reimbursement.

Ultrasound Inaudible high frequency sounds whose vibrations can be used to create a heat response in the internal structures of the body.

Ultraviolet "Modality used to stimulate a variety of chemical reactions in the skin and mucous membranes. Used in cases of psoriasis, and other skin conditions, and in assisting the healing process of open wounds. This ultraviolet treatment is not the same as photochemotherapy treatment, commonly called goeckerman or PUVA (petrolatum and ultraviolet a)." - *AMA CPT Assistant; Summer 1995*

Unassigned Claim A claim in which the provider did not agree to accept only the allowed amount as payment for services. Generally, the third party payment goes directly to the patient, not the provider.

Unbundling Billing for a package of healthcare procedures on an individual basis when a single procedure code could be used to describe the combined (complete) service.

United States Department of Justice (DOJ) The federal agency which prosecutes crimes against the nation, such as filing false claims.

United States Public Health Service (PHS) The federal agency which provides public health promotion and disease prevention services. Considered one of the United States uniformed services, agents are responsible for rapid and effective responses to public health situations.

Usual, Customary, and Reasonable (UCR) Provider's typical charge for, or payer's reimbursement rate of, a healthcare service.

Utilization Use of services and/or supplies.

Utilization Review (UR) or Management (UM) Evaluation of quality and appropriateness (e.g., necessity, frequency, efficacy) of services, procedures, and facilities.

Utilization Review Accreditation Commission (URAC) Non-profit organization that establishes and applies healthcare industry standards to payer networks.

V

VA Patient-Centered Community Care (VAPCCC or VAPC3) Created by the Veterans Health Administration (VHA), this program provides eligible Veterans access to specialized services, which are not readily accessible through the regular VA system.

Vascular Headache Involve abnormal function of the brain's blood vessels or vascular system. Vascular headaches are more commonly defined as migraines or cluster headaches.

Vicarious Liability In Latin, "Respondeat Superior", the responsibility of an employer for the acts of their employees.

W

Wellness Care Supportive care given to maintain optimal health and wellness after an annual (initial or periodic) health and wellness encounter, or release of a patient from active/ rehabilitative care.

With Aura Neurological symptoms that usually appear prior to the onset of a migraine. May include: blind spots in vision, tunnel vision, temporary blindness, flashing lights before the eyes, ringing in the ears, dizziness, vertigo, weakness, difficulty with speech, and more.

Without Aura Without neurological symptoms prior to the onset of a migraine

Without Refractory Responds to pharmacological agents (standard preventative medications)

Workers' Compensation Program that covers all medical costs incurred, and replaces wages lost as a result of a work related illness or injury.

X

X-rays Electromagnetic radiation that can penetrate many objects and reveal their internal structure by recording the shadow cast on photographic plates.

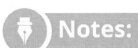

Notes:

Appendix H. Procedure Code Crosswalks

This appendix of some commonly billed procedure codes for behavioral health uses Medicare Adminstrative Contractor's Articles to list codes that are linked together as covered diagnoses in the LCD. Please note that in some cases, there were far too many codes to include here so the category or subcategory were listed instead. Also, note that some procedure codes like those for Evaluation and Management office visits are covered for most diagnosis codes. To review complete Medicare crosswalked code information by code, applicable to your specific location, visit FindACode.com.

90785, 90791, 90792, 90832, 90833, 90834, 90836, 90837

All F codes except:		F10.139	F10.929	F10.939	F11.929	F12.129	F12.929	F13.129	F13.929
F13.982	F14.129	F14.929	F14.982	F15.129	F15.929	F15.982	F16.129	F16.929	F18.129
F18.929	F19.129	F19.139	F19.929	F40.9	F48.9	F79	F84.2	F84.9	

All of the following:		A50.40	A50.42	A50.43	A50.45	A52.17	B20	C71-	E66.0-
E66.1	E66.8	E66.9	G10	G20- G21.3		G21.8	G21.9	G23.1	G24.0-
G24.2	G24.4	G24.8	G25.0-G25.2		G25.7-	G25.81	G25.89	G25.9	G26
G30-	G31.01	G31.09	G31.1	G31.83	G31.84	G31.85	G31.9	G35-G37	G40-
G44.209	G45-	G47.00	G47.21-G47.26		G47.31	G47.33-G47.37		G47.411-G47.429	
G47.51	G47.52	G47.53	G56.41	G56.42	G56.91	G56.92	G57.71	G57.72	G57.91
G57.92	G80.3	G89.21		G89.28-G89.4		G91.2	G93.1	H90.0-H90.8	
H91.0-	H91.3	H91.8-	H93.25	I69.00-I69.034		I69.041-I69.044		I69.051-I69.054	
I69.061-I69.064		I69.09-		I69.10-I69.134		I69.141-I69.144		I69.151-I69.154	
I69.161-I69.165		I69.190-I69.234		I69.241-I69.244		I69.251-I69.254		I69.261-I69.265	
I69.290-I69.334		I69.341-I69.344		I69.351-I69.354		I69.361-I69.365		I69.390-I69.834	
I69.841-I69.844		I69.851-I69.854		I69.861-I69.865		II69.890-I69.934		I69.941-I69.944	
I69.951-I69.954		I69.961-I69.965		I69.99-	L98.1	M54.16	N94.3	R06.3	R07.0
R37	R40.0	R40.1	R41-	R45-	R46-	R47-	R48.0	R48.1	R48.2
R48.8	R49.1	R56.1	R56.9	S06.0X0A-S06.1X5S		S06.1X9A-S06.2X5S		S06.2X9A-S06.305S	
S06.309A-S06.315S		S06.319A-S06.325S		S06.329A-S06.335S		S06.339A-S06.345S		S06.349A-S06.355S	
S06.359A-S06.365S		S06.369A-S06.375S		S06.379A-S06.385S		S06.389A-S06.4X5S		S06.4X9A-S06.5X5S	
S06.5X9A-S06.6X5S		S06.6X9A-S06.815S		S06.819A-S06.825S		S06.829A-S06.895S		S06.899_	T14.91-
T43.205_	T50.905_	T74.0-	T74.1-	T74.2-	T74.3-	T74.4-	T74.51-	T74.52-	T74.61-
T74.62-	T76.0-	T76.1-	T76.2-	T76.3-	T76.51-	T76.52-	T76.61-	T76.62-	Z01.818
Z60.0-Z60.8		Z62.81-	Z63.4	Z65.4	Z65.5	Z65.8	Z69.010-Z69.82		Z70.0
Z70.1	Z70.3	Z71.0	Z71.7	Z87.890	Z91.410-Z91.5				

Articles: A56685, A56850, A56937, A57053, A57065, A57130, A57520

90839

All F codes except:	F10.139	F10.929	F10.939	F11.929	F12.129	F12.929	F13.129	F13.929
F13.982	F14.129	F14.929	F14.982	F15.129	F15.929	F15.982	F16.129	F16.929	F18.129
F18.929	F19.129	F19.139	F19.929	F40.9	F48.9	F51.9	F79	F84.2	F84.9

All of the following:	A50.40	A50.42	A50.43	A50.45	A52.17	B20	C71.0-C71.9	
E66.01	E66.09	E66.1	E66.8	E66.9	G10	G20-G21.3	G21.8	G21.9	G23.1
G24.0-	G24.2	G24.4	G24.8	G25.0	G25.1	G25.2	G25.7-	G25.81	G25.89
G25.9	G26	G30-	G31.01	G31.09	G31.1	G31.83-G31.85		G31.9	G35-G37.9
G40-	G44.209	G45-	G47.00	G47.21-G47.26		G47.31		G47.33-G47.37	
G47.411-G47.429		G47.51-G47.53		G80.3	G89.21	G89.28-G89.4		G91.2	G93.1
H90.0-H90.8		H91.0-	H91.3	H91.8-	H93.25	I69.00-I69.034		I69.041-I69.044	
I69.051-I69.054		I69.061-I69.064		I69.09-	I69.10-I69.134		I69.141-I69.144		
I69.151-I69.154		I69.161-I69.165		I69.190-I69.234		I69.241-I69.244		I69.251-I69.254	
I69.261-I69.265		I69.290-I69.334		I69.341-I69.344		I69.351-I69.354		I69.361-I69.365	
I69.390-I69.834		I69.841-I69.844		I69.851-I69.854		I69.861-I69.865		II69.890-I69.934	
I69.941-I69.944		I69.951-I69.954		I69.961-I69.965		I69.99-	L98.1	M54.16	N94.3
R06.3	R07.0	R37	R40.0	R40.1	R41-	R45-	R46-	R47-	R48.0
R48.1	R48.2	R48.8	R49.0	R49.1	R56.1	R56.9		S06.0X0A-S06.1X5S	
S06.1X9A-S06.2X5S		S06.2X9A-S06.305S		S06.309A-S06.315S		S06.319A-S06.325S		S06.329A-S06.335S	
S06.339A-S06.345S		S06.349A-S06.355S		S06.359A-S06.365S		S06.369A-S06.375S		S06.379A-S06.385S	
S06.389A-S06.4X5S		S06.4X9A-S06.5X5S		S06.5X9A-S06.6X5S		S06.6X9A-S06.815S		S06.819A-S06.825S	
S06.829A-S06.895S		S06.899_	T14.91-	T43.205_	T50.905_	T74.0-	T74.1-	T74.2-	T74.3-
T74.4-	T74.51-	T74.52-	T74.61-	T74.62-	T76.0-	T76.1-	T76.2-	T76.3-	Z01.818
Z60.0-Z60.8 Z62.81-		Z63.4	Z65.4	T76.51-	T76.52-	T76.61-	T76.62-	Z65.5	Z65.8
Z69.010-Z69.82		Z70.0	Z70.1	Z70.3	Z71.0	Z71.7	Z87.890	Z91.410-Z91.5	

Articles: A56937, A57065, A57130, A57520

90846, 90847

All F codes except:	F10.139	F10.929	F10.939	F11.929	F12.129	F12.929	F13.129	F13.929
F13.982	F14.129	F14.929	F14.982	F15.129	F15.929	F15.982	F16.129	F16.929	F18.129
F18.929	F19.129	F19.139	F19.929	F40.9	F48.9	F79	F84.2	F84.9	

All of the following:	A50.40	A50.42	A50.43	A50.45	A52.17	B20	C71.0-C71.9	E66.01
E66.09	E66.1	E66.8	E66.9	G10	G20-G21.3	G21.8	G21.9	G23.1	G24.0-
G24.2	G24.4	G24.8	G25.0	G25.1	G25.2	G25.7-	G25.81	G25.89	G25.9
G26	G30-	G31.01	G31.09	G31.1	G31.83-G31.85		G31.9	G35-G37.9	G40-
G44.209	G45-	G47.00	G47.21-G47.26		G47.31	G47.33-G47.37		G47.411-G47.429	
G47.51-G47.53		G80.3	G89.21	G89.28-G89.4		G91.2	G93.1	H90.0-H90.8	
H91.0-	H91.3	H91.8-	H93.25	I69.00-I69.034		I69.041-I69.044		I69.051-I69.054	
I69.061-I69.064		I69.09-	I69.10-I69.134		I69.141-I69.144		I69.151-I69.154		
I69.161-I69.165		I69.190-I69.234		I69.241-I69.244		I69.251-I69.254		I69.261-I69.265	
I69.290-I69.334		I69.341-I69.344		I69.351-I69.354		I69.361-I69.365		I69.390-I69.834	
I69.841-I69.844		I69.851-I69.854		I69.861-I69.865		II69.890-I69.934		I69.941-I69.944	
I69.951-I69.954		I69.961-I69.965		I69.99-	L98.1	M54.16	N94.3	R06.3	R07.0
R37	R40.0	R40.1	R41-	R45-	R46-	R47-	R48.0	R48.1	R48.2
R48.8	R49.0	R49.1	R56.1	R56.9		S06.0X0A-S06.1X5S		S06.1X9A-S06.2X5S	
S06.2X9A-S06.305S		S06.309A-S06.315S		S06.319A-S06.325S		S06.329A-S06.335S		S06.339A-S06.345S	
S06.349A-S06.355S		S06.359A-S06.365S		S06.369A-S06.375S		S06.379A-S06.385S		S06.389A-S06.4X5S	
S06.4X9A-S06.5X5S		S06.5X9A-S06.6X5S		S06.6X9A-S06.815S		S06.819A-S06.825S		S06.829A-S06.895S	
S06.899_	T14.91-	T43.205_	T50.905_	T74.0-	T74.1-	T74.2-	T74.3-	T74.4-	T74.51-
T74.52-	T74.61-	T74.62-	T76.0-	T76.1-	T76.2-	T76.3-	T76.51-	T76.52-	T76.61-
T76.62-	Z01.818	Z60.0-Z60.8 Z62.81-		Z63.4	Z65.4	Z65.5	Z65.8	Z69.010-Z69.82	
Z70.0	Z70.1	Z70.3	Z71.0	Z71.7	Z87.890	Z91.410-Z91.5			

Articles: A56937, A57065, A57130, A57520

90853

All F codes except:
F10.139	F10.929	F10.939	F11.929	F12.129	F12.929	F13.129	F13.929
F13.982	F14.129	F14.929	F14.982	F15.129	F15.929	F15.982	F16.129	F16.929	F18.129
F18.929	F19.129	F19.139	F19.929	F40.9	F48.9	F79	F84.2	F84.9

All of the following: A50.40 A50.42 A50.43 A50.45 A52.17 B20 C71.0-C71.9 E66.01 E66.09 E66.1 E66.8 E66.9 G10 G20-G21.3 G21.8 G21.9 G23.1 G24.0-G24.2 G24.4 G24.8 G25.0 G25.1 G25.2 G25.7- G25.81 G25.89 G25.9 G26 G30- G31.01 G31.09 G31.1 G31.83 G31.84 G31.85 G31.9 G35-G37.9 G40- G44.209 G45- G47.00 G47.21-G47.26 G47.31 G47.33-G47.37 G47.411-G47.429 G47.51-G47.53 G80.3 G89.21 G89.28-G89.4 G91.2 G93.1 H90.0-H90.8 H91.0- H91.3 H91.8- H93.25 I69.00-I69.034 I69.041-I69.044 I69.051-I69.054 I69.061-I69.064 I69.09- I69.10-I69.134 I69.141-I69.144 I69.151-I69.154 I69.161-I69.165 I69.190-I69.234 I69.241-I69.244 I69.251-I69.254 I69.261-I69.265 I69.290-I69.334 I69.341-I69.344 I69.351-I69.354 I69.361-I69.365 I69.390-I69.834 I69.841-I69.844 I69.851-I69.854 I69.861-I69.865 II69.890-I69.934 I69.941-I69.944 I69.951-I69.954 I69.961-I69.965 I69.99- L98.1 M54.16 N94.3 R06.3 R07.0 R37 R40.0 R40.1 R41- R45- R46- R47- R48.0 R48.1 R48.2 R48.8 R49.0 R49.1 R56.1 R56.9 S06.0X0A-S06.1X5S S06.1X9A-S06.2X5S S06.2X9A-S06.305S S06.309A-S06.315S S06.319A-S06.325S S06.329A-S06.335S S06.339A-S06.345S S06.349A-S06.355S S06.359A-S06.365S S06.369A-S06.375S S06.379A-S06.385S S06.389A-S06.4X5S S06.4X9A-S06.5X5S S06.5X9A-S06.6X5S S06.6X9A-S06.815S S06.819A-S06.825S S06.829A-S06.895S S06.899_ T14.91- T43.205_ T50.905_ T74.0- T74.1- T74.2- T74.3- T74.4- T74.51- T74.52- T74.61- T74.62- T76.0- T76.1- T76.2- T76.3- T76.51- T76.52- T76.61- T76.62- Z01.818 Z60.0-Z60.8 Z62.81- Z63.4 Z65.4 Z65.5 Z65.8 Z69.010-Z69.82 Z70.0 Z70.1 Z70.3 Z71.0 Z71.7 Z87.890 Z91.410-Z91.5

Articles: A56850, A56937, A57053, A57065, A57130, A57520

90870

All F codes except:
F10.139 F10.229 F10.929 F10.939 F11.21 F11.929 F12.129 F12.21 F12.929 F13.129 F13.929 F13.982 F14.129 F14.21 F14.929 F14.982 F15.129 F15.929 F15.982 F16.129 F16.929 F17.201 F17.211 F17.221 F17.291 F18.129 F18.929 F19.129 F19.139 F19.929 F40.9 F48.9 F51.9 F59 F65.9 F69 F79 F80.4 F84.2 F84.9 F93.9 F98.9 F99

All of the following: A50.40 A50.42 A50.43 A50.45 A52.17 B20 C71.0-C71.9 E66.01 E66.09 E66.1 E66.8 E66.9 G10 G20-G21.3 G21.8 G21.9 G23.1 G24.0- G24.2 G24.4 G24.8 G25.0 G25.1 G25.2 G25.7- G25.81 G25.89 G25.9 G26 G30- G31.01 G31.09 G31.1 G31.83-G31.85 G31.9 G35-G37.9 G40- G44.209 G45- G47.00 G47.21-G47.26 G47.31 G47.33-G47.37 G47.411-G47.429 G47.51-G47.53 G80.3 G89.21 G89.28-G89.4 G91.2 G93.1 H90.0-H90.8 H91.0- H91.3 H91.8- H93.25 I69.00-I69.034 I69.041-I69.044 I69.051-I69.054 I69.061-I69.064 I69.09- I69.10-I69.134 I69.141-I69.144 I69.151-I69.154 I69.161-I69.165 I69.190-I69.234 I69.241-I69.244 I69.251-I69.254 I69.261-I69.265 I69.290-I69.334 I69.341-I69.344 I69.351-I69.354 I69.361-I69.365 I69.390-I69.834 I69.841-I69.844 I69.851-I69.854 I69.861-I69.865 II69.890-I69.934 I69.941-I69.944 I69.951-I69.954 I69.961-I69.965 I69.99- L98.1 M54.16 N94.3 R06.3 R07.0 R37 R40.0 R40.1 R41- R45- R46- R47- R48.0 R48.1 R48.2 R48.8 R49.1 R56.1 R56.9 S06.0X0A-S06.1X5S S06.1X9A-S06.2X5S S06.2X9A-S06.305S S06.309A-S06.315S S06.319A-S06.325S S06.329A-S06.335S S06.339A-S06.345S S06.349A-S06.355S S06.359A-S06.365S S06.369A-S06.375S S06.379A-S06.385S S06.389A-S06.4X5S S06.4X9A-S06.5X5S S06.5X9A-S06.6X5S S06.6X9A-S06.815S S06.819A-S06.825S S06.829A-S06.895S S06.899_ T14.91- T43.205_ T50.905_ T74.0- T74.1- T74.2- T74.3- T74.4- T74.51- T74.52- T74.61- T74.62- T76.0- T76.1- T76.2- T76.3- T76.51- T76.52- T76.61-

Continued on next page

| T76.62- | Z60.0-Z60.8 | Z62.81- | Z63.4 | Z65.4 | Z65.5 | Z65.8 | Z69.010-Z69.82 | Z70.0 |
| Z70.1 | Z70.3 | Z71.0 | Z71.7 | Z87.890 | Z91.410-Z91.5 | | | |

Articles: A56937, A57065, A57130

96116

All F codes except:		F10.139	F10.229	F10.929	F10.939	F11.929	F12.129	F12.929	F13.129
F13.929	F13.982	F14.129	F14.929	F14.982	F15.129	F15.929	F15.982	F16.129	F16.929
F17.201	F18.129	F18.929	F19.129	F19.139	F19.929	F40.9	F48.9	F65.9	F69
F79	F84.2	F84.9	F93.9	F98.9	F99				

All of the following:		A50.40	A50.42	A50.43	A50.45	A52.17	A81.0-	B20	C71.0-C71.9
E66.01	E66.09	E66.1	E66.8	E66.9	E75.0-	E75.11	E75.19	E75.4	E83.01
E83.09	G10	G20-G21.3	G21.8	G21.9	G23.1	G24.0-	G24.2	G24.4	G24.8
G25.0	G25.1	G25.2	G25.7-	G25.81	G25.89	G25.9	G26	G30-	G31.01
G31.09	G31.1	G31.83-G31.85		G31.9	G35-G37.9	G40-	G44.209	G45-	G47.00
G47.21-G47.26		G47.31	G47.33-G47.37		G47.411-G47.429		G47.51-G47.53		G51-
G52.1	G70-	G71.1-	G71.2-	G72.0-G72.3		G73.1	G80-	G81.01-G81.04	
G81.11-G81.14		G81.91-G81.94		G83.5	G83.8-	G83.9	G89.21	G89.28-G89.4	
G91.2	G93.1	H90.0-H90.8		H90.A-	H91.0-	H91.3	H91.8-	H93.221-H93.223	
H93.241-H93.243		H93.25		H93.291- H93.293		I69.00-I69.034		I69.041-I69.044	
I69.051-I69.054		I69.061-I69.064		I69.09-		I69.10-I69.134		I69.141-I69.144	
I69.151-I69.154		I69.161-I69.165		I69.190-I69.234		I69.241-I69.244		I69.251-I69.254	
I69.261-I69.265		I69.290-I69.334		I69.341-I69.344		I69.351-I69.354		I69.361-I69.365	
I69.390-I69.834		I69.841-I69.844		I69.851-I69.854		I69.861-I69.865		II69.890-I69.934	
I69.941-I69.944		I69.951-I69.954		I69.961-I69.965		I69.99-	J37.0	J37.1	J38.01-J38.7
J39.0-J39.2	K14.8	L98.1		M26.20-M26.213		M26.220-M26.29		M26.50	M30.0
M30.2	M30.8	M31.7	M54.16	N94.3	Q31.1-Q31.9		Q32-	Q35.1-Q35.7	Q36-
Q37.0-Q37.5		Q38.1	Q38.2	Q38.3	R06.3	R06.89	R07.0	R13-	R37
R40.0	R40.1	R41-	R45-	R46-	R47-	R48.0	R48.1	R48.2	R48.8
R49.0-R49.8		R56.1	R56.9	R62.0	R63.3	S01.522S	S01.531S	S01.532S	S01.541S
S01.542S		S06.0X0A-S06.1X5S		S06.1X9A-S06.2X5S		S06.2X9A-S06.305S		S06.309A-S06.315S	
S06.319A-S06.325S		S06.329A-S06.335S		S06.339A-S06.345S		S06.346S		S06.349A-S06.355S	
S06.359A-S06.365S		S06.369A-S06.375S		S06.379A-S06.385S		S06.389A-S06.4X5S		S06.4X9A-S06.5X5S	
S06.5X9A-S06.6X5S		S06.6X9A-S06.815S		S06.819A-S06.825S		S06.829A- S06.895S		S06.899_	S06.9X0S
S06.9X1S	S06.9X2S	S06.9X3S	S06.9X4S	S06.9X5S	S06.9X9S	S11.012S	S11.014S	S11.019S	S11.022S
S11.029S	S11.032S	S11.034S	S11.22XS	S11.24XS	S12.8XXS	T14.91-	T17.3 _ 8S	T17.4 _ 8S	T17.5 _ 8S
T43.205_	T50.905_	T74.01-	T74.02-	T74.11-	T74.12-	T74.21-	T74.22-	T74.31-	T74.32-
T74.4-	T74.51-	T74.52-	T74.61-	T74.62-	T76.01-	T76.02-	T76.11-	T76.12-	T76.21-
T76.22-	T76.31-	T76.32-	T76.51-	T76.52-	T76.61-	T76.62-	Z43.0	Z44.8	Z60.0-Z60.8
Z62.81-	Z63.4	Z65.4	Z65.5	Z65.8	Z69.010-Z69.82		Z70.0	Z70.1	Z70.3
Z71.0	Z71.7	Z85.21	Z87.890	Z91.410-Z91.5		Z96.3	Z97.4		

Articles: A56685, A56850, A56868, A56937, A57053, A57065, A57130

96130, 96131

All F codes except:		F10.139	F10.939	F19.139	F84.2				

All of the following:		A50.40	A50.42	A50.43	A50.45	A52.17	B20	C71-	E66.01
E66.09	E66.1	E66.8	E66.9	G10	G13.2	G13.8	G20- G21.3		G21.8
G21.9	G23.1	G24.0-	G24.2	G24.4	G24.8	G25.0-G25.2		G25.7-	G25.81
G25.89	G25.9	G26	G30-	G31.01	G31.09	G31.1	G31.2	G31.89	G31.83
G31.84	G31.85	G31.9	G35-G37	G40-	G44.209	G45-	G47.00	G47.21-G47.26	
G47.31	G47.33-G47.37		G47.411-G47.429		G47.51	G47.52	G47.53	G56.41	G56.42
G56.91	G56.92	G57.71	G57.72	G57.91	G57.92	G80.3	G89.21	G89.28-G89.4	
G91.0-G91.9		G93.1	G94	H90.0-H90.8		H91.01-H91.8X9		H93.25	I60-

Continued on next page

I61-	I62-	I63-		I65-	I66-		I69.00-I69.034	I69.041-	
I69.044	I69.051-I69.054	I69.061-I69.064			I69.09-		I69.10-I69.134	I69.141-I69.144	
I69.151-I69.154		I69.161-I69.165			I69.190-I69.234		I69.241-I69.244	I69.251-I69.254	
I69.261-I69.265		I69.290-I69.334			I69.341-I69.344		I69.351-I69.354	I69.361-I69.365	
I69.390-I69.834		I69.841-I69.844			I69.851-I69.854		I69.861-I69.865	II69.890-I69.934	
I69.941-I69.944		I69.951-I69.954			I69.961-I69.965		I69.99-	L98.1	
R06.3	R37	R40.0		R40.1	R41-	R45-	R46-	R47-	M54.16 N94.3 R48.0 R48.1
R48.2	R48.8	R48.9		R49.1	R56.1	R56.9	S06.0X0A-S06.1X5S		S06.1X9A-S06.2X5S
S06.2X9A-S06.305S		S06.309A-S06.315S			S06.319A-S06.325S		S06.329A-S06.335S	S06.339A-S06.345S	
S06.349A-S06.355S		S06.359A-S06.365S			S06.369A-S06.375S		S06.379A-S06.385S	S06.389A-S06.4X5S	
S06.4X9A-S06.5X5S		S06.5X9A-S06.6X5S			S06.6X9A-S06.815S		S06.819A-S06.825S	S06.829A-S06.895S	
S06.899_		T14.91-		T43.205_	T50.905_	T74.0-	T74.1-	T74.2-	T74.3- T74.4-
T74.51-	T74.52-	T74.61-		T74.62-	T74.91-	T74.92-	T76.0-	T76.1-	T76.2- T76.3-
T76.51-	T76.52-	T76.61-		T76.62-	T76.91-	T76.92-	Z60.0-Z60.8	Z62.81-	Z63.4
Z65.4	Z65.5	Z65.8		Z69.010-Z69.82		Z70.0	Z70.1	Z70.3	Z71.0 Z71.7
Z87.890	Z91.410-Z91.5								

Articles: A56685, A56850, A56937, A57053, A57065, A57130, A57780

96132, 96133

All F codes except: F10.139 F10.939 F19.139 F84.2

All of the following:	A50.40	A50.42	A50.43	A50.45	A52.17	B20	C71-	G10
G13.2	G13.8	G20- G21.3		G21.8	G21.9	G23.1	G24.0-	G24.2 G24.4
G24.8	G25.0-G25.2		G25.7-	G25.81	G25.89	G25.9	G26	G30- G31.01
G31.09	G31.1	G31.2	G31.89	G31.83	G31.84	G31.85	G31.9	G35-G37 G40-
G44.209	G45-	G47.00	G47.21-G47.26		G47.31	G47.33-G47.37		G47.411-G47.429
G47.51	G47.52	G47.53	G56.41	G56.42	G56.91	G56.92	G57.71	G57.72 G57.91
G57.92	G80.3	G89.21		G89.28-G89.4		G91.0-G91.9		G93.1 G94
H91.3	H93.25	I60-	I61-	I62-	I63-	I65-	I66-	I69.00-I69.034
I69.041-I69.044		I69.051-I69.054		I69.061-I69.064		I69.09-		I69.10-I69.134
I69.141-I69.144		I69.151-I69.154		I69.161-I69.165		I69.190-I69.234		I69.241-I69.244
I69.251-I69.254		I69.261-I69.265		I69.290-I69.334		I69.341-I69.344		I69.351-I69.354
I69.361-I69.365		I69.390-I69.834		I69.841-I69.844		I69.851-I69.854		I69.861-I69.865
II69.890-I69.934		I69.941-I69.944		I69.951-I69.954		I69.961-I69.965		I69.99- L98.1
M54.16	N94.3	R06.3	R37	R40.0	R40.1	R41-	R45-	R46- R47-
R48.0	R48.1	R48.2	R48.8	R49.1	R56.1	R56.9	R48.9	S06.0X0A-S06.1X5S
S06.1X9A-S06.2X5S		S06.2X9A-S06.305S		S06.309A-S06.315S		S06.319A-S06.325S		S06.329A-S06.335S
S06.339A-S06.345S		S06.349A-S06.355S		S06.359A-S06.365S		S06.369A-S06.375S		S06.379A-S06.385S
S06.389A-S06.4X5S		S06.4X9A-S06.5X5S		S06.5X9A-S06.6X5S		S06.6X9A-S06.815S		S06.819A-S06.825S
S06.829A-S06.895S		S06.899_		T14.91-	T43.205_	T50.905_	T74.0-	T74.1- T74.2-
T74.3-	T74.4-	T74.51-	T74.52-	T74.61-	T74.62-	T74.91-	T74.92-	T76.0- T76.1-
T76.2-	T76.3-	T76.51-	T76.52-	T76.61-	T76.62-	T76.91-	T76.92-	Z01.818 Z60.0-Z60.8
Z62.81-	Z63.4	Z65.4	Z65.5	Z65.8	Z69.010-Z69.82		Z70.0	Z70.1 Z70.3
Z71.7	Z87.890	Z91.410-Z91.5						

Articles: A56685, A56850, A56937, A57130, A57780

96136, 96137, 96138, 96139

All F codes except: F10.139 F10.939 F19.139 F84.2

All of the following:	A50.40	A50.42	A50.43	A50.45	A52.17	B20	C71-	E66.01
E66.09	E66.1	E66.8	E66.9	G10	G13.2	G13.8	G20- G21.3	G21.8
G21.9	G23.1	G24.0-	G24.2	G24.4	G24.8	G25.0-G25.2	G25.7-	G25.81
G25.89	G25.9	G26	G30-	G31.01	G31.09	G31.1	G31.2	G31.89 G31.83
G31.84	G31.85	G31.9	G35-G37	G40-	G44.209	G45-	G47.00	G47.21-G47.26

Continued on next page

G47.31	G47.33-G47.37		G47.411-G47.429	G47.51	G47.52	G47.53	G56.41	G56.42
G56.91	G56.92	G57.71	G57.72	G57.91	G57.92	G80.3	G89.21	G89.28-G89.4
G91.0-G91.9		G93.1	G94	H90.0-H90.8	H91.01-H91.8X9		H93.25	I60-
I61-	I62-	I63-	I65-	I66-	I69.00-I69.034		I69.041-I69.044	
I69.051-I69.054		I69.061-I69.064		I69.09-		I69.10-I69.134	I69.141-I69.144	
I69.151-I69.154		I69.161-I69.165		I69.190-I69.234		I69.241-I69.244	I69.251-I69.254	
I69.261-I69.265		I69.290-I69.334		I69.341-I69.344		I69.351-I69.354	I69.361-I69.365	
I69.390-I69.834		I69.841-I69.844		I69.851-I69.854		I69.861-I69.865	II69.890-I69.934	
I69.941-I69.944		I69.951-I69.954		I69.961-I69.965		I69.99-	L98.1	M54.16	N94.3
R06.3	R37	R40.0	R40.1	R41-	R45-	R46-	R47-	R48.0	R48.1
R48.2	R48.8	R48.9	R49.1	R56.1	R56.9	S06.0X0A-S06.1X5S		S06.1X9A-S06.2X5S
S06.2X9A-S06.305S		S06.309A-S06.315S		S06.319A-S06.325S		S06.329A-S06.335S	S06.339A-S06.345S
S06.349A-S06.355S		S06.359A-S06.365S		S06.369A-S06.375S		S06.379A-S06.385S	S06.389A-S06.4X5S
S06.4X9A-S06.5X5S		S06.5X9A-S06.6X5S		S06.6X9A-S06.815S		S06.819A-S06.825S	S06.829A-S06.895S
S06.899_		T14.91-	T43.205_	T50.905_	T74.0-	T74.1-	T74.2-	T74.3-	T74.4-
T74.51-	T74.52-	T74.61-	T74.62-	T74.91-	T74.92-	T76.0-	T76.1-	T76.2-	T76.3-
T76.51-	T76.52-	T76.61-	T76.62-	T76.91-	T76.92-	Z60.0-Z60.8		Z62.81-	Z63.4
Z65.4	Z65.5	Z65.8	Z69.010-Z69.82		Z70.0	Z70.1	Z70.3	Z71.0	Z71.7
Z87.890	Z91.410-Z91.5							

Articles: A56685, A56850, A56937, A57053, A57065, A57130, A57780

96146

All F codes except:		F10.139	F10.229	F10.929	F10.939	F11.929	F12.129	F12.929	F13.129
F13.929	F13.982	F14.129	F14.929	F14.982	F15.129	F15.929	F15.982	F16.129	F16.929
F17.201	F18.129	F18.929	F19.129	F19.139	F19.929	F40.9	F48.9	F65.9	F69
F79	F84.2	F84.9	F93.9						
All of the following:		A50.40	A50.42	A50.43	A50.45	A52.17	B20	C71-	E66.0-
E66.1	E66.8	E66.9	G10	G20-	G21.3	G21.8	G21.9	G23.1	G24.0-
G24.2	G24.4	G24.8	G25.0-G25.2		G25.7-	G25.81	G25.89	G25.9	G26
G30-	G31.01	G31.09	G31.1	G31.83	G31.84	G31.85	G31.9	G35-G37	G40-
G44.209	G45-	G47.00	G47.21-G47.26		G47.31	G47.33-G47.37		G47.411-G47.429
G47.51	G47.52	G47.53	G56.41	G56.42	G56.91	G56.92	G57.71	G57.72	G57.91
G57.92	G80.3	G89.21		G89.28-G89.4		G91.2	G93.1	H90.0-H90.8	
H91.0-	H91.3	H91.8-	H93.25	I69.00-I69.034		I69.041-I69.044	I69.051-I69.054	
I69.061-I69.064		I69.09-		I69.10-I69.134	I69.141-I69.144		I69.151-I69.154	
I69.161-I69.165		I69.190-I69.234		I69.241-I69.244		I69.251-I69.254	I69.261-I69.265	
I69.290-I69.334		I69.341-I69.344		I69.351-I69.354		I69.361-I69.365	I69.390-I69.834	
I69.841-I69.844		I69.851-I69.854		I69.861-I69.865		II69.890-I69.934	I69.941-I69.944	
I69.951-I69.954		I69.961-I69.965		I69.99-	L98.1	M54.16	N94.3	R06.3	R07.0
R37	R40.0	R40.1	R41-	R45-	R46-	R47-	R48.0	R48.1	R48.2
R48.8	R49.1	R56.1	R56.9	S06.0X0A-S06.1X5S		S06.1X9A-S06.2X5S		S06.2X9A-S06.305S
S06.309A-S06.315S		S06.319A-S06.325S		S06.329A-S06.335S		S06.339A-S06.345S	S06.349A-S06.355S
S06.359A-S06.365S		S06.369A-S06.375S		S06.379A-S06.385S		S06.389A-S06.4X5S	S06.4X9A-S06.5X5S
S06.5X9A-S06.6X5S		S06.6X9A-S06.815S		S06.819A-S06.825S		S06.829A-S06.895S	S06.899_	T14.91-
T43.205_	T50.905_	T74.0-	T74.1-	T74.2-	T74.3-	T74.4-	T74.51-	T74.52-	T74.61-
T74.62-	T76.0-	T76.1-	T76.2-	T76.3-	T76.51-	T76.52-	T76.61-	T76.62-	Z60.0-Z60.8
Z62.81-	Z63.4	Z65.4	Z65.5	Z65.8	Z69.010-Z69.82		Z70.0	Z70.1	Z70.3
Z71.0	Z71.7	Z87.890	Z91.410-Z91.5						

Articles: A56850, A56937, A57053, A57065, A57130

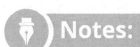
Notes:

Notes:

Indices

Indices Content

General Index 545

Code Index 551

General Index

A

Abbreviations 166
ABN 106, 98
Abuse 99, 473, 128
Abuse vs. Dependence vs. Use 500
Accountable Care Organizations (ACOs) 91
Adaptive Behavior Services 228
Add-On Codes 220
adjudication 39
Adjustment Disorders 476
Advance Beneficiary Notice of Noncoverage (ABN) 98
Advance Care Planning 375
Alcohol abuse counseling 503
Alcohol and/or Substance Abuse Screening 364
Allowed Amount 106, 88, 99, 88
Amnesia 488
Anorexia 489
Anticoagulant Management 361
Anti-Kickback Statute 130
Anxiety Disorders 477
Aphasia Assessment 204
Appeal 26, 69, 70, 71
Assessment
  Adaptive Behavior 228
  Alcohol Use 231, 238
  Cognitive 248
  Drug 231, 233, 238
  Emotional/behavioral 245
  Functional 249
  Substance Use 231, 238
Assessment and Testing Services 240
Assessments
  Adaptive Behavior 228
Attention Deficit Hyperactivity Disorder (ADHD) 478
Audit 123, 140
Autism Spectrum Disorder 479

B

Basic Life and/or Disability Evaluation 368
Behavioral Health Integration 375
Billing 24
Billing Patterns 125
Binge eating 489
Bipolar Disorder 480
Boarding Home 356
Borderline Personality Disorder 482
Bulimia nervosa 489
Buprenorphine 234, 389

C

Cannabis 471, 500
Cannabis Products 137
Care Management Services 371
  Behavioral Health Integration 375
  Collaborative 374
  Psychiatric 374
  Transitional 374
Care Plan Oversight Services 362
Care Plan Services 370
Case Management Services 361
Cash , 17, 77
Certifications 145
CHAMPUS 36
CHAMPVA 36
Chief Complaint (CC) 327
Chronic Care Management Services , 370
Civil Money Penalties (CMP) 132
Claim Form 41, 42, 45
Claim Scrubbing 143
Cloning 165
Clustering 144
Code of Conduct 136
Codes 379
Coding Scenario 324, 343
Cognitive Impairment Services 248
Cognitive rehabilitation 250
Cognitive Skill Training 251
Collections 22
Complex Chronic Care Management Services 372
Compliance Manual 128, 134
Compliance Officer 126
Compliance Program 123, 124, 126, 128, 140
Conduct Disorders 483
Consultation 352
  Electronic health record 366
  Internet 366
  Office or outpatient 352
  Telephone 366
Consumer Directed Healthcare Plans (CDHP) 32
Contracts 137
Conversion Factor (CF) 76
Coordination of Benefits 89, 99
Copayment 99
Copyright Violations 137
Counseling 231, 238, 341, 363
  Alcohol/substance Use 364
  Smoking/tobacco Use 364
COVID 494

CPT 379
Critical Care Services 354
Custodial Care 356

D

Data Mining 40, 63, 125, 144, 147
Deductible 99
Delivery/Birthing Room Attendance and Resuscitation Services 369
Denials 66, 68
Dependence 239
Depressive Disorders 484
Developmental
  Screening 243
  Testing 243
Developmental Disorders 486
Developmental Testing 201
Developmental Testing/Screening 201
Diagnosis 40, 320
Diagnostic Evaluation Documentation 202
Digitally Stored Data Services 367, 368
Disability Evaluation 368, 369
Disallowed Amounts 26
Discounts 35
Discrimination 135
  Language 135
Disruptive mood dysregulation disorder 486
Disruptive Mood Dysregulation Disorder 486
Dissociative Disorders 488
DME Modifiers 385
Documentation 153, 156
  Pharmacologic Management 208
  Psychotherapy 211
  Testing Services 209
Domiciliary, Rest Home (eg, Assisted Living Facility), or Home Care Plan Oversight Services 357
Domiciliary, Rest Home (eg, Boarding Home), or Custodial Care Services 356
Downcoding 67
Drug Abuse Counseling 503
Drug Delivery Implants 390
Drug Testing 240
Durable Medical Equipment 147, 380, 384
Dyslexia 486
Dysthymia 485

E

Eating Disorders 489
EFT 85
EHR 160
Electronic Protected Health Information (EPHI) 134
Eligibility 93
Emergency Department Services 354
Emotional/behavioral assessment 245
Emotional/behavioral Assessment, Brief 245

Established Patient: 312
Evaluation and Management (E/M) 253, 146, 164, 314, 339
  Scoring 314, 318, 325
  Telephone Service 365
Evergreen Contracts 65
Examination 325, 344
Examination and observation 491
Exclusions Database 131
Experimental 147
Explanation of Benefits (EOB) , 23
External Causes 203
Extrapolation 140

F

Factitious Disorder 493
False Claims Act 129
Family Psychotherapy 207
Family therapy 265
Federal Employees 35
Fee for Service 29
Fees 73
Financial Hardship 16, 78
Fines 126
Flowcharts
  Medicare fees decision chart 107
  Psychotherapy Coding Flowchart 263
Fraud 100, 127, 128, 129, 132

G

Group Psychotherapy 207
Group therapy 265

H

Hair-pulling 493
Hamilton Depression Rating Scale 209
Harassment 136
HCPCS 379
Health Behavior
  Intervention 206
Health History 15
Health Insurance Exchanges , 19
Health Reimbursement Arrangement (HRA) 33
Health Savings Accounts (HSA) 33
HIPAA 16, 42, 128, 132, 133, 134
History 324, 330, 344
HITECH 134
Hoarding 493
Home Services 357
Hospital
  Discharge Services 351
  Inpatient Services 350
Hypnotherapy 208

I

Incident to 94
Informed Consent 16
Initial Nursing Facility Care 355
Initial Observation Care 349
Initial Visit 14
Intellectual Disabilities 486
Intensive Care Services 370
Intensive Outpatient Treatment (IOP) 256
Interactive complexity 257
Interactive Complexity 257

L

Language Access Plan 136
Limiting Charge 104, 100, 105, 106, 108, 88
Local Coverage Determination (LCD) 92
Locum Tenens 312

M

Maintenance 106
Major Depressive Disorder 485
Maltreatment 473
Managed Care 31
Medicaid 37
Medical
   Decision Making (MDM) 318, 344
Medical Decision Making (MDM) 335
Medical Disability Evaluation 368
Medical History 15
medical necessity 70
Medical Necessity 155, 18, 154, 146
Medical Record 154
Medical Team Conferences 361
Medicare Administrative Contractors (MACs) 87, 92, 103, 113, 155
Medicare Advantage 83, 91, 100, 93
Medicare Appeals 114
Medicare Conversion Factor (CF) 105
Medicare Enrollment 84
Medicare Fees Decision Chart 107
Medicare Medical Savings Accounts (MSA) 33
Medicare Part B 83
Medicare Physician Fee Schedule (MPFS) 103, 104
Medicare Secondary Payer (MSP) 90
Medicare Summary Notice 23
Medication
   Assisted Treatment for Substance Use Disorder 388
Medication Assisted Treatment 232
Medication Management 232, 250, 258
Medigap 90, 100
Merit-Based Incentive Payment System (MIPS) 110
Methadone 234, 389
Methadone Maintenance 232, 236

Military 36
Mini Mental Status Exam 246
Minnesota Multiphasic Personality Inventory 2 (MMPI-2) 209
Mobile Devices 134
Modifiers 96, 97, 145, 220, 419
   Modifier 25 422
   Modifier 59 446

N

National Correct Coding Initiative (NCCI) 66, 222
National Provider Identifier (NPI) 85, 134
National Uniform Claim Committee (NUCC) 45
Neglect 473
Neonatal Intensive Care Services 369
Neurobehavioral Status Examination 206, 245
Neuropsychological Testing 204
New Patient 312, 347
Non-Participating (Non-PAR) 104, 87, 90, 100, 105, 106, 108, 88
NPPES 85

O

Observation Care Discharge Services 349
Obsessive-Compulsive Disorder (OCD) 493
Office of Inspector General (OIG) 127
Office Policies 13
On-Line Medical Evaluation 365
Open Enrollment 87
Opioid Treatment Program 234
Oppositional defiant disorder 483
Opt Out 100
OSHA 132
OTP 233
Outcomes Assessment Tool (OATs) 169
Out-of-Network 31
Out-of-Pocket 30
Overpayments 100, 25, 63, 95

P

Paperwork Segment (PWK) 43
Participating (PAR) 31, 105, 87, 90, 100, 84, 106, 108, 105, 313
Patient Protection and Affordable Care Act (PPACA) 32, 33, 71, 128
Payment Offset 67, 68
PECOS 84
Pharmacologic Management 258
   Documentation 208
Physician Quality Reporting System (PQRS) 110, 218
Pica 489
Piggy-Back Audits 138

Postpartum Depression and Psychosis 495
Post-Traumatic Stress Disorder (PTSD) 496
Pre-Authorizations 19
Premenstrual dysphoric disorder 486
Preventive Medicine Services 362
Principal Care Management 227
Principal Care Management Services 373
Privacy 136
Profiling 144
Program Integrity Reviews 129
Prolonged Services 264, 316
Prompt Pay Laws 64, 68, 78
Protected Health Information (PHI) 134, 161
Psychiatric Collaborative Care 259
Psychoanalysis 207
Psychological Testing 207
Psychotherapy 266
  Documentation 211
Psychotherapy coding flowchart 262
Psychotherapy Coding Flowchart 263
Psychotherapy for crisis 267
Psychotherapy for Crisis Documentation 211
Psychotherapy Notes 213
PTAN 85, 101

Q

Quality Payment Program 109

R

Random Text Generator 165
Referring Provider 51
Refunds 67, 68
Reimbursement Life Cycle , 13, 39, 63
Relative Value Units (RVUs) , 75
Remittance Advice (RA) , 89, 23
Remote Monitoring 367, 368
Reserved for Local Use 53
Resource-Based Relative Value Scale (RBRVS) 75
Rest Home 356
Review of Systems (ROS) 328
Rorschach 209

S

SBIRT 238
Schizoaffective Disorder 497
Schizophrenia 498
Screening 491
  Alcohol and/or substance 364
  Alcohol Use 231
  Developmental 201, 243
  Substance Use 231
Secondary Payer , 18, 97, 101
Security Rule 134

Self-Audit 140, 141
Sexual Misconduct 136
Signature 117, 161, 163
Signature on File 49
Skilled nursing facility visits 254
Skin Picking 493
Smoking/Tobacco Use Counseling 364
Social Determinants of Health (SDoH) 499
Social pragmatic communication disorder 486
Special Evaluation and Management Services 368, 369
Special Report 221
Standby Services 361
Stark Law 130
Subsequent Nursing Facility Care 356
Subsequent Observation Care 350
Subsequent Treatment Visits 167
Substance Use Disorders 499
Substance Use Medication-Assisted Treatment 388
Superbill 21
Supplies 379
Sustainable Growth Rate (SGR) , 76

T

Table of Risk 323
Telephone
  Consultation 366
  Evaluation and management service 365
Telephone Calls 166
Testing
  Administration and scoring 246
  Developmental 201, 243
  Evaluation services 247
  Neurobehavioral Status 245
Testing Documentation 209
Thematic Apperception Test (TAT) 209
Time 341
Timed Codes 270
Time of Service 35, 77
Tobacco abuse counseling 503
Transcranial Magnetic Stimulation (TMS) 270
Treatment
  Adaptive Behavior 228
Treatment Plan 21
TRICARE 36
Trichotillomania 493

U

Unbundling 144
Underpayments 25
Unlisted Codes 221
Upcoding 144
Usual and Customary 29
Usual, Customary, and Reasonable (UCR) 74

V

Verification of Insurance Coverage 14, 19
Veterans Administration 36
Voice Recognition 164

W

Welcome Letter 14
Wellness 362
Workers' Compensation 18
Work Plan 127, 144

X

X-Ray Report 162

Notes:

Code Index

A

Absorption dressing, A6251-A6256
Adaptive Behavior
   assessments, 97151-97152, 0362T
   treatment
      family, 97156-97157
      group, 97154, 97158
      one patient, 0373T, 97153, 97155
Adhesive, A4364
   bandage, A6413
   remover, A4455, A4456
Administration
   health risk assessment
      caregiver-focused, 96161
      patient-focused, 96160
Air travel and nonemergency transportation, A0140
Alert device, A9280
Analysis
   chromosome, 88245-88289
   implant
      neurostimulator pulse generator, 95970-95984
Ankle
   application
      strapping, 29540
   strapping, 29540
Antigen
   detection, 87260-87899
   tumor, 86294-86316
Application
   modality, 97010-97036
Aripiprazole lauroxil, (aristada), J1944
   aristada initio, J1943
Aripiprazole, J0400, J0401, J1942
Assays
   therapeutic drug, 80150-80299
Assessment
   speech, V5362-V5364
Assessment
   adaptive behavior, 97151-97152, 0362T
   emotional/behavioral, 96127
   health risk, 96160-96161
   interprofessional internet/telephone, 99446-99449
Auditory canal
   foreign body, 69200-69205

B

Baclofen, J0475, J0476
Bacteria
   culture
      aerobic, 87040-87071
      other, 87070-87075
      screening, 87081
      urine, 87086-87088
Battery, L7360, L7364-L7368
   replacement for TENS, A4630
Bilirubin (phototherapy) light, E0202
Biofeedback device, E0746
Biofeedback training, 90875-90876, 90901-90911
Bleeding
   nasal
      cauterization, 30901-30906

Blood
   cell
      count
         differential WBC, 85004-85007, 85009
         hematocrit, 85014
         hemoglobin, 85018
         hemogram
            automated, 85025-85027
            manual, 85032
         red blood cell (RBC), 85032-85041
         smear, 85007-85008
         white blood cells, 85032, 85048, 89055
      sedimentation rate
         manual, 85651
   coagulation
      factor
         III
            partial time, 85730-85732
   collection
      capillary, 36416
      venipuncture, 36415
   complete count (CBC), 85025-85027
   leukocyte
      count, 85032, 85048, 89055
      differential, 85004-85007, 85009
   platelet
      count, 85008
      manual, 85032
   pressure, 2000F
      analysis, 99091
   red blood cell (RBC)
      count, 85032-85041
      hematocrit, 85014
      morphology, 85007
      platelet estimation, 85007
      sedimentation rate
         manual, 85651
   test
      complete, 85025-85027
      erythrocyte, 85032
      glucose, 82947-82948, 82962
      hematocrit, 85014
      hemoglobin, 85018
      leukocyte, 85032, 84048
      panels
         general health, 80050
         hepatic function, 80076
         lipid, 3011F, 3278F, 80061
         metabolic, 80047-80048, 80053
      platelet, 85032, 85049
      thromboplastin time, 85730
      white blood (WBC), 85004-85009
   white blood cell
      count, 85032, 85048, 89055
      differential, 85004-85007, 85009
Bone
   facial
      fracture
         closed, 21310-21320
   nasal
      fracture
         closed, 21310-21320
Brain
   electrode
      stimulation, 95961-95962
   magnetic resonance imaging (MRI), 70551-70559

stimulation
electrode, 95961-95962
surface electrode, 95961-95962
Brush
border, 86308-86310
Buprenorphine/Naloxone, J0571-J0575
Burn
treatment, 16000-16036
debridement, 01951-01953, 15002-15005, 16020-16030
dressings, 16020-16030
initial, 16000
Bus, nonemergency transportation, A0110

C

Canal, auditory
foreign body
removal, 69200-69205
Care
custodial
subsequent, 99307-99310
physician
telephone, 99441-99443
therapy
activities
of daily living, 97535, 99509
therapeutic, 97530
community/work reintegration, 97537
contrast baths, 97034
diathermy treatment, 97024
direct, 97032-97039
electric stimulation
attended, 97032
unattended, 97014
evaluation
occupational, 97165-97168
exercises, 4240F-4242F, 97110
group
education and training, 98961-98962
group therapeutic, 97150
hot or cold pack, 97010
individual
home management training, 97535, 98960
infrared light treatment, 97026
iontophoresis, 97033
kinetic therapy, 97530
massage therapy, 97124
microwave therapy, 97024
sensory integration, 97533
supervised procedure, 97010-97028
ultrasound, 97035
ultraviolet light, 97028
whirlpool therapy, 97022
work reintegration, 97537
Case management, T1016, T1017
Cauterization
nasal, 30901-30906
Cell
blood
count
differential WBC, 85004-85007, 85009
hematocrit, 85014
hemoglobin, 85018
hemogram
automated, 85025-85027
manual, 85032
red blood cell (RBC), 85032-85041
smear, 85007-85008
white blood cell, 85032, 85048, 89055
sedimentation rate
manual, 85651

count
blood
differential WBC, 85004-85007, 85009
hematocrit, 85014
hemoglobin, 85018
hemogram
automated, 85025-85027
manual, 85032
red blood cell (RBC), 85032-85041
smear, 85007-85008
white blood cells, 85032, 85048, 89055
Change
dressing
burn, 15852, 16020-16030
Chemotherapy
drugs (see also drug by name), J9000-J9999
Chemotherapy administration, 0519F
intramuscular, 96372, 96401-96402
subcutaneous, 96369-96372, 96401-96402
Cholesterol
test, 80061, 82465, 83718-83722
Chorionic
gonadotropin
test, 84702-84704
Chromosome analysis, 88230-88239, 88245-88269, 88280-88289
Cinefluorographies, 70371, 74230
Cineradiography, 70371, 74230
Cleanser, wound, A6260
Clonidine, J0735
Coagulation
factor
III
partial time, 85730-85732
Coagulin, 85347, 85705, 85730-85732
Cognitive, 3720F
assessment and care, 99483
performance, 96125
Cold
pack, 97010
Collection
blood, 36415-36416, 36591-36592
Complete blood count (CBC)
differential WBC, 85004-85007, 85009
hematocrit, 85014
hemoglobin, 85018
hemogram
automated, 85025-85027
manual, 85032
red blood cell (RBC), 85032-85041
smear, 85007-85008
white blood cell, 85032, 85048, 89055
Computer-aided, -assisted
analysis
stored clinical data, 99091
navigation
cranial procedure, 61781-67782
testing
neuropsychological, 96146
psychological, 96146
Consultation
psychiatric, 90887
Consultation, S0285, S0311, T1040, T1041
Contact layer, A6206-A6208
Contrast
bath, 97034
Cortical mapping, 95961-95962
Counseling
genetic, 96040
marriage counseling, 99510
psychotherapy, 90832-90853

Count
blood
  cell
    differential WBC, 85004-85007, 85009
    hematocrit, 85014
    hemoglobin, 85018
    hemogram
      automated, 85025-85027
      manual, 85032
    red blood cell (RBC), 85032-85041
    smear, 85007-85008
    white blood cell, 85032, 85048, 89055
  platelet, 85008
complete blood count
  differential WBC, 85004-85007, 85009
  hematocrit, 85014
  hemoglobin, 85018
  hemogram
    automated, 85025-85027
    manual, 85032
  red blood cell (RBC), 85032-85041
  smear, 85007-85008
  white blood cell, 85032, 85048, 89055
erythrocyte, 85032-85041
leukocyte, 85032, 85048, 89055
Cover, wound
  hydrogel dressing, A6242-A6248
  specialty absorptive dressing, A6251-A6256
Cranial
  nerve
    implantation
      electrode, 64553, 64568
Culture
  bacteria, 87040-87077, 87081, 87086-87088
  pathogen, 87084
Cutaneous
  electrostimulation, 97014, 97032
  tissue
    burns, 16000-16030
    introduction, 11900-11977, 11981, 11983
    removal, 11982-11983
Cytogenetic study, 88271-88275, 88291, 88364-88366

D

Dalalone, J1100
Debridement
  skin, 11000-11047
    burns, 16020-16030
Deoxyribonucleic acid (DNA), 86225-86226
  probe
    molecular, 88271-88275, 88291
Desipramine, 80335-80337
Developmental screening, 96110
Developmental testing, 96112, 96113
Dexamethasone sodium phosphate, J1100
Diagnostic
  injection, 20501
    intramuscular, 96372
    subcutaneous, 96372
  psychiatric interview, 90791-90792
Diaper, T1500, T4521-T4540, T4543, T4544
Diathermy
  retina
    modality, 97024
Diazepam, J3360
Diclofenac, J1130
Dipropylacetic acid, 80164-80165
Doxepin, 80335-80337
Dressing (*see also* **Bandage**), A6020-A6406
  contact layer, A6206-A6208
  gauze, A6216-A6230, A6402-A6406
  hydrogel, A6242-A6248

specialty absorptive, A6251-A6256
transparent film, A6257-A6259
Dressings, 15852, 16020-16030
Drug
  antidepressants
    tricyclic, 80335-80337
  assay/testing
    amitriptyline, 80335-80337
    desipramine, 80335-80337
    dipropylacetic acid, 80164-80165
    doxepin, 80335-80337
    haloperidol, 80173
    imipramine, 80335-80337
    lithium, 80178
    nortriptyline, 80335-80337
  delivery, 96365-96379
  management
    psychiatric, 90863
  screen, 80305-80307
Drugs (*see also* **Table of Drugs**)
  administered through a metered dose inhaler, J3535
  not otherwise classified, J3490, J7599, J7699, J7799, J7999, J8499, J8999, J9999
  prescription, oral, J8499, J8999

E

Ear, 00120-00126
  canal, 4130F-4132F
    foreign body
      removal, 69200-69205
  collection, 36415-36416
  wax, removal, 62909-69210
Elbow
  strapping, 29260
Electric
  stimulation
    cortical, 95961-95962
    modality, 97014, 97032
    transcutaneous, 97014, 97032
Electroconvulsive therapy, 90870
Electrode
  implantation, 63650-63655, 64553-64561, 64568, 64575-64581
Electroencephalogram (EEG), 3650F, 95812-95827, 95830, 95950-95958
Electronic analysis
  neurostimulator pulse generator, 95970-95984
Electrophoresis, 84165-84166, 86320-86327, 86334-86335
EMG, E0746
Encephalon
  electrode
    stimulation, 95961-95962
  magnetic resonance imaging (MRI), 70551-70559
  stimulation
    electrode, 95961-95962
  surface electrode
    stimulation, 95961-95962
Epistaxis, 30901-30906, 31238
Erythrocyte
  count, 85032-85041
  hematocrit, 85014
  morphology, 85007
  platelet estimation, 85007
  sedimentation rate, 85651-85652
Evaluation
  occupational therapy, 97165-97168
  psychiatric, 90791-90792, 90885
Evoked
  potential
    somatosensory, 95925-95928
    visual, 95930, 0333T, 0464T

F

Facial
   bone, 00190-00192
      fracture
         closed
            nasal, 21310-21320
Factor
   blood coagulation
      III
         partial time, 85730-85732
Ferric chloride, 81005
Filler, wound
   hydrogel dressing, A6248
   not elsewhere classified, A6261, A6262
Film, transparent (for dressing), A6257-A6259
Fixation
   latex, 86403-86406
Fluid
   cerebrospinal, 86325, 78630-78650
Foot, 01462-01486
   cast, 29345-29358, 29405-29445, 29505-29515
      strapping, 29540-29580
Foreign body
   removal
      ear, 69200-69205
Fracture
   closed treatment
      head
         nose, 21310-21320, 21337, 21345

G

Glucose
   blood test, 82947-82950, 82960
Glycohemoglobin, 83036
Gonadtropin
   chorionic, 84702-84704
Goserelin acetate implant (*see also* **Implant**), J9202
Group health education, 98961-98962

H

Haloperidol, 80173
Haloperidol, J1630
   decanoate, J1631
Hand, 01810-01860
   strapping, 29280
Hanganutziu Deicher antibody, 86308-86310
Head
   fracture treatment, 21310-21497
Heat
   application, E0200-E0239
   lamp, E0200, E0205
   pad, A9273, E0210, E0215, E0237, E0249
Heel
   collection, 36415-36416
Hemoglobin, 3044F-3046F, 3279F-3281F
   glycosylated, 83036
Hemogram
   automated, 85025-85027
   manual, 85014-85018, 85032
Hemorrhage, control of
   cauterization
      nose, 30901-30906
   nasal
      cauterization, 30901-30906
Hepatitis, 3215F-3220F, 4150F-4159F
   A
      vaccine, 90632-90634
   B
      antigen
         surface, 87340-87341
Herpes
   simplex
      antigen detection
         immunofluorescence, 87273-87374
Heteroantibody, 86308-86310
Hinton positive, 86592-86593
Home services
   ADL, 99509
   counseling
      family, 99510
      individual, 99510
Hormone
   thyroid stimulating, 3278F, 80418, 80438-80439, 84443
Hot pack treatment, 97010
Human
   chorionic
      gonadotropin, 80414-80415, 84702-84703
Hydrogel dressing, A6242-A6248, A6231-A6233
Hypnotherapy, 90880

I

Icthyosis, 86592-86593
Imaging
   echography
      physical therapy, 97035
   magnetic resonance
      imaging (MRI)
         brain, 70551-70555, 70557-70559
Imipramine, 80335-80337
Immunoassay
   infectious agent, 86317-86318, 87301-87451
Immunoelectrophoresis, 86320-86327, 86334-86335
immunofluorescence, single antibody stain, 88346, 88350
Immunogen
   detection, 87260-87899
   tumor, 86294-86316
Implant
   buprenorphine implant, J0570
Implantation
   drug delivery device, 11981, 11983, 61517
   electrode (array)
      cranial nerve, 64553, 64568
   nerve, 64553-64561, 64575-64581
Infection
   immunoassay, 86317-86318
   rapid test, 86403-86406
Infectious
   agent
      antigen detection
         immunoassay technique
            hepatitis B surface antigen (HBsAg), 87340-87341
            multiple step method, 87301-87449, 87451
Infrared light treatment, 97026
Inhalation solution (*see also* **drug name**), J7608-J7699, Q4074
Injection
   diagnostic, 96372-96379
   intramuscular, 96372
   prophylactic, 96365-96379
   subcutaneous, 96372
   therapeutic, 96365-96379
Injections (*see also* **drug name**), J0120-2504, J2794, J2798, J1303, J1942-J1944, J2506, J3031, J7311, J7313, J7314, J7320, J7332, J7208, J9032, J9036, J9039, J9044, J9057, J9153, J9118, J9173, J9199, J9201, J9210, J9229, J9269, J9271, J9299, J9308, J9309, J9313, J9355, J9356, Q5112-Q5118, Q9950, Q9991, Q9992
   supplies for self-administered, A4211

Insertion
nerve
electrode, 64553-64581
skin
drug delivery implant, 11981, 11983
vein
catheter, 36011-36012, 36400-36410, 36420-36425, 36500-36510
venipuncture, 36400-36410, 36420-36425
Insurance
basic life/disablilty
examination, 99450-99456
Integumentary system, 00300, 00400-00410
burns, 16000-16030
introduction, 11900-11977, 11981, 11983
removal, 11200-11201, 11982-11983
Internet
assessment/management, interprofessional, 99446-99449
Interprofessional telephone/internet/EHR services, 99446-99449, 99451-99452
Intramuscular injection, 96372, 96379, 99506
Introduction
drug delivery, 11981, 11983
Ionization, 89230, 97033

K

Kinetic therapy, 97530
Knee, 01320-01444
strapping, 29530

L

Larynx, 00320-00326
x-ray, 70370-70371
Latex fixation, 86403-86406
Lead investigation, T1029
Lead, 83655
Lithium, 80178
Lodging, recipient, escort nonemergency transport, A0180, A0200
Lorazepam, J2060
Loxapine, for inhalation, J2062

M

Magnetic resonance
imaging (MRI), 3319F-3320F
brain, 70551-70555, 70557-70559
Mantoux test, 86580
Massage, 97124
Medical
genetic counseling, 96040
testimony, 99075
Medical and surgical supplies, A4206-A8999
Microbiology, 87003-87999
Microsomal antibody, 86376
Mini-bus, nonemergency transportation, A0120
Moderate sedation, 99151-99157
Monitoring
electroencephalogram (EEG), 95812-95813, 95950-95954, 95956, 95958
Monospot test, 86308
Mosenthal test, 81002
Multidisciplinary services, H2000-H2001, T1023-T1028

N

Naloxone HCl, J2310
Naltrexone, J2315
Narcosynthesis, 90865

Nasal
bleeding, 30901-30906, 31238
epistaxis, 30901-30906, 31238
fracture
treatment, 21310-21337, 21343-21344
Needle, A4215
with syringe, A4206-A4209
Nerve(s)
cranial
implantation
electrode, 64553, 64568, 64575-64581
electrode
insertion, 64553-64581
Neurobehavioral status, 96116, 96121
Neurofunctional test, 96020
Neurology procedures
cerebral
function testing
aphasia, 96105
neuropsychological, 96132-96133, 96136-96139, 96146
mapping, 96020
performance, 96125
stimulation
electrode, 95961-95962
electroencephalogram (EEG), 95816, 95965-95967
coma, 95822
functional mapping, 95961-95962
monitoring, 95812-95813, 95950-95953, 95956
sleep, 95822, 95827
standard, 95819
evoked potentials
short latency, 95925-95927
visual, 95930
mapping, functional brain, 96020
somatosensory testing, 95925-95927
Neuromuscular stimulator, E0745
Neuropsychology testing, 96132-96133, 96136-96139, 96146
Neurostimulator
application, 64566, 97014, 97032
electronic analysis
brain/cranial nerve, 95970, 95976-95977, 95983-95984
spinal cord, 95970-95972
implantation, electrode
cranial, 64553, 64568
New patient care
office
initial visit, 99201-99205
Nonchemotherapy drug, oral, NOS, J8499
Noncovered services, A9270
Nonemergency transportation, A0080-A0210
Nonimpregnated gauze dressing, A6216-A6221, A6402-A6404
Nonprescription drug, A9150
Nortriptyline, 80335-80337
Nose, 00160-00164
cauterization, 30801-30802, 30901-30906, 31238
fracture treatment, 30930
closed, 21310-21320, 21337, 21345
Not otherwise classified drug, J3490, J7599, J7699, J7799, J8499, J8999, J9999, Q0181
Nucleases (DNA), 86225-86226
probe
molecular, 88271-88275, 88291

O

Occupational therapy, 97165-97168
Olanzapine, J2358
OnabotulinumtoxinA, J0585
Onychia
excision, 11750-92242

Organ
  panel, 80050
    hepatic, 80074-80076
Outpatient services
  consultation, 99201-99215
  established patient, 99211-99215
  new patient, 99201-99205
  office visit, 99201-99215

P

Packing
  nasal hemorrhage, 30901-30906
Pad
  heat, E0210, E0215, E0217, E0238, E0249
Paliperidone palmitate, J2426
Panel
  general health, 80050
  hepatic function, 80076
  lipid, 3011F, 3278F, 80061
  metabolic, 80047-80048, 80053
Parking fee, nonemergency transport, A0170
Particle agglutination, 86403-86406
Pathology
  immunofluorescence, single antibody stain, 88346, 88350
Percutaneous
  electric nerve stimulation, 64566, 97014, 97032
  venipuncture, 36400-36410
Performance measures
  documentation
    results, 3006F-3763F
    screening, 3006F-3763F
Performance test
  cognitive, 96125
  psychological, 96130-96131, 96136-96139, 96146
Pharynx
  cineradiography, 70371, 74230
  video study, 70371, 74230
Phototherapy light, E0202
Physical examination measures, 2000F-2060F
  activities
    daily living, 97535, 99509
    therapeutic, 97530
  community reintegration, 97537
  contrast baths, 97034
  diathermy treatment, 97024
  direct, 97032-97039
  electric stimulation
    attended, 97032
    unattended, 97014
  evaluation
    occupational therapy, 97165-97168
  exercises, 4240F-4242F, 97110
  group, 97150
  hot or cold pack, 97010
  infrared light treatment, 97026
  iontophoresis, 97033
  kinetic, 97530
  massage, 97124
  microwave, 97024
  sensory integration, 97533
  supervised procedure, 97010-97028
  ultrasound, 97035
  ultraviolet light, 97028
  whirlpool, 97022
Physician services
  telephone, 99441-99443
Platelet
  blood, 85025
  count, 85032, 85049

Potential
  evoked
    sensory, 95925-95927
    visual, 95930, 0333T, 0464T
Pregnancy
  test, 84702-84704
Preparatory prosthesis, L5510-L5595
  nonchemotherapy, J8499
Procoagulant activity
  partial time, 85730-85732
Prothrombin, 85210
  time, 85610-85611
Psychiatric services
  biofeedback training, 90875-90876
  collaborative care, 99492-99494
  consultation with family, 90887
  drug management, 90863
  electroconvulsive therapy, 90870
  environmental intervention, 90882
  evaluation of records or reports, 90885
  family, 90846-90849
  group, 90853
  hypnotherapy, 90880
  individual, 90832-90838
  interactive complexity, 90785
  interview and evaluation, 90791-90792
  narcosynthesis analysis, 90865
  pharmacologic management, 90863
  psychoanalysis, 90845
  psychological testing, 96130-96131, 96136-96139, 96146
  psychotherapy
    crisis, 90839-90840
    family, 90846-90849
    group, 90853
    interactive complexity, 90785
    patient, 90832-90838
  report preparation, 90889
Pulse
  generator, neurostimulator
    electronic anaylsis, 95970-95984
Puncture
  venipuncture, 36410, 36425
  routine, 36415

Q

Quick test, 85610-85611

R

Radiocinematography
  evaluation, 70371, 74230
  pharynx, 70371, 74230
Rapid
  test
    infection, 86308, 86403-86406
    plasma reagent, 86592-86593
Red blood cell(s)
  count, 85032-85041
  hematocrit, 85014
  morphology, 85007
  platelet estimation, 85007
  sedimentation rate, 85651-85652
Reinsertion
  drug delivery implant, 11983
Removal
  device
    drug delivery implant, 11982-11983
  drug delivery implant, 11982-11983
  foreign body
    arm, 24200-24201, 25248 ear canal, 69200-69205

Replacement
battery, A4630
Results documentation, 3006F-3725F
Risperidone (risperdal consta), J2794
(perseris), J2798
Ross
assessment, 96125

S

Screening
developmental, 96110
Sedation
conscious (moderate)
different physician, 99155-99157
same physician, 99151-99153
Semiquantitative, 81005
Serologic test, 86592-86593
Sex
ichtyoses, 86592-86593
Skin
allergy, 86485-86490, 86510, 86580
burn, 16000
debridement, 01951-01953, 16020-16030
dressing, 16020-16030
debridement, 11000-11001
burn, 16020-16030
implant
device, 11981-11983
insertion
drug delivery, 11981
removal
drug delivery, 11982-11983
Sleep studies
unattended, 95806, 95800-95801
Sling, A4565
Smears
developmental, 96110
documentation, 3006F-3725F
drug test(s), 80305-80307
Social worker, nonemergency transport, A0160
Somatosensory testing
head, 95927
lower limbs, 95926
trunk, 95927
upper limbs, 95925
Specialty absorptive dressing, A6251-A6256
Specimen
handling, 99000-99001
Speech
evaluation, 92521-92523
cine, 70371
video, 70371
Speech assessment, V5362-V5364
Splint, A4570, L3100, L4350-L4380
Stimulation
cortical, 95961-95962
electrical
brain, 95961-95962
physical therapy, 97014, 97032
magnetic, 90867-90868
nerve
peripheral, 95925-95927
neurostimulation, transcutaneous
application, 97014, 97032
subcortical, 95961-95962
transcranial
magnetic, 90867--90869, 95939
Stimulators
neuromuscular, E0744, E0745

Strapping
ankle, 29540
elbow, 29260
finger, 29280
foot, 29540
hand, 29280
knee, 29530
wrist, 29260
Syphilis
test, 86592-86593
Syringe, A4213
with needle, A4206-A4209

T

T-7 index
thyroxine, 84436
Taxi, non emergency transportation, A0100
TB test
skin test, 86580
Telehealth transmission, T1014
Telehealth, Q3014
Telephone
assessment/management, interprofessional, 99446-99449, 99451-99452
evaluation and management services, 99441-99443
TENS, 97014, 97032
TENS, A4595, E0720-E0749
Test
blood
complete, 85025-85027
erythrocyte, 85032
glucose, 82947-82948, 82962
hematocrit, 85014
hemoglobin, 85018
leukocyte, 85032, 84048
panels
general health, 80050
hepatic function, 80076
lipid, 3011F, 3278F, 80061
metabolic, 80047-80048, 80053
platelet, 85032, 85049
thromboplastin time, 85730
WBC, 85004-85009
cholesterol, 80061, 82465, 83718-83722
developmental, 96112-96113
function
neurological
aphasia, 96105
neuropsychological, 96132-96133, 96136-96139, 96146
gonadotropin, 84702-84704
infection, 86403-86406
Mantoux, 86580
monospot, 86308
Mosenthal, 81002
neurofunctional, 96020
neuropsychology, 96132-96133, 96136-96139, 96146
performance
cognitive, 96125
pregnancy, 84702-84704
psycological, 96130-96131, 96136-96139, 96146
quick, 85610-85611
rapid
infection, 86308, 86403-86406
plasma reagent, 86592-86593
serologic, 86592-86593
somatosensory, 95925-95927
syphilis, 86592-86593
tuberculosis, 86480, 86580
Wintrobe, 85651-85652
Therapeutic lightbox, A4634, E0203

Thrombocyte
 count, 85008
  manual, 85032
Thromboplastin
 partial time, 85730-85732
Thyroid, 00320-00322
 hormone binding, 84479
 hormone stimulation, 84443
  uptake, 84479
Thyroxine
 total, 84436
Time
 prothrombin, 85610-85611
 thromboplastin, 85730-85732
Tissue
 factor, 85705
  time, 85730-85732
TMS, 90867-90869
Toll, non emergency transport, A0170
Toxicology screening, 80305-80307
Training
 biofeedback, 90901-90911
 integration
  sensory, 97533
 management
  home, 97535, 99509
 reintegration
  community, 97537
  work, 97537
 self care, 97535, 98960-98962, 99509
Transcranial
 stimulation
  magnetic, 90867-90869
Transcutaneous electrical nerve stimulator (TENS), E0720-E0770
Transparent film (for dressing), A6257-A6259
Transportation
 handicapped, A0130
 non emergency, A0080-A0210, T2001-T2005
 taxi, non emergency, A0100
 toll, non emergency, A0170
 volunteer, non emergency, A0080, A0090
Triacylglycerol, 84478
Triglycerides, 84478
Tuberculosis
 skin test, 86580

U

Ultrasound, 3319F-3320F
 physical therapy, 97035
Ultraviolet light therapy system, A4633, E0691-E0694
Unclassified drug, J3490
Urinalysis
 automated, 81001, 81003
 non-automated, 81002
 qualitative, 81005
 routine, 81002
Urine
 colony count, 87086
 test, 81001

V

Vaccines/Toxoids
 hepatitis
  A and B, 90636
  A, 90632-90634
**Valproic acid, 80164-80165*
Venipuncture
 percutaneous, 36400-36410
 routine, 36415

Video
 pharynx, 70371, 74230
 speech, 70371
Vitamin B-12 cyanocobalamin, J3420

W

Wheelchair, E0950-E1298, K0001-K0108
 van, non-emergency, A0130
Whirlpool therapy, 97022
White blood cell
 count, 85032, 85048, 89055
 differential, 85004-85007, 85009
Whitman
 astragalectomy, 97022
Wintrobe test, 85651-85652
Wound cleanser, A6260
Wound cover
 hydrogel dressing, A6242-A6247
 specialty absorptive dressing, A6251-A6256
Wound filler
 hydrogel dressing, A6248
 not elsewhere classified, A6261, A6262
Wrist, 01810-01860
 strapping, 29260

X

Xenoantibody, 86308-86310

Notes:

Notes: